CUTANEOUS MEDICINE AND SURGERY

Self Assessment and Review

CUTANEOUS MEDICINE AND SURGERY
Self Assessment and Review

Edited by

JEFFREY S. DOVER, MD, FRCPC

Chief, Division of Dermatology
New England Deaconess Hospital
Assistant Professor of Dermatology
Harvard Medical School
Boston, Massachusetts

In Consultation with

KENNETH A. ARNDT, MD

Dermatologist-in-Chief
Beth Israel Hospital
Professor of Dermatology
Harvard Medical School
Boston, Massachusetts

JUNE K. ROBINSON, MD

Professor of Dermatology and Surgery
Department of Dermatology and Surgery
Northwestern University Medical School
Chicago, Illinois

PHILIP E. LeBOIT, MD

Associate Professor of Pathology and
  Dermatology
University of California, San Francisco
San Francisco, California

BRUCE U. WINTROUB, MD

Professor and Chairman
Department of Dermatology
Associate Dean
School of Medicine
University of California, San Francisco
San Francisco, California

W.B. SAUNDERS COMPANY
A Division of Harcourt Brace & Company
Philadelphia • London • Toronto • Montreal • Sydney • Tokyo

W.B. SAUNDERS COMPANY
A Division of Harcourt Brace & Company

The Curtis Center
Independence Square West
Philadelphia, Pennsylvania 19106

Library of Congress Cataloging-in-Publication Data

Cutaneous medicine and surgery : self assessment and review / edited by Jeffrey S. Dover, in consultation with Kenneth A. Arndt . . . [et al.].—1st ed.

p. cm.

ISBN 0-7216-5408-8

1. Dermatology—Examinations, questions, etc. 2. Dermatology—Outlines, syllabi, etc. 3. Skin—Surgery—Examinations, questions, etc. 4. Skin—Surgery—Outlines, syllabi, etc. I. Dover, Jeffrey S. [DNLM: 1. Skin—surgery—examination questions. 2. Skin Diseases—pathology—examination questions. WR 18 C9876 1996]

RL74.2.C88 1996

616.5′0076—dc20
DNLM/DLC   94-21584

CUTANEOUS MEDICINE AND SURGERY: SELF ASSESSMENT AND REVIEW   0-7216-5408-8

Copyright © 1996 by W.B. Saunders Company

All rights reserved. No part of this publication may be reproduced or transmitted in any form or by any means, electronic or mechanical, including photocopy, recording, or any information storage and retrieval system, without permission in writing from the publisher.

Printed in the United States of America.

Last digit is the print number: 9   8   7   6   5   4   3   2   1

To Mark Robert Dover

For

      A. Endless encouragement
      B. Fostering inquisitiveness
      C. Love
      D. Friendship
      E. All of the above.

(Correct answer, **E**)

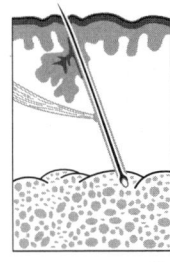

Contributors

RHODA M. ALANI, M.D.
Resident in Dermatology, Harvard Medical School; Research Fellow, Department of Pathology, Harvard Medical School, Boston, Massachusetts, United States
Inflammation, Pruritus, Percutaneous Absorption, and Topical Therapy

LORNE ALBRECHT, M.D., F.R.C.P.(C.)
Resident in Dermatology, University of British Columbia, Vancouver, British Columbia, Canada
Keratinocyte-Derived Tumors

MARC AVRAM, M.D.
Assistant Professor of Dermatology, New York University School of Medicine, New York, New York, United States
Disorders of Hair, Nails, and Sweat

ARTHUR P. BERTOLINO, M.D., Ph.D.
Associate Clinical Professor of Dermatology, New York University School of Medicine; Director, Hair Consultation Unit, New York University Medical Center, New York, New York, United States
Disorders of Hair, Nails, and Sweat

JEAN BOLOGNIA, M.D.
Associate Professor, Department of Dermatology, Yale University School of Medicine; Attending Physician, Yale-New Haven Hospital, New Haven, Connecticut, United States
Disorders of Pigmentation and Pigment Cell Biology

RINO CERIO, F.R.C.P., Dip.R.C.Path.
Senior Lecturer in Dermatopathology, Tutor in Dermatology, London Hospital Medical School, University of London, Royal London Hospital; Consultant and Clinical Director of Dermatology, Royal Hospital's Trust, Dermatology Department, Royal London Hospital, White Chapel, London, England, United Kingdom
Mesenchymal Tumors

PAUL COLLINS, D.C.H., M.R.C.P.I.
Senior Registrar, Department of Dermatology, Ninewells Hospital and Medical School, Dundee, Scotland, United Kingdom
Photodermatoses

MICHAEL J. DANNENBERG, M.D.
Resident in Dermatology, Medical College of Virginia, Richmond, Virginia, United States
Panniculitis, Fibrosing Disorders, and Atrophies

R. DAWE, M.B.Ch.B. (Glasg.), M.R.C.P. (U.K.)
Registrar, Photobiology Unit, Department of Dermatology, Ninewells Hospital and Medical School, Dundee, Scotland, United Kingdom
Photodermatoses

JULIE K. DESCH, M.D.
Dermatopathology Fellow, Stanford University Medical Center, Stanford, California, United States
Dermatopathology

PETER G. EHRNSTROM, M.D.
Chief of Dermatology, 3rd Medical Operations Squadron, United States Air Force, Elmendorf AFB, Arkansas, United States
Zoonoses, Protozoal and Helminthic Infections, Bites and Stings

JAMES FERGUSON, M.B.Ch.B., M.R.C.P.
Honorary Senior Lecturer, University of Dundee Medical School; Consultant Dermatologist, Photobiology Unit, Department of Dermatology, Ninewells Hospital and Medical School, Dundee, Scotland, United Kingdom
Photodermatoses

JO-DAVID FINE, M.D., M.P.H.
Professor of Dermatology and Adjunct Professor of Epidemiology, University of North Carolina at Chapel Hill, Schools of Medicine and Public Health; Attending Physician, University of North Carolina Hospitals, Chapel Hill, North Carolina, United States
Bullous Diseases

PHILLIP K. HALL, M.D.
Resident in Dermatology, Medical College of Virginia, Richmond, Virginia, United States
Panniculitis, Fibrosing Disorders, and Atrophies

CONTRIBUTORS

JAN V. HIRSCHMANN, M.D.
Professor of Medicine, University of Washington School of Medicine; Assistant Chief of Medicine, Veterans Affairs Medical Center, Seattle, Washington, United States
Bacterial and Rickettsial Infections

VINCENT C. HO, B.Sc.(Pharm.), M.D., F.R.C.P.(C.)
Associate Professor of Medicine (Dermatology), University of British Columbia; Head, Department of Dermatology, British Columbia Cancer Agency, Vancouver, British Columbia, Canada
Melanocytic Disorders

MICHELE HOLDER, M.D.
Resident in Dermatology, University of Iowa Hospitals and Clinics, Iowa City, Iowa, United States
Vasculitis and Disorders of Vascular Reactivity

ROBERT JACKSON, M.D., F.R.C.P.(C.)
Clinical Professor of Dermatology, School of Health Sciences, University of Ottawa; Consultant, Ottawa Civic Hospital, Ottawa, Ontario, Canada
Psoriasiform Dermatitis, Lichen Simplex Chronicus, Prurigo, and Psychocutaneous Disorders

LINA F. KANJ, M.D.
Instructor, Department of Dermatology, Boston University School of Medicine, Boston, Massachusetts, United States
What Is Normal Skin? What Does Normal Skin Do? How Are Abnormalities of the Skin Described?

GEORGIA A. KANNON, M.D.
Resident in Dermatology, Medical College of Virginia, Richmond, Virginia, United States
Panniculitis, Fibrosing Disorders, and Atrophies

LARISA KELLEY, M.D.
Resident in Dermatology, Department of Dermatology, Harvard Medical School, Boston, Massachusetts, United States
Inherited Diseases and Malformations of the Skin

STEVEN R. KOHN, M.D.
Deceased
Zoonoses, Protozoal and Helminthic Infections, Bites and Stings

SANDRA J. LANDOLT, M.D., F.R.C.P.(C.) Medicine, F.R.C.P.(C.) Dermatology
Instructor, University of Toronto Faculty of Medicine; Courtesy Staff, Women's College Hospital; Visiting Staff, Sunnybrook Health Science Centre, Toronto, Ontario, Canada
Interface Dermatitides

DAVID J. LEFFELL, M.D.
Associate Professor, Dermatology, Plastic Surgery, and Otolaryngology, Yale University School of Medicine; Attending Physician, Yale-New Haven Hospital, New Haven, Connecticut, United States
What Basic Surgical Concepts and Procedures Are Required for the Practice of Cutaneous Medicine and Surgery?

AMY B. LEWIS, M.D.
Clinical Assistant Professor, Kings County Hospital and SUNY Health Science Center, Brooklyn, New York, United States
What Basic Surgical Concepts and Procedures Are Required for the Practice of Cutaneous Medicine and Surgery?

MARK H. LOWITT, M.D.
Assistant Professor, Department of Dermatology—Residency Program Director, University of Maryland School of Medicine; Chief of Dermatology, Baltimore Veterans Affairs Hospital, Baltimore, Maryland, United States
Diseases with Dermal Inflammation

TOBY A. MAURER, M.D.
Clinical Instructor, University of California, San Francisco, San Francisco, California, United States
Viral and Fungal Infections

SUSAN M. MENARD, M.D.
Resident in Dermatology, University of Iowa Hospitals and Clinics, Iowa City, Iowa, United States
Vasculitis and Disorders of Vascular Reactivity

JAMES W. PATTERSON, M.D., F.A.C.P.
Clinical Professor of Pathology, Medical College of Virginia, Richmond, Virginia, United States
Panniculitis, Fibrosing Disorders, and Atrophies

TANIA J. PHILLIPS, M.D., F.R.C.P.C.
Associate Professor of Dermatology, Boston University School of Medicine; Attending Physician, Boston University Medical Center, Boston, Massachusetts, United States
What is Normal Skin? What Does Normal Skin Do? How Are Abnormalities of the Skin Described?

WARREN W. PIETTE, M.D.
Professor of Dermatology, University of Iowa College of Medicine, Iowa City, Iowa, United States
Vasculitis and Disorders of Vascular Reactivity

FRANK PINTO, M.D.
Head, Dermatology Department, Naval Hospital Beufort, Beufort, South Carolina, United States
Disorders of Pigmentation and Pigment Cell Biology

RONALD PRUSSICK, M.D., F.R.C.P.(C.)
Clinical Instructor, Division of Dermatology, Department of Medicine, University of Toronto Faculty of Medicine; Clinical Instructor, Sunnybrook Health Science Centre, Toronto, Ontario, Canada
Drug Eruptions and Skin Manifestations of Immune Suppression

DIANE QUINTAL, M.D., F.R.C.P.(C.)
Assistant Professor of Medicine, School of Health Sciences, University of Ottawa; Consultant and Staff Division of Dermatology, Ottawa General Hospital, Ottawa, Ontario, Canada
Psoriasiform Dermatitis, Lichen Simplex Chronicus, Prurigo, and Psychocutaneous Disorders

JASON K. RIVERS, M.D., F.R.C.P.(C.)
Assistant Professor, Department of Medicine, Division of Dermatology, University of British Columbia; Vancouver, British Columbia; National Director, Canadian Dermatology Association's Skin Awareness Program, Canada
Keratinocyte-Derived Tumors

DONALD ROSENTHAL, M.D., F.R.C.P.(C.)
Professor of Medicine, Head, Division of Dermatology, McMaster University School of Medicine, Faculty of Health Sciences; Chief of Service, Dermatology, Chedoke-McMaster Hospital, Hamilton, Ontario, Canada
Mast Cell and Langerhans Cell Proliferative Disorders, Lymphocytic Proliferative Disorders, and Metastatic Disease

RICHARD K. SCHER, M.D., F.A.C.P.
Professor, Department of Dermatology, Columbia University College of Physicians and Surgeons; Attending Physician, Dermatology, Presbyterian Hospital, New York, New York, United States
Disorders of Hair, Nails, and Sweat

JOHN SEXTON, D.M.D., M.S.D.
Instructor, Oral and Maxillofacial Surgery, Harvard Medical School; Chief, Department of Oral and Maxillofacial Surgery and Director, Maxillofacial Trauma Service, Beth Israel Hospital, Boston, Massachusetts, United States
Oral Diseases

NEIL H. SHEAR, M.D., F.R.C.P.(C.), F.A.C.P.
Director, Clinical Pharmacology; Deputy Director, Dermatology; and Associate Professor, University of Toronto Faculty of Medicine; Head, Clinical Pharmacology and Director, Adverse Drug Reaction Clinic, Sunnybrook Health Science Centre, Toronto, Ontario, Canada
Drug Eruptions and Skin Manifestations of Immune Suppression

ELIZABETH R. SHURNAS, M.D.
Resident in Dermatology, University of Colorado School of Medicine; Pediatrician, Children's Hospital, Denver, Colorado, United States
Spongiotic and Intraepidermal Pustules

R. GARY SIBBALD, M.D., F.R.C.P.(C.) (Medicine), F.R.C.P.(C.) (Dermatology), M.D.C.P., D.A.A.D.
Associate Professor of Medicine, University of Toronto Faculty of Medicine; Active Staff, Womens College Hospital, Toronto; Active Staff, Mississauga Hospital, Toronto, Ontario, Canada
Interface Dermatitides

BRUCE R. SMOLLER, M.D.
Associate Professor, Pathology and Dermatology and Director, Dermatopathology, Stanford University Medical Center, Stanford, California, United States
Dermatopathology

ELIZABETH M. SPIERS, M.D.
Assistant Professor of Dermatology, University of Pennsylvania School of Medicine, Philadelphia, Pennsylvania, United States
Bullous Diseases

LESLIE STEWART, M.D.
Assistant Professor of Dermatology, Department of Dermatology, University of Colorado School of Medicine; Head, Division of Dermatology, National Jewish Center for Immunology and Respiratory Medicine, Denver, Colorado, United States
Spongiotic and Intraepidermal Pustules

JEFFREY B. TRAVERS, M.D., Ph.D.
Resident in Dermatology, University of Colorado School of Medicine, Denver, Colorado, United States
Spongiotic and Intraepidermal Pustules

VICTOR TRON, M.D., F.R.C.P.(C.)
Associate Professor, Department of Pathology, University of British Columbia, Vancouver, British Columbia, Canada
Keratinocyte-Derived Tumors

MARIA L. TURNER, M.D.
Clinical Professor, Dermatology, George Washington University School of Medicine and Health Sciences, Washington, D.C.; Medical Officer, Dermatology, National Institutes of Health, Bethesda, Maryland, United States
Genital Diseases

NICHOLAS J. WAINWRIGHT, M.A. (Oxon), M.B.B.S., M.R.C.P. (U.K.)
Honorary Lecturer, University of Dundee Medical School; Senior Registrar, Department of Dermatology, Ninewells Hospital and Medical School, Dundee, Scotland, United Kingdom
Photodermatoses

HEIDI ANN WALDORF, M.D.
Department of Dermatology, Harvard Medical School, Boston, Massachusetts, United States
Follicular Inflammation and Inflammation of Cartilage

KAREN WISS, M.D.
Assistant Professor, University of Massachusetts Medical School; Director of Pediatric Dermatology, University of Massachusetts Medical Center, Worcester, Massachusetts, United States
Inherited Diseases and Malformations of the Skin

DAVID M. ZLOTY, M.D., F.R.C.P.(C.)
Division of Dermatology, University of British Columbia, Vancouver, British Columbia, Canada
Melanocytic Disorders

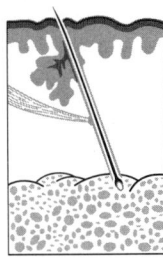

Preface

Cutaneous Medicine and Surgery: An Integrated Program in Dermatology is a new approach to the study of the specialty. It consists of a flagship textbook *Cutaneous Medicine and Surgery* and three related texts: the *Atlas of Cutaneous Surgery;* the *Pocket Guide to Cutaneous Medicine and Surgery;* and the *Self Assessment and Review*. The main text serves as the backbone of the program, and the other publications either complement or supplement it.

Residents and practitioners in dermatology will find that the *Self Assessment and Review* serves as an excellent review of the basic science and clinical aspects of dermatology. This text is an ideal means of testing knowledge—for examination preparation for residents in training (both for the mock boards and for the American Board of Dermatology Certification Examinations) and for dermatologists in practice (for recertification). In addition, the book can be used alone as an enjoyable way to learn dermatology. Each of the answers is a précis of an individual topic and not simply an explanation of the answer to the question at hand.

A well-respected group of 50 dermatologists from the United States, Canada, Scotland, and England composed the 2,000 questions and answers in this book. It is divided into 25 comprehensive chapters based on the table of contents of the main text, ensuring that every topic is extensively covered. For those interested in a more detailed discussion of any particular topic, each answer supplies a reference to the appropriate chapter of the main text. The chapters are organized with the questions appearing first, followed by the answers and a concise, but detailed, discussion. Although the text of the *Self Assessment and Review* follows the direction of the main text in order and general content, the questions and answers were composed by an independent group of contributors, thus ensuring a varied approach to each topic and an avoidance of repetition. References to other sources are also provided within chapters for those who wish to pursue further reading outside the integrated program.

Six different styles of multiple choice questions are used throughout the book to provide readers with the experience of answering the different types of questions included in the various national and local examinations. These question types include single correct answer; true and false; matching; associations with one or two answers, both, or neither; and type K, in which one or more answers complete an incomplete statement.

JEFFREY S. DOVER, M.D., F.R.C.P.C.

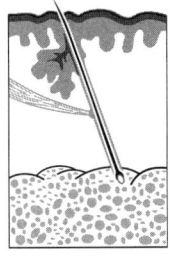

Acknowledgement

I would like to acknowledge all those who were helpful in preparing this text. In particular, I would like to thank Dr. Jean Pierre des Grosseilliers, a dermatologist and Director of the Office of Training and Evaluation for the Royal College of Surgeons of Canada, for his guidance in establishing the style and types of multiple choice questions to include in this text.

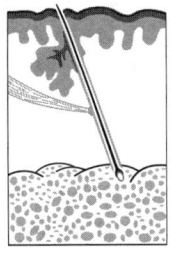

Contents

section one

What Fundamental Information Is Necessary to Understand Cutaneous Medicine and Surgery? 1

chapter 1
What Is Normal Skin? What Does Normal Skin Do? How Are Abnormalities of the Skin Described? 2
TANIA J. PHILLIPS, and LINA F. KANJ

chapter 2
What Basic Surgical Concepts and Procedures Are Required for the Practice of Cutaneous Medicine and Surgery? 13
AMY B. LEWIS, and DAVID J. LEFFELL

section two

What Disorders Present with Inflamed Skin? 25

chapter 3
Inflammation, Pruritus, Percutaneous Absorption, and Topical Therapy 26
RHODA M. ALANI, and JEFFREY S. DOVER

chapter 4
Spongiotic and Intraepidermal Pustules 37
LESLIE STEWART, ELIZABETH R. SHURNAS, and JEFFREY B. TRAVERS

chapter 5
Interface Dermatitides 51
R. GARY SIBBALD, and SANDRA J. LANDOLT

chapter 6
Psoriasiform Dermatitis, Lichen Simplex Chronicus, Prurigo, and Psychocutaneous Disorders 64
ROBERT JACKSON, and DIANE QUINTAL

chapter 7
Diseases with Dermal Inflammation 79
MARK H. LOWITT

chapter 8
Follicular Inflammation and Inflammation of Cartilage 89
HEIDI ANN WALDORF

chapter 9
Vasculitis and Disorders of Vascular Reactivity 102
WARREN W. PIETTE, MICHELE HOLDER, and SUSAN M. MENARD

chapter 10
Panniculitis, Fibrosing Disorders, and Atrophies 117
MICHAEL J. DANNENBERG, PHILLIP K. HALL, GEORGIA A. KANNON, and JAMES W. PATTERSON

chapter 11
Drug Eruptions and Skin Manifestations of Immune Suppression 129
NEIL H. SHEAR, and RONALD PRUSSICK

section three

What Diseases Cause Blistering of the Skin? 143

chapter 12
Bullous Diseases 144
JO-DAVID FINE, and ELIZABETH M. SPIERS

section four

What Diseases Are Caused by Environmental Exposure or Physical Trauma? 157

chapter 13
Photodermatoses 158
N. J. WAINWRIGHT, P. COLLINS, R. DAWE, and J. FERGUSON

section five

What Infections and Infestations Affect the Skin? ... 171

chapter 14
Bacterial and Rickettsial Infections ... 172
JAN V. HIRSCHMANN

chapter 15
Viral and Fungal Infections ... 181
TOBY A. MAURER

chapter 16
Zoonoses, Protozoal and Helminthic Infections, Bites and Stings ... 190
PETER G. EHRNSTROM, and STEVEN R. KOHN

section six

What Diseases Alter Skin Color, Hair, Nails, Sweat Glands, and Mucous Membranes? ... 197

chapter 17
Disorders of Pigmentation and Pigment Cell Biology ... 198
FRANK PINTO, and JEAN BOLOGNIA

chapter 18, part I
Oral Diseases ... 211
JOHN SEXTON

chapter 18, part II
Genital Diseases ... 220
MARIA L. TURNER

chapter 19
Disorders of Hair, Nails, and Sweat ... 224
MARC AVRAM, ARTHUR P. BERTOLINO, and RICHARD K. SCHER

section seven

What Benign and Malignant Proliferations of Cells Affect the Skin and How Are They Treated? ... 233

chapter 20
Keratinocyte-Derived Tumors ... 234
JASON K. RIVERS, LORNE ALBRECHT, and VICTOR TRON

chapter 21
Mesenchymal Tumors ... 247
RINO CERIO

chapter 22
Melanocytic Disorders ... 260
DAVID M. ZLOTY, and VINCENT C. HO

chapter 23
Mast Cell and Langerhans Cell Proliferative Disorders, Lymphocytic Proliferative Disorders, and Metastatic Disease ... 274
DONALD ROSENTHAL

section eight

What Diseases of the Skin Are Malformations or Are Predominantly Inherited? ... 283

chapter 24
Inherited Diseases and Malformations of the Skin ... 284
LARISA KELLEY, and KAREN WISS

section nine

What Are the Pathologic Findings in Skin Disease? ... 299

chapter 25
Dermatopathology ... 300
JULIE K. DESCH, and BRUCE R. SMOLLER

section one

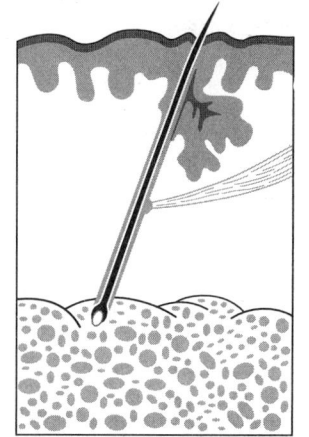

What Fundamental Information Is Necessary to Understand Cutaneous Medicine and Surgery?

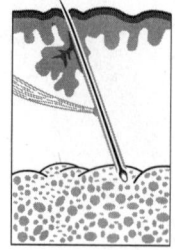

chapter 1

What Is Normal Skin? What Does Normal Skin Do? How Are Abnormalities of the Skin Described?

TANIA J. PHILLIPS, and LINA F. KANJ

Choose the ONE best answer to each of the following questions.

1. All of the following characteristics are true of keratinocytes EXCEPT
   A. Basal keratinocytes are 10 to 14 nm in diameter
   B. All keratinocytes contain keratin filaments in the cytoplasm
   C. The stratum spinosum has numerous hemidesmosomal connection plaques
   D. The stratum granulosum contains numerous intracellular basophilic granules of keratohyalin
   E. Terminally differentiated keratinocytes are nonviable.

2. Each of the following statements is true EXCEPT
   A. Mitoses are found in the normal human epidermis, largely in the basal cell layer
   B. The average normal epidermal germinative cell has a DNA synthesis time of 16 hours
   C. In normal skin, the average time required for transit of a cell from the basal cell layer to the surface of the granular cell layer is between 26 and 42 days
   D. The passage of horny cells through the normal stratum corneum requires approximately 35 days
   E. The germinative cell population in normal human epidermis is principally in the basal layer.

3. Each of the following statements is true EXCEPT
   A. The epithelial keratins can be divided into basic and acidic groups
   B. Simple epithelia are characterized by the keratin pair 6 and 16
   C. The major keratins in the basal layer are keratins 5 and 14
   D. Keratins 1 and 10 are characteristic of epidermal differentiation
   E. Keratin 19 is found in hair follicles.

Decide whether EACH of the following statements is TRUE or FALSE. Any combination of answers, from all true to all false, may occur.

4. Regarding the basement membrane zone,
   A. The lamina lucida separates the trilaminar plasma membrane from the lamina densa
   B. The lamina lucida contains the sub-basal cell dense plate
   C. Anchoring filaments extend from the basal cell plasma membrane to the lamina lucida
   D. The lamina lucida is 30 to 60 nm wide
   E. Type 4 collagen and the KF1 antigen are found within the lamina densa.

5. Regarding the lamina lucida and anchoring fibrils, decide which of the following statements are TRUE and which, FALSE:
   A. The distal part of anchoring fibrils inserts into the lamina lucida
   B. Anchoring fibrils contain type 7 collagen
   C. In junctional epidermolysis bullosa, blisters arise within the lamina lucida
   D. Anchoring fibril antigens 1 and 2 are deficient or totally absent in patients with recessively inherited dystrophic epidermolysis bullosa.

6. Odland bodies
   A. Are discharged from the granular cells into the intercellular space
   B. Establish a barrier to water loss
   C. Mediate stratum corneum adhesion
   D. Measure 300 to 500 nm in diameter.

7. Regarding integrins,
   A. Integrins are cell surface glycoproteins that form receptors
   B. They mediate interactions between cells and extracellular matrix protein
   C. They are important in intercellular adhesion
   D. They consist of 3 subunits: alpha, beta, and gamma
   E. They are important in wound healing and immune defense mechanisms.

8. Melanocytes can be identified with which of the following stains?
   A. Bloch dopa reaction
   B. Silver stains
   C. Fontana Masson stain
   D. Congo red.

Regarding melanocytes

9. The highest concentration of melanocytes is found on the trunk.
10. The lowest concentration of melanocytes is found on the face and the male genitalia.
11. Black skin contains larger and more dendritic melanocytes than white skin.
12. In black skin, there is increased density and numbers of melanocytes for any given area compared with white skin.
13. In black skin, the melanocytes are uniformly reactive.
14. A single exposure to ultraviolet light in white skin results in increased numbers of dopa-positive melanocytes.
15. Repeated exposure to ultraviolet light causes an increase in the concentration of dopa-positive melanocytes.
16. A single exposure to ultraviolet light in vivo causes increased size and functional activity of melanocytes.
17. Multiple exposures of white skin to ultraviolet light cause an increase in the size and functional activity of melanocytes.
18. Tyrosinase
    A. Catalyzes the conversion of tyrosine to dihydroxyphenylalanine
    B. Catalyzes the oxidation of dopa to dopa quinone
    C. Requires the conversion of cupric to cuprous atoms before it can act upon tyrosine
    D. Converts tyrosine to melanin
    E. Requires dopa as a cofactor in its action.
19. Stage I melanosomes
    A. Are round
    B. Measure 0.3 microns in diameter
    C. Possess intense tyrosinase activity
    D. Contain melanin.
20. In black skin,
    A. Melanosomes can be found throughout the epidermis
    B. Melanosomes can be found in the stratum corneum
    C. Melanosomes and keratinocytes are aggregated within membrane-bound melanosome

complexes containing two or three melanosomes

D. Melanosomes are larger in size than in white skin

E. Melanosomes are degraded more rapidly than in white skin.

21. Langerhans cells may be identified with the following stains
    A. Adenosine triphosphatase
    B. Aminopeptidase
    C. OKT 6
    D. Argentaffin
    E. Gold chloride.

22. Langerhans cells
    A. Constitute 2% to 4% of the total epidermal cell population
    B. Express immune response–associated antigens IA and HLA DR
    C. Express S100 protein
    D. Possess actin-like filaments
    E. Possess vimentin filaments.

23. Langerhans cells
    A. Present antigen to B lymphocytes
    B. Play an important role in contact sensitization
    C. Are important in skin graft rejection
    D. Increase in number in skin after ultraviolet radiation.

24. Eccrine glands are present in the following sites
    A. The labia minora
    B. The palms and soles
    C. The vermilion border of the lip
    D. The inner aspect of the prepuce
    E. The axillae.

25. Apocrine glands
    A. Originate from the hair germ
    B. Contain PAS-negative diastase-resistant granules
    C. Possess eosinophilic cytoplasm
    D. Have a larger lumen than that of eccrine glands
    E. Secrete sialomucin.

26. Sebaceous glands produce the following lipids:
    A. Triglycerides
    B. Phospholipids
    C. Esterified cholesterol
    D. Free cholesterol
    E. Waxes.

27. Regarding hair biology,
    A. The hair matrix gives rise to hair and the inner root sheath
    B. The outer root sheath represents a downward extension of the epidermis
    C. The keratin of the inner root sheath represents hard keratin
    D. The inner root sheath contains melanin
    E. The three layers of the inner root sheath keratinize by means of trichohyaline granules.

28. Ground substance contains
    A. Glycosaminoglycans
    B. Proteoglycans
    C. Hyaluronic acid
    D. Collagen.

29. Regarding Meissner's corpuscles, they
    A. Are located in the deep dermis
    B. Mediate the sense of touch
    C. Occur on the trunk
    D. Are found in more numbers on the hands than on the feet
    E. Average 200 microns in size.

In the following question, a set of lettered headings accompanies a list of numbered words or phrases. For each numbered word or phrase, choose

A. If the item is associated with A only
B. If the item is associated with B only
C. If the item is associated with both A and B
D. If the item is associated with neither A nor B.

30. For each of the following characteristics, choose whether it describes clear cells of eccrine glands, dark cells of eccrine glands, both, or neither.

    i. Broader at the base than near the lumen of the gland
    ii. Contain PAS-positive diastase-labile glycogen
    iii. Contain PAS-positive diastase-

    A. Clear cells of eccrine glands
    B. Dark cells of eccrine glands
    C. Both

iv. Secrete abundant amounts of aqueous material and glycogen

D. Neither.

v. Secrete sialomucin.

For each of the following numbered items, choose the one lettered item with which it is most closely associated. Each lettered item may be used once, more than once, or not at all.

31. For the following types of collagen, indicate in which location each is found.

    i. Type I collagen
    ii. Type III collagen
    iii. Type IV collagen
    iv. Type II collagen
    v. Type VII collagen.

    A. Subepidermal regions
    B. Reticular dermis
    C. Basement membrane zones and perivascular regions
    D. Anchoring fibrils
    E. Cartilage.

For each of the following questions, one or more completions correctly finish the incomplete statement; choose the letter that indicates the correct completion of that statement.

A. If only 1, 2, and 3 are correct
B. If only 1 and 3 are correct
C. If only 2 and 4 are correct
D. If only 4 is correct
E. If all are correct.

32. Cells involved in the immune response in the skin include
    1. Langerhans cells
    2. Keratinocytes
    3. Indeterminate dendritic cells
    4. Melanocytes.

33. The main barriers to passage of water and electrolytes in the skin are the
    1. Epidermis
    2. Dermis
    3. Stratum corneum
    4. Subcutaneous tissue.

34. Which of the following statements regarding Odland bodies in the skin are true?
    1. They are also called membrane-coating granules, or lamellar bodies
    2. They are present only in the granular cell layer
    3. They discharge their contents into the intercellular spaces to form intercellular cement
    4. They contain lipids only.

35. Specific androgen targets in the skin are
    1. Sebaceous glands
    2. Some hair follicles
    3. Apocrine sweat glands
    4. Eccrine sweat glands.

36. Estrogens have the following effects on skin:
    1. Maintain dermal collagen
    2. Increase the synthesis of ground substance
    3. In the long term, if given in pharmacologic doses, they can inhibit sebaceous gland secretion
    4. Estradiol binds to cytosolic receptors in human skin.

37. Which of the following is (are) true of epidermal growth factor (EGF)?
    1. EGF is a polypeptide which stimulates epidermal cell proliferation in some animals
    2. Receptors for EGF are mainly found in the basal cell layer
    3. Receptors for EGF may also occur in mitotically inactive cells such as those of sweat ducts
    4. In mice, production of EGF may be affected by estrogen and testosterone.

38. Heat can be lost through the skin surface by
    1. Radiation
    2. Convection
    3. Conduction
    4. Evaporation.

39. The following can be considered primary lesions of the skin:
    1. Nodule
    2. Lichenification
    3. Pustule
    4. Excoriation.

40. Which of the following are true about nails?
    1. The matrix is primarily responsible for the production of the nail plate
    2. Keratinization in the matrix occurs without a granular layer
    3. Absence of subcutaneous tissue, allowing close association with the vasculature, is a unique feature of the dermal component of the nail structure
    4. The rate of growth of the thumbnail is around 0.1 mm/day.

41. Which of the following are true about vitamin D synthesis in the skin?
    1. Vitamin D_3 synthesis occurs mainly in stratum basale and stratum spinosum
    2. It is synthesized from 7-dehydrocholesterol through the intermediate previtamin D_3
    3. A plateau of vitamin D_3 is reached when around 15% of 7-dehydrocholesterol has been converted
    4. Vitamin D_3 is synthesized in the skin mainly as a result of exposure to UVA.

Choose the ONE best answer to each of the following questions:

42. The mechanical properties of the skin depend primarily on the
    A. Epidermis
    B. Dermis
    C. Subcutaneous tissue
    D. Stratum corneum.

43. Each of the following is true about apocrine glands EXCEPT
    A. They usually open directly into the surface of the skin
    B. Their secretion is odorless
    C. Their secretion is pulsatile
    D. Their secretion is controlled by adrenergic nerves.

44. Each of the following is true about hair EXCEPT
    A. Anagen lasts around 3 years; catagen, 3 weeks; and telogen, 3 months
    B. On the scalp, the average daily growth is approximately 0.4 mm
    C. A loss of around 100 scalp hairs daily is considered normal
    D. *Isthmus* refers to the upper portion of the hair follicle extending from the entrance of the sebaceous duct to the surface of the skin.

45. All the following are true about granulomas EXCEPT
    A. They are chronic proliferative lesions containing mononuclear cells (lymphocytes, monocytes, macrophages) as well as epithelioid and/or multinucleated giant cells
    B. Foreign body granulomas usually show many epithelioid cells
    C. Zirconium, beryllium, and tattoos can produce allergic granulomas
    D. Allergic granulomas are characterized by the presence of epithelioid and multinucleated giant cells.

46. All the following are true about parakeratosis EXCEPT
    A. It refers to retention of nuclei by keratinocytes in the horny layer
    B. It is usually associated with an increased granular cell layer
    C. It is usually focal in psoriasis
    D. It is a physiologic phenomenon in the oral mucosa.

47. Which statement about hydropic degeneration of the basal layer of the epidermis is FALSE?
    A. It occurs in lupus erythematosus, lichen sclerosus et atrophicus and poikiloderma atrophicans vasculare
    B. It is a distinctive feature in lichen planus and acute dermatitis
    C. It may lead to pigment incontinence
    D. It may lead to formation of bullae.

48. Which one of the following statements is TRUE about colloid bodies?
    A. They are seen only in the epidermis
    B. They are round, basophilic, homogeneous bodies
    C. They should not be confused with Civatte's bodies, which are primarily found in poikiloderma of Civatte
    D. They commonly occur in lupus erythematosus and lichen planus.

Decide whether EACH of the following statements is TRUE or FALSE. Any combination of answers from all true to all false may occur.

49. Melanocytes constitute approximately 50% of the epidermal cell population.
50. Meissner's corpuscles mediate the sense of heat. Their concentration is highest on the ventral aspect of hands and feet.
51. Vater-Pacini corpuscles are located in the subcutis. They mediate the sense of pressure.
52. Merkel's cells constitute less than 1% of the epidermal cell population and basically are slowly adapting mechanoreceptors.

Regarding hair,

53. The change from vellus to terminal hair starts in the axillae in both men and women.
54. Usually < 1% of hairs are in catagen in the human scalp.

Regarding layers of the skin,

55. The dermis is the major component responsible for protection against damage from low voltage electric current.
56. The stratum corneum is responsible for prevention of water loss and protection against chemical assault.

In each of the following questions, a set of lettered headings accompanies a set of numbered words or phrases. For each numbered word or phrase, choose

A. If the item is associated with A only
B. If the item is associated with B only
C. If the item is associated with both A and B
D. If the item is associated with neither A nor B

57. For each of the following pathology findings, choose whether it describes an allergic granuloma, is a peripheral arrangement of nuclei in a horseshoe pattern, both, or neither.

    i. Langhans giant cell   A. Allergic granuloma
    ii. Foreign body giant cell.   B. Peripheral arrangement of nuclei in a horseshoe pattern
                                    C. Both
                                    D. Neither.

58. For each pattern, choose whether it is found in fibrous tumors, non-Hodgkin's lymphoma, both, or neither.

    i. Cartwheel pattern   A. Fibrous tumors
    ii. Indian filing of cells. B. Non-Hodgkin's lymphoma
                                 C. Both
                                 D. Neither.

59. For each type of hair, choose whether it is medullated, pigmented, both, or neither.

    i. Lanugo hair   A. Medullated
    ii. Vellus hair   B. Pigmented
    iii. Terminal hair.   C. Both
                          D. Neither.

60. For each cell type, choose whether it is found in the epidermis, dermis, both, or neither.

    i. Melanocyte   A. Epidermis
    ii. Langerhans cell B. Dermis
    iii. Mast cell   C. Both
    iv. Macrophages   D. Neither.
    v. Merkel cell.

61. For each statement, choose whether it describes testosterone, 5α-dihydrotestosterone, both, or neither.

    i. Can bind to receptors in the skin   A. Testosterone
    ii. Needed for development of pubic and axillary hair   B. 5α-Dihydrotestosterone
                                                       C. Both
    iii. Needed for development of facial and body hair.   D. Neither.

ANSWERS

1. C (F) The epidermis is divided into four layers: basal, spinous, granular, and horny (stratum basale, stratum spinosum, stratum granulosum, and stratum corneum). The basal layer consists of small cuboidal cells that are 10 to 14 nm in diameter and have deeply basophilic cytoplasm. The basal cells are connected by hemidesmosomes to the basal lamina. The cells of the stratum spinosum, or spinous layer, are polygonal in shape and are connected by desmosomes that act as intercellular bridges. In the upper spinous layer, cells tend to become flatter and larger. Cells of the spinous layer contain large bundles of keratin filaments. The granular layer contains numerous intracellular basophilic granules of keratohyaline, associated with epidermal differentiation. The stratum corneum acts as the major barrier of the skin and is composed of flat polyhedral cells containing a high percentage of keratins stabilized by disulfide bonds. The cells are anucleate and nonviable (Chapters 1, 2 and 3).

2. D (F) Mitoses are mainly found in the basal layer of the epidermis. The normal epidermal stem cell, or germinative cell, has a DNA synthesis time of 16 hours and divides approximately every 19 days. The epidermal transit time is the time required for a cell to pass from the basal layer to the granular layer. In normal skin, this is between 26 and 42 days. Using radioactive labels or fluorescent dyes, the transit time through the horny layer has been estimated as approximately 14 days. In conditions such as psoriasis, the epidermal transit time is much more rapid (Chapters 1, 2, and 3).

3. B (F) The epithelial keratins can be divided into two groups: the basic group (keratins 1-8) and the acidic group (keratins 9-19). The basic keratins are also known as type 1 keratins, and those in the acidic group are known as type 2 keratins. In epithelia, keratins are expressed in pairs with one member of each group (basic and acidic) required for keratin filament assembly. In simple epithelia, the keratin pair 8 and 18 is expressed. In the skin, keratins 5 and 14 are predominantly expressed in the basal layer. In the suprabasal layer, keratins 1 and 10 are expressed and are characteristic of epidermal differentiation. In hyperproliferative conditions such as psoriasis, the keratin pair 6 and 16 is expressed (Chapter 3).

4. A (T); B (T); C (F); D (T); E (T)

5. A (F); B (T); C (T); D (T) Hemidesmosomes are found at the lower surface of basal cells. They contain an intracellular attachment plaque, to which tonofilaments are attached, and an extracellular component known as the sub-basal dense plate, which is found in the lamina lucida. The hemidesmosomes help maintain attachment between the dermis and epidermis. Below the plasma membrane of the basal cell is the basement membrane. This consists of a lucent zone called the lamina lucida and a more electron-dense zone, the lamina densa.

Anchoring filaments are fine filaments that extend from the basal cell plasma membrane through the lamina lucida to the lamina densa. The anchoring fibrils are short, curved structures that insert into the lamina densa and can extend into the dermis or curve back to reinsert into the lamina densa. They have irregular cross-striations and fan out at either end. They contain type 7 collagen. In blistering disorders, there may be defective anchoring fibril formation. For example, in recessively inherited dystrophic epidermolysis bullosa, anchoring fibril antigens 1 and 2 are deficient or totally absent. In junctional epidermolysis bullosa, decreased numbers of hemidesmosomes and blisters arise within the lamina lucida (Chapters 3 and 72).

6. A (T); B (T); C (T); D (T) Odland bodies are also known as membrane-coating granules or lamellar granules. They are found within the granular layer of the epidermis and are rich in lipids, which include phospholipids, glycolipids, and free sterols. They discharge their contents into the intercellular spaces, helping to establish a barrier to water loss within the stratum corneum and mediate adhesion of the cells. Odland bodies measure 300 to 500 nm in diameter (Chapters 1 and 2).

7. A (T); B (T); C (T); D (F) The integrins are glycoproteins found on the cell surface that form receptors and mediate interactions between cells and extracellular matrix protein. They consist of two subunits: alpha and beta. They are important in immune defense mechanisms, wound healing, and skin development (Chapter 2).

8. A (T); B (T); C (T); D (F) Melanocytes can be stained with the Bloch dopa reaction, the silver, and Fontana Masson stains. The dopa reaction requires incubation of fresh skin in a 0.01% solution of 3,4-dihydroxyphenylalanine (dopa). The melanocytes stain black with this procedure. Melanin can be treated with silver nitrate solution and then reduced with hydroquinone to stain melanocytes black. This method also stains nerve fibers and reticulum fibers. Fontana Masson with ammoniated silver nitrate also stains melanocytes. Congo red is used to stain amyloid tissue (Chapters 1 and 129).

9. (F); **10.** (F); **11.** (T); **12.** (F); **13.** (T); **14.** (F); **15.** (T); **16.** (T); **17.** (T) The highest concentration of melanocytes has been found on the face and on the male genitalia. The lowest concentration is found on the trunk. In black skin, the density and distribution of melanocytes is the same as for white skin. However, in black skin, the melanocytes are larger and more highly dendritic. In white skin, after a single exposure to ultraviolet light, melanocytes tend to increase in size and functional activity, but there is no increase in melanocyte numbers. This requires multiple exposures to ultraviolet light, and also results in increased size and functional activity of these cells (Chapters 1 and 129).

18. A (T); B (T); C (T); D (T); E (T) (Chapter 129.)

19. A (T); B (T); C (T); D (F) (Chapter 129.)

20. A (T); B (T); C (F); D (T); E (F) Conversion of tyrosine to dopa and the oxidation of dopa to dopa quinone is catalyzed by the enzyme tyrosinase. The reduction of the cupric atoms in tyrosinase to cuprous atoms must occur before the enzyme can act. Dopa is believed to be a cofactor in this reaction.

Four stages of melanosomes have been described; stage I melanosomes do not contain any melanin. They measure approximately 3 microns in diameter, have a round shape, and have high tyrosinase activity; stage II melanosomes are elliptical in shape and measure 0.5 microns in width. Melanin deposition has begun at this stage, and enzyme activity persists; stage III melanosomes have more melanin deposition with little tyrosinase activity. They, too, are elliptical in shape and measure 0.5 microns in width; stage IV melanosomes have no tyrosinase activity and are filled with melanin.

Melanosomes are found in the basal layer as well as throughout the epidermis and in the stratum corneum. However, in skin, particularly in non–sun-exposed areas, melanosomes tend to be concentrated in the basal layer of the epidermis. In black skin, most melanosomes are dispersed singly. Few melanosome complexes are found. This is in contrast to white skin, in which the melanosomes tend to be aggregated within membrane-bound melanosome complexes (Chapter 129).

21. A (T); B (T); C (T); D (F); E (T) (Chapter 1.)

22. A (T); B (T); C (T); D (T); E (T) (Chapter 1.)

23. A (T); B (T); C (T); D (F) Langerhans cells are bone marrow–derived cells that are important in antigen processing and recognition. They constitute 2% to 4% of the total epidermal cell population and express Ia and HLA-DR antigen as well as S100 protein and actin-like and vimentin filaments. They can be identified with adenosine triphosphatase, aminopeptidase, OKT6, and gold chloride. Argentaffin stains melanocytes but not Langerhans cells. Because of their ability to present antigen to T cells, Langerhans cells are important in contact sensitization, skin graft rejection, and immune surveillance. Their numbers in the skin decrease after ultraviolet radiation (Chapter 1).

24. A (F); B (T); C (F); D (F); E (T) Eccrine, or sweat, glands are present in all areas of the body except the vermilion border of the lips, the nail beds, the labia minora, the glans penis, and the inner aspect of the prepuce. Large numbers of eccrine glands are found in the palms, soles, and axillae (Chapters 1 and 137).

25. A (T); B (F); C (T); D (T); E (T) Apocrine glands represent scent glands and differ from eccrine glands in location, size, and origin. They contain PAS-positive diastase-resistant granules and originate from the hair germ. They are found in the axillae, eyelid, breast, and anogenital areas. They are tubular glands in which secretion occurs by "decapitation-secretion," a process in which the cytoplasm of the secretory cell is pinched off. The secretory cells possess eosinophilic cytoplasm and have a larger lumen than that of eccrine glands (Chapters 1 and 137).

26. A (T); B (T); C (T); D (F); E (T) Sebaceous glands are found throughout the skin with the exception of the palms and soles. They secrete a variety of lipids, including triglycerides, phospholipids, and esterified cholesterol, but no free cholesterol. Waxes are also present (Chapter 1).

27. A (T); B (T); C (F); D (F); E (T) The bulk of a hair is formed by the hair cortex within which is the core, or medulla. The cortex is surrounded by a cuticle composed of the inner root sheath cuticle, the Huxley layer, the Henley layer (which stains dark because of the presence of trichohyalin granules), and the outer root sheath. The outer root sheath is continuous with the superficial epidermis. During hair growth, the hair exhibits a hair bulb at its inferior end. The dermal papilla protrudes into the bulb and maintains the growth of the hair follicle. Within the hair bulb, the cells of the hair matrix produce hair and the inner root sheath. The outer root sheath, however, is a downward extension of the epidermis. The hair cortex contains hard keratin, that is, keratinization occurs without the formation of keratohyaline granules. In contrast, in the inner root sheath, keratohyaline granules form. Thus, the inner root sheath represents soft keratin, whereas the cortex represents hard keratin. The inner root sheath does not contain melanin. Melanin is produced by melanocytes between the basal cells of the hair matrix superior to and lateral to the dermal hair papilla (Chapters 1 and 133).

28. A (T); B (T); C (T); D (F) The dermis consists of protein fibers, principally collagen and elastin, embedded in a supporting matrix of ground substance. The composition of ground substance includes polysaccharides, also known as glycosaminoglycans. These are usually linked to proteins to form proteoglycans. This molecule has remarkable water-holding capacity and is the principal component of the connective tissue matrix. The principal glycosaminoglycans found in ground substance are hyaluronic acid, chondroitin, dermatan sulfate (chondroitin sulfate B), chondroitin 4 sulfate (chondroitin sulfate A), and chondroitin 6 sulfate (chondroitin sulfate C) (Chapters 1, 2, and 97).

29. A (F); B (T); C (F); D (T); E (T) Meissner's corpuscles mediate a tactile sensation. They are found in the dermal papillae of the hands and feet, particularly on the fingertips. They are elongated in shape, and the average size is 30 × 80 microns. The corpuscle is surrounded by Schwann's cells, and the center of the corpuscle is probably composed of modified Schwann's cells (Chapter 1).

30. i A; ii A; iii B; iv A; v B Two types of cells line the lumen of the eccrine glands—dark cells and clear cells. The clear cells are broadest at their base, whereas the dark cells are broadest near the lumen. The dark cells contain PAS-positive diastase-resistant mucopolysaccharides, but the clear cells contain PAS-positive diastase labile glycogen. The dark cells secrete sialomucin, whereas the clear secrete aqueous material and glycogen (Chapters 1 and 137).

31. i B; ii A; iii C; iv E; v D Type I collagen is mainly found in the reticular dermis. Type II collagen is found in cartilage. Type III collagen is found mainly in early fetal life, whereas in adult life it is limited to the subepidermal and periappendicular regions. Type IV collagen is found in the basement membrane zone. Type V collagen is found in vascular tissue, and Type VII collagen is found in basement membranes, particularly in the anchoring fibrils (Chapters 1 and 97).

32. A The three types of cells that are known to be involved in the immune response in the skin are the Langerhans cell, the indeterminate dendritic cell and the keratinocyte. Langerhans cells are bone marrow–derived cells that are functionally and immunologically related to the monocyte-macrophage-histiocyte series. They are important for antigen processing and presentation to lymphocytes. Among other things, they express immune response–associated antigens Ia and HLA-DR as well as Fc and C3 receptors. With electron microscopy, they are seen to contain characteristic racquet-shaped Birbeck granules. They are believed to play an important role in contact sensitization, graft rejection, and immune surveillance against viral infections and tumors of the skin. The indeterminate dendritic cells are much less well defined. They occur in the dermis and the epidermis and can only be seen by electron microscopy. They demonstrate several of the molecules found on the surface of Langerhans cells but lack Birbeck granules. Keratinocytes participate in the immune response by producing thymus-like hormones, α-interferon, prostaglandins, colony-stimulating factors, and a thymocyte-activating factor (Chapter 1).

33. B A major function of the skin is to protect the body, be it against mechanical injury, radiation, fluid loss, or penetration of unwanted material. The barrier to inward or outward passage of water and electrolytes resides mainly in the epidermis and more specifically in the stratum corneum. This is achieved by the tight packaging of the cornified cells as well as by the lipid-rich intercellular material produced by the Odland bodies. The barrier properties of the skin vary, depending on the permeability constant of the substance involved (permeability constant equals the ratio of flux to the concentration applied), body site, age, and environmental conditions (Chapters 1 and 2).

34. B Odland bodies are also referred to as membrane-coating granules, lamellar bodies, and keratinosomes. These small (0.2 to 0.3 micrometers in diameter), ovoid organelles are first identifiable in the spinous cell layer. In the granular cell layer, they fuse with the plasma membrane and discharge their contents into the intercellular space. They are thus responsible for maintaining cell cohesion and providing a barrier to water loss in the stratum corneum. As they move up in the epidermis, the content of Odland bodies changes significantly. Originally, they contain neutral sugars linked to lipids, and/or proteins, hydrolytic enzymes, and free sterols. Later, phospholipids diminish, and neutral lipids and sphingolipids increase. Cholesterol sulfate increases from the spinous to the granular layer but decreases in the stratum corneum (Chapters 1 and 2).

35. A Specific androgen receptors in the skin include sebaceous glands, apocrine glands, some hair follicles, and fibroblasts. The superficial epidermis seems to be a specific target for androgens too, since testosterone stimulates epidermal cell division in rodents. Dehydroepiandrosterone is converted to testosterone, which is rapidly metabolized to dihydrotestosterone (DHT) through the action of the enzyme 5α-reductase. DHT binds to intracellular receptors. Because of this influence of androgens on various skin elements, several skin disorders such as acne vulgaris and hidradenitis suppurativa are androgen-dependent. In addition, several genetic disorders such as male pseudohermaphroditism and testicular feminization result from deficiency or abnormality in 5α-reductase or androgen receptors. Eccrine gland function, which is dependent on sympathetic, mainly cholinergic, nerve supply, is controlled by thermal, mental, and gustatory stimuli (Chapters 1 and 181).

36. E Although the level of estrogen receptors in skin is low (highest in face and lowest in breast and thigh), these hormones seem to affect various components of the skin. They increase the epidermal mitotic rate in humans; stimulate synthesis, maturation, and turnover of collagen; increase the synthesis of hyaluronic acid; and slow the rate of hair growth. Although initially they may have a stimulatory effect on sebaceous glands, when given in pharmacologic doses, their long-term effect is inhibition of sebaceous gland size and activity. Like androgens, these hormones also bind to cytosolic receptors (Chapters 1 and 181).

37. E Epidermal growth factor (EGF) was originally isolated from submaxillary glands of adult mice, in which it seemed to accelerate the eruption of incisors and opening of eyelids in neonatal animals. In humans, a homologous polypeptide with identical functions was isolated from urine. EGF increases the mitotic rate and proliferation of epidermal cells. Its receptors in human skin seem to be highest in the mitotically active basal keratinocytes and to diminish as cells become more differentiated. However, they are also found in mitotically inactive cells such as sweat ducts. In mice, the production of EGF is stimulated by testosterone and inhibited by estrogen (Chapter 1).

38. E Maintenance of a constant core temperature of the body is essential for human life. Skin plays a major role in thermoregulation. In a cold environment, heat is lost from the skin through convection, conduction, and radiation. Convection refers to the transfer of heat to moving air, which has a lower temperature than the body surface. It depends on blood flow to the skin and varies with the level of vasodilatation or constriction as well as with the vascular supply to different areas of the body. Conduction is the transfer of heat by direct contact. It is affected by the underlying tissue. Adipose tissue has a low conductivity and is thus a good heat insulator. Air is a poor conductor of heat. A "dead-air" layer (of about 0.2 cm in a quiet environment) on the surface of the skin acts as an insulator and is enhanced by clothing and disrupted by wind. Loss of heat by radiation is proportional to the difference in absolute temperatures of the cutaneous surface and the colder object receiving heat. At high environmental temperatures, sweat evaporation plays a crucial role in cooling down the skin (Chapter 1).

39. B Primary lesions are the basic lesions that first appear on the skin. They are important for description as well as diagnosis of different dermatologic diseases. Examples include macules, papules, patches, plaques, nodules, tumors, wheals, and vesicles. Secondary lesions appear later on in the course of the disease and can be induced by rubbing, scratching, or infection. Examples are lichenification, erosions, ulcers, and excoriations (Chapter 5).

40. E The four epidermal components of the nail organ are the matrix, the nail bed, the proximal nail fold, and the hyponychium. The nail plate is primarily synthesized by the matrix, in which keratinization occurs without a granular cell layer. A few horny cells are, however, added to the undersurface of the nail plate from the nail bed and hyponychium. The dermal component of the nail unit is in close association with its vasculature because of the absence of subcutaneous tissue. The rate of growth of the nail plate depends on the rate of turnover of the matrix cells. Fingernails grow faster than toenails. The average daily rate of growth for the thumbnail is 0.1 to 0.2 mm (Chapter 136).

41. A Specific receptors for 1,25-dihydroxyvitamin D_3, the active form of vitamin D, have been found in the skin. This hormone is synthesized mainly in the basal and spinous cell layers of the epidermis upon exposure to ultraviolet light B (UVB). 7-Dehydrocholesterol is converted to the intermediate previtamin D_3. When isolated skin is exposed to UVB radiation, a plateau in previtamin D_3 synthesis is reached when about 15% of the original dehydrocholesterol has been utilized. Further exposure leads to the conversion of previtamin D_3 to two biologically inactive isomers: lumisterol$_3$ and lachysterol$_3$ (Chapter 1).

42. B The mechanical properties of the skin depend mainly on the dermis. This is achieved by the collagen and elastic fibers as well as the ground substance. Initially, skin stretches easily, primarily as a result of reorientation of collagen fibers toward the load axis and a reduction in their convolution. Elastic fibers maintain the tone of the skin and are responsible for restoring the extensibility of slack skin. After the initial slack has been taken up, skin becomes much harder to extend. However, under continued stretch, further irreversible extension does occur through the process of viscous slip/extension. This is mainly dependent on collagen fibrils, which are believed to slip either relative to each other or within the related ground substance. This viscous slip is ordinarily restrained by the highly viscous interfibrillar substance. When compressed by a small object, skin seems to mould around that object, thus reducing the pressure at any one point—achieved by a flow of ground substance through the dermal collagen fibers. Although the stratum corneum has a relatively high tensile strength, it offers little protection against mechanical forces. The subcutaneous tissue helps by providing a cushion against blunt trauma (Chapters 1 and 97).

43. A Apocrine glands are scent glands found mainly in the axillae and perineal region. Although occasionally apocrine glands may open directly to the skin surface, they usually open into the pilosebaceous follicles at the level of the infundibulum, above the entry of the sebaceous duct. Histologically, they are composed of three segments: a secretory portion, constituted of a single layer of secretory cells and an outer layer of myoepithelial cells; intradermal and epidermal ducts, both of which are composed of a double layer of basophilic cells; and a periluminal eosinophilic cuticle. Apocrine glands become functional at puberty. Their secretion, which is pulsatile, is controlled by adrenergic nerves. They release their secretion through "decapitation," i.e., part of the cytoplasm of secretory cells is pinched off and released into the ductal lumen during secretion (Chapters 1 and 137).

44. D Hair grows at different rates in different regions of the body. On the human scalp, the daily growth rate is around 0.4 mm. In women, scalp hair grows faster and body hair, slower than in men. The activity of hair follicles is intermittent. Anagen is the active period, which may last for 3 or more years. Telogen is the resting phase, usually lasting about 3 months. Catagen is the transition or regression phase, usually approximately 3 weeks in duration. In the human scalp, at any one point approximately 84% of hair is in anagen, 14% in telogen, and 2% in catagen. Assuming that the scalp contains about 100,000 hairs, it can reasonably be expected that 100 hairs will be molted daily.

Histologically, the hair follicle consists of three parts: The lower portion, which extends from the base of the follicle to the insertion of the arrector pili muscle; the isthmus, which extends from the insertion of the arrector pili muscle to the entrance of the sebaceous duct; and the infundibulum, which extends from the entrance of the sebaceous duct to the follicular orifice (Chapters 1 and 133).

45. B Granulomas are chronic proliferative lesions containing mononuclear cells (lymphocytes, monocytes, macrophages) as well as epithelioid cells and/or multinucleated giant cells. They can occur as a foreign body reaction (foreign body granuloma) in response to exogenous (e.g., oils or starch powder) or endogenous (e.g., keratin) substances or as an allergic granuloma in individuals previously sensitized to various chemicals (e.g., zirconium, beryllium), microorganisms (e.g., *Mycobacterium tuberculosis, M. leprae, Treponema pallidum*), or fungi. Foreign body granulomas usually show macrophages and multinucleated giant cells with few or no epithelioid cells. Allergic granulomas are characterized by the presence of epithelioid cells but may also contain multinucleated giant cells (Chapter 5).

46. B Parakeratosis refers to retention of nuclei by keratinocytes in the horny layer, usually associated with an underdeveloped or absent granular cell layer. It is physiologic in mucous membranes. The pattern of parakeratosis may be helpful diagnostically. In psoriasis for example, it is focal and scattered. In porokeratosis, it occurs as a column in a keratin-filled invagination (cornoid lamella) (Chapter 5).

47. B Hydropic, or liquefactive, degeneration is a type of degeneration leading to vacuolation of the basal cells of the epidermis. It occurs in several entities, including lupus erythematosus, dermatomyositis, poikiloderma atrophicans, erythema dyschromicum perstans, lichen sclerosus et atrophicus, and early lichen planus, in which it usually progresses to complete disappearance of the basal cell layer. This degeneration is commonly associated with pigment incontinence. If severe enough, it may result in the formation of subepidermal bullae. In acute spongiotic dermatitis, intraepidermal vesiculation, bullae, spongiosis, exocytosis, and parakeratosis may occur but not hydropic degeneration (Chapter 5).

48. D Formation of colloid or Civatte's bodies results from the degeneration of epithelial cells and their extrusion into the dermis through apoptosis. They are round or ovoid eosinophilic, homogeneous bodies, approximately 10 micrometers in diameter. They are usually seen in the dermis and lower epidermis. They are nonspecific but occur most commonly in lichen planus and lupus erythematosus (Chapter 5).

49. F Melanocytes are dendritic cells that constitute about 5% to 10% of the epidermal cell population. Their main function is melanin synthesis through a tyrosinase-dependent pathway. Derived from the neural crest, they are present in the skin, mucous membranes, eye (uveal tract and retina), and central nervous system (leptomeninges). Together with the associated keratinocytes (approximately 36 in number), melanocytes form the epidermal melanin unit (Chapters 1 and 129).

50. F Meissner's corpuscles are special nerve end-organs that mediate the sense of touch. They are present in the dermal papillae on the palms and soles. Their number is highest in the fingertips. Their size averages 30 to 80 micrometers in diameter (Chapter 1).

51. T Vater-Pacini corpuscles are large nerve end-organs that mediate the sense of pressure. Located in the subcutis, they average 1 mm in diameter and can thus be seen under light microscopy. They are present most commonly in the volar aspect of palms and soles and also in the subcutis of the nipple and the anogenital region (Chapter 1).

52. T Merkel cells are scarce, irregularly distributed, slow-adapting mechanoreceptors. They are present in the epidermis, oral mucosa, and outer root sheath of hair follicles. On electron microscopy, they show characteristic membrane-bound granules with dense cores (Chapter 1).

53. F Lanugo hair is produced by fetal follicles. It is fine, soft, unpigmented, and unmedullated. Normally, it is shed in utero by the seventh or eighth month of gestation. Post-natal hair is divided into vellus or terminal hair. Vellus hair is soft, unmedullated, usually unpigmented, rarely more than 2 cm in length. Terminal hair is longer, coarse, medullated, and pigmented. At puberty, vellus hair is transformed into terminal hair. In both males and females, this starts in the pubic region. Axillary hair usually appears approximately 2 years later and facial hair in males begins growth at around the same time (Chapters 1 and 133).

54. F See answer to Question 44.

55. F; **56.** T The stratum corneum acts as an effective barrier against water and electrolyte loss as well as the penetration of toxic agents and ultraviolet radiation. Because of its relatively low water content, it has a high electrical resistance and thus is the main component of the skin to offer some protection against damage from low-voltage electric current (Chapters 1 and 2).

57. i C; ii D Langhans giant cells are multinucleated giant cells often found in allergic granulomas. In general, they are smaller than foreign body giant cells and often show a peripheral horseshoe, rather than irregular, arrangement of their nuclei (Chapter 5).

58. i A; ii B The cartwheel pattern, a histologic description, refers to the whorl-like radiation of elongated cells and collagen bundles from a central small blood vessel. It usually occurs in fibrous tumors. Indian filing of cells is most commonly seen in specific infiltrates of leukemia and metastatic adenocarcinoma, especially of the breast. It refers to the extension of single rows of cells between and around collagen bundles (Chapter 5).

59. i D; ii D; iii C (See answer to Question 53.)

60. i A; ii C; iii B; iv B; v A The epidermis (malpighian layer) contains keratinocytes (80%), melanocytes (5–10%), and Merkel's cells (<1%). Langerhans cells can be found in the epidermis or the dermis. Mast cells and macrophages are usually found only in the dermis (Chapter 1).

61. i C; ii A; iii B Both testosterone and 5α-dihydrotestosterone can bind to androgen receptors, but dihydrotestosterone shows a higher affinity. Testosterone is needed for the development of pubic and axillary hair, muscle development, and breaking of the voice; thus 5α-reductase activity is not essential. Facial and other body hair as well as prostate development, on the other hand, need dihydrotestosterone and are thus 5α-reductase activity–dependent (Chapter 181).

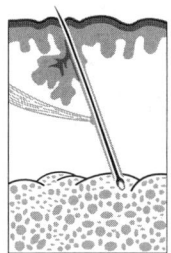

chapter 2

What Basic Surgical Concepts and Procedures Are Required for the Practice of Cutaneous Medicine and Surgery?

AMY B. LEWIS, and DAVID J. LEFFELL

For the following questions, ONE or MORE of the following completions correctly finishes the incomplete statement. Choose

- A. If only 1, 2, and 3 are correct
- B. If only 1 and 3 are correct
- C. If only 2 and 4 are correct
- D. If only 4 is correct
- E. If all are correct.

1. Chlorhexidine (Hibiclens), an antiseptic surgical scrub,
   1. Has both gram-negative and gram-positive activity
   2. Has a prolonged duration of action of several hours
   3. May irritate the eyes and therefore should not be used in this area
   4. Has slow onset of action (approximately 60 minutes).

2. The iodophors, e.g., betadine,
   1. Have both gram-negative and gram-positive activity
   2. Have a duration of action that may be as long as 1 hour
   3. Have an onset of action that is moderate to fast
   4. May be used around the eyes without irritation.

3. Hexachlorophene
   1. Is bacteriostatic against gram-positive organisms only
   2. Has an onset of action that is faster than chlorhexidine
   3. Lasts for several hours and remains on skin even after rinsing
   4. Is not absorbed through skin and is safe for use in pregnancy.

4. Ethanol and isopropyl alcohol are used as skin preparation solutions. Their properties include
   1. Activity against gram-negative organisms
   2. Activity against gram-positive organisms
   3. Sustained antimicrobial action of at least 1 hour
   4. Extremely fast onset of action.

5. Benzalkonium chloride (Zephiran) is a surfactant that is occasionally used as an antiseptic. Its properties include

1. Activity against gram-positive organisms
2. Activity against gram-negative organisms
3. Its nonirritating nature and its safe use around the eyes
4. The slow onset of activity and short duration of action.

Decide whether EACH of the following questions is TRUE or FALSE. Any combination of answers from all true to all false may occur.

6. The chemical structure of local anesthetics
    A. Is divided into three parts—aromatic portion, intermediate chain, and amine portion
    B. The lipophilic property, determined by the aromatic portion, determines the time required for onset of action
    C. The amine portion, which is responsible for the hydrophilic properties, determines the duration of action
    D. The intermediate chain is linked by either an amide or an ester group, thus forming the two major categories of local anesthetics
    E. Lidocaine is from the ester group
    F. Procaine is an amide anesthetic.
7. The ester group of anesthetics
    A. Cross-reacts with para-aminobenzoic acid (PABA)
    B. Contains the anesthetic agent procaine (Novocaine)
    C. Is metabolized by the liver
    D. Is metabolized in the plasma via pseudocholinesterase
    E. Cross-reacts with lidocaine.
8. Bupivacaine (Marcaine)
    A. Is longer acting than lidocaine
    B. Has a long onset of action; therefore its use is limited as a solitary agent in skin surgery
    C. Is an amide anesthetic
    D. Is metabolized in the liver.

For each numbered item, choose the most likely associated lettered item. Each numbered item has ONLY ONE answer. Within each group, each lettered item may be the answer to one, more than one, or none of the numbered items.

9. Supplies the medial forehead
10. Supplies the central chin and lower lip
11. Supplies the cheek and the side of the nose
12. Does not exit a foramen near the mid-pupillary line
13. Supplies the forehead and scalp superiorly as far as the vertex

    A. Supratrochlear nerve
    B. Infraorbital nerve
    C. Mental nerve
    D. Zygomaticotemporal nerve
    E. Supraorbital nerve.

14. Injury causes inability to lift the ipsilateral eyebrow
15. Injury causes inability to completely close the eye
16. Injury causes elevation of the lip with inward rotation on the affected side when smiling
17. Injury causes an inability to elevate the shoulder on the affected side
18. Injury causes sensory loss to the lower anterior portion of the ear.

    A. Temporal branch of the facial nerve
    B. Zygomatic branch of the facial nerve
    C. Marginal mandibular nerve branch
    D. Spinal accessory nerve
    E. Greater auricular nerve
    F. Zygomaticotemporal nerve.

Choose the ONE BEST answer to each of the following questions.

19. The mental nerve can be blocked via direct infiltration
    A. At the mental foramen
    B. In a preauricular location
    C. Via an intraoral approach through the gums
    D. And is an excellent means of anesthesia for surgical treatment of actinic chelitis
    E. All of the above.
20. The preferred solution for use in nerve blocks is
    A. Lidocaine 2%
    B. Lidocaine 1%

C. Lidocaine 1% with epinephrine

D. Lidocaine 2% with epinephrine

E. Bupivacaine with epinephrine.

21. The spinal accessory nerve
    A. Courses through the anterior triangle of the neck
    B. Is very superficial and therefore may be at high risk of injury
    C. Is always protected by the platysma muscle and is therefore of no great concern to the cutaneous surgeon
    D. Provides sensory innervation to the mid-portion of the neck
    E. All of the above.

22. Figure 2–1* shows a nerve block of which of these?
    A. Supratrochlear nerve
    B. Supraorbital nerve
    C. Lacrimal nerve
    D. External nasal nerve
    E. Infraorbital nerve.

23. The artery depicted in Figure 2–2† is the
    A. Labial artery
    B. Angular artery
    C. Infraorbital artery
    D. Buccal artery
    E. Nasal artery.

For the following questions, ONE or MORE of the following completions correctly finishes the statement. Choose

A. If only 1, 2, and 3 are correct
B. If only 1 and 3 are correct
C. If only 2 and 4 are correct
D. If only 4 is correct
E. If all are correct.

24. Ligation of one side of the labial artery
    1. Should be avoided so that necrosis of the lip does not occur
    2. Is not of great concern because of the excellent collateral flow from the contralateral side

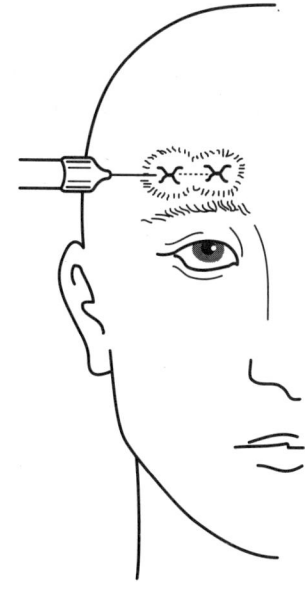

FIGURE 2–1.

    3. Is almost never needed in any lip surgery procedure
    4. Is of no great concern because of the collateral supply from the angular artery above.

For each numbered item, choose the most likely associated lettered item. Each numbered item has ONLY ONE answer. Within the group, each lettered item may be the answer to one, more than one, or none of the numbered items.

25. Low amperage, low voltage
    A. Electrocoagulation
    B. Electrodesiccation

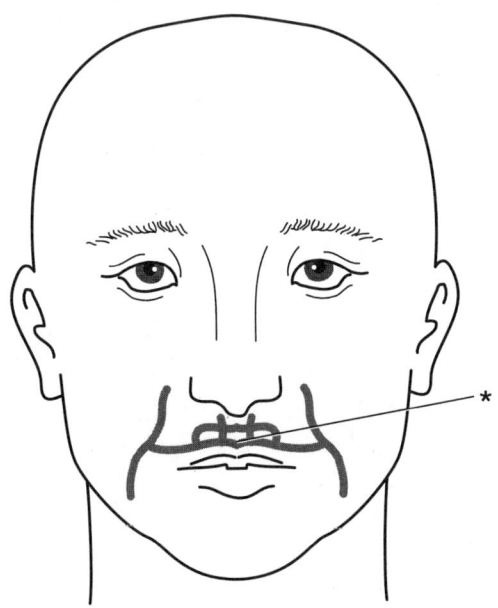

FIGURE 2–2.

---

* Modified and redrawn from Auletta MJ, Grekin RC. Local Anesthesia for Dermatologic Surgery. New York: Churchill Livingstone, 1990:58.

† Redrawn from Breisch EA, Greenway HT, Jr. Cutaneous Surgical Anatomy of the Head and Neck. New York: Churchill Livingstone, 1992:61.

26. Low voltage, high amperage, biterminal
27. Heat only, no current passes through tissue
28. High voltage, low amperage, no spark gap
29. High voltage, low amperage, spark gap
30. Safe to use in patients with pacemakers.

C. Electrolysis
D. Electrocautery
E. Electrofulguration.

Choose the ONE best answer to each of the following questions.

31. The following may cause a cutaneous tattoo
    A. Monsel's solution
    B. Aluminum chloride
    C. Tincture of benzoin
    D. Mastisol
    E. Drysol.
32. Monsel's solution contains which element?
    A. Iron
    B. Zinc
    C. Bromine
    D. Oxygen
    E. Potassium.
33. To help with hemostasis, the cutaneous surgeon can use the following EXCEPT
    A. Epinephrine with the anesthetic agent
    B. Direct pressure with gauze for 10 minutes
    C. Ferric subsulfate
    D. Aluminum chloride
    E. Tincture of benzoin.
34. Which of the following suture materials is monofilament?
    A. Prolene
    B. Polyester
    C. Vicryl
    D. Dexon
    E. Silk.

For each numbered item, choose the most likely associated lettered item. Each numbered item has ONLY ONE answer. Within the group, each lettered item may be the answer to one, more than one, or none of the numbered items.

35. Is used to better evert the edges
36. Will help in areas of tension
37. Can be used at the ends of a bilateral M-plasty
38. Eliminates the risk of "railroad track" suture marks
39. For hemostasis on a well-vascularized area such as the helix of the ear.

A. Horizontal mattress suture
B. Vertical mattress suture
C. Running locking suture
D. Tip stitch
E. Running subcuticular suture.

Choose the ONE best answer to each of the following questions.

40. "Railroad track suture" marks are likely because of
    A. Size of the needle used
    B. Sutures being left in too long
    C. Diameter of the suture used
    D. Type of suture used
    E. All of the above.
41. A pulley stitch
    A. Is used to evert the edges
    B. Is used to elevate the edges for better visualization
    C. Is used in areas of tension to stretch the skin
    D. Should never be used on the back
    E. All of the above.
42. A patient presents with a nodular growth on the helix of the ear. The major differential diagnosis includes a basal cell carcinoma and chondrodermatitis nodularis helicis. On biopsy, it would be most helpful to include
    A. Bone
    B. Cartilage
    C. A wide superficial shave of epidermis

D. Papillary dermis

E. Muscle.

43. The major branches of the facial nerve include all of the following EXCEPT

   A. Temporal

   B. Zygomatic

   C. Marginal mandibular

   D. Cervical

   E. Parotid.

For each of the following questions, decide whether EACH choice is TRUE or FALSE:

44. The area of highest vulnerability of the buccal branch of the facial nerve is from the anterior border of the parotid gland to a line drawn from the lateral canthus to the oral commissure.

45. The zygomatic branch of the facial nerve is highly vulnerable at it branches from the main stem of the facial nerve.

46. The marginal mandibular branch of the facial nerve is present on the external surface of the masseter muscle and may be vulnerable to damage there.

47. The marginal mandibular branch is covered by the platysma as it innervates the lip depressors.

Choose the ONE best answer to each of the following questions.

48. Monofilament sutures are

   A. Stiffer than braided sutures

   B. Require more knots for security

   C. Have more memory

   D. Have a relatively low risk of infection

   E. All of the above.

49. Braided sutures

   A. Include Vicryl and Dexon

   B. Have less memory than monofilament

   C. Include some nylon sutures such as Surgilon

   D. Have a higher incidence of infection compared with monofilament

   E. All of the above.

For each of the following numbered items, choose the most likely associated lettered item. Each numbered item has ONLY ONE answer. Within the group, each lettered item may be the answer to one, more than one, or none of the numbered items.

50. Absorbable, extremely tissue-reactive

51. Absorbable, synthetic, monofilament, and may last up to 6 months

52. Good for running subcuticular sutures

53. High tensile strength but may corrode or cut through tissue

54. Used almost exclusively on mucosal surfaces.

   A. PDS (polydioxanone)

   B. Surgical cat gut

   C. Stainless steel

   D. Silk

   E. Prolene.

For the following, ONE or MORE of the completions correctly finishes the incomplete statement. Choose

   A. If only 1, 2, and 3 are correct

   B. If only 1 and 3 are correct

   C. If only 2 and 4 are correct

   D. If only 4 is correct

   E. If all are correct.

55. Vasoconstrictors are added to anesthetic solutions in order to

   1. Decrease the bleeding at the operative site

   2. Prolong the duration of the longer-acting anesthetic agents mostly

   3. Prolong the duration of the shorter-acting anesthetic agents mostly

   4. Hasten the onset of action of the anesthetic agents.

56. Epinephrine

   1. Is the most commonly used vasoconstrictor in anesthetic solutions

   2. Is found commercially at a concentration of 1:100,000

   3. Usually takes 7 to 15 minutes to exert its full vasoconstrictor effect

   4. Is found commercially at a concentration of 1:500,000.

57. Sodium bicarbonate

   1. Is often added to lidocaine with epinephrine to decrease the pain of the injection

2. Has no effect on the pain of the injection
3. May cause a decrease in the efficacy of the epinephrine over time
4. May cause a decrease in the efficacy of the lidocaine over time.

58. The tumescent technique
    1. Is used often with liposuction
    2. Involves large volumes of dilute anesthetic solutions
    3. Provides prolonged anesthesia
    4. Is the preferred type of anesthesia for Mohs' microscopically controlled surgery.

59. Epinephrine should be avoided
    1. Mostly on the ears and nasal tip
    2. Mostly on the fingers and toes
    3. Anywhere on the hands and feet
    4. In patients with hyperthyroidism.

Choose the ONE best answer to each of the following questions.

60. For direct immunofluorescence, the optimal site for biopsy would be perilesional skin in
    A. Pemphigus
    B. Cicatricial pemphigoid
    C. Bullous pemphigoid
    D. Herpes gestationis
    E. All of the above
    F. None of the above.

61. For lepromatous leprosy, a punch biopsy site should be
    A. Perilesional only
    B. Lesional only
    C. Anesthetic skin only
    D. Sun-exposed skin only
    E. Anywhere.

62. If panniculitis is suspected, the preferred biopsy technique is
    A. Shave biopsy
    B. Saucerization
    C. Incisional biopsy
    D. Curettage
    E. All of the above.

63. Clinically, a patient has a purpuric eruption that is suspected to be Henoch-Schönlein purpura. The biopsy shows leukocytoclastic vasculitis. For positive direct immunofluorescence
    A. The biopsy should be done within 24 hours
    B. The biopsy should be done within 3 days
    C. Direct immunofluorescence would not be helpful
    D. The biopsy will show positive immunofluorescence within only 6 hours of the appearance of a new lesion
    E. The biopsy should be done within 7 days.

64. Figure 2–3* shows a block of the
    A. Infraorbital nerve
    B. Zygomaticotemporal nerve
    C. Maxillary nerve
    D. Facial nerve
    E. Mental nerve.

65. Figure 2–4† shows a nerve block of the
    A. Supraorbital nerve
    B. Mandibular nerve
    C. Infraorbital nerve
    D. Angular nerve
    E. Mental nerve.

66. Erb's point may help to locate the
    A. Superficial temporal nerve
    B. Parotid gland
    C. Supratrochlear nerve
    D. Eleventh cranial nerve
    E. Infraorbital nerve.

67. A patient has a large plantar wart on the posterior aspect of his sole. To anesthetize this area, the clinician attempts a block of the
    A. Posterior tibial nerve
    B. Sural nerve
    C. Anterior tibial nerve
    D. Deep peroneal nerve
    E. Superficial peroneal nerve.

---

*,† Modified and redrawn from Auletta MJ, Grekin RC: Local Anesthesia for Dermatologic Surgery, New York: Churchill Livingstone, 1990:60, 63.

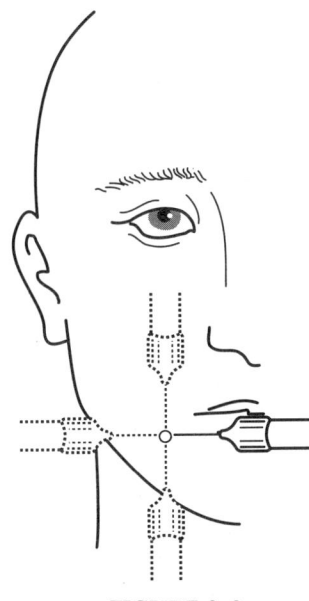

FIGURE 2–3.

68. In Question 67, the clinician infiltrates the anesthesia
    A. Behind the medial malleolus
    B. Anterior to the medial malleolus
    C. Midline on the dorsum of the foot
    D. Anterior to the lateral malleolus
    E. Posterior to the lateral malleolus.

69. A patient has an eccrine poroma on the plantar surface of the large toe. The clinician attempts to anesthetize this area with a block of the
    A. Posterior tibial nerve

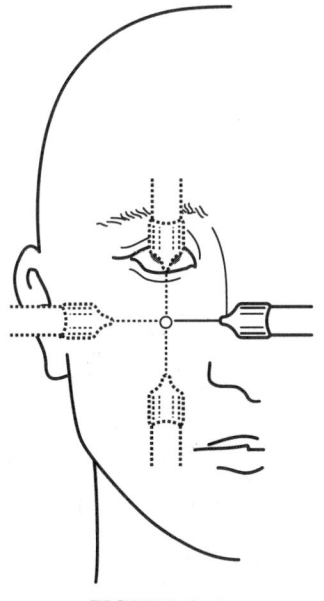

FIGURE 2–4.

B. Sural nerve
C. Anterior tibial nerve
D. Deep peroneal nerve
E. Superficial peroneal nerve.

70. In Question 69, the clinician infiltrates the anesthesia
    A. Posterior to the medial malleolus
    B. Anterior to the medial malleolus
    C. Midline on the dorsum of the foot
    D. Anterior to the lateral malleolus
    E. Posterior to the lateral malleolus.

71. Eutectic mixture of local anesthesia (EMLA)
    A. Is a topical anaesthetic agent
    B. Contains 2.5% lidocaine cream
    C. Contains 2.5% prilocaine cream
    D. Is used after occlusion for 1 to 2 hours
    E. All of the above.

For the following question, ONE or MORE of the following correctly finishes the incomplete statement. Choose

A. If only 1, 2, and 3 are correct
B. If only 1 and 3 are correct
C. If only 2 and 4 are correct
D. If only 4 is correct
E. If all are correct.

72. To block the entire dorsum of the foot, the nerves that need to be anesthetized include the
    1. Superficial peroneal nerve
    2. Deep peroneal nerve
    3. Saphenous nerve
    4. Anterior tibial nerve.

For each numbered word or phrase, choose the most likely associated lettered item. Each numbered item has ONLY ONE answer. Within the group, each lettered item may be the answer to one, more than one, or none of the numbered items.

73. Division of the trigeminal nerve
74. Branch of the maxillary nerve
75. Branch of the cervical plexus

A. Supratrochlear nerve
B. Maxillary nerve
C. Auriculotemporal nerve
D. Infraorbital nerve

76. Branch of the ophthalmic nerve
77. Branch of the mandibular nerve.

E. Great auricular nerve.

Choose the ONE BEST answer to each of the following questions.

78. Surgicel is
    A. A gelatin sponge
    B. Made of thrombin
    C. Made of fibrin
    D. Made of cellulose
    E. None of the above.

79. Gelfoam is
    A. A gelatin sponge
    B. Made of thrombin
    C. Made of fibrin
    D. Made of cellulose
    E. None of the above.

80. A tourniquet is often helpful for performing surgery on the nail. Generally, it should not be left in place for longer than
    A. 2 minutes
    B. 6 minutes
    C. 15 minutes
    D. 30 minutes
    E. 1 hour.

ANSWERS

1. A; **2.** A; **3.** B; **4.** C; **5.** E

Chlorhexidine (Hibiclens) is the most advantageous of all of the currently used surgical scrubs. It has broad-spectrum activity and is fast acting with a long duration of action. There is little skin absorption; however, it may cause irritation around the eyes.

The iodophors are a combination of the poorly water-soluble iodines complexed with a surface-active agent. This forms a solubilized compound with a longer duration of action than iodine alone. If it is not wiped off after application, the effects may last up to 1 hour. The iodophors have fewer side effects than iodine, such as staining, sensitizing, and irritation. However, when used on broken skin, iodophors may produce tissue damage and decrease the wound's ability to resist infection.

Hexachlorophene (pHisohex) is active against gram-positive organisms but is characterized by its long duration of action. It forms a bacteriostatic film similar to that of chlorhexidine. The major disadvantage to hexachlorophene is that it is absorbed through skin with handwashing. Excessive use by pregnant female hospital personnel leads to an unexpectedly high incidence of teratogenic effects in the fetus. Hexachlorophene may cross the blood–brain barrier and may be dangerous if used in premature infants.

Benzalkonium chloride is not irritative to mucous membranes and is useful around the eyes (Chapter 6).

6. A (T); B (T); C (T); D (T); E (F); F (F)

7. A (T); B (T); C (F); D (F); E (F)

8. A (T); B (T); C (T); D (T)

The chemical structure of local anesthetics affects their function:

1. The *aromatic portion* is responsible for the lipophilic properties and therefore the time required for onset of activity.
2. The *intermediate chain* contains either an amide or an ester linkage
3. The *amine* portion with hydrophilic properties determines the duration of action.

Alteration in any one component may significantly modify the anesthetic properties.

Local anesthetics are separated into two major groups, the amides and the esters. The amides include lidocaine, mepivacaine, prilocaine, bupivacaine, and etidocaine. These are metabolized by the liver and excreted by the kidney. Both bupivacaine and etidocaine have a significantly longer duration of action than lidocaine, but only etidocaine has a short onset of action like that of lidocaine.

The ester group includes cocaine, procaine (Novocain), benzocaine, butethamine, tetracaine, and propoxycaine. These all cross-react with the entire para-amino group (PABA) and are metabolized in the plasma by

AGENT	ACTIVITY	ONSET	DURATION
Alcohol (isopropyl)	Gram +	Fast	None
Iodine	Gram +, gram −	Fast	None
Iodophors (Betadine, povidone-iodine)	Gram +, gram −	Moderate/fast	Up to 1 hour
Hexachlorophene (pHisohex)	Gram +	Slow	Hours
Chlorhexidine (Hibiclens)	Gram +, gram −	Fast	Hours
Benzalkonium chloride	Gram +, gram −	Slow	None

the enzyme pseudocholinesterase. Some people have a deficiency of this enzyme and therefore should not be given anesthetic agents in this class.

Bupivacaine (Marcaine) is an amide anesthetic agent that is slower in onset than lidocaine but has a longer duration of action. It is used in some prolonged surgical cases such as Mohs' surgery and dental procedures. However, it is often mixed with lidocaine so that the duration of onset of anesthesia is not delayed (Chapter 6).

9. A; **10.** C; **11.** B; **12.** D; **13.** E The trigeminal nerve has three divisions: the ophthalmic, maxillary, and mandibular nerves. Branches of the ophthalmic nerve (V1) include the supraorbital, supratrochlear, infratrochlear, lacrimal, and external nasal nerves. The maxillary division (V2) has three branches: the infraorbital, zygomaticotemporal, and zygomaticofacial nerves. The mandibular nerve (V3) branches into the mental, auriculotemporal, and buccal nerves.

The supratrochlear nerve exits the orbit approximately 1 cm lateral to the midline and courses upward over the supraorbital rim, creating a supratrochlear notch. Branches of this nerve supply the medial upper eyelid, the medial anterior forehead, and the scalp.

The supraorbital nerve exits about 2.5 cm lateral to the midline through the supraorbital foramen. It supplies the upper eyelid, the forehead, and the scalp as far back as the vertex.

The infraorbital nerve emerges from the infraorbital foramen, which is approximately 2.5 cm lateral to the midline, about 1 cm below the infraorbital rim. This supplies the lower eyelid, the ala and nasal side wall, the upper lip, and the medial cheek.

The zygomaticotemporal nerve exits through a small foramen on the frontal process of the zygomatic bone on the lateral orbital margin to supply the temple and part of the scalp.

The mental nerve emerges through the mental foramen and supplies the chin and lower lip.

The supraorbital, infraorbital, and mental foramina are all aligned along the midpapillary line (Chapter 6).

14. A; **15.** B; **16.** C; **17.** D; **18.** E Injury to the zygomatic, buccal, and marginal mandibular branches of the facial nerve may occur anterior to the parotid gland. They are at risk here and as they continue to cross the buccal region of the cheek until they are arborized or extend deep to the surface of the muscles they supply.

Damage to the temporal branch leads to paralysis of the frontalis muscle. This causes flattening of the forehead and an inability to wrinkle the forehead or elevate the eyebrow. Paralysis of the zygomatic branch of the facial nerve innervating the orbicularis oculi muscle may result in ectropion of the lower eyelid. Damage to the transverse cervical nerve results in lack of sensation to the midportion of the neck. The greater auricular nerve ascends to the ear and is not covered by the platysma muscle. Damage will result in sensory loss to the lower anterior portion of the ear. Injury to the marginal mandibular nerve has a characteristic defect. When the patient attempts to smile, the lower lip cannot be pulled laterally or downward, and thus remains elevated. The pull from the unaffected side causes it to flatten and rotate inward. There is no deformity at rest (Chapter 6).

19. E The supraorbital nerve is anesthetized by injection above the supraorbital notch. Attempting to enter the foramen may cause damage to the nerve.

The infraorbital nerve can be blocked by either an external or intraoral approach. The external approach involves infiltration of anesthesia just medial to the infraorbital foramen. In the intraoral approach, the needle is inserted high in the labial sulcus at the apex of the canine fossa and is advanced superiorly toward the foramen.

The mental nerve can be anesthetized by an external approach adjacent to the mental foramen or in a preauricular location. In addition, it can be accomplished by an intraoral approach. The needle is inserted inside the lower lip, below the second bicuspid. A finger is used to palpate the mental foramen, and the injection is aimed in its direction. Since the mental nerve supplies the chin and lower lip, a mental nerve block is advantageous for procedures in this area (Chapter 6).

20. A Anesthetics of the amide type, similar to those used in infiltration anesthesia, are most commonly used for nerve blocks. Vasoconstrictors are usually not added because the anesthesia is not usually placed directly into the operative site and would therefore not be helpful for hemostasis. Higher concentrations of anesthetics such as 2% lidocaine are useful because they provide a greater concentration gradient and promote diffusion. Thus smaller amounts of anesthesia are needed when performing nerve blocks (Chapter 6).

21. B The spinal accessory nerve divides the posterior triangle into upper and lower parts of similar size. It supplies the sternocleidomastoid and trapezius muscles. The skin and the superficial cervical fascia are the only structures that cover the nerve during its course through the posterior cervical triangle. It is at risk for injury there. The platysma muscle does not extend far enough to cover this nerve. Damage to this nerve results in loss of function of the trapezius muscle with winging of the scapula and chronic inability to elevate the shoulder (Chapter 6).

22. B (See answer to Question 19.)

23. B The arterial supply to the external nose is from the superior labial, angular, ophthalmic, and infraorbital arteries. The angular artery is a branch of the facial artery, which runs adjacent to the nose up to the medial canthus. It terminates here and connects with the dorsal nasal artery (Chapter 6).

24. C In minor surgical procedures involving the labial mucosa, the labial arteries are frequently severed. The labial arteries anastomose with each other across the midline. A labial artery which has been cut will bleed freely from either end and often requires suturing. In addition, collaterals from the angular artery superomedially provide additional blood flow (Chapter 6).

25. C; **26.** A; **27.** D; **28.** B; **29.** E; **30.** D *Electrocautery* uses an electric current to heat a metal element that is in direct contact with the tissue to produce its effects. No electrical current passes through the tissue. *Electrofulguration and electrodesiccation* are very similar. They are high voltage and low amperage (current). They differ because in electrodesiccation the electrode is in direct contact with the treated surface. In electrofulguration there is a spark gap. A spark of energy jumps from the electrode to the tissue. This allows for more superficial tissue damage.

Electrocoagulation uses a low-voltage, high-amperage current and is biterminal. It is used with a grounding plate which is held by the patient. The high current from the active electrode causes sufficient heat to coagulate the larger vessels. *Electrolysis* uses low amperage and low voltage.

Most modern *pacemakers* are normally well shielded and filtered to avoid interference, but high-frequency electrosurgery should be avoided in patients with pacemakers. Limited electrodesiccation of small lesions usually presents no risk. However, electrocautery is safe since no electrical current passes to the patient (Chapter 6).

31. A; **32.** A Monsel's solution, ferric subsulfate, which contains iron (Fe) is used as a hemostatic chemical agent. However, it may cause pigmentation with or without a granulomatous reaction. This is often called Monsel's tattoo (Chapter 6).

33. E Various modalities are used during surgical procedures for the control of bleeding. These include vasoconstriction with the use of epinephrine in the anesthetic agent. (See answers for Questions 55 to 59.)

Direct pressure with gauze is often adequate for hemostasis. Drysol (aluminum chloride) can be used for hemostasis without the risk of pigmentation that can be seen with ferric subsulfate (Monsel's solution). The hemostatic effect is probably due to protein precipitation by the aluminum ion and the acidic nature of the solution. Tincture of benzoin, however, is not a hemostatic agent and is used as a liquid adhesive (Chapter 6).

34. A Sutures are either braided or monofilament. The monofilaments include Prolene, some nylon sutures, polydioxanone (PDS), and glycolic acid (Maxon). The widely used, braided sutures include Vicryl, Dexon, some nylon sutures, and polyester. The monofilaments are harder, stiffer, have more memory and therefore require more knots. In addition, there is a lower risk of infection. The braided sutures are more flexible, softer, and stronger. However, there is a higher incidence of infection with their use (Chapter 6).

35. B; **36.** A; **37.** D; **38.** E; **39.** C A horizontal mattress suture is used primarily in areas of tension. A vertical mattress suture is used to aid in eversion of the wound edges. A running subcuticular suture eliminates the risk of "railroad tracking" because sutures pierce the epidermal surface only at each end of the wound.

A tip stitch, also known as a corner stitch, is a variation of the half-buried horizontal mattress suture. It allows for gentle approximation of a V-shaped corner with low risk of tip strangulation. It is an excellent suture for an M-plasty. The suture has three bites, one through the epidermal edge, a small bite through the dermis at the tip of the M, and then one through the other epidermal edge. This allows for advancement of the tip and keeps it level with the surrounding tissue.

A running locking suture, often called a blanket stitch, is useful with wounds under moderate tension. It is often used on the ear and is especially helpful with hemostasis in this area (Chapter 6).

40. B "Railroad tracking" refers to suture marks that are permanently imprinted scars on the skin surface. Some of the factors that determine the severity of the suture marks are the length of time a suture is left in place, tension, relation of suture to the body, infection, and propensity for keloid formation. However, studies show that the largest suture marks have invariably occurred when sutures were left in place for approximately 14 days. The sizes of suture and needles was unimportant (Chapter 6).

41. C A pulley stitch is a modification of the vertical mattress suture. It is used to pull together the ends of a wound that are under tension. It can be used to allow the skin to stretch for a while before continued closure of the wound. Essentially, it is a mild intraoperative tissue expansion technique. The disadvantage is that the suture may tear through the skin if the tissue is very thin. This suture is often used on the back (Chapter 6).

42. B With both basal cell carcinoma and chondrodermatitis nodularis helicis, the patient may present with a nodule on the ear. Both may show superficial ulceration on clinical examination. On histologic examination, chondrodermatitis demonstrates degenerated collagen along with granulation tissue. In addition, there are often changes in the cartilage. Although the latter is not needed for the diagnosis, it helps if present (Chapter 6).

43. E

44. (T); **45.** (F); **46.** (T); **47.** (T) Classically, there are five branches of the facial nerve. These include the temporal, zygomatic, buccal, marginal mandibular, and cervical nerves. The branches most at risk are the temporal and marginal mandibular nerves. The temporal branch is at highest risk where it is the most superficial, as it crosses the zygomatic arch. Injury causes inability to raise the eyebrow or wrinkle the forehead.

The marginal mandibular branch of the facial nerve exits the parotid gland at the angle of the jaw and is found there on the external surface of the masseter muscle. At this site, it is vulnerable to damage because it is covered only by skin, subcutaneous fat, and fascia. As it advances forward to innervate the depressors of the lip, it is covered by the platysma muscle.

The zygomatic and buccal branches lie deeper in the tissue after exiting the parotid gland and are at less risk. Their highest area of vulnerability is from the anterior border of the parotid to a line drawn from the lateral canthus to the oral commissure (Chapter 6).

48. E

49. E (See answer to Question 34.)

50. B; **51.** A; **52.** E; **53.** C; **54.** D Absorbable sutures include surgical gut, polyglactin (Vicryl), polyglycolic acid (Dexon), glycolic acid (Maxon), and polydioxanone (PDS). Vicryl is completely absorbed in approximately 60 to 90 days. The most absorbent and tissue reactive of these is surgical cat gut. PDS is a monofilament synthetic suture and may not be completely absorbed for up to 6 months.

Nonabsorbable sutures include silk, nylon, polypropylene (Prolene and Surgilene), polyester (Mersilene and Ethibond), and stainless steel. Silk is used primarily on mucosal surfaces because it is soft and pliable. It is avoided in other areas because it may generate an intense tissue reaction and has poor tensile strength.

Nylon is available in both monofilament and braided forms. It is widely used because of its low reactivity and high tensile strength. Prolene has high tensile strength, is a monofilament, and is inert. It resists infection and can be used in contaminated wounds. It has an extremely smooth surface and low coefficient of friction. It is therefore often used as a running subcuticular suture.

Polyester is braided and may last indefinitely. It is a good suture for skin surgery but is relatively expensive. Stainless steel has a very high tensile strength and low tissue reactivity. However, it may corrode and cut through tissue, and it may be difficult to handle. It may be monofilament or braided (Chapter 6).

55. B; **56.** A; **57.** B; **58.** A; **59.** C Vasoconstrictors, usually epinephrine, are added to anesthetic solutions because they decrease the absorption of the anesthetic agent, enabling the use of smaller amounts of drug with prolonged duration. However, with the more lipophilic, longer-acting agents such as bupivacaine and etidocaine, they are not prolonged significantly with vasoconstrictors because the agents are themselves tightly tissue-bound. In addition, most anesthetics cause vasodilatation by direct relaxation of the vascular smooth muscle, thus enhancing bleeding. A vasoconstrictor helps decrease the bleeding at the operative site.

Epinephrine is commercially available with anesthetics at a concentration of 1:100,000. Concentrations higher than 1:200,000 may be associated with an increased risk of side effects. The vasoconstrictive effect of epinephrine usually takes 7 to 15 minutes and usually shows obvious blanching of the skin.

Sodium bicarbonate is added to lidocaine with epinephrine to neutralize the acidic solution and cause less stinging on injection. The concentration of the epinephrine in these solutions decreases approximately 25% per week, and the solutions are usually discarded after that time. However, the lidocaine itself does not lose its effectiveness.

The tumescent technique of local anesthesia is used widely for liposuction. Large volumes of extremely dilute solutions of lidocaine and epinephrine in saline are infiltrated into the subcutaneous fat. This technique has dramatically decreased the morbidity of liposuction by obviating the need for general anesthesia. In addition, it provides prolonged anesthesia and replenishes fluid loss during the procedure.

Tissue necrosis due to vasoconstrictors has been reported. It is usually seen on the digits, particularly in patients with peripheral vascular disease. It is therefore recommended that epinephrine should not be used on the fingers or toes. The tip of the nose and the ears have an extensive vascular supply and therefore hyperthyroid patients are extremely sensitive to small doses of epinephrine. If epinephrine is injected into a patient on propranolol, a beta blocker, resultant hypertension, bradycardia, and even cardiac arrest may occur (Chapter 6).

60. E; **61.** E; **62.** C Perilesional skin is the preferred site for a biopsy for direct immunofluorescence for pemphigus, cicatricial and bullous pemphigoid, herpes gestationis, and epidermolysis bullosa. Lepromatous leprosy involves all the skin diffusely and therefore a skin biopsy may be done anywhere. Panniculitis is localized to the fat, which is deep. A shave biopsy, curettage, or saucerization would all be too superficial. A deep punch, a double-punch, or an incisional biopsy are adequate. Double punch is use of a second punch biopsy through the defect caused by the initial punch biopsy (Chapter 6).

63. B Direct immunofluorescence of early lesions ideally less than 4 hours old but usually less than 24 hours old often shows complement components, frequently in association with immunoglobulin. The absence of complement and immunoglobulin in many lesions older than 24 hours is the result of their lysosomal destruction (Chapter 6).

64. E; **65.** C (See answer to Question 19.)

66. D Erb's point is located along the posterior border of the sternocleidomastoid muscle. A vertical line dropped 6 cm down from the midpoint of a line connecting the mastoid process with the angle of the jaw identifies Erb's point. The spinal accessory nerve, which is the 11th cranial nerve, can be found in this area and is vulnerable to injury there (Chapter 6).

67. B; **68.** E; **69.** A; **70.** A The sural nerve runs lateral to the Achilles tendon to innervate the posterior and lateral aspect of the sole. It is superficial at the level of the lateral malleolus and lies between it and the Achilles tendon. Infiltration is directed from the lateral aspect of the Achilles tendon to the border of the lateral malleolus. The posterior tibial nerve runs medial to the Achilles tendon to innervate the anterior and medial aspect of the sole. At the ankle, the nerve lies posterolateral to the posterior tibial artery. The posterior tibial nerve is located by first palpating the posterior tibial artery just behind the medial malleolus. The needle should be positioned two fingerbreadths posterior to the medial malleolus and directed posteriorly and lateral to the pulsations (Chapter 6).

71. E EMLA is a mixture of 2.5% lidocaine cream with 2.5% prilocaine cream in their base forms. Application under occlusion for 1 to 2 hours is needed to obtain superficial anesthesia to pinprick. EMLA is extremely useful for surgical procedures performed on children. Its use is somewhat limited by the fact that it requires prolonged occlusion prior to the procedure. It causes partial but not complete anesthesia (Chapter 6).

OPHTHALMIC NERVE BRANCHES	MAXILLARY NERVE BRANCHES	MANDIBULAR NERVE BRANCHES
Supraorbital nerve Supratrochlear nerve Infraorbital nerve Lacrimal nerve External nasal nerve	Infraorbital nerve Zygomaticotemporal nerve Zygomaticofacial nerve	Mental nerve Auriculotemporal nerve Buccal nerve

72. A To block the entire dorsum of the foot, three nerves must be anesthetized: the superficial peroneal nerve, the deep peroneal nerve, and the saphenous nerve. However, the largest component of this area is innervated by the superficial peroneal nerve (Chapter 6).

73. B; 74. D; 75. E; 76. A; 77. C The trigeminal nerve supplies part of the sensory innervation to the head and neck. The trigeminal nerve has three divisions: the ophthalmic (V1), the maxillary (V2), and the mandibular (V3). Their branches are as shown in the chart at the top of the page.

The cervical nerve plexus also participates in sensory innervation to the head and neck. Branches include the great auricular nerve, the greater and lesser occipital nerves, and the third occipital nerve (Chapter 6).

78. D; 79. A Gelfoam is a sterile, nonantigenic, pliable surgical sponge made from animal skin gelatin. It is a gelatin sponge that is porous and can absorb many times its weight in blood. After being implanted, the gelatin sponge is completely absorbed in 4 to 6 weeks.

Surgicel or Oxycel is an absorbable material made from cellulose that has been oxidized by nitrous oxide. It absorbs uncoagulated blood as does Gelfoam. It also possesses mild bactericidal properties (Chapter 6).

80. C A tourniquet is often helpful during surgical procedures on the fingers, especially when involving the nail. It should generally not be left in place for longer than 15 minutes (Chapter 6).

Bibliography

Auletta MJ, Grekin RC. Local Anesthesia for Dermatologic Surgery. New York: Churchill Livingstone, 1990.
Bennett, RG. Fundamentals of Cutaneous Surgery. St. Louis: CV Mosby Co., 1988.
Breisch EA, Greenway HT, Jr. Cutaneous Surgical Anatomy of the Head and Neck. New York: Churchill Livingstone, 1992.
Dahl MV. Clinical Immunodermatology. Chicago: Year Book Medical Publishers, 1988.
Lever WF, Schawmburg-Lever G. Histopathology of the Skin, 7th ed. Philadelphia: JB Lippincott, 1990.
Salasche SJ, Bernstein G, Senkarik M. Surgical Anatomy of the Skin. East Norwalk, CT: Appleton & Lange, 1988.
Smith JW, Sherrell AJ, eds. Plastic Surgery, 4th ed. Boston: Little, Brown & Company, 1991.
Snow SN, Dortzbach R, Moyer D. Managing Common Suturing Problems. J Dermatol Surg Oncol 1991; 17:502–508.
Wheeland RG. Cutaneous Surgery. Philadelphia: WB Saunders Co., 1994.

section two

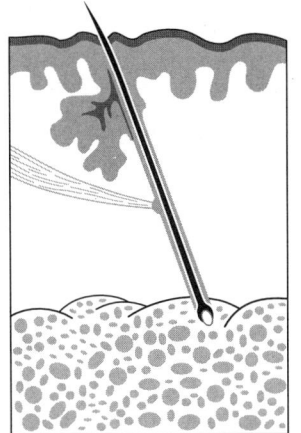

What Disorders Present with Inflamed Skin?

chapter 3

Inflammation, Pruritus, Percutaneous Absorption, and Topical Therapy

RHODA M. ALANI, and JEFFREY S. DOVER

For the following questions, ONE or MORE of the following completions may correctly finish the incomplete statements; choose

- A. If only 1, 2, and 3 are correct
- B. If only 1 and 3 are correct
- C. If only 2 and 4 are correct
- D. If only 4 is correct
- E. If all are correct.

1. Which of the following are true regarding integrins?
   1. They are composed of α- and β-heterodimers
   2. They mediate cell-cell interactions
   3. They mediate cell-matrix interactions
   4. Most cells express a single integrin.

2. In acute inflammation, leukocytes are induced to roll on vascular endothelium by increased endothelial cell expression of
   1. P-selectin
   2. E-selectin
   3. Intercellular adhesion molecule-1 (ICAM-1)
   4. Very late activation antigen-4 (VLA-4).

3. Human cutaneous mast cells release histamine in response to
   1. C3a
   2. C5a
   3. IgE
   4. Substance P.

4. Which of the following molecules are directly involved in cell adhesion?
   1. Integrins
   2. Immunoglobulin superfamily
   3. Cadherins
   4. Selectins.

5. Cytokines synthesized and expressed in skin include
   1. GM-CSF
   2. TNF-α
   3. TGF-β
   4. IL-1.

6. Substance P has which of the following properties?
   1. Potent degranulator of mast cells
   2. It is naturally derived from chili peppers
   3. It is a neuropeptide
   4. It is a potent neutrophil chemoattractant.

7. Phenotypic characteristics of Langerhans cells include
   1. HLA-DR
   2. OKT6
   3. Vimentin
   4. S-100.

8. T lymphocytes
   1. Recognize antigens attached to MHC molecules on the surface of antigen-presenting cells
   2. Contain receptors for the Fc portion of immunoglobulins
   3. Secrete cytokines
   4. Contain CD3 cell markers.

For each of the following numbered items, choose the most likely associated lettered item. Each numbered item has ONLY ONE correct answer. Within each group, each lettered item may be the answer to one, more than one, or none of the numbered items.

For the following questions, choose from the list the T-cell marker most closely associated with the cell(s) described:

9. Cytotoxic/suppressor T cells   A. CD1a
10. Pan–T-cell marker   B. CD3
11. T helper cells   C. CD4
12. Langerhans cells   D. CD6
13. Part of T-cell receptor complex.   E. CD8.

From the following list, choose the cytokine best described in each of the following questions:

14. Induces fever, activates resting T cells, induces B-cell proliferation   A. IL-1
15. Growth factor for activated T cells, induces lymphocyte-activated killer (LAK) cells   B. IL-2
                                                                                   C. IL-4
                                                                                   D. IL-8
                                                                                   E. Tumor necrosis factor (TNF).
16. Activates macrophages, growth factor for mast cells
17. Induces granulocytosis
18. Endogenous pyrogen activates coagulation system, induces cachexia.

Choose the ONE BEST answer to the following question:

19. All of the following statements are true regarding human T cells EXCEPT
    A. They induce graft rejection
    B. They mediate delayed-type hypersensitivity reactions
    C. They provide defense against viral and fungal infections
    D. They possess immunologic "memory"
    E. They mediate the development of serum sickness.

For the following questions the set of lettered headings accompanies a list of numbered words or phrases. For each numbered word or phrase, choose

   A. If the item is associated with A only
   B. If the item is associated with B only
   C. If the item is associated with both A and B
   D. If the item is associated with neither A nor B.

20. Composed of kappa or lambda light chains   A. IgG
21. Contains a J-region   B. IgM
22. Able to fix complement   C. Both
23. Can be transferred transplacentally.   D. Neither.

24. Responsible for immediate hypersensitivity reactions
25. Found preformed in mast cells   A. PGD2
26. Increases vascular permeability   B. Histamine
27. Contracts smooth muscle   C. Both
28. Promotes platelet aggregation.   D. Neither.

Choose the one best answer to each of the following questions.

29. The classic complement cascade is initiated primarily by which ONE of the following molecules?
    A. Oligosaccharides
    B. Antibody-antigen complexes
    C. Bacterial cell walls
    D. Nucleic acids
    E. Radiographic contrast medium.

30. All of the following are true regarding prostaglandins EXCEPT
    A. PGE2, PGD2, and PGI2 are potent proinflammatory agents in the skin
    B. They are formed by cyclooxygenase conversion of arachidonic acid
    C. Nonsteroidal anti-inflammatory agents inhibit their formation
    D. Their levels in skin are increased by ultraviolet radiation
    E. Their levels are decreased in the physical urticarias.

31. The main cyclooxygenase product of human skin mast cells is

A. PGE2
B. PGD2
C. PGI2
D. LTB4
E. 5-HPETE.

32. All of the following are true regarding IL-1 EXCEPT
    A. It is a constitutive product of the epidermis
    B. It is encoded by two genes, IL-1α and IL-1β
    C. The bioactive form in skin is IL-1β
    D. There is only one receptor for IL-1α and IL-1β
    E. It is partly responsible for fever associated with sunburns.

33. All of the following are true regarding natural killer (NK) cells EXCEPT
    A. They possess T-cell and B-cell markers
    B. They are CD16-positive
    C. They are able to lyse tumor cells
    D. They are able to lyse virally infected cells
    E. They constitute 20% of peripheral blood lymphocytes.

34. Which ONE of the following is true regarding antigen presentation by macrophages?
    A. Ia (class II) antigen expression is not necessary for antigen presentation
    B. Foreign antigens are processed extracellularly
    C. IL-1 is secreted by macrophages
    D. IL-2 is secreted by macrophages
    E. Processed antigen is presented to B cells.

35. Which one of the following is true regarding cytokines?
    A. They include interleukins, interferons, and antibodies
    B. They are long-acting
    C. They mediate cell–cell communication in an autocrine and paracrine manner
    D. They are of high molecular weight
    E. They possess unique functions.

36. Which one of the following is true regarding pruritus?
    A. Pruritus is produced primarily within the subcutaneous tissues
    B. Itch and pain sensations are carried to the central nervous system via the same sensory afferents
    C. The reflex response to itch is the same as the reflex response to pain
    D. Itch cannot be elicited when the dermis and epidermis have been removed
    E. Itch and pain cannot be experienced in the same site simultaneously.

37. The free nerve endings that serve as the point of initiation of itch sensation are
    A. Located in the lower dermis
    B. Formed into an epidermal nerve net
    C. Formed from nerve termini of myelinated cutaneous nerves
    D. Composed mainly of A-δ sensory fibers
    E. Found to project into the granular layer of the epidermis.

38. Which one of the following statements is true regarding histamine?
    A. There are three types of histamine receptors in the body
    B. Dermal blood vessels contain only H1 receptors
    C. Itch is mediated by H2 receptors
    D. H1 receptors are found only in the skin
    E. H2 receptors are found primarily in the brain.

39. All of the following substances have been shown to mediate pruritus EXCEPT
    A. Histamine
    B. Interleukins
    C. Opioids
    D. Temperature
    E. Substance P.

40. Which of the following diseases has been associated with systemic pruritus?
    A. Biliary cirrhosis
    B. Anemia
    C. Uremia
    D. Polycythemia vera
    E. All of the above.

For each numbered item, choose the most likely associated lettered item. Each numbered item has ONLY ONE correct answer. Within each group, each lettered item may be the answer to one, more than one, or none of the numbered items.

41. Cholestasis-related pruritus
42. Uremic pruritus
43. Dermographism
44. Prurigo nodularis
45. Lichen simplex chronicus.

A. UVB therapy
B. Cholestyramine
C. Topical or intralesional steroids
D. Antihistamines
E. Dialysis.

Choose the ONE BEST answer to each of the following questions:

46. The major barrier to drug absorption in human skin is
    A. The stratum corneum
    B. The granular layer
    C. The basal layer
    D. The papillary dermis
    E. Dermal vessel walls.

47. Drug absorption across the stratum corneum is calculated using
    A. Murphy's law
    B. Fitzpatrick's law
    C. Fick's law
    D. Koebner's law
    E. Civatte's law.

48. Hydration of the stratum corneum results in
    A. Increased permeability of lipophilic molecules only
    B. Increased permeability of hydrophilic molecules only
    C. Increased permeability of hydrophilic and lipophilic molecules
    D. Increased permeability of charged molecules only
    E. Decreased permeability of lipophilic molecules.

49. Increased cutaneous penetration of topical steroid therapies is achieved by
    A. Increasing skin temperature
    B. Stripping the stratum corneum
    C. Wetting the skin before using the medication
    D. Occluding the steroid treatment with an airtight dressing
    E. All of the above.

For the following questions, ONE or MORE of the following completions may correctly finish the incomplete statements; choose

A. If only 1, 2, and 3 are correct
B. If only 1 and 3 are correct
C. If only 2 and 4 are correct
D. If only 4 is correct
E. If all are correct.

50. Because of regional variation in skin properties, superpotent topical steroids should be avoided in the
    1. Periorbital/facial region
    2. Palms and soles
    3. Axillary skin
    4. Elbows and knees.

51. Adverse effects of long-term usage of superpotent topical steroids include
    1. Epidermal atrophy
    2. Striae
    3. Rosacea
    4. Suppression of the hypothalamic-pituitary-adrenal axis.

52. Traditional methods for determining topical steroid potency include
    1. Thermal measurements
    2. Epidermal thickness changes
    3. Vasodilator assay
    4. Vasoconstrictor assay.

53. Changes in the structure of the basic steroid moiety (Fig. 3–1) that have led to increased potency include
    1. Fluorination at the 9 position of the steroid ring
    2. Introduction of a double bond between carbons 1 and 2 of the steroid ring
    3. Alteration of the side chains at C-21
    4. Alkylation at position 6 of the steroid ring.

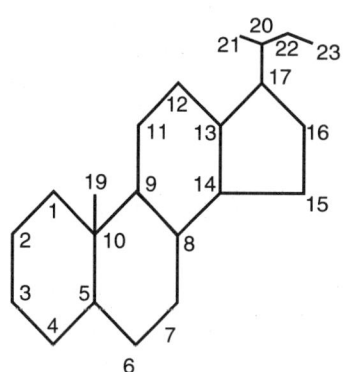

FIGURE 3–1.

54. In order to combine two immiscible liquids it is necessary to
    1. Emulsify one product into the other
    2. Add a surfactant to the two agents
    3. Reduce the surface tension at the interface between the two agents
    4. Have an excess of the hydrophobic agent.

55. Characteristics of ointments include
    1. Lipophilic preparations
    2. Usually oil-in-water emulsions
    3. Composed of microcrystalline hydrocarbons
    4. Ability to absorb water.

56. The rate of topical drug absorption depends on
    1. Concentration of drug in the vehicle
    2. The lag phase of drug absorption
    3. The steady-state phase of drug absorption
    4. The vehicle used.

57. Which of the following is (are) true regarding the partition coefficient of a topical drug?
    1. It describes the movement of a drug out of its vehicle into the stratum corneum
    2. It is determined by the relative solubility of the drug in the vehicle versus the stratum corneum
    3. A drug that is twice as soluble in its vehicle as in the stratum corneum has a partition coefficient of 1:2
    4. A drug that is twice as soluble in the stratum corneum as in its vehicle has a partition coefficient of 1:2.

58. Which of the following factors significantly and positively influence absorption of topically applied drugs?
    1. Lipophilic molecule
    2. Increased frequency of application greater than three times per day
    3. Increased hydration of skin
    4. Increased density of hair follicles.

59. Factors that favor topical therapy over systemic therapy for a particular disease process include
    1. Target site of therapeutic agent in the skin
    2. Small area of skin involved
    3. High first-pass effect in the liver
    4. Hydrophilic drug.

60. Lipophilic topical steroid agents are generally more effective than hydrophilic agents because of
    1. Increased absorption across the stratum corneum
    2. Increased receptor binding of such agents within the cytoplasm of viable epidermal cells
    3. Increased active transport across cell membranes of epidermal cells
    4. Increased penetration across viable cells within the epidermis.

Choose the ONE BEST answer to each of the following questions:

61. Long-term topical steroid use that results in subsequent decreased efficacy over time is termed
    A. Anaphylaxis
    B. Tachyphylaxis
    C. Habituation
    D. Tachydermia
    E. Koebnerization.

62. Tachyphylaxis against a potent topical steroid may occur
    A. Within a day of initiating treatment
    B. Within a week of initiating treatment
    C. Only years after initiating treatment
    D. Never occurs
    E. Is rarely reversible.

63. Dermal effects of long-term topical steroid use include
    A. Reduced collagen synthesis
    B. Increased ground substance
    C. Increased elastin synthesis
    D. Inhibition of melanogenesis
    E. Vasoconstriction.

64. In order for corticosteroids to exert their physiologic effects, they must bind to
    A. Specific receptors on cell membranes
    B. Specific receptors within target cell cytoplasm
    C. Specific nuclear membrane receptors
    D. Ribosomes
    E. Mitochondria.

65. The form of topical corticosteroid that is generally most potent is

A. Cream
B. Lotion
C. Ointment
D. Foam
E. Gel.

For each numbered item, choose the most likely associated lettered item. Each numbered item has ONLY ONE correct answer. Within each group, each lettered item may be the answer to one, more than one, or none of the numbered items.

66. Tincture
67. Lotion
68. Cream
69. Paste
70. Gel.

A. Oil-in-water
B. Water-in-oil
C. Alcohol-based
D. Propylene glycol–based
E. Powder in ointment.

Choose ONE BEST answer to each of the following questions:

71. The average amount of ointment required to cover an entire adult skin surface is
    A. 1 gram
    B. 10 grams
    C. 45 grams
    D. 75 grams
    E. 100 grams.

72. Class I topical steroids should be limited to
    A. One day of therapy
    B. One week of therapy
    C. Two weeks of therapy
    D. One month of therapy
    E. Six months of therapy.

73. The effect of a particular topical agent on a specific cutaneous disorder depends on
    A. The availability of the drug for absorption
    B. The penetration of the drug through the skin
    C. The interaction of the drug with target receptors
    D. Degradation of the active ingredient in the topically applied agent
    E. All of the above.

74. Topical steroids can be used for all of the following EXCEPT
    A. Inflammatory lesions
    B. Hyperplastic lesions
    C. Infiltrative lesions
    D. Infectious lesions
    E. Pruritic lesions.

75. All of the following regarding intralesional steroid therapy are true EXCEPT
    A. It achieves high-dose local treatment with rare systemic effects
    B. It is useful for treating keloids
    C. It may result in local skin atrophy
    D. It is useful for generalized pruritic eruptions
    E. It is useful for treating acne cysts.

For questions 76 to 80 choose the one steroid moiety from the illustration that best matches the following descriptions (Fig. 3–2, *A* to *E*):

76. The active form of cortisol
77. A class VII steroid
78. A halogenated steroid
79. A class II steroid
80. Prednisone.

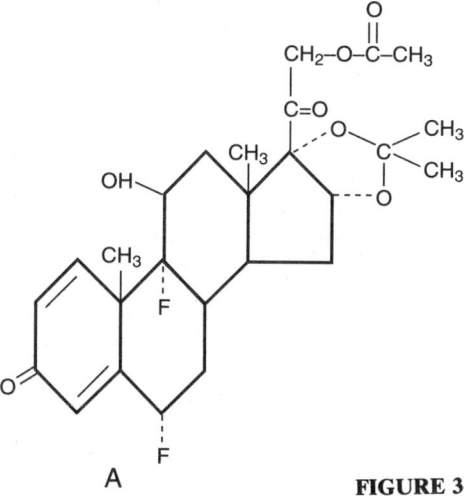
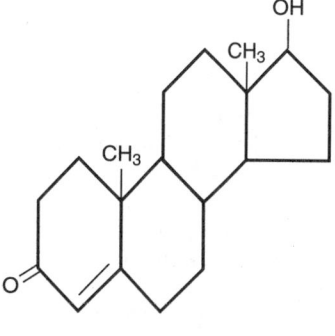

FIGURE 3–2.

Illustration continued on following page

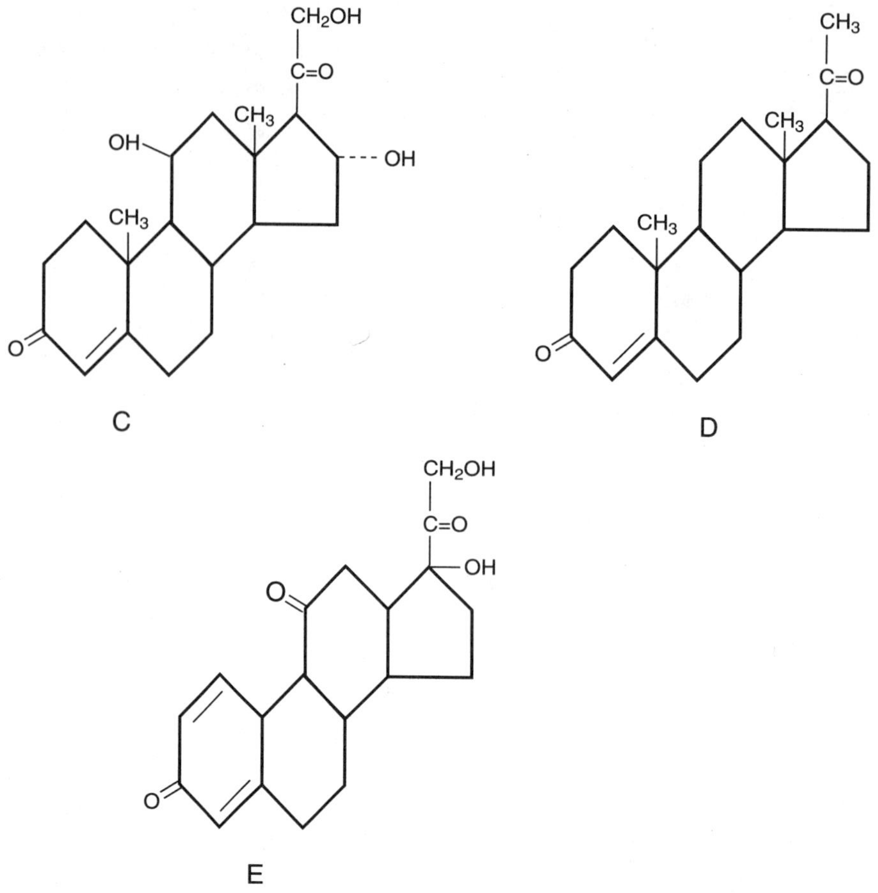

FIGURE 3–2 *Continued*

ANSWERS

1. A Integrins are adhesion receptors on cells that mediate cell-cell and cell-matrix interactions. They are composed of α- and β-heterodimers that possess distinct ligand specificity. Integrin receptor families are classified according to their β subunits. β_1 integrins may be expressed by leukocytes or fibroblasts and show specificity for binding to collagens, laminin, and fibronectin. Most cells express several integrins and can therefore bind to several extracellular matrix proteins (Chapters 1, 2, and 3).

2. A A great deal of information has been obtained in recent years regarding mechanisms of leukocyte homing and migration in acute inflammation. Much of our understanding of these processes stems from work on cellular adhesion molecules involved in cell-cell and cell-matrix interactions. There are currently four families of cell adhesion molecules that have been classified: cadherins, immunoglobulin superfamily, selectins, and integrins. During acute inflammation, endothelial cells are induced to express P-selectin. Neutrophils attach to P-selectin at sites of inflammation and are caused to roll along the vascular endothelium. Later expression of E-selectin by vascular endothelium contributes to this process. Full adhesion and extravasation of neutrophils at vascular endothelium requires the expression of a VLA (β_1) integrin by leukocytes that binds to ICAM-1 (an immunoglobulin superfamily member) on endothelial cells. The correct answer here therefore is A. VLA-4 is expressed by leukocytes, *not* by endothelial cells (Chapter 7).

3. E Human mast cells release histamine in response to numerous stimuli. Mast cells possess receptors for the Fc portion of IgE and for the anaphylatoxins C3a, C4a, and C5a. Additionally, numerous hormones and endogenous opiate peptides can cause mast cell degranulation. Known mast cell activators include IgE, C3a, C5a, opiates, and substance P (Chapter 7).

4. E (See answer to Question 2.)

5. E While there are many cytokines expressed in the skin, little is known about their precise relationships to cutaneous disorders. Interleukins (IL-1, -3, -6, -8); colony-stimulating factors, including granulocyte-macrophage colony–stimulating factor (GM-CSF), granulocyte colony–stimulating factor (G-CSF), macrophage colony–stimulating factor (M-CSF); tumor necrosis factor (TNF); and nerve, tumor, and fibroblast growth factors (NGF, TGFα, TGFβ, bFGF) have all been localized to skin (Chapter 7).

6. B Substance P is a neuropeptide that is localized to sensory nerve terminals. It is a potent degranulator of cutaneous mast cells. Substance P is released in association with cutaneous sensory nerve firing and is involved in generation of the sensation of cutaneous pain. Capsaicin, a derivative of chili peppers, depletes sensory nerves of neuropeptides and prevents their reaccumulation. It has been used clinically to treat the cutaneous pain of postherpetic neuralgia. Substance P is *not* derived from chili peppers, nor does it possess neutrophil chemoattractant properties (Chapter 7).

7. E Langerhans cells are responsible for suprabasal antigen presentation in skin. They contain numerous phenotypic markers, including HLA-DR, CD1a, HLA-DS, OKT6, vimentin, S-100, Fc receptors, and C3 receptors. These cells are mesenchymal and are derived from bone marrow precursor cells (Chapter 7).

8. E Human T cells are composed of helper, cytotoxic, and suppressor cells. They have distinct cell surface receptors that enable them to recognize processed antigens on the surface of antigen-presenting cells in association with major histocompatibility complex (MHC) molecules. They secrete numerous cytokines which are involved in cell-cell communication. CD3 is a pan–T cell marker and is part of the T-cell receptor complex. T cells contain receptors for immunoglobulins that enable them to induce immune responses to foreign antigens (Chapters 7 and 10).

9. E; **10.** B; **11.** C; **12.** A; **13.** B The current designation of T-cell markers is based on the CD designation. CD1a is a marker for Langerhans cells. It is particularly useful in evaluating the histiocytoses; CD3 is part of the T-cell receptor complex and therefore is a pan–T cell marker; CD6 is a marker for malignant T cells; CD8 is present on cytotoxic and suppressor T cells (Chapters 7 and 10).

14. A; **15.** B; **16.** C; **16.** C; **17.** D; **18.** E Cytokines are non–antibody soluble molecular mediators of cell-cell communication. They include interleukins, interferons, and growth factors. These molecules are generally of low molecular weight, produced transiently by the body, act by binding to specific receptors, function in immune-mediated processes, and have overlapping functions. IL-1 induces fever, activates resting T cells, and induces B-cell proliferation. IL-2 is a growth factor for activated T cells and induces LAK cells. IL-4 activates macrophages and is a growth factor for mast cells. IL-8 induces granulocytosis. Tumor necrosis factor (TNF) is referred to as endogenous pyrogen; it also activates the coagulation system and induces cachexia (Chapter 7).

19. E T cells are responsible for recognizing non–self-antigens as a function of an organism's immune surveillance capacities. They must recognize foreign antigens in the context of cellular MHC molecules in order to function appropriately. Although B cells are primarily responsible for antibody production and immune defense against bacterial infections, T cells are primarily involved in defense against mycobacterial, fungal, intracellular viral and protozoal infections. T cells are the primary mediators of delayed-type hypersensitivity reactions, which involve "memory" T cells. T cells also mediate graft rejection and graft-versus-host disease. B cells and subsequent antibody production with antigen–antibody complex formation and tissue deposition are responsible for the development of serum sickness reactions (Chapter 10).

20. C; **21.** B; **22.** C; **23.** A; **24.** D There are five distinct classes of immunoglobulins—IgG, IgM, IgA, IgD, and IgE. IgM and IgA can exist as multimers that are joined by J-regions. All immunoglobulins are composed of two heavy chains and two light chains that contain variable and constant regions. Only IgG and IgM antibodies are able to fix complement, and only IgG antibodies can be transferred across the placenta. Immediate hypersensitivity reactions are mediated by IgE binding to mast cells (Chapters 7 and 10).

25. B; **26.** C; **27.** C; **28.** D Mast cells contain preformed and newly formed mediators that are released during degranulation and subsequent activation. Preformed mediators contained within mast cell granules include histamine, heparin, trypsin, chymotrypsin, and arylsulfatases. Arachidonic acid metabolites, including the prostaglandins, thromboxanes, and leukotrienes, are synthesized following mast cell activation. Both histamine and PGD2 cause increased vascular permeability and smooth muscle contraction. Neither histamine nor PGD2 are involved in promoting platelet aggregation. PGD2 is an inhibitor of platelet aggregation. Platelet-aggregating factor, an additional mast cell product, is responsible for mast cell–induced platelet aggregation (Chapter 7).

29. B The classical complement cascade is activated by many factors, including IgG, IgM, antigen-antibody complexes, proteolytic enzymes, C-reactive protein, and RNA viruses. In contrast, the alternative complement cascade is activated by bacterial cell walls, endotoxic polysaccharides, aggregated immunoglobulins, and radiographic contrast medium (Chapter 7).

30. E PGE2, PGD2, and PGI2 are highly potent proinflammatory agents in skin, causing erythema, edema, and pain in nanomolar concentrations. Nonsteroidal anti–inflammatory agents inhibit formation of prostaglandins by direct inhibition of cyclooxygenase and, therefore, conversion of arachidonic acid to prostaglandins. Increased levels of prostaglandins in skin are seen in response to UV irradiation, in allergic contact dermatitis, and in the physical urticarias (Chapter 7).

31. B The main cyclooxygenase product of human skin mast cells is PGD2, which along with histamine is responsible for much of the inflammatory response of mast cells. PGE2 and PGI2 are found in skin but at lower concentrations than PGD2. LTB4 and 5-HPETE are products of the lipoxygenase pathway in human skin (Chapter 7).

32. C Interleukin-1 (IL-1) is a cytokine produced constitutively by the epidermis. There are two forms of IL-1, alpha and beta. Both forms bind to the same receptor; however, the bioactive form in skin is IL-1α. Elevated levels of IL-1 are associated with fevers following increased UV exposure of skin (Chapter 7).

33. A Natural killer cells are CD16-positive cells capable of natural killer (NK) and antibody-dependent cell cytotoxicity (ADCC). They are important cells in host defense against viral infections and tumors. They constitute 20% of peripheral blood lymphocytes; however, they lack T-cell and B-cell markers (Chapter 7).

34. C Macrophages take up and internalize foreign antigens, which are then processed intracellularly. Macrophages then secrete IL-1, which induces T-cell recognition of the foreign antigen *only* in association with 1a (Class II MHC) antigens. IL-2 is secreted by activated T cells following recognition of processed antigens on macrophage cell surfaces (Chapters 7 and 10).

35. C Cytokines are low-molecular-weight nonantibody mediators of cell-cell interactions. Included in this group of molecules are interleukins, interferons, and growth factors. They are short-acting mediators that function in an autocrine or paracrine manner. Cytokines possess multiple overlapping functions (Chapter 7).

36. D Pruritus is produced primarily at the dermoepidermal junction; consequently, itch cannot be elicited without an intact dermis and epidermis. The sensory fibers transmitting pain and itch sensation from the skin to the central nervous system are unique and are composed of two distinct populations of primary sensory afferents. Because there are two unique sensory afferents for itch and pain, these two sensations can be experienced at the same site simultaneously. The reflex response to itch is scratching, whereas the reflex response to pain is withdrawal (Chapter 8).

37. E The free nerve endings that serve as a point of initiation of itch sensation are located primarily in the upper dermis. They form a subepidermal nerve network. These free nerve endings are terminals of unmyelinated cutaneous nerves that are composed mainly of type C fibers. Free nerve endings that project into the epidermis reach the granular layer and then spread laterally (Chapter 8).

38. A There are three types of histamine receptors in the human body: H1 receptors are found in the skin and brain; H2 receptors mediate gastric acid secretion; and H3 receptors are found in brain, lung, and other tissue. Dermal blood vessels contain both H1 and H2 receptors, which cause vasodilation when stimulated. Itch is mediated through the H1 receptor (Chapter 8).

39. B Histamine, opioids, thermal stimuli, and substance P have all been demonstrated to mediate pruritus either by direct effects on itch receptors or through effects on mast cells. While interleukins are known products of keratinocytes and are mediators of the inflammatory response, they have not been demonstrated to induce pruritus (Chapter 8).

40. E Pruritus may be a prominent feature of several systemic disease processes. Frequent causes include malignancies (especially malignant lymphoma), uremia, obstructive biliary disease, polycythemia vera, hypothyroidism, hyperthyroidism, carcinoid, and anemia. Oftentimes, a workup for chronic generalized pruritus includes a complete history and physical examination, CBC with differential; thyroid, liver, and renal function laboratory studies; fasting blood sugar; and a chest x-ray (Chapter 8).

41. B; **42.** A; **43.** D; **44.** C; **45.** C Multiple therapies have been tried for cholestasis pruritus. Although there is no correlation between the levels of serum-conjugated bile acids and pruritus, substantial relief has been obtained with bile acid–sequestering agents, e.g., cholestyramine. Uremic pruritus appears to be best controlled by ultraviolet B (UVB) therapy. There is no correlation between level of uremia or serum creatinine and pruritus; furthermore, dialysis has not been shown to substantially reduce pruritus in these patients. Dermographism involves an accentuated wheal and flare response to stroking the skin. It is primarily histamine-mediated and is therefore responsive to antihistamine therapy. Prurigo nodularis and lichen simplex chronicus are both types of neurodermatitides. Oftentimes, these disorders are associated with a patient's excessive stress and anxiety. The pruritus here is often severe. Once systemic causes for the pruritus have been ruled out, successful treatment of these lesions usually requires potent topical or intralesional steroids. A consideration of mild systemic anxiolytic therapy or improved stress management techniques might also be useful in this situation (Chapter 8).

46. A In stratified squamous epithelium, the major barrier to drug absorption is the stratum corneum. There is no active transport across the stratum corneum; therefore, drug transport across this skin layer is dependent on Fick's law of diffusion (Chapter 9).

47. C Because there is no active transport across the stratum corneum, transport across it is dependent on passive diffusion, or Fick's law. In Fick's law,

$$J = \frac{K \times D \times \Delta C}{d}$$

J = flux, or flow of diffusing drug, K = partition coefficient between the stratum corneum and the vehicle, D = diffusion coefficient of the stratum corneum, ΔC = concentration gradient between the skin surface and the epidermis, and d = the thickness of the stratum corneum (Chapter 9).

48. C Water in the stratum corneum may be "bound" or "free." As the stratum corneum becomes hydrated, more free water is available, allowing water molecules to move more freely through the skin. This increased water content of the stratum corneum gives it a larger diffusion constant in Fick's law as a result of increased movement of molecules across a fixed concentration gradient (Chapter 9).

49. E Increased skin temperature, wetting the skin, and occlusive therapy all contribute to increased permeability of the stratum corneum to topical steroids. Stripping the skin of the stratum corneum increases penetration by topical steroids through elimination of the largest barrier to skin absorption (Chapter 9).

50. B Because of variability in skin permeability, potent topical steroids should be avoided at certain skin sites.

In particular, adverse effects from potent topical steroid use are seen more frequently in these areas that include the face, the groin, and perineum—all intertriginous areas—and mucosal surfaces (Chapter 9).

51. E Superpotent topical steroids, when used long-term, may have serious and lasting side effects. Among the more commonly encountered side effects are steroid-induced rosacea and epidermal atrophy and subsequent striae. Rarely is suppression of the hypothalamic-pituitary-adrenal axis seen with topical steroid treatment, although this may occur (Chapter 9).

52. D In 1962 the vasoconstrictor assay was presented as a novel method for determining percutaneous absorption of topical steroids. Since that time, the assay has undergone some modifications but has essentially remained the "gold standard" for determining topical steroid potency (Chapter 9).

53. E Increased steroid glucocorticoid potency is achieved by halogenation at the 6 or 9 positions of the steroid ring, introduction of a double bond between carbons 1 and 2 of the steroid ring, alteration of the side chains at C-21, and alkylation at position 6 or 16 of the steroid ring (Chapter 9).

54. A Emulsions are composed of two immiscible liquids—usually oil and water. When forming a vehicle for a particular topical therapeutic agent oftentimes a water-in-oil or oil-in-water emulsion is used. The internal phase is said to be dispersed in the external or continuous phase. This can only occur with the use of a surfactant to reduce surface tension at the interface of the two phases. Whether the emulsion is oil-in-water or water-in-oil is determined by the amount of oil and water in the compound and the surfactant used. Most creams are oil-in-water–based. It is not necessary to have excess of either the hydrophilic or hydrophobic phase in order to form an emulsion (Chapter 9).

55. B Ointments are lipophilic preparations that, if prepared as an emulsion, are usually water-in-oil mixtures. They are often composed of a petrolatum base comprising a complex mixture of various hydrocarbons, including microcrystalline hydrocarbons. Because of the hydrophobic nature of ointments, they tend to repel, not absorb, water unless an emulsifying agent is present to form an absorption base (Chapter 9).

56. E The rate of topical drug absorption is related to Fick's law as previously described. The rate of absorption depends on the concentration gradient from the stratum corneum to the dermal vasculature. Initially, the absorption of a topically applied agent as the drug moves from the vehicle to the stratum corneum through the epidermis to the dermal vessels is slow. This initial phase of absorption is the lag phase. Once the amount of drug absorption per unit time is constant, we have reached the steady-state phase of absorption. The vehicle used is also important for drug absorption, more water-impermeable (i.e., hydrophobic) vehicles allowing more absorption of drug through a hydrated stratum corneum. In addition, the vehicle used is important in determining the partition coefficient of a particular drug as relates to Fick's law (Chapter 9).

57. A See the preceding answers regarding Fick's law for further details. The partition coefficient in Fick's law is equal to the ratio of concentration of drug in the stratum corneum to concentration of drug in the vehicle (Chapter 9).

58. B Increased absorption of topically applied agents is achieved by lipophilic substances and a hydrated skin surface. Increased frequency of topical application does not significantly influence transcutaneous drug absorption beyond three times a day treatment, since maximal flux is reached by most drugs at one to three times daily applications. The transfollicular route of drug absorption is not very significant, and density of hair follicles in a given region does not influence absorption to a great extent (Chapter 9).

59. A Factors that favor the use of topical treatment of a disease process include skin as the target site, involvement of a small area of skin, and a high first-pass effect on the therapeutic agent in the liver. Hydrophilic drugs tend to be better absorbed by the oral route and therefore favor systemic administration (Chapter 9).

60. C The stratum corneum favors increased absorption of lipophilic agents. Increased absorption of lipophilic agents is seen within the viable cell layers of the epidermis. In addition, there is increased cytoplasmic binding of such lipophilic steroid molecules within viable epidermal cells. There is no appreciable active transport of these molecules across cell membranes (Chapter 9).

61. B Long-term continuous use of topical steroid agents results in tachyphylaxis and decreased efficacy. It is thought that intermittent application of topical steroid agents may decrease the incidence of tachyphylaxis to a particular agent (Chapter 9).

62. B Tachyphylaxis may begin within one week of initiating treatment with a potent topical steroid. The ability to fully respond to the same medication usually returns within a week of stopping the topical therapy. It therefore is best to treat disorders with potent agents over a short period of time with "rest" periods, either without steroid treatment or with use of a substantially weaker steroid (Chapter 9).

63. A Dermal effects of long-term topical steroid use include decreased collagen synthesis with reduction in ground substance, which leads to decreased vascular support and subsequent striae. Although immediate effects of topical steroids include vasoconstriction, long-term use promotes vasodilation, often as a rebound phenomenon. Inhibition of melanocyte function is an effect of topical steroid use on the epidermis (Chapter 9).

64. B Corticosteroids exert their effects by diffusing through cell membranes, binding to specific cytosolic receptors, and subsequently migrating to the cell nucleus, where the steroid-receptor complex binds to cellular DNA to initiate transcription of various effector molecules (Chapter 9).

65. C The ointment form of a topical corticosteroid is generally more potent than other forms of the same drug. This is largely related to the occlusive effects of ointments, which tend to prevent water evaporation from the skin surface and enhance drug absorption (Chapter 9).

66. C; 67. A; 68. A; 69. E; 70. D Ointments are generally considered water-in-oil formulations, whereas creams and lotions are oil-in-water formulations. Solutions and tinctures are alcohol-based with solutions containing variable amounts of propylene glycol. Gels are propylene glycol–based agents. Pastes are creams or ointments to which powder has been added (Chapter 9).

71. C The average adult individual requires 30 to 60 grams of ointment to cover the entire cutaneous surface area (Chapter 9).

72. C Because of the superpotent nature of class I steroids, their use should generally be limited to 2 weeks of continuous therapy with a subsequent rest period to reduce the likelihood of side effects and tachyphylaxis of the agent used. Generally, a 1- to 2-week rest period is sufficient to avoid severe side effects of the stronger topical steroid therapies. Retreatment with more potent topical steroids should then be initiated for exacerbation of the disease process being treated (Chapter 9).

73. E The effect of any topically applied agent depends on drug availability from the vehicle in which it is prepared, penetration of the agent through the skin, interactions of the agent with various cellular receptors, and its degradation in the skin (Chapter 9).

74. D Topical steroids possess both an antiinflammatory effect and an antimitotic effect. Pruritic lesions, depending on their cause, can often be relieved by topical steroids. Topical steroids have no antimicrobial effects; rather, because they affect various cytokines, they may make persons MORE prone to infections (Chapter 9).

75. D Intralesional steroid therapy is useful for treating well-circumscribed, localized, inflammatory, or hyperplastic lesions. It rarely produces systemic effects if used correctly. Local side effects of this treatment include atrophy, hypopigmentation, localized increased hair growth, infection, and ulceration of treated lesions (Chapter 9).

76. C; 77. C; 78. A; 79. A; 80. E The steroid ring has the following basic structure, with carbon atoms numbered as illustrated (Fig. 3–2). Oxygen is necessary at position 11 in order for corticoid function to exist. A hydroxyl or C=O at position 17 leads to increased glucocorticoid activity, as does a double bond between C1 and C2; halogenation at C6 or C9; or alkylation of C6 or C16.

In Figure 3–2, the structure in *A* is fluocinonide, a class II fluorinated topical steroid; in *B* the structure is testosterone; in *C*, hydrocortisone. *D* represents progesterone and *E*, prednisone (Chapter 9).

Bibliography

Anderson PJ, Tedder TF. Lymphocytes. In: Fitzpatrick TB, Eisen AZ, Wolff K, et al., eds. Dermatology in General Medicine, 4th edition. New York: McGraw-Hill, 1993:436–444.

Arndt KA. Manual of Dermatologic Therapeutics, 3rd edition. Boston: Little, Brown, 1985.

Arndt KA, Jorizzo JL. Which topical corticosteroid—and when. Patient Care May 30, 1992:115–136.

Arndt KA, Mendenhall PV, Sloan KB, et al. The pharmacology of topical therapy. In: Fitzpatrick TB, Eisen AZ, Wolff K, et al., eds. Dermatology in General Medicine, 4th edition. New York: McGraw-Hill, 1993:2837–2845.

Gigli I. Human complement system. In: Fitzpatrick TB, Eisen AZ, Wolff K, et al., eds. Dermatology in General Medicine, 4th edition. New York: McGraw-Hill, 1993:454–463.

Goldstein SM, Wintroub BU. The cellular and molecular biology of the human mast cell. In: Fitzpatrick TB, Eisen AZ, Wolff K, et al., eds. Dermatology in General Medicine, 4th edition. New York: McGraw-Hill, 1993:359–374.

Greaves MW. Pathophysiology and clinical aspects of pruritus. In: Fitzpatrick TB, Eisen AZ, Wolff K, et al., eds. Dermatology in General Medicine, 4th edition. New York: McGraw-Hill, 1993:413–423.

Hynes RO. Integrins: Versatility, modulation, and signaling in cell adhesion. Cell 1992; 69:11–25.

Jamoulle JJ, Schaefer H. Pharmacokinetics and topical applications of drugs. In: Fitzpatrick TB, Eisen AZ, Wolff K, et al., eds. Dermatology in General Medicine, 4th edition. New York: McGraw-Hill, 1993:2829–2836.

Kupper TS. Adhesion molecules, matrix, and cytokines: Integration during leukocyte migration. In: Fitzpatrick TB, Eisen AZ, Wolff K, et al., eds. Dermatology in General Medicine, 4th edition. New York: McGraw-Hill, 1993:145–149.

Lawley TJ. Immunoglobulin structure and function. In: Fitzpatrick TB, Eisen AZ, Wolff K, et al., eds. Dermatology in General Medicine, 4th edition. New York: McGraw-Hill, 1993:429–435.

Lowitt MH, Bernhard JD. Pruritus. Semin Neurol 1992; 12:374–384.

Rubin EH, Cannistra SA. Regulation of the production and activation of polymorphonuclear leukocytes, eosinophils, and basophils. In: Fitzpatrick TB, Eisen AZ, Wolff K, et al., eds. Dermatology in General Medicine, 4th edition. New York: McGraw-Hill, 1993:445–453.

Stoughton RB, Cornell RC. Corticosteroids. In: Fitzpatrick TB, Eisen AZ, Wolff K, et al., eds. Dermatology in General Medicine, 4th edition. New York: McGraw-Hill, 1993:2846–2850.

chapter 4

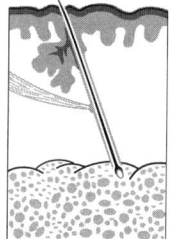

Spongiotic and Intraepidermal Pustules

LESLIE STEWART, ELIZABETH R. SHURNAS,
and JEFFREY B. TRAVERS

CONTACT DERMATITIS: CELL-MEDIATED IMMUNITY, LANGERHANS CELL BIOLOGY

Choose the ONE best answer to each of the following questions.

1. Which ONE of the following statements is TRUE of Langerhans cells?
   A. They probably play a major role in scavenging dyskeratotic keratinocytes in the epidermis
   B. They actively produce interleukin-2 (IL-2) on appropriate stimuli
   C. They are embryologically derived from neural ectoderm
   D. They are thought to be terminally differentiated T lymphocytes
   E. They have receptors for Fc and C3b.

2. Which ONE of the following statements is TRUE of Langerhans cells?
   A. They are characterized by cytoplasmic organelles known as Birbeck granules
   B. They express class II major histocompatibility (MHC) antigens
   C. After becoming sensitized to an antigen, Langerhans cells are thought to migrate to the draining lymph nodes, where they present antigen to unsensitized T lymphocytes
   D. Langerhans cells in the epidermis have dendrites
   E. All of the above statements are true.

For the following question, ONE or MORE of the completions given correctly finishes the incomplete statement; choose

A. If only 1, 2, and 3 are correct
B. If only 1 and 3 are correct
C. If only 2 and 4 are correct
D. If only 4 is correct
E. If all are correct.

3. Characteristics of allergic contact allergens include
   1. Ability to penetrate the epidermis
   2. Ability to form covalent bonds with proteins
   3. Ability to act as haptens
   4. Ability to act as polyclonal T-lymphocyte mitogens in vitro.

CONTACT DERMATITIS AND OCCUPATIONAL DERMATOLOGY

Choose the ONE best answer to each of the following questions.

4. Which ONE of the following statements is TRUE regarding occupationally related skin disease?

   A. Atopic persons with a history of childhood eczema are not at an increased risk for the development of occupational dermatoses

   B. Irritant contact dermatitis of the hands is the most common occupationally related skin disease

   C. Occupationally related skin diseases account for less than 20% of occupational illnesses

   D. All of the above statements are TRUE

   E. None of the above statements are TRUE.

5. All of the following compounds potentially are cross-reactive with poison ivy (rhus) EXCEPT

   A. Rhubarb stalks and leaves

   B. Oil of cashew

   C. Mango rind

   D. Furniture lacquer from the Japanese lacquer tree

   E. Poison sumac.

6. All of the statements regarding cosmetic allergic contact dermatitis are true EXCEPT

   A. Allergens applied to the scalp can often produce dermatitis of the eyelids, ears, and hands, whereas the scalp remains normal

   B. Earlobe dermatitis is often a sign of nickel allergy

   C. Fragrance ingredients are the most frequently identified allergens causing cosmetic allergic contact dermatitis

   D. Unilateral facial dermatitis is often due to allergic contact reactions to facial cosmetics

   E. Eyelid dermatitis can be due to allergic contact reactions to nail products.

7. A registered nurse presents with a 2-month history of itching, redness, and urticaria on her hands approximately 5 to 10 minutes after she wears latex gloves. The patient also describes rhinitis for the past 6 weeks. Physical examination reveals patches of mild dermatitis on the dorsum of her hands bilaterally. Which ONE of the following statements is TRUE regarding management of this patient?

   A. The patient should be started on oral (H-1) antihistamines and topical midpotency corticosteroids, and diagnostic studies should be planned only if the patient does not respond to this treatment

   B. The patient should be advised either to wear latex gloves for only short periods of time or to use only hypoallergenic latex gloves

   C. Closed patch testing of formaldehyde and formaldehyde releasers found in latex gloves should be initiated

   D. Prick testing should be initiated to evaluate the possibility of a Type 1 IgE–mediated response to the water-soluble latex protein

   E. The patient should be instructed to avoid only powdered latex gloves.

8. Topical exposure to which ONE of the following agents followed by ingestion of alcohol can result in an Antabuse-like reaction consisting of itching, redness, and hives.

   A. Musk ambrette

   B. Quaternium-15

   C. Thiuram

   D. Paratertiary butylphenol formaldehyde resin

   E. Glutaraldehyde.

For the following questions, ONE or MORE of the completions given correctly finishes the incomplete statement; choose

   A. If only 1, 2, and 3 are correct
   B. If only 1 and 3 are correct
   C. If only 2 and 4 are correct
   D. If only 4 is correct
   E. If all are correct.

9. An orthopedic surgeon is referred to you for evaluation of a suspected allergic contact dermatitis. Closed patch testing revealed sensitivity to an acrylic monomer found in bone cement. Which of the following statements are TRUE regarding acrylic bone cement allergies?

   1. This allergen can pass through rubber and vinyl gloves

   2. Patients with this disorder often complain of persistent paresthesias of their fingers

   3. This patient should still be able to conduct operations involving artificial joints but should have an associate mix and apply the bone cement

   4. Allergies to bond cement ingredients are thought to be the leading cause of artificial joint rejection.

10. A 38-year-old otherwise healthy female factory worker is referred to you with a 6-month history of depigmentation of her face and hands. Because she is exposed to hydroquinones found in photographic developers, you suspect contact vitiligo. Which of the following statements are TRUE regarding contact vitiligo?

    1. Contact vitiligo and idiopathic vitiligo can be readily distinguished from each other by histologic findings
    2. Repigmentation occurs within 1 to 2 weeks after patient ends exposure to causative agent
    3. Closed patch testing for 48 to 72 hours using the suspected agent is the diagnostic test of choice to diagnose contact vitiligo
    4. In addition to hydroquinones, exposure to paratertiary butylphenol and phenol detergents can also result in contact vitiligo.

11. A hairdresser is found to be sensitized to paraphenylenediamine. What other compounds should this patient be instructed to avoid for fear of cross-sensitization?

    1. Benzocaine
    2. Para-aminobenzoic acid (PABA)
    3. Sulfanilamide
    4. Cinnamic aldehyde.

12. Which of the following statements regarding beautician-associated contact allergens is (are) TRUE?

    1. A hairdresser, sensitive to the hair dye allergen paraphenylenediamine, can cut previously dyed hair without risk of causing an allergic contact dermatitis
    2. A potential allergen in salon (hot, acid) perms is glycerylmonothioglycolate (GMTG)
    3. A potential allergen in home (cold, alkaline) perms is ammonium thioglycolate (ATG)
    4. A hairdresser, sensitive to glycerylmonothioglycolate (GMTG), can cut hair that has been permed one month ago without risk of causing an allergic contact dermatitis.

13. A 32-year-old female is referred to you with a facial rash. Closed patch testing reveals allergy to released formaldehyde found in her cosmetics. What other cosmetic preservatives should the patient be advised to avoid?

    1. Imidazolidinyl urea
    2. Propylene glycol
    3. Quaternium-15
    4. Ethylenediamine tetraacetate (EDTA)

For each numbered item choose the most likely associated lettered item. Each numbered item has ONLY ONE answer. Within each group, each lettered item may be the answer to one, more than one, or none of the numbered items.

For each substance, select the associated contact allergen.

14. After-shave lotions
15. Toothpaste
16. Cement
17. Rubber gloves.

    A. Cinnamic aldehyde
    B. Potassium dichromate
    C. Musk ambrette
    D. Formaldehyde
    E. Thiuram.

Choose the indicator test used to determine the presence of the possible allergen:

18. Formaldehyde
19. Nickel sulfate
20. Chromates.

    A. Diphenylcarbazide spot test
    B. Lutidine (acetylacetate) test
    C. Dimethylglyoxime test
    D. None of the above.

HAND AND FOOT DERMATITIS

Choose the ONE BEST answer to each of the following questions.

21. The following palmoplantar eruptions are associated with sterile neutrophilic pustules EXCEPT

    A. Acrodermatitis continua of Hallopeau (dermatitis repens)
    B. Pustular psoriasis of the Barber type (pustular palmoplantar psoriasis)
    C. Vesicular hand and foot dermatitis (pompholyx)
    D. Infantile acropustulosis
    E. Pustular bacterid.

22. Recommended or optional treatments of pustular palmoplantar psoriasis includes all of the following EXCEPT

    A. Potent topical corticosteroids
    B. Oral corticosteroids
    C. Oral retinoids (etretinate or isotretinoin)
    D. Topical psoralens and ultraviolet A radiation (PUVA)
    E. All of the above are acceptable treatments.

23. Which ONE of the following statements is TRUE regarding acrodermatitis continua of Hallopeau?
    A. Histology is similar to acute allergic contact dermatitis
    B. Lesions start on palms and progress distally to involve digits and can be associated with nail loss and bone resorption
    C. Oral corticosteroids are the treatment of choice
    D. Often associated with a peripheral eosinophilia
    E. Usually has a chronic course lasting many years.

24. Which ONE of the following statements is TRUE of infantile acropustulosis?
    A. Lesions consist of intensely pruritic pustules that recur in crops
    B. Seen predominantly in black male infants
    C. Direct immunofluorescent findings are not specific for this disorder
    D. All of the above are TRUE
    E. None of the above are TRUE.

25. Treatment of infantile acropustulosis has included all of the following EXCEPT
    A. Topical corticosteroids
    B. Topical and oral antipruritics
    C. Dapsone
    D. Minocycline
    E. All of the above are acceptable treatments.

Decide whether EACH of the following statements is TRUE or FALSE. Any combination of answers from all true to all false may occur.

Decide whether EACH of the following statements about hand dermatitis is TRUE or FALSE.

26. It is often impossible to clinically distinguish between irritant and allergic contact dermatitis.

27. The use of bactericidal soaps is often helpful for patients with severe hand dermatitis to treat concurrent bacterial infections.

28. Finger dermatitis localized under a ring is almost always due to allergic contact sensitization to the metal nickel.

29. The majority of patients with hand dermatitis will respond to a nickel-free diet.

For the following questions, ONE or MORE of the completions given correctly finishes the incomplete statement; choose
   A. If only 1, 2, and 3 are correct
   B. If only 1 and 3 are correct
   C. If only 2 and 4 are correct
   D. If only 4 is correct
   E. If all are correct.

30. Which statements are TRUE of juvenile plantar dermatosis?
    1. Tinea pedis often mimics juvenile plantar dermatosis
    2. Redness, cracking, and dryness of the dorsum of the feet are characteristically seen
    3. Involvement is usually bilateral and symmetrical
    4. Treatment consists of drying agents such as aluminum chloride hexahydrate.

31. Which of the following laboratory tests should be obtained before initiating psoralen and ultraviolet A radiation (PUVA) therapy?
    1. Antinuclear antibodies (ANA)
    2. Glucose-6-phosphate dehydrogenase (G-6-PD) level in blacks and patients of Mediterranean descent
    3. Complete blood count (CBC)
    4. Reticulocyte count.

PITYRIASIS ROSEA

Choose the ONE BEST answer to each of the following questions.

32. All of the following statements are true of pityriasis rosea EXCEPT
    A. It is least common during the months of June, July, and August
    B. Lesions are characteristically distributed along skin lines of cleavage on the trunk and proximal extremities
    C. Sunlight often exacerbates the lesions
    D. Oral lesions can occur
    E. All of the above.

33. All of the following have been used as treatments for symptomatic pityriasis rosea EXCEPT
    A. Midpotency topical corticosteroids
    B. Oral H1 antihistamines

C. Short course of oral corticosteroids

D. Short course of oral retinoids (isotretinoin)

E. Ultraviolet B (UVB) radiation.

34. A pityriasis rosea–like eruption can occur as a reaction to all of the following drugs EXCEPT

    A. Captopril
    B. Barbiturates
    C. Psoralens
    D. Clonidine
    E. β-blocking agents.

Decide whether each of the following statements is TRUE or FALSE. Any combination of answers from all true to all false may occur.

Decide whether EACH of the following statements about pityriasis rosea is TRUE or FALSE.

35. "Inverse pityriasis rosea" is characterized by lesions distributed perpendicular to skin lines of cleavage on the trunk and proximal extremities.

36. The papular variant of pityriasis rosea is often found in black children.

37. Herpes virus type 6 is thought to be the causative agent.

For the following question, ONE or MORE of the completions given correctly finishes the incomplete statement; choose

A. If only 1, 2, and 3 are correct
B. If only 1 and 3 are correct
C. If only 2 and 4 are correct
D. If only 4 is correct
E. If all are correct.

38. Which of the following is (are) histologic characteristics of pityriasis rosea?

    1. Focal epidermal spongiosis associated with lymphocytic exocytosis
    2. Lymphohistiocytic perivascular infiltrates in the dermis
    3. Occasional dyskeratotic, eosinophilic keratinocytes (colloid bodies) in the epidermis
    4. Extravasated erythrocytes in dermal papillae.

PARAPSORIASIS (SMALL PLAQUE)

Choose the ONE BEST answer to each of the following questions.

A 30-year-old white female is referred to you with a 12-month history of an asymptomatic rash. It consisted of small (less than 3-4 cm) oval patches and barely raised plaques with a small amount of fine scale distributed following skin lines of cleavage on her trunk and proximal extremities. The patient claims that the rash is essentially unchanged from when it first appeared. A biopsy taken 10 months ago was read as consistent with pityriasis rosea.

39. What is the probable diagnosis?

    A. Pityriasis rosea
    B. Pityriasis lichenoides, acute type
    C. Pityriasis lichenoides, chronic type
    D. Small-plaque parapsoriasis
    E. Lymphomatoid papulosis.

40. What percentage of patients with this condition will progress to cutaneous lymphoma?

    A. Less than 1%
    B. 5 to 10%
    C. 20%
    D. 50%
    E. 100%.

For the following questions, ONE or MORE of the completions correctly finishes the incomplete statement; choose

A. If only 1, 2, and 3 are correct
B. If only 1 and 3 are correct
C. If only 2 and 4 are correct
D. If only 4 is correct.

41. Which of the following statements is (are) characteristic of small-plaque parapsoriasis?

    1. The lesions may persist for years to decades
    2. Most lesions occur on the head, neck, and proximal extremities
    3. Most lesions are less than 5 cm in diameter
    4. There is a 20% chance of progression to large-plaque parapsoriasis.

42. Which of the following is (are) histologic characteristics of small-plaque parapsoriasis?

    1. Interface dermatitis with vacuolar degeneration and occasional colloid bodies

2. Lymphocytic perivascular infiltrate in the superficial dermis
3. Pautrier's microabscesses
4. Focal epidermal exocytosis, spongiosis, mild acanthosis, and parakeratosis.

43. Which of the following is (are) acceptable treatments for small-plaque parapsoriasis?
    1. Lubrication with emollients
    2. Systemic retinoids (isotretinoin, etretinate)
    3. Ultraviolet B (UVB) radiation
    4. Methotrexate.

ATOPIC DERMATITIS, DIAPER DERMATITIS, SEBORRHEIC DERMATITIS, NUMMULAR DERMATITIS, INCONTINENTIA PIGMENTI

Choose the ONE best answer to each of the following questions.

44. Which feature is associated with atopic dermatitis?
    A. Nipple dermatitis
    B. Isolated adult hand eczema
    C. Follicular accentuation
    D. Normal serum IgE level
    E. All of the above are associated with atopic dermatitis.

45. Which of the following conditions is associated with incontinentia pigmenti?
    A. Retinal detachment
    B. Dwarfism
    C. Cataracts and strabismus
    D. Syndactyly
    E. All of the above are associated with incontinentia pigmenti.

46. Of all infants who develop atopic dermatitis, what proportion will continue to have problems as adolescents?
    A. One half
    B. One ninth
    C. One third
    D. Two thirds
    E. 100%.

47. The distribution of infantile atopic dermatitis is typically
    A. Flexor surfaces, face, and trunk
    B. Hands and feet
    C. Cheek, face, trunk, and extensor surfaces
    D. Flexor surfaces, hands, and feet
    E. Scalp, face, and flexor surfaces.

48. Which of the following statements are not characteristic of incontinentia pigmenti?
    A. Infants are generally systemically ill
    B. Significant leukocytosis may be present
    C. Linear vesiculation is usually present at birth or shortly thereafter
    D. Pigmentation stage fails to follow the location and shape of bullous and verrucous lesions
    E. Whorled pigmentation usually fades by adolescence.

49. A true statement regarding seborrheic dermatitis is
    A. Fluorinated topical steroids are the treatment of choice for facial involvement
    B. Incidence is increased in Parkinson's disease
    C. Blepharitis is never an associated feature
    D. Seborrheic dermatitis appears to be equally prevalent in males and females
    E. None of the above are true.

50. All of the following syndromes are associated with an eczematous dermatitis EXCEPT
    A. Ataxia-telangiectasia
    B. Histiocytosis X
    C. Hypereosinophilic syndrome
    D. Phenylketonuria
    E. Cronkhite's syndrome.

51. Which of the following is most characteristic of infantile atopic dermatitis?
    A. Flares in summer are a concern
    B. A "dry-type" dermatitis is most common
    C. Usually begins at 1 to 4 months of age
    D. *Staphylococcus aureus* infection is not thought to play a role in the pathogenesis
    E. In most infants, skin symptoms disappear at around 6 to 9 months of age.

Decide whether EACH of the following statements is TRUE or FALSE. Any combination of answers from all true to all false may occur.

52. Seborrheic dermatitis is usually not different histologically or clinically in HIV seropositive patients when compared with seronegative patients.

53. Ammonia is the main agent responsible for inducing the irritant contact dermatitis of diaper dermatitis.

54. The inguinal and suprapubic folds are not classically involved early on in uncomplicated diaper dermatitis.

55. Atopic dermatitis is more common in premature infants.

56. The dermal infiltrate in atopic dermatitis consists exclusively of mast cells and eosinophils.

57. Pityrosporum ovale may influence the course of seborrheic dermatitis.

58. Prolonged breast feeding can aggravate atopic dermatitis.

In each of the following questions, a set of lettered headings accompanies a list of numbered words or phrases. For each numbered word or phrase, choose

- A. If the item is associated with A only.
- B. If the item is associated with B only.
- C. If the item is associated with both A and B.
- D. If the item is associated with neither A nor B.

For each of the following characteristics, choose whether it describes seborrheic dermatitis, nummular dermatitis, both, or neither.

59.	May be an early sign of AIDS in the pediatric age group	A.	Seborrheic dermatitis
60.	Common cause of otitis externa	B.	Nummular dermatitis
61.	Frequently associated with hay fever and asthma	C.	Both
62.	Cause of desquamative erythroderma in infants	D.	Neither.
63.	Topical antifungals achieve good results.		

For EACH numbered word or phrase, select the ONE lettered heading that is most closely associated with it. Each lettered heading may be selected once, more than once, or not at all.

64.	Reactive red-brown nodules after potent topical steroid treatment	A.	Chafing diaper dermatitis
65.	Most frequently observed type of diaper dermatitis	B.	Perianal diaper dermatitis
66.	Most frequently seen in children with diarrhea and newborns	C.	Genital ulceration type diaper dermatitis
67.	Seen most often secondary to *Candida albicans* infection	D.	Red confluent erythema with satellitosis
68.	Observed most frequently at the age when infants' urine volume exceeds diaper absorbing capacity.	E.	Granuloma gluteale infantum.

69.	The skin lesions typically follow lines of Blaschko	A.	Nummular dermatitis
70.	Commonly seen in patients with a history of atopic dermatitis	B.	Incontinentia pigmenti
71.	Skin biopsy demonstrates subcorneal vesicles filled with numerous eosinophils	C.	Seborrheic dermatitis
72.	May be a cause of pruritus ani.	D.	Isolated eyelid dermatitis.
73.	Red-haired females with cold abscesses and eczema	A.	Wiskott-Aldrich syndrome
74.	Hemorrhagic crusted eczematous dermatitis	B.	Job's syndrome
75.	Ichthyosis linearis circumflexa, trichorrhexis invaginata, and later onset of atopic diathesis.	C.	Netherton's syndrome
		D.	All of the above
		E.	None of the above.

For the following questions, ONE or MORE of the following completions correctly finishes the incomplete statement. Choose

- A. If only 1, 2, and 3 are correct
- B. If only 1 and 3 are correct
- C. If only 2 and 4 are correct
- D. If only 4 is correct
- E. If all are correct.

76. The differential diagnosis of diaper dermatitis includes

   1. Letterer-Siwe disease
   2. Psoriasis
   3. Perianal cellulitis
   4. HIV-associated eruption.

77. The histologic phenomenon of eosinophilic spongiosis is consistent with which of the following diseases?
    1. Incontinentia pigmenti
    2. Pemphigus foliaceus
    3. Bullous pemphigoid
    4. Pemphigus vegetans.

78. True statements regarding incontinentia pigmenti include
    1. Overlapping of the various clinical stages can occur
    2. Pigmentary changes are consistent with postinflammatory hyperpigmentation
    3. Retinal vascular abnormalities in some patients may result in blindness
    4. Pattern of inheritance is X-linked recessive.

79. Associated signs of atopic dermatitis may include
    1. Geographic tongue
    2. Pityriasis alba
    3. Anterior neckfolds
    4. Keratoconus.

80. You receive a call to consult on a 6-week-old infant regarding a generalized eczematous eruption. Your differential diagnosis should include
    1. Acrodermatitis enteropathica
    2. Leiner's disease
    3. Histiocytosis X
    4. Multiple carboxylase deficiency.

ANSWERS

CONTACT DERMATITIS: CELL-MEDIATED IMMUNITY, LANGERHANS CELL BIOLOGY

1. E; **2.** E The role of the Langerhans cell is to process antigens absorbed through the epidermis and present them to lymphocytes. Langerhans cells function similarly to macrophages and have many of the same surface markers found on macrophages (Mac-1, Mac-2, Ia antigens [class II MHC] and receptors for Fc and C3b). Like macrophages, Langerhans cells are produced in the bone marrow. Langerhans cells process and present antigens to lymphocytes in the epidermis and dermis. Recent evidence indicates that they also travel to draining lymph nodes to present antigens to unsensitized lymphocytes. Langerhans cells are dendritic and have cytoplasmic organelles known as Birbeck granules. Interleukin-2 (IL-2) is produced by activated lymphocytes, not Langerhans cells (Chapters 1 and 10).

3. A Allergic contact allergens share several properties, including the abilities to penetrate the epidermis, to act as haptens, and to form covalent bonds with proteins. This latter property is necessary because haptens are not allergens by themselves. Immune system recognition occurs only after combination with a carrier protein. Unlike polyclonal T-lymphocyte mitogens (phytohemagglutinin, concanavalin-A) that nonspecifically activate lymphocytes, allergic contact allergens characteristically induce a mitogenic (monoclonal) response only in previously sensitized lymphocytes (Chapter 10).

CONTACT DERMATITIS AND OCCUPATIONAL DERMATOLOGY

4. B Skin diseases account for a disproportionately large percentage of occupational diseases with estimates ranging from 24% to 37%. The true number of occupationally related dermatoses is thought to be 10 to 50 times higher because of underdiagnosing, underreporting, and misclassification of cutaneous disease. Irritant contact dermatitis of the hands is felt to be the most common work-related dermatosis. Atopy has been shown to be a significant risk factor for the development of occupational skin disorders (OSD). Studies have suggested that the risk of OSD is 13 times greater for atopic individuals (Chapter 10).

5. A The rhus group of plants includes poison ivy, poison oak, and sumac. Pentadecylcatechols found in the plant oleoresin are the sensitizers in these plants. The entire rhus group contains identical antigens and produces indistinguishable eruptions. The rhus group of plants is related to the mango, the Japanese lacquer, cashew nut, and ginkgo trees; they are all members of the Anacardiaceae plant family (Chapter 10).

6. D Sensitization to ingredients in cosmetics is not uncommon; one study indicated 5.4% of patients were identified by patch testing as having reactions caused by cosmetic ingredients. The top three causes of cosmetic allergic reactions are perfume, preservatives, and hair dyes. Cosmetic dermatitis is usually patchy and is bilateral on the face. Common causes of unilateral facial dermatitis include nail polish and consort dermatitis. Eyelid dermatitis from cosmetics is usually due to those applied elsewhere, like fingernail polish, rather than by direct application of periocular cosmetics (Chapter 10).

7. D This case describes latex surgical glove allergic contact urticaria, an example of immediate type 1 hypersensitivity. Clues to this diagnosis include the immediate nature of the reaction and associated respiratory symptoms. Because of the possibility of a potentially life-threatening anaphylactic reaction, the patient should be cautioned to avoid the suspected allergen, and prick (scratch) testing should be initiated to evaluate the possibility of allergic contact urticaria. Inasmuch as severe allergic reactions, including anaphylaxis, may occur with skin testing, epinephrine and resuscitation equipment should always be available (Chapter 10).

8. C Antabuse (disulfiram) is a tetraethylthiuram. An "Antabuse reaction" consisting of erythema, urticaria, and pruritus may develop shortly after the consumption of alcohol in persons exposed to either systemic or topical thiurams. This reaction is nonallergenic and results from the accumulation of toxic ethanol breakdown products (acetaldehyde) because of thiuram's inhibition of the enzyme aldehyde dehydrogenase (Chapter 10).

9. A Acrylic bone cement is used for the attachment of prostheses to bone and is commonly used by orthopedic surgeons. It is a powerful solvent that penetrates all types of gloves and can produce inflammation of nerve endings in the fingers, resulting in distressing paresthesias. The use of acrylic bone cement is not associated with an increased incidence of graft rejection (Chapter 10).

10. D Contact leukoderma (vitiligo) may result from exposure to certain phenolic compounds and the monobenzyl ether of hydroquinone. The depigmentation produced by these chemicals may or may not be preceded by dermatitis. The leukoderma can clinically mimic "idiopathic" vitiligo by becoming widespread and occurring on areas other than those directly exposed to the agent. A biopsy usually is not helpful in distinguishing idiopathic from contact vitiligo because both types have similar histologic findings, consisting of degenerated melanocytes. Inasmuch as the depigmentation caused by chemicals is a toxic rather than an allergic process, closed patch testing for 48 to 72 hours is not useful. However, closed patch testing of suspected chemicals for long (2-week) periods of time may reproduce the leukoderma through its toxic effect on melanocytes (Chapter 10).

11. A Patients sensitive to topical paraphenylenediamine found in hair and fur dyes can react to other para-amino compounds such as benzocaine, procaine, butacaine, para-aminobenzoic acid (PABA), and sulfonamides (Chapter 10).

12. A Paraphenylenediamine (PPD) found in permanent hair dyes is a common sensitizing agent. Patients allergic to PPD do not react to previously dyed hair because during the dying process PPD becomes oxidized to nonallergenic products. Glycerylmonothioglycolate (GMTG) is an allergen found in salon (hot, acid) perms. Ammonium thioglycolate is an allergen found in home (cold, basic) perms. Unlike PPD, allergenicity of the thioglycolates are not altered by the perming process and thus can persist in hair for at least 3 months after perming (Chapter 10).

13. B Formaldehyde-donating compounds actually release small amounts of formaldehyde through hydrolysis. This production of formaldehyde is a temperature- and pH-dependent process. These compounds are commonly used as preservatives in cosmetics and medicines. Examples of formaldehyde-releasing preservatives include Bronopol, quaternium-15, diazolidinyl urea, imidazolidinyl urea and tris(hydroxymethyl)nitromethane. Positive closed patch test results to these compounds can be due to sensitivity to the native compound or to the released formaldehyde (Chapter 10).

14. C; 15. A; 16. B; 17. E Cinnamic aldehyde is a potent sensitizer that is chemically related to cinnamon and cassia oils. This compound is commonly used as a flavoring agent in many toothpastes. Potassium dichromate is a common industrial sensitizer used in tanning leather, staining wood, safety matches, fireworks, waxes, and waterproofing fabrics. It is also frequently used as an oxidizer in the manufacture of organic chemicals and electric batteries. The most common contact is seen in construction workers reacting to the hexavalent chromium found in cement. Fragrances in aftershave preparations are probably the most common shaving-associated allergens. Musk ambrette used to be commonly found in aftershave lotions and is a potent photosensitizer. Chemical additives used to speed up the process of rubber vulcanization ("accelerators") such as thiurams and benzothiazole derivatives along with antioxidants are the main sensitizers found in association with rubber products (Chapter 10).

18. B; 19. C; 20. A Indicator tests are commercially available kits that can be used to test for the presence of a specific ingredient. Indicator tests are available for nickel, formaldehyde, and chromate (Chapter 10).

HAND AND FOOT DERMATITIS

21. C With the exception of vesicular hand and foot dermatitis (pompholyx), all of the palmoplantar eruptions listed are characterized by sterile neutrophilic pustules. Pompholyx is characterized by spongiotic vesicles containing lymphocytes (Chapter 12).

22. B Pustular palmoplantar psoriasis can be extremely difficult to treat. Potent topical corticosteroids, often under occlusion, are used with only some success. Oral dapsone and colchicine, because of antineutrophil effects, have also been used with some success. Topical or systemic psoralens and UVA (PUVA) is one of the best treatments, often leading to clearing and even resulting in long-lasting remissions. Oral retinoids have also been shown to be useful, although relapses often occur when patients are taken off the drug. Severe disabling disease is sometimes treated with methotrexate. As with other types of psoriasis, oral corticosteroids are of questionable value. Large doses of oral prednisone (40 to 60 mg per day) can often suppress pustulation, but withdrawal is commonly followed by a severe relapse of disease activity. For this reason, oral corticosteroids are not considered a recommended treatment for pustular palmoplantar psoriasis (Chapter 12).

23. E Acrodermatitis continua is a rare pustular dermatosis that often starts on the tips of fingers and slowly extends proximally. The nails are involved early, and often both destruction of the nails and atrophy of the distal phalanx occurs. Like pustular palmoplantar psoriasis, acrodermatitis continua is thought to be a type of psoriasis. The treatment of this chronic disorder is similar to that of pustular palmoplantar psoriasis (Chapter 12).

24. D; **25.** D Infantile acropustulosis is a pruritic vesiculopustular eruption found mostly on the palms and soles of infants. The lesions consist of intensely pruritic pustules that start as vesicles that become purulent. The lesions last 1 to 2 weeks but recur at weekly to monthly intervals. The disease is seen primarily in male black infants but onset can occur between birth and several years of age. Direct immunofluorescence findings are negative or nonspecific. Infantile acropustulosis runs a benign and self-limited course, with spontaneous resolution by age 2 to 3 years. For this reason, treatment is usually symptomatic. Topical corticosteroids and antipruritics often provide symptomatic relief. Dapsone treatment has been shown to result in rapid clearing of the lesions. It has been used for patients with symptomatic disease unresponsive to topical treatment. Antibiotics are not very helpful. Tetracyclines should not be used in infants because of their effects on developing teeth (Chapter 12).

26. (T); **27.** (F); **28.** (F); **29.** (F) It is often impossible clinically to distinguish between irritant and allergic contact hand dermatitis. Although the majority of hand dermatitis is irritant or endogenous in nature, patch testing can be beneficial to evaluate the possibility of an allergic component (found in approximately 20% of patients). Examination of the patient with hand dermatitis should always include the feet to evaluate the possibility of a systemic disease such as psoriasis or infectious etiology such as tinea. The management of irritant hand dermatitis includes avoidance of irritants such as harsh detergents, soaps, and antiseptics. Patients should be instructed to use vinyl or rubber gloves (with cotton liners) when exposed to irritants. Corticosteroids in bland emollient creams or ointments often result in improvement of the dermatitis. Because bactericidal soaps are often irritants, secondarily infected hand dermatitis should be treated with oral antibiotics or antibacterial ointments such as mupirocin. Although nickel allergy is common, finger dermatitis localized under a ring is more often the result of trapped irritants such as soaps, detergents, waxes, and polishes. A nickel-free diet is often impossible to achieve and probably does not play a role in the vast majority of hand dermatitis, even in individuals allergic to this ubiquitous metal (Chapters 10 and 12).

30. B Juvenile plantar dermatosis is characterized by redness, cracking, and dryness of the weight-bearing surface of the feet. Although it is uncommon in children, tinea pedis can mimic juvenile plantar dermatosis. Because dryness and chapping are the underlying cause, treatment of this condition consists of lubrication. An ointment base such as petroleum jelly is helpful for mild disease. Topical corticosteroids are often used for cases that have severe inflammation. Drying agents may actually exacerbate this condition (Chapters 10 to 12).

31. B Adverse effects of oral PUVA therapy have been divided into acute and chronic. Acute side effects include erythema, pruritus, transient nausea, and headache. Chronic adverse effects encompass the possibility of ocular damage, including cataracts, nuclear disease, and posterior subcapsular opacities. Induction of cutaneous carcinoma has also been suggested in studies of patients receiving long-term therapy (more than 260 treatments). Lupus erythematosus has also been reported to develop during PUVA therapy. Other rare, systemic reactions include hepatotoxicity, preleukemia, acute myeloid leukemia, and nephrotic syndrome. PUVA monitoring guidelines consist of a baseline ocular examination (gross, funduscopic, slit-lamp, and visual acuity), skin examination, and laboratory examinations (complete blood count, liver and renal function tests, ANA, and urinalysis). Follow-up consists of repeat ocular (after 6 months, after 1 year, and yearly), complete skin (at least every 6 to 12 months), and laboratory (after 6 months, after 1 year, and yearly) examinations. Glucose-6-phosphate dehydrogenase levels are important for systemic drugs with oxidant properties such as dapsone (Chapters 12 and 27).

PITYRIASIS ROSEA

32. C Pityriasis rosea (PR) is a common, self-limited dermatosis of unknown but suspected viral etiology. PR is typically found in children and young adults. The disease is more common during the fall, winter, and spring months. Lesions are round to oval, erythematous to salmon-colored papules and plaques with an inner collarette of fine scale. Lesions are characteristically distributed along skin lines of cleavage on the trunk and proximal extremities. Oral lesions can occur. Prodromal symptoms are uncommon (approximately 5%), and the rash often begins with the appearance of a "herald patch" 3 to 14 days before onset of the generalized exanthem. New lesions continue to appear over several weeks, and gradually resolve over a time course of 3 to 8 weeks. Sunlight actually improves the rash, and areas that receive significant sun exposure are often free of lesions. Approximately 10% to 20% of PR does not follow the classic course. Variations consisting of papular, vesicular, purpuric, and urticarial lesions in both the characteristic and "inverse" distributions (extremities and intertriginous areas) have been described. Children often have more widespread lesions than adults, and involvement of face and extremities is not uncommon. Rashes that can clinically mimic PR include psoriasis (especially guttate), small-plaque parapsoriasis, secondary syphilis, and tinea versicolor (Chapter 17).

33. D PR is often asymptomatic, and thus treatment is often not necessary. However, for symptomatic PR, topical corticosteroids and oral H1 antihistamines can be used. Severe cases have been treated with oral corticosteroids, although there have been reports of PR worsening with this therapy. Erythemogenic exposure to either sunlight or UVB is effective in decreasing the pruritus and hastening the resolution of this dermatosis (Chapter 17).

34. C A pityriasis rosea–like eruption can occur as a reaction to captopril, barbiturates, clonidine, beta-adrenergic receptor antagonists, bismuth-containing compounds, and metronidazole. Unlike idiopathic PR,

PR-like drug eruptions are not characterized by a herald patch (Chapters 17 and 43).

35. (F); **36.** (T); **37.** (F) "Inverse" pityriasis rosea (PR) is characterized by lesions found on extremities and intertriginous areas and is more commonly found in dark-skinned races. Herpes virus type 6 is thought to be responsible for roseola (Chapter 17).

38. E (Chapter 17).

PARAPSORIASIS (SMALL PLAQUE)

39. D; **40.** A; **41.** B; **42.** C This case history describes one of the many presentations of small-plaque parapsoriasis (SPP). SPP is characterized by small (5-cm or smaller), asymptomatic, oval patches or thin plaques with discrete margins and fine (pityriasis-type) scale. Lesions are found primarily on the trunk and proximal extremities. SPP is differentiated from the otherwise clinically similar pityriasis rosea by the long history (greater than 3 months) and the absence of evolving and resolving individual lesions. The histologic picture of SPP is usually nonspecific, consisting of perivascular lymphocytic infiltrates. Focal epidermal involvement with exocytosis, spongiosis, mild acanthosis, and parakeratosis is occasionally present. Because the histologic picture of pityriasis rosea and other subacute or chronic dermatoses can be somewhat similar, the diagnosis of SPP cannot be made based upon histologic findings alone. SPP can be confused with other conditions including nummular eczema. Although it is chronic in nature, less than 1% of patients with this condition will progress to cutaneous lymphoma (Chapter 18).

43. B Although small-plaque parapsoriasis is a chronic disorder, the benign and often asymptomatic nature of this dermatosis dictates that safe therapies be used. Lubrication with emollients for mild disease and UVB for more extensive or symptomatic disease are commonly used (Chapter 18).

ATOPIC DERMATITIS, DIAPER DERMATITIS, SEBORRHEIC DERMATITIS, NUMMULAR DERMATITIS, INCONTINENTIA PIGMENTI

44. E Atopic dermatitis can have a number of associated findings. These include either a moist oozing and crusting nipple eczema or a chronic dry and scaly nipple dermatitis. Patients frequently have hyperlinear palms, follicular accentuation, and bilateral hand eczema (especially common in adults and adolescents). Increased IgE serum levels and normal values have been documented in atopic patients. Additionally, elevated IgE levels are not unique to atopic dermatitis patients, since increased serum IgE levels have also been reported in patients with contact dermatitis and psoriasis. Most investigators believe that increased IgE levels are not a specific feature of atopic dermatitis (Chapter 13).

45. E Incontinentia pigmenti is a rare X-linked dominant genodermatosis that usually is lethal to males. It is characterized by an acral linear vesicobullous erythematous rash occurring at birth or within 6 weeks after delivery. This is followed within weeks to months by verrucous growths, most apparent on the extremities. These lesions spontaneously resolve, sometimes leaving areas of atrophy, depigmentation, or both. The final pigmentary stage consists of slate gray to brown whorls or streaks on the torso and occasionally on the extremities. These gradually resolve and fade by adolescence. Other developmental abnormalities include problems with hair, eyes, teeth, and central nervous system. Some of the specifically mentioned problems include retinal detachment, cataracts, strabismus, and syndactyly (Chapter 165).

46. B Of all infants who develop atopic dermatitis, one third still have problems during childhood. Of those childhood eczema patients, one third continue into adolescence with atopic dermatitis. Therefore, only one ninth of patients with infantile atopic dermatitis still have problems as adolescents. Of note, by adolescence more than 90% of patients with atopic dermatitis manifest the disorder (Chapter 13).

47. C Atopic dermatitis can be divided into three stages:

> Infantile eczema (2 months to 2 years)
> Childhood eczema (2 to 10 years)
> Adolescent and adult stage.

The distribution of atopic dermatitis is mostly age-dependent. Infantile atopic dermatitis distribution is mostly on the face, cheeks, trunk, and extensor surfaces of the extremities. In the childhood phase, the distribution is in the flexural areas, neck, and feet. In the adult and the adolescent, the distribution is bilateral flexural involvement, including the hands. Eyelid dermatitis is also common and can be seen in all stages of atopic dermatitis (Chapter 13).

48. A (See answer for Question 45). Infants generally are not systemically ill, in fact their general health is good. Patients have no fevers in spite of a significant leukocytosis (counts as high as 45,000) and eosinophilia. In the pigmentary phase, the brown pigmentation has a whorled appearance and is found in areas in which blisters and verrucous lesions did not occur. This whorled pigmentation usually fades by adolescence. There may be considerable overlap among the three stages. For example, infants have been born with verrucous lesions or pigmented streaks (Chapter 165).

49. B Seborrheic dermatitis consists of a dry form (dandruff) with dry scales and little erythema as well as an oily form with greasy scales on an erythematous base. It tends to occur in seborrheic areas, including eyelid margins (seborrheic blepharitis) and may have an associated conjunctivitis. Seborrheic dermatitis has a predilection for males and is usually more severe in the winter. The incidence is increased in Parkinson's disease, although the mechanism is poorly understood. Usually, low-potency topical corticosteroids are adequate for facial involvement. Fluorinated steroids should never be used on areas such as the face as they may lead to cutaneous atrophy and acneiform eruptions (Chapter 16).

50. E In infants, several disorders are associated with an eczematous dermatitis, such as ataxia-telangiectasia, histiocytosis X, phenylketonuria and the hypereosinophilic syndrome. Hypereosinophilic syndrome usually affects middle-aged men with peripheral eosinophilia and a pruritic, atopic, dermatitis-like rash. Cutaneous problems associated with ataxia-telangiectasia include an eczematous dermatitis as well as a telangiectatic eruption that appears in the flexural surfaces of the upper extremities. The eruption in histiocytosis X classically involves the scalp, neck, and abdomen. In late stages of the disease, weeping eczematoid dermatitis becomes evident. Skin manifestations in phenylketonuria are seen in about 50% of patients and have a predilection for the flexural areas. This eczematous dermatitis may be sclerodermatous in nature and interestingly, these patients are also sensitive to light (Chapters 35, 135, and 175).

51. C Usually, a partial or complete remission of infantile atopic dermatitis occurs in the summer and flares during the winter or colder months. The latter is usually secondary to low humidity and increased exposure to irritating clothing (i.e., wool). Lesions typically exhibit polymorphism; exudative or ''moist-type'' dermatitis is the most frequently observed type. ''Dry-type'' dermatitis is seen more often in older children and adolescents. Most infants develop atopic dermatitis at about the ages of 1 to 4 months, and the skin symptoms tend to disappear toward the end of the second year. *Staphylococcus aureus* is a frequent inhabitant of normal skin as well as of the skin of the atopic dermatitis patients. It appears that patients with atopic dermatitis have a higher rate and density of colonization with *S. aureus*. Since the skin's barrier function is frequently disrupted in these patients, they acquire superinfection more readily (Chapter 13).

52. (F) Seborrheic dermatitis (SD) in HIV-positive patients differs histologically from classic SD. In patients with AIDS, the histology is fairly distinctive, consisting of spotty keratinocyte necrosis, leukoexocytosis, and plasma cells. Classic seborrheic dermatitis may have features of both psoriasis and chronic dermatitis. The major difference histologically between psoriasis and seborrheic dermatitis is the occurrence of more spongiosis in seborrheic dermatitis (Chapter 16).

53. (F) It is now thought that ammonia by itself is not responsible for diaper dermatitis. For example, diaper dermatitis does not result without maceration and prolonged contact with water. Prolonged diaper occlusion of feces and urine against the skin enhances irritation and penetration of these alkaline substances through the epidermal barrier. Irritating fecal enzymes probably also play a role. If diaper dermatitis is present for approximately 3 days, *Candida albicans* then also plays a role as a secondary invader (Chapter 11).

54. (T) The distribution of diaper dermatitis becomes important in helping to differentiate between other dermatoses that can involve the napkin area. It seems likely that friction may play a role in which areas are affected by diaper dermatitis. This is supported by the frequent predilection for sites where friction is maximal, i.e., buttocks, inner thighs, and convex surfaces of the genitalia. The inguinal and suprapubic folds tend not to be as frequently involved in simple diaper dermatitis as they are in intertrigo, inverse psoriasis, seborrheic dermatitis, and secondary infection with *Candida albicans* (Chapter 11).

55. (F) Atopic dermatitis is actually less common in premature infants and usually begins at about 1 to 4 months. Frequently, the dermatitis at this age is subacute with significant oozing (Chapter 13).

56. (F) Although it is true that the inflammatory infiltrate in atopic dermatitis may contain an increased number of mast cells, eosinophils are rare. The dermal infiltrate more often consists of lymphocytes and monocytes (Chapter 13).

57. (T) The influence of *Pityrosporum ovale* on seborrheic dermatitis (SD) appears to have been explained by clinical studies showing a good therapeutic response of SD to oral or topical antifungals such as ketoconazole. Studies have shown profuse numbers of *P. ovale* organisms in the scalp lesions of patients with SD; however, others have shown an abundance of this organism in the scalps of patients without SD (Chapter 16).

58. (F) Prolonged breast feeding has not been shown to be an aggravating factor associated with atopic dermatitis. A number of studies have actually suggested that breast feeding may be protective. Other studies have shown neither protective nor aggravating effects with prolonged breast feeding (Chapter 13).

59. A Pediatric HIV infections are the cause of disease in an increasing number of children. Like adults, children often have cutaneous manifestations. There is no particularly pathognomonic rash associated with HIV disease in children; however, the course of routine common dermatoses is usually abnormal. Severe seborrheic dermatitis, severe herpes zoster, recurrent oral HSV infection, and unusual dermatophyte infections of nails and diaper area are among several examples seen in HIV-positive children (Chapters 16 and 125).

60. A Although it is frequently unrecognized, seborrheic dermatitis is a common cause of otitis externa. The skin in and around the external auditory meatus and ear becomes red, fissured, and swollen. The differential diagnosis includes otitis externa from other causes, such as bacterial and fungal infections or contact dermatitis (Chapter 16).

61. D Neither seborrheic dermatitis nor nummular dermatitis appears to be related to an atopic diathesis. Patients who are considered atopic have a personal or family history of hay fever, asthma, and/or atopic dermatitis (Chapters 13 and 16).

62. **A** Seborrheic dermatitis may progress to a generalized exfoliative condition in infants. When this occurs, it is known as erythroderma desquamativum (Leiner's disease). Infants are severely ill with anemia, diarrhea, adenopathy, vomiting, and secondary infection. In a few patients, defects in leukocyte chemotaxis and C5 inhibitor have been reported (Chapter 16).

63. **A** (See answer to Question 57). Topical antifungals such as ketoconazole 2% cream have been shown in numerous studies to be effective both in the acute treatment of seborrheic dermatitis and in lowering the relapse rate after their use (Chapter 16).

64. **E** Granuloma gluteale infantum is a rare condition characterized by cherry-sized red-brown nodules in the diaper area of infants. The etiology remains obscure; however, there may be an association with prolonged use of fluorinated topical corticosteroids. The nodules usually resolve after the discontinuation of the corticosteroid (Chapter 11).

65. **A**; 68. **A** Of the four types (perianal, chafing, ulcerated, and candidal dermatitis), chafing dermatitis is the most frequently observed form. It involves the convex surfaces of the diapered area, usually in 7- to 12-month-olds. This is also the time period when an infant's urine volume usually exceeds the absorbent capacity of the diaper. The genital ulceration form is characterized by shallow and discrete ulcers primarily in the genitalia and diaper area (Chapter 11).

66. **B** Perianal diaper dermatitis is more common in newborns and infants with diarrhea. It is usually limited most often to this area (Chapter 11).

67. **D** This is a classic description of *Candida albicans* diaper dermatitis. It usually involves the inguinal creases with satellite lesions at the periphery. In other types of diaper dermatitis, such as chafing dermatitis, it is often a secondary invader after approximately 3 days of preceding inflammation (Chapter 11).

68. **A** See the answer to Question 65.

69. **B** Incontinentia pigmenti (IP) usually begins as a vesicular eruption that evolves into linear streaks of confluent vesicles and these classically follow the lines of Blaschko. These lines do not appear to follow any known vascular or nervous structures in the skin. They are assumed to be derived from embryonic migration patterns, forming linear patterns on the extremities and more curvilinear patterns on the torso (Chapter 165).

70. **D** Isolated eyelid dermatitis is frequently observed in patients with a history of atopic dermatitis. The differential diagnosis should also include psoriasis, tinea faciale, and allergic contact dermatitis from nail polish or eye makeup. Lichenification, poorly circumscribed lesions, and excoriations help differentiate atopic disease from psoriasis. Seborrheic dermatitis frequently involves the eyelid margin (Chapter 13).

71. **B** Histologically, the vesicles that develop during the first stage of incontinentia pigmenti are usually intraepidermal and are associated with spongiosis. Numerous eosinophils are seen within the vesicles and surrounding epidermis and dermis (Chapter 165).

72. **C** Seborrheic dermatitis of the anal area can be a cause of pruritus ani. It can also involve other areas such as the groin, face, scalp, chest, and axillae (Chapter 16).

73. **B** In Job's syndrome, the key laboratory finding is a great elevation of serum IgE (usually >2000 IU/mL). This syndrome has cutaneous manifestations resembling atopic dermatitis, but it tends to involve the scalp, axillae, and groin. Other features include severe lung damage, cold abscesses (abscesses lacking the usual warmth, erythema, and fluctuance), frequent *S. aureus* infections, impaired neutrophil chemotaxis and clinically coarse facial features in a fair, red-headed female (Chapter 105).

74. **A** Wiskott-Aldrich syndrome is an X-linked recessive disorder characterized by a triad of thrombocytopenia, atopic-like eczematous dermatitis, and recurrent infections. Because of the thrombocytopenia and abnormal platelet function, hemorrhage and hemorrhagic-crusted dermatitis aid in making the diagnosis. It is exclusively seen in young boys in whom death by age 6 usually occurs secondary to infection, bleeding, or associated malignancies. These patients can present in the first few weeks of life with bloody diarrhea and persistent epistaxis. Later, the eczematous dermatitis mostly involves the scalp, face, and flexural areas. Recurrent infections such as pyoderma or suppurative otitis media occur frequently. Levels of IgM are low, whereas IgA and IgE are usually elevated. Hepatosplenomegaly is common, and these patients are prone to develop lymphoreticular malignancies, especially lymphoma (Chapter 13).

75. **C** Netherton's syndrome is a rare autosomal recessive disorder characterized by ichthyosis linearis circumflexa, hair-shaft abnormalities, and an atopic diathesis. The syndrome occurs more often in females. At birth, a generalized erythroderma or collodion-baby phenotype may be present. The hair abnormality leading to short brittle hairs is known as trichorrhexis invaginata, or bamboo hairs. These bamboo hairs may be present on the scalp, eyebrows, or eyelashes but rarely in other hairy areas. The bamboo hair defect is caused by intussusception of the hair shaft at the zone of beginning keratinization. Ichthyosis linearis circumflexa is an ichthyosis in which migratory annular and polycyclic patches occur. The lesions may involute without evidence of scarring, atrophy, or pigmentation abnormalities. The eruption usually clears in the summer and is asymptomatic. Other reported findings include pili torti, trichorrhexis nodosa, moniliform hairs, and mental retardation (Chapters 133 and 163).

76. **E** The differential diagnosis of diaper dermatitis includes inverse psoriasis, Letterer-Siwe disease, perianal cellulitis (usually *Streptococcus pyogenes*), HIV-associated eruptions, allergic contact dermatitis, congenital syphilis, and intertriginous fungal or yeast infections. The inguinal and suprapubic folds are involved

early in intertrigo, inverse psoriasis, and seborrheic dermatitis, in contrast to diaper dermatitis. In Letterer-Siwe disease, the lesions are widespread in the scalp, face, trunk, and groin with involvement of other organs. A hemorrhagic, seborrhea-like dermatitis with chronic genitocrural ulceration should suggest this diagnosis. Congenital syphilis cutaneous lesions are characterized by a bright red maculopapular eruption with significant scaling and involvement of the face, arms, buttocks, legs, palms, and soles (Chapter 11).

77. E Eosinophilic spongiosis consists of eosinophilic invasion of a spongiotic epidermis before acantholysis becomes evident. By itself, it is considered not diagnostic but suggestive of all diseases listed in the answer as well as herpes gestationis, arthropod reaction, and allergic contact dermatitis (Chapters 10, 74, 75, 77, and 165).

78. B In about 90% to 95% of the cases of incontinentia pigmenti (IP), eruptions begin at 2 to 6 weeks of life and usually are vesicular (87% of the patients). However, the peak age for the onset of the verrucous stage is also about 2 to 6 weeks of life, the onset of the pigmentary stage following closely at 12 to 26 weeks of life. Therefore, overlapping of the stages may occur. Infants may be born with any of the mentioned stages, implying that lesions may also begin and progress in utero. Usually, the pigmentary stage persists for years and fades, sometimes leaving atrophic or hypopigmented areas. Severe ocular abnormalities can occur with loss of vision or blindness. Vascular abnormalities of the retina seen with IP may also ultimately lead to blindness. Incontinentia pigmenti is an X-linked dominant disorder. The pigment in IP is histologically manifested by melanin in melanophages in the upper dermis, dyskeratotic cells, and vacuolar degeneration of the basal layer. In postinflammatory hyperpigmentation, there may be an increase in free melanin or melanophages in the dermis without a significant epidermal alteration (Chapter 165).

79. E All of the listed are associated signs of atopic dermatitis. Specifically, elongation of the corneal surface is known as keratoconus, which is an uncommon disorder seen in about 1% of atopic persons and is present during the second or third decade of life. Pityriasis alba is a condition found in normal as well as atopic individuals. It is characterized by ill-defined hypopigmented scaly patches usually on the cheeks, upper arms, or shoulders and may represent a subclinical dermatitis. Geographic tongue can be a manifestation of atopy in some patients; however, in most patients it is an isolated finding. It consists of a benign inflammatory disorder characterized by multiple annular, smooth patches with gray elevated borders on the tongue. The patterns of involvement change from day to day and spontaneous remissions can occur. Anterior neckfolds are redundant skin that are occasionally seen in association with atopic dermatitis. These skinfolds are only an associated feature and not necessarily pathognomonic of atopic dermatitis (Chapter 13).

80. E The differential diagnosis of eczematous disorders in the newborn is rather extensive but extremely important when considering the spectrum of diagnostic possibilities and therapeutic options. The list includes acrodermatitis enteropathica, atopic dermatitis, Leiner's disease, and multiple carboxylase deficiency. Acrodermatitis enteropathica is an autosomal recessive disorder of zinc metabolism. It is usually apparent at 1 to 2 months of age with acral, perioral, and perineal erosions; diarrhea; and failure to thrive. Leiner's disease is seen in infants at 6 to 20 weeks of age. It is characterized by a generalized exfoliative dermatitis with marked erythema, and scaling. The infants usually have diarrhea, failure to thrive, and intercurrent infections. Multiple carboxylase deficiency occurs late in the newborn period and is associated with eczematous skin lesions, diarrhea, respiratory infections, and failure to thrive. Other disorders to include in the differential diagnosis are scabies, diaper dermatitis, seborrheic dermatitis, histiocytosis X, candidiasis, and contact dermatitis (Chapter 13).

Bibliography

Abramson JS, Dahl MV, Walsh G, et al. Antistaphylococcal immunoglobulin levels in patients with atopic dermatitis. J Am Acad Dermatol 1982; 7:105–110.
Adams RM, Maibach HI. A five-year study of cosmetic reactions. J Am Acad Dermatol 1985; 13:1062.
Carney RG. Incontinentia pigmenti. Arch Dermatol 1976; 112:535–539.
Dahl MH. Clinical Immunodermatology, 2nd edition. Chicago: Year Book Medical Publishers, 1988.
Engasser PG, Maibach HI. Dermatitis due to cosmetics. In: Fisher AA, ed. Contact Dermatitis, 3rd edition. Philadelphia: Lea & Febiger, 1986:368.
Fisher AA. Contact Dermatitis, 3rd edition. Philadelphia: Lea & Febiger, 1986.
Fisher AA, Adams RM. Occupational dermatitis. In: Fisher AA, ed. Contact Dermatitis, 3rd edition. Philadelphia: Lea & Febiger, 1986:486.
Frieden IJ. The dermatologist in the newborn nursery: Approach to neonates with blisters, pustules, and ulcerations. Current Probs Dermatol 1992; 4:160–161.
Hurwitz S. Cutaneous disorders of the newborn. In: Hurwitz S. Clinical Pediatric Dermatology. Philadelphia: WB Saunders Co., 1981:30.
Kramer MS, Moroz B. Do breastfeeding and delayed introduction of solid foods protect against subsequent atopic eczema? J Pediatr 1981; 98:546–550.
Leung DM. Immune mechanism and relevance to treatment in atopic dermatitis. Allergy Proc 1991; 12:342–343.
Matthew DJ, Norman AP, Taylor B, et al. Prevention of eczema. Lancet 1977; 1:321–324.
Rajka, G. Histopathologic and laboratory findings. In: Essentials of Atopic Dermatitis. New York: Springer-Verlag, 1989:70–71.
Roth D. Atopic dermatitis revisited. Int J Dermatol 1987; 26:141.
Skinner RB. Psoralens. In: Wolverton SE, Wilkin JK, eds. Systemic Drugs for Skin Diseases. Philadelphia: WB Saunders Co., 1991: 219.
Spraker MK. Pediatric dermatology. Prog Dermatol 1989; 23:1–2.
Taylor JS. Rubber. In: Fisher AA, ed. Contact Dermatitis, 3rd edition. Philadelphia: Lea & Febiger, 1986:603.
Weston WL, Lane AT: Dermatitis. In: Color Textbook of Pediatric Dermatology. St. Louis: Mosby Year Book, 1991:26–39.

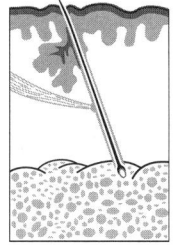

chapter 5

Interface Dermatitides

R. GARY SIBBALD, and SANDRA J. LANDOLT

Choose the ONE BEST answer to each of the following questions:

1. All of the following are features of lichen planus EXCEPT
   A. Can cause a scarring alopecia
   B. Frequently exhibits the Koebner phenomenon
   C. The majority of patients who present with cutaneous disease have evidence of oral mucosal involvement
   D. Involvement of genitalia is unusual
   E. May manifest with associated gastrointestinal symptomatology.

2. Lichen planus has been described in association with all of the following EXCEPT
   A. Primary biliary cirrhosis
   B. Abnormal hepatic transaminase levels in a significant number of patients
   C. Chronic active hepatitis in approximately 10% of cases
   D. Increased incidence of glucose intolerance
   E. Underlying infectious etiology.

3. Clinical features of lichen planus include all of the following EXCEPT
   A. A hypertrophic variant with predominant involvement of the scalp
   B. Symmetrical, flexural distribution of lesions
   C. Pruritus in the majority of patients
   D. Annular variant with localization to the glans penis
   E. Wickham's striae thought to be areas of focal hypergranulosis.

4. Oral disease in lichen planus is characterized by
   A. Eventual progression to oral epidermoid malignancy as the rule
   B. Presence only with coexisting cutaneous involvement
   C. Erosive involvement that may preferentially predispose to malignant degeneration
   D. Preferential localization to the tongue
   E. Resolution with pigmentary change.

5. Nail findings of lichen planus include all of the following EXCEPT
   A. Incidence in approximately 10% of patients with lichen planus
   B. Pterygium formation as a classic finding
   C. Hyperkeratosis and onycholysis typically seen
   D. Atrophic changes, including distal friability and anonychia
   E. Association with 20-nail dystrophy.

51

6. Lichen striatus is an acquired pediatric dermatosis
   A. That follows Blaschko's lines with linear erythematous papules
   B. That is typically pruritic
   C. That is persistent into adulthood
   D. That is likely a forme fruste of psoriasis.

7. All of the following are true of Nekam's disease EXCEPT
   A. It is also known as keratosis lichenoides chronica
   B. It tends to be highly resistant to most therapeutic measures
   C. Pathologically it resembles lichen planus
   D. It typically spares the head and neck
   E. It may be responsive to PUVA.

8. Erythema multiforme minor
   A. Is often the result of Eaton agent of *Mycoplasma pneumoniae*
   B. Cannot be treated with prophylactic acyclovir
   C. May involve more than two mucosal sites as long as the eyes are spared
   D. Appears in many cases to be hypersensitivity reaction to herpes simplex virus (HSV)
   E. Is treated with prednisone as the method of choice.

9. All of the following are true of erythema multiforme EXCEPT
   A. There is abrupt onset of the eruption with acral predominance
   B. It usually presents with monomorphous lesions in a given patient
   C. It is coincident with a herpetic outbreak and thus should, if herpes simplex virus–related, have active lesions with positive culture
   D. It is unusual in infants and the elderly
   E. It does not always show epidermal necrosis on histopathology.

10. The following is true of Stevens-Johnson syndrome EXCEPT
    A. Sulfonamides may be a precipitating factor
    B. It may have mucosal involvement with significant scarring sequelae
    C. It is best treated by high-dose and pulse corticosteroid therapy
    D. It involves two or more mucosal sites
    E. It may have internal mucosal involvement, although internal organ involvement is rare.

11. Pityriasis lichenoides
    A. Is an inflammatory dermatosis that responds well to topical steroids
    B. Is a condition that typically resolves with no pigmentary change
    C. Can evolve from the acute stage (PLEVA) to the chronic stage, pityriasis lichenoides chronica
    D. Is unresponsive to all treatment modalities, including ultraviolet light
    E. Has no supporting evidence for an infectious cause.

12. All of the following are true of pityriasis lichenoides et varioliformis acuta (PLEVA) EXCEPT
    A. It may manifest with constitutional symptoms and fever
    B. It may result in ulceration and significant scarring
    C. It may be confused on clinical grounds with lymphomatoid papulosis
    D. It is typically asymptomatic
    E. It responds to oral erythromycin.

For the following questions, ONE or MORE of the following completions correctly finishes the incomplete statement; choose

A. If only 1, 2, and 3 are correct
B. If only 1 and 3 are correct
C. If only 2 and 4 are correct
D. If only 4 is correct
E. If all are correct.

13. An individual with lichen planus has
    1. An increased likelihood of being HLA-A3 and HLA-DR1–positive
    2. A high likelihood of a family history of the disorder
    3. The possibility of having a clinical picture that could be confused with lupus erythematosus
    4. A typically chronic, unremitting course.

14. Pathologic findings in lichen planus include
    1. Parakeratosis
    2. Sawtooth-patterned acanthosis with hypergranulosis
    3. IgG staining of colloid bodies as a typical finding

4. Basement membrane abnormalities and clefting known as Max Joseph's spaces.

15. Drugs implicated in lichen planus–type eruptions include
    1. Antimalarials
    2. Gold
    3. Angiotensin-converting enzyme inhibitors
    4. Oral hypoglycemics

16. Typical features of lichen planus–like drug eruptions include
    1. Severe involvement of the oral mucosa
    2. Severe involvement of the scalp
    3. Clinical findings easily distinguished from lichen planus
    4. Marked follicular involvement with morphology of lichen planopilaris.

17. Lichen planus can
    1. Have a zosteriform presentation
    2. Manifest with a vesicular variant having similarities to bullous pemphigoid
    3. Occur with a desquamative gingivitis with clinical similarity to cicatricial pemphigoid
    4. Result in eventual hypopigmentation.

18. Erythema dyschromicum perstans is
    1. A form of pinta
    2. A condition described primarily in individuals of darker skin type
    3. Is usually seen in conjunction with a clear active border
    4. Has histopathologic changes similar to lichen planus and is occasionally called lichen planus pigmentosus.

19. The risk of malignant transformation in lichen planus is
    1. In oral lichen planus, 0.5% to 2.5%
    2. More prominent in erosive disease of the oral cavity
    3. Affected significantly by tobacco use and chronic superinfection
    4. Is not well documented in cutaneous lesions.

20. Lichen nitidus is similar to lichen planus in that
    1. Histopathology features a lichenoid infiltrate
    2. Mucosal involvement is a prominent feature
    3. It exhibits the Koebner phenomenon
    4. It is easily controlled with fluorinated topical steroids.

21. The differential diagnosis of lichen striatus includes
    1. Inflammatory linear verrucous epidermal nevus
    2. Zosteriform lichen planus
    3. Linear porokeratosis
    4. Verruca plana.

22. Which of the following are true of erythema multiforme?
    1. It may present as a chronic picture
    2. It has an association to HLA-DQ3 in recurrent disease
    3. It manifests with targetoid lesions called iris lesions of Bateman
    4. It is called erythema multiforme because lesions are polymorphic in the same patient.

23. The pathology in erythema multiforme shows
    1. Marked papillary edema
    2. Satellite keratinocyte necrosis
    3. Widespread keratinocyte necrosis
    4. Minimal dermal inflammatory infiltrate.

24. The following drugs have frequently been implicated in association with erythema multiforme-major and toxic epidermal necrolysis:
    1. Beta-blockers
    2. Trimethoprim-sulfamethoxazole
    3. Erythromycin
    4. Phenytoin.

25. Which of the following are true of the Stevens-Johnson syndrome?
    1. Lesions tend to be relatively asymptomatic
    2. The treatment of choice is high-dose systemic corticosteroids
    3. Leukopenia is a marker of poor prognosis
    4. Acute tubular necrosis of the kidney is a common complicating event.

26. In pityriasis lichenoides,
    1. There is some suggestion of an Epstein-Barr virus role
    2. There is evidence of clinical progression to lymphomatoid papulosis in some patients
    3. Scarring is never evident
    4. The acute form is usually self-limited.

27. The use of ultraviolet light in pityriasis lichenoides
    1. Is of no known benefit
    2. Is useful both with UVB and PUVA
    3. May cause the Koebner phenomenon if used aggressively
    4. Has a potential risk of increasing pigmentary changes.

Decide whether each choice in the following questions is TRUE or FALSE. Any combination of answers from all true to all false may occur.

Regarding lichen planus,

28. Hypertrophic lichen planus is a risk factor for malignant transformation.
29. Lichen planus may occur as a contact reaction to color film developer.
30. Lichen planus requires high-dose cyclosporin to attain remission.
31. Lichen planus can be treated with both systemic and topical retinoids.
32. Lichen planus may be indistinguishable from drug-induced lichen planus.
33. Lichen planus is associated with primary biliary cirrhosis only in individuals taking D-penicillamine.

Regarding erythema multiforme,

34. It is characterized in all patients by target lesions.
35. It can be triggered by ultraviolet (UV) exposure.
36. It can be easily distinguished from urticaria.
37. HSV-associated disease tends to be severe and extensive.
38. It accounts for approximately 1% of outpatient dermatology visits.
39. It is more common in elderly patients because of increased drug exposure.
40. It can be treated with intravenous acyclovir.

Regarding lupus erythematosus,

41. Which of the following statements regarding the relationship of discoid lupus erythematosus (DLE) to systemic lupus erythematosus (SLE) are true and which, false?
    A. The risk of conversion of DLE to SLE is higher if discoid lesions are confined to the head and neck
    B. A biopsy of *non-involved* skin from a patient with DLE reveals immunoglobulins and complement in a granular pattern at the dermal-epidermal junction
    C. There is a greater female preponderance of young patients with SLE compared with patients affected with DLE
    D. The presence of serologic abnormalities in patients with DLE usually indicates they are at risk of converting to SLE
    E. Excessive ultraviolet exposure is usually responsible for DLE patients converting to SLE.

42. Histopathologic findings of lupus lesions include
    A. Keratotic plugs in hair follicle openings
    B. Liquefactive degeneration of the epidermal basal layer
    C. Degenerative change of the superficial dermal collagen
    D. A patchy to dense lymphocytic infiltrate that may be centered around appendages
    E. Thinning of the basement membrane zone.

43. The following are morphologic types of DLE.
    A. Hyperkeratotic papular or nodular lesions
    B. Annular lesions with a flattened or atrophic center
    C. An acne rosacea–like picture of the face
    D. Reticulate telangiectasia
    E. Pernio, or chilblain-like, lesions of the hands and feet
    F. Annular lesions resembling erythema multiforme.

44. Oral antimalarial therapy for DLE
    A. Usually shows a response within 6 weeks with use of chloroquine sulphate 200 mg bid
    B. Should be monitored by visual field examination if eye symptoms develop
    C. Can bleach the scalp hair
    D. May be associated with myasthenia
    E. Is not associated with neuropathy or mental disturbances.

45. A 35-year-old woman presented with annular polycyclic lesions on the face and arms that had evolved a few weeks after a sunburn with only minimal ultraviolet exposure. History revealed a gradually diffuse thinning of the hair and pains in the joints over the past 6 months. Physical examination demonstrated a 1.5-cm ulcer of the left buccal mucosa and periungual telangiectasias. There was noticeable swelling of three of the metacarpophalangeal joints. This patient:

A. Fulfils the American College of Rheumatology (formerly ARA) criteria for SLE

B. Most likely has subacute lupus erythematosus

C. Is more likely to have a positive Ro antibody than a positive La antibody.

D. Is more likely to have disease activity if the Ro antibody titer is high

E. Has an increased likelihood of positive HLA-B8 and HLA-Dw3.

46. Pemphigus erythematosus (Senear-Usher syndrome) is associated with

    A. Circulating pemphigus-like antibodies

    B. Anti-DNA antibodies

    C. ENA (extractable nuclear antigen) antibodies

    D. Positive antinuclear antibodies (ANAs)

    E. Prior systemic therapy with penicillamine, propranolol, or captopril.

47. Treatment of a 35-year-old woman with severe lupus nephritis may include

    A. High-dose oral corticosteroids (e.g., 60 mg per day)

    B. Pulse steroids (e.g., 1 g methylprednisolone daily for 3 days)

    C. Cyclophosphamide orally, 1 to 2 mg/kg per day or pulse therapy

    D. Oral contraceptives

    E. Barrier birth control methods.

48. Lupus lesions can be experimentally induced by UVB and UVA in

    A. DLE

    B. SLE

    C. Subacute cutaneous LE.

49. Lupus profundus

    A. Is associated with a deep lymphocytic infiltrate of the skin

    B. Is a frequent complication of discoid lupus

    C. Is occasionally associated with discoid lupus on the surface of the skin

    D. Is not as common on the cheeks as the arms, legs, or back

    E. May respond to oral antimalarials.

50. The following skin manifestations qualify as ARA criteria for the diagnosis of SLE.

    A. Malar rash

    B. Discoid lesions

    C. Photosensitivity

    D. Previous history of oral ulcers

    E. Periungual telangiectasia.

51. Extracutaneous manifestations of SLE that qualify as ARA criteria include

    A. Arthritis with soft tissue swelling in hands and wrists with radiologic erosions

    B. Transient pleurisy

    C. Proteinuria with sediment of 300 mg per day

    D. Neuropsychiatric features (seizures, psychosis) in the absence of a known cause.

52. Lesions in bullous LE

    A. Manifest clinically as blisters on a relatively noninflamed base

    B. Are associated with subepidermal neutrophilic microabscesses

    C. Demonstrate positive linear deposits of IgG, IgA, IgM, and to a lesser extent, C3 at the dermal-epidermal junction

    D. May have circulatory antibodies that localize in the sublamina densa

    E. Respond to prednisone but not to dapsone.

53. Neonatal lupus erythematosus is associated with

    A. Annular or discoid lesions that are always present at birth

    B. Skin rash that improves in the first few weeks of life

    C. Heart block due to ribonucleoprotein antibodies

    D. Active or previous systemic lupus in the neonate's mother

    E. Antibodies that cross the placenta and disappear within the first few weeks of life.

54. The lupus anticoagulant syndrome

    A. Is associated with elevated partial thromboplastin time (PTT)

    B. Is present in about one seventh of patients with SLE

    C. Can be associated with fetal death

    D. Is associated with thrombocytosis

    E. In pregnant women can be treated with prednisone 40 to 80 mg daily and aspirin 75 mg daily, increasing neonatal survival.

For each of the following numbered items, choose the most likely associated lettered item. Each numbered item has ONLY ONE answer. Within each group, each lettered item may be the answer to one, more than one, or none of the numbered items.

55. Heart block in neonatal lupus
56. Thrombosis, recurrent abortion, and thrombocytopenia
57. Drug-induced lupus
58. High levels reflect disease activity in SLE
59. Mixed connective tissue disease
60. Found only in SLE.

A. Anti–double stranded DNA
B. Antinuclear histone antibodies
C. Anti-Ro antibody
D. Antiphospholipid antibody
E. Anti-RNP
F. Anti-Sm antibody
G. None of the above.

For each of the following questions, the set of lettered headings accompanies a list of numbered words or phrases. For each numbered word or phrase choose

A. If the item is associated with A only.
B. If the item is associated with B only.
C. If the item is associated with both A and B.
D. If the item is associated with neither A nor B.

For each of the following characteristics, choose whether it describes childhood dermatomyositis, adult dermatomyositis, both, or neither.

61. Cutaneous calcinosis is common
62. Urinary 24-hour creatine is the best index of disease activity
63. High incidence of associated malignancy
64. Jo-1 antibody found with overlap syndromes
65. Increased incidence of HLA-B8 in whites.

A. Childhood dermatomyositis
B. Adult dermatomyositis
C. Both
D. Neither.

Decide whether EACH of the following questions is TRUE or FALSE. Any combination of answers from all true to all false may occur.

Skin eruptions characteristically associated with dermatomyositis include

66. Erythema between the knuckles of the hands
67. Discoid lesions with follicular plugging
68. Patches of telangiectatic erythema
69. Violaceous hue of eyelids.
70. Decide which of the following statements regarding dermatomyositis treatment are TRUE and which are FALSE:

   A. Prednisone in low doses of 10 to 20 mg per day is often useful to control myositis
   B. Combined therapy with azathioprine and prednisone is more likely to improve myositis in dermatomyositis than prednisone
   C. Oral cyclosporine has sometimes been successful when prednisone and an immunosuppressive combination have not controlled disease activity
   D. Systemic steroids are more likely to clear cutaneous erythematous patches of dermatomyositis than antimalarials
   E. Steroid and immunosuppressive dose reduction can be monitored by watching creatine phosphokinase and urinary creatinine decrease.

For each of the following questions, the set of lettered headings accompanies a list of numbered words or phrases. For each numbered word or phrase choose

A. If the item is associated with A only.
B. If the item is associated with B only.
C. If the item is associated with both A and B.
D. If the item is associated with neither A nor B.

For each of the following characteristics, choose whether it describes acute graft-versus-host disease, chronic graft-versus-host disease, both, or neither.

71. Toxic epidermal necrolysis
72. Cyclosporine reduces incidence
73. Lichen planus–like change
74. Coexisting liver disease
75. 50% 10-year mortality rate.

A. Acute graft-versus-host disease
B. Chronic graft-versus-host disease
C. Both
D. Neither.

For each numbered item, choose the most likely associated lettered item from those provided. Each numbered item has ONLY ONE answer. Within each group, each lettered item may be the answer to one, more than one, or none of the numbered items.

76. Schamberg's disease (progressive pigmented purpuric dermatosis)
77. Gravitational purpura
78. Pigmented purpuric dermatosis of Gougerot and Blum
79. Lichen aureus
80. Majocchi's disease.

A. Especially men with venous disease
B. Predominantly in females
C. Frequent in young adults of either sex at any site
D. Cayenne pepper spots on the legs of males
E. Solitary lesion resembling a bruise
F. Lichenoid papules with purpuric areas.

ANSWERS

1. D Flat-topped violaceous papules with white surface lines known as Wickham's striae are characteristic of lichen planus. Lesions exhibit the Koebner phenomenon, and have a flexural predilection. Oral involvement is common in 15% to 35% of cases being the sole manifestation and 65% of individuals presenting with cutaneous lesions having concomitant oral involvement. The highest incidence is on the buccal mucosa with a lacy reticulate white pattern, although the tongue, oropharynx, and rest of the gastrointestinal tract may be involved. A desquamative gingivitis can be seen. Other variants of morphology on oral mucosa include plaque, atrophic, papular, erosive, and bullous lesions.
Genital mucosal involvement is seen, 25% of male patients usually presenting with lesions on the glans penis, although the glabrous skin is sometimes involved. The annular variant is commonly seen on the glans penis. Vulvovaginal involvement, occasionally erosive and desquamative, is also seen with frequently associated symptoms of dyspareunia, pruritus, and burning.
Lichen planopilaris, also known as Graham Little syndrome, consists of follicular involvement more prominent on hair-bearing skin. This can eventuate in a cicatricial alopecia (Chapter 20).

2. E There is some association of autoimmune hepatic disease in patients with lichen planus. It is thought that the incidence of chronic active hepatitis varies from 9.5% to 13.5% and that there may also be an association of primary biliary cirrhosis with lichen planus. Various investigators have noted in addition that abnormal glucose tolerance is more common in individuals with lichen planus. There is no underlying infectious cause.

3. A Lichen planus was originally described by Wilson in 1869. This clinical cutaneous entity is characterized by a typically pruritic papulosquamous eruption, symmetrically distributed with a predilection to the flexural areas. Wickham's striae are thought to be areas of focal hypergranulosis and accentuated hyperkeratosis by some. There is no hypertrophic variant with predominant involvement of the scalp (Chapter 20).

PATTERN VARIATION IN LICHEN PLANUS	
Variation in Configuration	**Variation in Morphology**
Linear or zosteriform	Hypertrophic
Annular, often on glans penis	Follicular
	Bullous lichen planus
Variation of Location	Pemphigoides
Oral/GI mucosa	Erosive
Genitals	Atrophic
Nails	Actinicus
Scalp	Erythematosus
	Exfoliative
	Guttate
	LE/LP overlap

4. C Oral involvement of lichen planus may occasionally progress to squamous cell carcinoma, but erosive involvement preferentially predisposes to malignant degeneration. Oral involvement may be the sole manifestation in 15% to 35% of lichen planus patients (Chapter 20).

5. C Nail involvement can be seen in 10% of patients. Classic findings are longitudinal grooving and ridging with thinning of the distal nail plate and friability. There may be pterygium formation or atrophy, leading to anonychia. These changes are often permanent. Twenty-nail dystrophy seen as a childhood-acquired syndrome may be a forme-fruste of nail involvement of lichen planus. Hyperkeratosis and onycholysis is not characteristically seen (Chapter 20).

6. A Lichen striatus is a childhood-acquired linear dermatosis featuring a generally asymptomatic erythematous linear papular eruption following Blaschko's lines. The configurations are linear on the extremities, V-shaped over the spine, and S-shaped on the lateral trunk. Lichen striatus is more common in children with atopic dermatitis and appears to be self-limited, having a mean duration of 9.5 months. Hypopigmentation, known as lichen striatus alba, is a sequela in 50% of cases. There is no association with psoriasis, and it is not typically pruritic (Chapter 21).

7. D Keratosis lichenoides chronica, also known as Nekam's disease, consists of keratotic papules and plaques, often in linear or reticulate distribution on the extremities. There may be oral and acral involvement and a seborrheic dermatitis–like eruption involving the head and neck. Histopathologic features sometimes resemble those of hypertrophic lichen planus, and it has been proposed to be an unusual variant of that condition. Also unusual is the high degree of resistance to therapeutic modalities. Levamisole and PUVA have been reported to have some success (Chapter 20).

8. D; **9.** C Erythema multiforme (EM) minor, defined originally by Hebra in 1866, is a relatively common disorder, accounting for approximately 1% of outpatient dermatology consultations. It is uncommon in children under the age of 3 and in the elderly. Peak incidence is in the second to third decade, and there is a slight dominance in males. Seasonal epidemics and recurrences are common; this can be accounted for by the seasonal and/or epidemic nature of some of the more common triggers such as HSV, other infections, and UV irradiation. It may even be that triggers such as other viral infections, menstruation, and UVL may actually have a common pathway of subclinical HSV activation.

Clinically, EM minor has an abrupt onset of lesions, usually with acral predilection, often symmetrical. In a given patient, lesions are usually monomorphous, although the clinical picture is polymorphic. Clinical lesions may be maculopapulourticarial to vesicular, the classic iris lesion of Bateman being within the spectrum. Mucosal lesions are mild and are limited to oral mucosae. However, there is a lag period of approximately 2 weeks between the herpes simplex virus (HSV) outbreak and the onset of EM minor, so one would not expect to see active herpetic lesions.

Pathologic correlation ranges from a "dermal" type with papillary edema and scant epidermal necrosis to a mixed type and an "epidermal type," showing minimal inflammatory changes and many necrotic keratinocytes. Erythema multiforme is actually a single pathologic process, and the epidermis is always affected somewhere in the lesion (Chapter 22).

10. C Erythema multiforme (EM) major, also known as Stevens-Johnson syndrome, has an estimated incidence of 0.8 per million per year. Although mycoplasmal infections (Eaton agent of *Mycoplasma pneumoniae*) are documented as a precipitating cause, there is little good evidence to support other infectious causes. EM major precipitated by HSV is reported but unusual. Drug exposures to antibiotics, anti-inflammatories, and anticonvulsants are more commonly implicated. Extensive drug associations can be found in many large texts; however, sulfonamides and phenytoin are most frequent.

Clinically, a flu-like prodromal illness is followed by an acute onset of worsening constitutional symptoms and cutaneous and visceral involvement. Lesions tend to be asymptomatic, similar to those of EM-minor; however, they typically are larger, tending to be vesicular, hemorrhagic, and necrotic, and involving a variable body surface area. There is involvement of at least two mucosal surfaces: oral, ocular, or anogenital. Late complications include mucosal scarring and stricture; the ocular scarring occasionally leads to tragic blindness. There may be acute systemic complications of GI bleeding, pneumonia, and acute tubular necrosis, although these are rare as opposed to TEN in which internal organ involvement is not infrequent. In the situation of EM major, there is controversy with respect to the role, if any, of systemic steroids. No controlled clinical study has shown that systemic corticosteroids are of benefit in EM (Chapter 22).

11. C; **12.** D Pityriasis lichenoides may manifest as an acute dermatosis, pityriasis lichenoides et varioliformis acuta (PLEVA), or it may follow a chronic course, pityriasis lichenoides chronica (PLC). It is a dermatosis of unknown etiology that however is suspected to be a hypersensitivity reaction to an infectious antigen. The predominance in immunopathologic studies of T cytotoxic-suppressor lymphocytes supports the role of cell-mediated immunity in vessel damage and keratinocyte destruction. Although one study has shown clonal rearrangement of the T cell receptor β-chain gene, most authors do not consider it to be a lymphoproliferative disorder.

Clinically, PLC is the chronic and more common variety presenting with multiple small lichenoid papules typically sparing face, palms, and soles. The scale is mica-like and adherent, and lesions may be purpuric in appearance. Resolution often occurs with hyperpigmentation, although ulceration and true scarring are rare compared with PLEVA. The evolution of new lesions gives the eruption a polymorphous appearance.

PLEVA is characterized by sudden onset of a generalized eruption, consisting of multiple papulovesicular lesions, often associated with constitutional symptomatology of fever, headache, malaise, and arthralgia. Lesions are purpuric and eventuate to necrotic and crusted centers. Often, they have a painful burning or itching symptomatology. Truncal and flexural predominance is typical although other areas, including the mucosa, may be involved. Natural history is that of resolution over weeks to a few months, although PLEVA may evolve to a chronic PLC. Healing may result in a varioliform scar. Treatment with ultraviolet light, erythromycin, or tetracycline in doses of 1 to 2 g per day is often useful (Chapter 23).

13. B Study of HLA class II antigens in lichen planus patients suggests an association with DR-1 and A3. In addition to sporadic lichen planus, there is a rare familial variant with earlier age of onset, increased severity and chronicity.

Lichen planus/lupus erythematosus overlap syndrome often has a protracted clinical course, lesions having clinical and pathologic similarities of morphology. Immunologic markers such as ANA may be only low titer-positive, patients may however complain of some symptoms suggestive of systemic involvement with lupus erythematosus. Most patients with lichen planus improve with time (Chapter 20).

14. C Light microscopy of lichen planus reveals hyperkeratosis, sawtooth pattern, irregular acanthosis, and focal hypergranulosis. Parakeratosis, which is a feature of psoriasis, is not seen. Dyskeratotic basal keratinocytes result in Civatte colloid bodies. Direct immunofluorescence reveals IgM and occasionally other immunoglobulins staining the colloid bodies in 87% of cases. There is a band-like, lichenoid, lymphocytic infiltrate at the dermal-epidermal junction. Areas of clefting known as Max Joseph's spaces can be seen; in the extreme situation they can lead to vesicular lesions (Chapter 20).

15. E; **16.** C Eruptions resembling lichen planus can be seen with a number of drugs and industrial exposures. Oral involvement is more unusual with drug-induced disease. The most common drug to cause oral lichen planus–like reactions is gold. Follicular involvement is often prominent, with resulting alopecia (Chapter 20).

AGENTS CAUSING LICHEN PLANUS–LIKE ERUPTIONS	
ACE inhibitors	Captopril, enalapril
Antiarrhythmics	Quinidine
Antiarthritics	Gold
Antibiotics	Streptomycin, tetracycline
Antimalarials	Chloroquine (quinacrine)
Antipsychotics	Phenothiazines
Chelators	Penicillamine
Diuretics	Hydrochlorothiazide
Oral hypoglycemics	Chlorpropamide
Others	Topical contact with color film developer

17. E *Lichen planus* variants include a zosteriform presentation and desquamative gingivitis.

Lichen planus pemphigoides is a clinical variant believed to be an overlap of bullous pemphigoid and lichen planus. Bullae are seen on lesional and nonlesional skin, with histopathologic findings of lichen planus. Immunofluorescence reveals linear basement membrane deposits of IgG and C3. It is thought the antigen may, however, be different from that found in bullous pemphigoid. This is different from vesiculobullous lichen planus, which reveals clinical bullae and pathologic Max Joseph's clefting, a pathologic finding seen in 17% of cases of lichen planus. Lichen planus causes dermal-epidermal junction disruption that can lead to postinflammatory hyperpigmentation or hypopigmentation (Chapter 20).

18. C Erythema dyschromicum perstans is a rare disorder also known as ashy dermatosis or lichen planus pigmentosis. Primarily described in patients from South America or India, this may be a variant of atrophic or actinic lichen planus seen predominantly in dark-skinned individuals. Clinical presentation is that of a bluish-gray macular pigmentation, often with an antecedent erythematous (not clear), raised, active border. Early pathology is similar to lichen planus. Infiltrating lymphocytes are OKT4 and OKT8, that is, helper-inducer and suppressor-cytotoxic–positive, as seen in lichen planus. Pathology of the late nonactive dusky areas shows only vacuolar alteration or pigmentary incontinence. It is not a form of pinta (Chapter 20).

19. A Malignant degeneration is most commonly seen with oral lichen planus, particularly erosive disease. The estimated risk of developing an oral squamous cell carcinoma in a patient with oral lichen planus is 0.5% to 2.5%. Hypertrophic cutaneous lesions also have some propensity to malignant transformation (Chapter 20).

20. B Lichen nitidus, translated literally as shiny papules, is a chronic eruption of small, well-defined, hypopigmented to fleshtone papules with a predilection for the penis, arms, and abdomen. The Koebner phenomenon is exhibited and has been seen to coexist with lichen planus in the same patient. However, it is generally not pruritic, and mucosal involvement is unusual. Histopathologic changes, although lichenoid, are predominantly granulomatous with an extension of rete ridges beneath the infiltrate in a ball-and-claw pattern. There is no evidence of immunoglobulin staining. Lichen nitidus is fairly resistant to therapy but usually is self-limited to 12 to 24 months. The use of potent topical steroids and PUVA is of limited success (Chapter 20).

21. E; **22.** A EM may manifest with acute or chronic forms. Target lesions are the most characteristic lesion of EM, but papules are more common. In a given patient lesions are usually monomorphous, although the clinical picture is polymorphous (Chapter 22).

23. E Pathologic correlation ranges from a dermal type with papillary edema and minimal to no epidermal necrosis to a mixed type and to a strict epidermal type, showing less to little inflammatory change and predominantly eosinophilic keratinocyte necrosis. The epidermal type is seen clinically as target lesions, erythema multiforme major, or even a TEN-type (Chapter 22).

24. C; **25.** B See answer to question 10 (Chapter 22).

26. D; **27.** C Pityriasis lichenoides may yet prove to have a viral association but there is no evidence of Epstein-Barr virus infection. Lymphomatoid papulosis may be confused clinically with pityriasis lichenoides, but it can be distinguished pathologically. Pityriasis lichenoides does not progress to lymphomatoid papulosis.

PLEVA is generally self-limited; however, it may lead to significant varioliform scarring. Response has been favorable to oral antibiotics such as erythromycin and tetracycline. Sulfones and methotrexate have been used in resistant cases. Both UVB and PUVA are effective in PLC; however, light treatment may increase the risk of postinflammatory pigmentation. PLC tends to have a chronic recurrent cyclic course (Chapter 23).

28. (T); **29.** (T); **30.** (F); **31.** (T); **32.** (T); **33.** (F) The treatment of lichen planus can be difficult (Chapter 20).

34. (F); **35.** (T); **36.** (F); **37.** (F); **38.** (T); **39.** (F); **40.** (F) EM is most commonly seen as urticarial papules, although target lesions are the most characteristic. Erythematous conditions such as urticarial vasculitis, chronic urticaria, and erythema multiforme may be indistinguishable clinically. Target lesions are not seen in all patients. EM may be triggered by viral infections, menstruation, and ultraviolet light. All these triggers may have a common pathway of subclinical herpes simplex virus (HSV) activation. HSV-associated EM does not tend to be severe or extensive. EM minor is a relatively common disorder, accounting for approximately

TOPICAL MODALITIES	SYSTEMIC MODALITIES
Potent topical steroids +/− occlusion Topical retinoids—Tretinoin 0.1% gel Oral-dental hygiene Oral-topical cyclosporin 100 mg/mL tid (swish and spit)	Short-term oral corticosteroids PUVA Griseofulvin Retinoids—etretinate or acetretin Cyclosporin up to 5 mg/kg/day (low-dose)

1% of patient dermatology consultations. It is uncommon under the age of 3 and in the elderly. EM usually follows a herpes simplex virus outbreak, and by the time the eruption appears, the herpes simplex virus is no longer replicating. Intravenous acyclovir works only on replicating herpes virus and therefore is not successful in treatment at this stage (Chapter 22).

41. A. (F); B. (F); C. (T); D. (F); E. (F) DLE patients convert to systemic lupus in 1.3% to 6.5% of cases. Individuals with DLE limited to head and neck are much less likely to convert to systemic lupus compared with patients with disseminated discoid lupus. Light exposure does not appear to be a risk factor in conversion. Biopsy of involved skin in DLE and SLE shows deposits of immunoglobulins and complement at the dermal-epidermal junction, but in discoid lupus patients, immunoreactants are present only in involved skin. Serologic abnormalities are seen in 20% to 50% of patients with DLE. Systemic lupus is more common in females. A female 8:1 predominance in the childbearing years is noted and is thought to be partly caused by increases in estrogen levels. The onset of discoid lupus is often later in life (Chapter 24).

42. A. (T); B. (T); C. (T); D. (T); E. (F) Histopathology of discoid lupus erythematosus characteristically demonstrates keratotic plugs in the hair follicles and liquefactive degeneration of the basal epidermal layer. The dermis shows a variable lymphocytic infiltrate, often centered around appendages. Degenerative changes of the dermal collagen is noted, and the basement membrane zone is thickened (Chapter 24).

43. A. (T); B. (T); C. (T); D. (T); E. (T); F. (T) Discoid lupus lesions can resemble thick papular or nodular lesions, annular lesions either with atrophic centers or resembling erythema multiforme, or telangiectatic lesions with a reticulate or acne rosacea–like morphology. These lesions may be associated with SLE, DLE, or SCLE (Chapter 24).

44. A. (T); B. (F); C. (T); D. (T); E. (F) Antimalarial therapy is often useful for DLE in cases when topical and intralesional steroids have been unsuccessful. Eye examinations *must* be ordered prior to therapy and then repeated every 4 to 6 months. Loss of the central red scotoma is usually a contraindication to antimalarials. Antimalarial deposits in the retina are reversible with early detection. Visual field examination (Ambler grid initially and every 4 to 6 months) detects damaging deposits with loss of the central red scotoma. A small percentage of patients with idiopathic loss of the central red scotoma and women who may become pregnant should not be given antimalarials. Baseline blood work should screen for significant liver and kidney disease as well as glucose-6-phosphate dehydrogenase (G6PD) deficiency. Antimalarials may precipitate porphyrias and aggregate psoriasis in susceptible individuals. Periodic blood monitoring is recommended. The usual dose of chloroquine is 250 mg (od/bid) or hydroxychloroquine 200 mg (od/bid). Response usually takes 4 to 6 weeks; nausea, diarrhea, and abdominal pain are common side effects, and headache, itchy skin eruptions, and blurred vision, rare.

Antimalarials can bleach scalp hair and may rarely be associated with myasthenia, neuropathy, or mental illness. They can also cause cutaneous hyperpigmentation, lichenoid eruptions, and a generalized exfoliative dermatitis (Chapter 24).

45. A. (F); B. (T); C. (T); D. (F); E. (T) The patient in this example has three ARA criteria for SLE:

> Photosensitivity
> Oral ulceration observed by a physician
> Arthritis of more than two joints

Annular lesions, diffuse thinning of the hair, and periungual telangiectasia are not ARA criteria for SLE because of their occurrence in many disorders other than lupus.

Subacute cutaneous lupus erythematosus often manifests with photosensitivity, annular or psoriasiform lesions, and arthritis. They are more likely to have Ro antibodies than La antibodies. The titer of the Ro antibody does not relate to disease activity. It often persists despite treatment. There is a high concordance of anti-Ro antibodies and the HLA-8B and HLA-DR3 phenotypes (Chapter 24).

46. A. (T); B. (F); C. (F); D. (T); E. (T) Pemphigus erythematosus (Senear-Usher syndrome) consists of erythematous or scaly eruptions with secondary hyperkeratotic crusting of the face and upper trunk. Patients have circulating pemphigus antibodies and a positive ANA. ENA and anti-DNA antibodies are absent. Drugs associated with a pemphigus erythematosus–like syndrome include penicillamine, propranolol, and captopril. Pemphigus erythematosus is usually treated with systemic steroids in initial doses that are usually lower than the 80 to 120 mg (often 40–60 mg per day) recommended for pemphigus vulgaris (Chapters 24 and 74).

47. A. (T); B. (T); C. (T); D. (F); E. (T) Lupus nephritis can be a life-threatening complication of SLE. High-dose oral corticosteroids along with pulse steroids may be necessary for control, but immunosuppressive therapy may also be necessary. Oral contraceptives can aggravate lupus and are contraindicated, whereas barrier types of birth control are preferred (Chapter 24).

48. A. (T); B. (T); C. (T) Both UVA and UVB can trigger DLE, SLE, and subacute cutaneous LE (Chapter 24).

49. A. (T); B. (F); C. (T); D. (F); E. (T) Lupus profundus appears clinically as nodules that heal with depressed scars. Lesions are most common on the cheeks but can occur elsewhere and are only occasionally associated with discoid lesions on the surface. Pathologically, a deep dermal and subcutaneous infiltrate is noted. Although intralesional steroids can be used in early lesions, oral antimalarials with or without oral steroids are often necessary to control nodular lesions and prevent atrophic, disfiguring residual lesions (Chapter 24).

50. A. (F); B. (T); C. (F); D. (F); E. (F); **51.** A. (F); B. (T); C. (F); D. (T) The ARA published criteria for the diagnosis of lupus in 1982. These criteria serve as a guide to information that is useful on history and physical examination. The following are criteria for the classification of systemic lupus erythematosus (SLE).*

1. Malar rash
2. Discoid lupus erythematosus lesions
3. Photosensitivity (by history or observation)
4. Oral ulcers, usually painless, observed by physician
5. Arthritis—nonerosive, involving two or more joints
6. Serositis—pleuritis or pericarditis
7. Renal disorder—proteinuria (>500 mg/day) or cellular casts
8. Central nervous system disorder—seizures or psychosis (absence of known cause)
9. Hematologic disorder—hemolytic anemia, leukopenia (<4000/mm^3); or thrombocytopenia (<100,000/mm^3)
10. Immunologic disorder—positive LE prep, abnormal titers of antinative (n) DNA, and anti-Sm, false-positive VDRL
11. Antinuclear antibody

If four or more criteria are present serially or simultaneously during any period of observation, the patient is considered to have SLE (Chapter 24).

52. A. (T); B. (T); C. (F); D. (T); E. (F) Bullous LE is an uncommon type of lupus that appears to have two subtypes. In the most common type, patients have no circulating antibasement membrane antibodies and respond to dapsone and sometimes to low-dose oral prednisone. In the second type, patients have circulating antibasement membrane antibodies directed against the epidermolysis bullosa acquisita (EBA) antigen (type 7 collagen) below the lamina densa. Patients with circulating antibodies may be more difficult to treat, sometimes requiring oral cyclosporine for control (Chapter 24).

53. A. (F); B. (F); C. (T); D. (T); E. (F) Neonatal LE is due to maternal anti-Ro antibodies that cross the placenta and are responsible for the heart block and skin rash. The rash and antibodies take 4 and 6 months to improve and disappear, respectively. Skin disease usually develops after birth, usually on first exposure to the sun, but heart block is present congenitally (Chapter 24).

54. A. (T); B. (F); C. (T); D. (T); E. (T) The lupus anticoagulant is seen in 25% to 50% of SLE patients but can be found in the antiphospholipid syndrome without the criteria for lupus. These patients suffer recurrent thromboses and livedo reticularis that can be associated with skin ulceration. The valvular heart vegetations (Libman-Sacks) may be associated with myocardial dysfunction. The PTT is elevated. Treating affected pregnant women with a combination of prednisone and aspirin reduces the fetal death rate (Chapter 24).

55. C; **56.** D; **57.** B; **58.** A; **59.** E; **60.** F The congenital heart block in neonatal LE is associated with Ro antibodies. The lupus anticoagulant is associated with thromboses, recurrent abortion, and thrombocytopenia. (See answers to Questions 53 and 54.)

Drug-induced lupus erythematosus (especially related to hydralazine) is associated with antihistone antibodies. They are also found in 30% to 70% of SLE patients. The anti-ribonucleoprotein (RNP) has a high frequency of association with Raynaud's disease and a low frequency of association with renal disease. Pulmonary disease, sclerodactyly, and esophageal dismotility may also be associated. The Smith antibody is found in only 20% of lupus patients but is specific for SLE (Chapter 24).

61. A; **62.** C; **63.** B; **64.** B; **65.** A Childhood dermatomyositis is associated with calcinosis (good prognosis), low incidence of malignancy, and vasculitis (poor prognosis). HLA-B8 is more common in affected whites.

The Jo-1 "antibody" is associated with adult dermatomyositis and an increase of pulmonary fibrosis. Adults also have an increase in HLA-B14.

Dermatomyositis is associated with a typical rash, muscle weakness, and increased creatine phosphokinase. However, serial estimates of urinary creatinine provide the best index of disease activity (Chapter 25).

66. (F); **67.** (F); **68.** (T); **69.** (T) The pathognomonic eruptions of dermatomyositis are Gottrons papules, which occur over bony prominences of the hands and elbows, and the violaceous heliotrope eruption on the eyelids. The erythema that occurs on the distal digits and spares the distal and proximal interphalangeal and metacarpophalangeal joints is more characteristic of SLE, whereas discoid lesions with follicular plugging

---

*Modified from Criteria for Classification of Systemic Lupus Erythematosus. Tan EM, Cohen AS, Fries JF, et al: Arthritis Rheum 25:1271–1277, 1982.

are typical of DLE. Patches of poikilodermatous telangiectatic erythema are characteristic of dermatomyositis. Other cutaneous findings include periungual telangiectasia, cuticular hypertrophy, and photosensitivity (Chapter 25).

70. A (F); B (T); C (T); D (F); E (T) Therapy for dermatomyositis often requires 60 to 120 mg of prednisone in the acute stage. Addition of azathioprine (1.5 to 3.0 mg/kg) may be necessary as an additional step in difficult cases. Cyclosporine 5 mg/kg/day has been added to prednisone and immunosuppressive drugs when combined therapy has still failed to induce remission. Oral antimalarials are often necessary to control the poikilodermal telangiectatic erythema that does not respond to oral steroids (Chapter 25).

71. A; **72.** A; **73.** B; **74.** C; **75.** B Graft-versus-host disease (GvHD) occurs when immunocompetent cells in the graft react to the immunocompetent host tissue. Acute graft-versus-host disease usually occurs 7 to 12 days post transplant but may occur up to 100 days later. A mild macular eruption to frank toxic epidermal necrolysis can be seen. Fever, hepatitis, and diarrhea may coexist. Chronic GvHD also involves the skin and liver. A lichen planus–like eruption (face, palms, soles) may be followed by scleroderma-like changes. Cyclosporine A reduces the incidence of acute but not chronic GvHD. Fifty per cent of chronic GvHD disease patients are dead after 10 years (the mortality rate is even higher if lichenoid eruption, liver disease, or thrombocytopenia persists) (Chapter 19).

76. D; **77.** A; **78.** F; **79.** E; **80.** C Pigmentary purpuras are local, nonpalpable purpuras of unknown etiology that are occasionally itchy. There is perivascular lymphocytic infiltrate around small vessels of the superficial dermis with surrounding hemorrhage in the absence of vasculitis (Chapter 26).

PIGMENTED PURPURAS			
Type	**Incidence**	**Location**	**Clinical Appearance**
Schamberg's disease (progressive pigmentary purpura)	Especially men	Legs (occasionally elsewhere or generalized)	Cayenne pepper patches with chronic lesions orange-brown color
Lichenoid purpura of Gougerot-Blum	Especially men Ages 40 to 60	Legs (occasionally elsewhere)	Lichenoid papules associated with localized Schamberg-type lesions
Lichen aureus (lichen purpuricus)	Younger individuals	Legs (occasionally elsewhere)	Solitary rust-yellow to purple patches
Majocchi's disease (purpura annularis telangiectoides)	Especially adolescents and young adults	Any site	1–3 cm; telangiectatic and purpuric plaques purple-yellow to brown ± cayenne pepper spots
Gravitational purpura (dermite ocre of favre)	Especially men with venous disease	Lower legs to dorsum of feet	Yellow-brown minute purpuric macules (sometimes perifollicular) may coalesce into larger lesions ± scale

The differential diagnosis of pigmentary purpura includes drug reactions (especially carbromal), food additive reactions, clothing dermatitis with purpura, and hyperglobulinemic purpura.

Bibliography

Alcorn-Segovia D, Deleze W, Oria CV, et al. Antiphospholipid antibodies and the antiphospholipid syndrome in systemic lupus erythematosus. Medicine (Baltimore) 1989; 68:353–365.

Asherson RA, Khamashta MA, Ordi-Ross J, et al. Primary antiphospholipid syndrome: Major clinical and serologic features. Medicine (Baltimore) 1989; 68:366–374.

Bielsa I, Herrero C, Ercilla G. Immunogenetic findings in cutaneous lupus erythematosus. J Am Acad Dermatol 1991; 25:251–257.

Boyd AS, Neldner KH. Lichen planus. J Am Acad Dermatol 1991; 25:593–619.

Fellner MJ. Lichen planus. Int J Derm 1980; 19:71–75.

Goltz RW. The graft-vs-host reaction. Arch Dermatol 1988; 124:1849–1850.

Howland WW, et al. Erythema multiforme: clinical, histopathologic, and immunologic study. J Am Acad Dermatol 1984; 10:438.

Huff JC. Erythema multiforme and latent herpes simplex infection. Semin Dermatol 1992; 11:207–210.

Lee LA, David KM. Cutaneous lupus erythematosus. Curr Probl Dermatol 1989; 44:93–151.

Lehmann P, Holzle E, Kind P, et al. Experimental reproduction of skin lesions in lupus erythematosus by UVA and UVB radiation.

McCarty GA. Autoantibodies in scleroderma and polymyositis: An update. Semin Dermatol 1991; 10:206–216.

Miyagawa S, et al. Erythema dyschromicum perstans. J Am Acad Dermatol 1989; 20:882–886.

Newton RC, Raimer SS. Pigmented purpuric eruptions. Dermatol Clin 1985; 3:165–169.

Sigurgeirsson B, et al. Lichen planus and malignancy. Arch Dermatol 1991; 127:1684–1688.

Toda K, Okamoto H, Horio T. Lichen striatus. Int J Med 1986; 25:584–585.

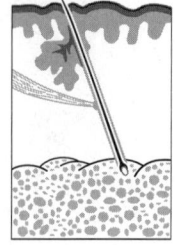

chapter 6

Psoriasiform Dermatitis, Lichen Simplex Chronicus, Prurigo, and Psychocutaneous Disorders

ROBERT JACKSON, and DIANE QUINTAL

Choose the ONE BEST answer to each of the following questions.

1. Epidermal keratinocytes undergo certain changes as they ascend from undifferentiated basal cells to fully differentiated cornified cells. All of the following statements are true EXCEPT

   A. Basal cells synthesize tonofilaments that later become aggregated into bundles of alpha keratins that contribute flexibility and elasticity to the cornified layer

   B. The amorphous protein that forms the matrix in which the tonofilaments are embedded is derived from keratinosomes

   C. This protein is degraded into filaggrin, which functions as an interfilamentous glue to aggregate and align keratin filaments within the cornified cells

   D. Keratinosomes appear near the top of the spinous zone

   E. The nuclei of keratinocytes and most of their cytoplasmic organelles disappear gradually as a result of the action of lysosomal enzymes.

2. All of the following statements are true of desmosomes EXCEPT

   A. Desmosomes are specialized intercellular contact zones of keratinocytes

   B. Desmosomes consist of intracytoplasmic tonofilaments connected to electron-dense plaques at the plasma membrane

   C. Desmosomes contain two groups of proteins: desmogleins and desmoplakins

   D. The intercellular attachments formed by desmosomes can be seen only by electron microscopy

   E. The intercellular attachments break and reform continuously as keratinocytes ascend and mature.

3. The mean turnover, or renewal, time of normal epidermis is estimated to be

    A. 36 hours
    B. 5 days
    C. 13 days
    D. 26 days
    E. 39 days.

Decide whether each of the following questions is TRUE or FALSE. Any combination of answers from all true to all false may occur.

4. Regarding the pathogenesis of psoriasis,

    A. Increased epidermal cell proliferation in psoriasis may be the result of increased recruitment of noncycling resting cells
    B. High levels of cyclic adenosine monophosphate (cAMP) within psoriatic epidermal cells could explain the accelerated cell division
    C. Both arachidonic acid and leukotriene B_4 are found in increased amounts within psoriatic epidermal cells. They may function partly by stimulating DNA synthesis
    D. Leukotrienes are chemotactic factors for polymorphonuclear leukocytes and may thus perpetuate the psoriatic lesions
    E. The dermal capillary loops of both involved and uninvolved skin of psoriatic patients are dilated and abnormally tortuous.

5. Regarding nail psoriasis,

    A. Toenails are more often affected than fingernails
    B. A thickened or onycholytic psoriatic nail may often contain *Candida* organisms
    C. Yellow discoloration and onycholysis, the "oil-drop sign," is the most common finding
    D. Splinter hemorrhages are a regular feature of nail psoriasis
    E. Classic psoriatic arthritis affecting the distal interphalangeal joints is usually associated with nail dystrophy.

6. Regarding the histopathologic features of psoriasis,

    A. Microabscesses of Munro and spongiform pustules of Kogoj are most diagnostic of psoriasis
    B. Microabscesses similar to those of psoriasis can also be seen in seborrheic dermatitis
    C. Increased mitoses are seen in multiple layers of the basal cells
    D. The granular layer is thickened because of the increased number of keratohyaline granules in the differentiating cells
    E. Increased tonofilament formation is seen on electron microscopy.

Choose the ONE BEST answer to each of the following questions.

7. The most common form of psoriatic arthritis is

    A. Distal interphalangeal arthritis
    B. Arthritis mutilans
    C. Spondylitis
    D. Arthritis indistinguishable from rheumatoid arthritis
    E. Asymmetric oligoarthritis.

8. All of the following may exacerbate psoriasis EXCEPT

    A. Chloroquine
    B. Hydrochlorothiazide
    C. Alcohol consumption
    D. Lithium
    E. Propranolol.

9. Diagnostic morphologic features of a psoriatic lesion include all of the following EXCEPT

    A. Surrounding clear peripheral zone
    B. Deep red color often referred to as "salmon pink."
    C. Well-defined borders
    D. Asymmetric distribution
    E. Silvery-white scaling.

For the following questions, ONE or MORE of the following completions correctly finishes the incomplete statement. Choose

A. If only 1, 2, and 3 are correct
B. If only 1 and 3 are correct
C. If only 2 and 4 are correct
D. If only 4 is correct
E. If all are correct.

10. Conditions that may cause diagnostic confusion with psoriasis are

    1. Lichen planus
    2. Drug eruptions

3. Congenital ichthyosiform erythroderma
4. Mycosis fungoides.

11. Generalized pustular psoriasis of von Zumbusch is associated with
    1. High fever, leukocytosis, and arthralgia
    2. Hypercalcemia
    3. Occasional involvement of tongue and buccal mucosa
    4. A poor prognosis when it occurs in young children.

12. Psoriatic spondylitis has been described in association with
    1. Aortic insufficiency
    2. HLA-B27
    3. Gastrointestinal amyloidosis
    4. Ocular inflammation.

In each of the following questions regarding the treatment of psoriasis, a set of lettered headings accompanies a list of numbered words or phrases. For each numbered word or phrase, choose

A. If the item is associated with A only
B. If the item is associated with B only
C. If the item is associated with both A and B
D. If the item is associated with neither A nor B.

13. For each statement below, choose whether it is associated with anthralin, crude coal tar, both, or neither.

   i. Suppresses epidermal synthesis of DNA   A. Anthralin
   ii. The product of the distillation of bituminous coal in the absence of oxygen   B. Crude coal tar
                                                     C. Both
                                                     D. Neither.
   iii. Discontinuation may be followed by a rebound phenomenon
   iv. Significantly increases the risk of developing skin cancer
   v. Can be combined with ultraviolet B light in the Ingram regimen for the treatment of stable plaque-type psoriasis.

14. Systemic drug therapy is occasionally necessary in the treatment of psoriasis. For each drug side effect, choose if it can be seen with retinoids, cyclosporine, both, or neither.

   i. Hyperlipidemia   A. Retinoids
   ii. Headaches   B. Cyclosporine
   iii. Renal dysfunction   C. Both
   iv. Liver function test abnormalities   D. Neither.
   v. Musculoskeletal pain.

15. For each drug side effect, choose if it can be seen with retinoids, methotrexate, both, or neither.

   i. Blepharoconjunctivitis   A. Retinoids
   ii. Bone marrow suppression   B. Methotrexate
   iii. Teratogenicity   C. Both
   iv. Malignancy   D. Neither.
   v. Alopecia.

16. For each of the types of psoriasis below, choose whether it responds best to etretinate, cyclosporine, both, or neither.

   i. von Zumbusch's generalized pustular psoriasis   A. Etretinate
                                                      B. Cyclosporine
   ii. Acrodermatitis continua of Hallopeau   C. Both
                                                      D. Neither.
   iii. Guttate psoriasis
   iv. Erythrodermic psoriasis
   v. Severe plaque-type psoriasis.

For the following questions, ONE or MORE of the following completions correctly finishes the incomplete statement. Choose

A. If only 1, 2, and 3 are correct
B. If only 1 and 3 are correct
C. If only 2 and 4 are correct
D. If only 4 is correct
E. If all are correct.

17. For a patient with von Zumbusch's generalized pustular psoriasis, the following therapeutic modality would be an appropriate consideration:
    1. Cyclosporine
    2. Etretinate
    3. Goeckerman's
    4. Methotrexate.

18. Which of the following groups of patients have an increased risk of developing hyperlipidemia during retinoid administration?
    1. Patients who smoke
    2. Patients who drink alcohol

3. Patients who are overweight
4. Patients who have evidence of diabetes mellitus.

19. When treating psoriatic patients with methotrexate, which of these factors increases the risk of liver toxicity?
    1. Previous use of hepatotoxic drug
    2. Diabetes mellitus
    3. A history of excessive alcohol intake
    4. A history of intravenous drug abuse.

Decide whether each of the following statements is TRUE or FALSE. Any combination of answers from all true to all false may occur.

20. Regarding the use of calcipotriol ointment in psoriasis treatment,
    A. Calcipotriol, a derivative of vitamin B_3, is indicated mainly for mild to moderate stable plaque psoriasis
    B. Calcipotriol does not affect immunologic and inflammatory mediators that may play a pathogenic role in psoriasis
    C. Calcipotriol may act directly on the keratinocyte to inhibit proliferation and promote differentiation
    D. The best results will be obtained after 2 to 4 weeks of therapy
    E. Safety of calcipotriol has not been established for children.

Choose the ONE BEST answer to each of the following questions.

21. Etretinate is absolutely contraindicated in which of the following conditions?
    A. Immunosuppression
    B. Diabetes mellitus
    C. Morbid obesity
    D. Pregnancy
    E. Hypertension.

22. Etretinate therapy is contraindicated in psoriatic patients who are at increased risk of developing
    A. Diabetes mellitus
    B. Pulmonary edema
    C. Cardiac arrhythmias
    D. Hyperlipidemia
    E. Urolithiasis.

23. All of the following should be recommended for patients with hyperlipidemia as a result of retinoid therapy EXCEPT
    A. Avoidance of excess dietary sugars
    B. Distribution of caloric intake over three meals
    C. Reduction of caloric intake if overweight
    D. Reduction of alcohol consumption
    E. Decreasing exercise activities.

24. After stopping etretinate, it is recommended that women avoid pregnancy for at least
    A. 3 months
    B. 6 months
    C. 9 months
    D. 1 year
    E. 2 years.

25. During treatment of plaque-type psoriasis with etretinate, the first change to be observed in about half the patients is
    A. Disappearance of superficial scale
    B. Reduction in size of plaques
    C. Increase in size of plaques
    D. Reduction in thickness of plaques
    E. Increase in thickness of plaques.

26. During etretinate therapy for psoriasis, nail growth rates
    A. Increase
    B. Decrease
    C. Stop
    D. At first increase, and then stop
    E. At first decrease, and then stop.

27. Methotrexate is contraindicated in the presence of the following situations EXCEPT
    A. Obesity
    B. Renal dysfunction
    C. Pregnancy
    D. Hepatitis
    E. Immunodeficiency.

28. According to recent guidelines, during therapy with methotrexate, a patient with normal liver func-

tion tests and no risk factors for hepatotoxicity should have a liver biopsy after a total cumulative dose of

A. 1.0 g
B. 1.5 g
C. 2.5 g
D. 5.0 g
E. 10.0 g.

29. These drugs may interact with methotrexate to increase its toxicity EXCEPT

A. Sulfonamides
B. Phenytoin
C. Salicylates
D. Beta-blockers
E. Retinoids.

30. When treating a male patient with methotrexate, current recommendations are to avoid conception

A. During therapy only
B. During therapy and 3 months after discontinuation
C. During therapy and 6 months after discontinuation
D. During therapy and 1 year after discontinuation
E. During therapy and 2 years after discontinuation.

31. The following drugs increase cyclosporine blood levels and can thus predispose to cyclosporine nephrotoxicity EXCEPT

A. Ranitidine
B. Macrolide antibiotics
C. Phenytoin
D. Calcium antagonists
E. Ketoconazole.

32. The following are common side effects of cyclosporine EXCEPT

A. Decreased glomerular filtration rate
B. Anemia
C. Hypertension
D. Gingival hyperplasia
E. Paresthesias and headaches.

33. In Reiter's disease all the following are true EXCEPT

A. There is a highly significant association with HLA-B27
B. The disease occurs predominantly in young men
C. In the urogenital form, mild urethritis usually occurs 4 to 20 days after sexual exposure
D. The arthritis resolves after 1 to 4 months
E. Recurrences after the acute episode can occur but are rare.

34. Multiple infective agents have been implicated in the provocation of Reiter's disease. In the urogenital form of the disease, the most common organism is

A. *Chlamydia trachomatis*
B. *Neisseria gonorrhoeae*
C. *Ureaplasma urealyticum*
D. *Gardnerella vaginalis*
E. *Treponema pallidum.*

35. All of the following statements about the cutaneous manifestations of Reiter's disease are true EXCEPT

A. Keratoderma blennorrhagicum tends to involve the palms more commonly than the soles
B. The keratoderma is usually self-limiting, lasting weeks or months
C. In circumcised men, the erosive lesions of the penis quickly become keratotic
D. Circinate erosions such as those seen on the glans penis can also be found on other mucosal surfaces, such as the vulva and the oral mucosa
E. The histology of the cutaneous lesions is psoriasiform.

Decide whether each of the following questions is TRUE or FALSE. Any combination of answers from all true to all false may occur.

36. The following are contraindications to the use of cyclosporine in psoriasis.

A. Patients with uncontrolled hypertension
B. Patients under treatment with ultraviolet B
C. Patients with malignancies

D. Patients with migraine headaches

E. Patients who abuse alcohol.

37. The following are clinical types of pityriasis rubra pilaris (PRP).

    A. Adult atypical
    B. Juvenile atypical
    C. Adult classic
    D. Juvenile circumscribed
    E. Juvenile classic.

For each numbered item, choose the most likely associated lettered item from those provided. Each lettered item has ONLY ONE answer. Within each group, each numbered item may be the answer to one, more than one, or none of the numbered items.

38. Match the best cutaneous finding for each disease.

    1. Pityriasis rubra pilaris
    2. Psoriasis
    3. Seborrheic dermatitis.

    A. Micaceous scale
    B. Keratoderma
    C. Located on face and scalp.

39. Match the best diagnostic feature for each of the following keratodermas:

    1. Pityriasis rubra pilaris
    2. Psoriasis
    3. Arsenic
    4. Tylotic eczema
    5. Vohwinkel's disease.

    A. Present since birth
    B. Orange hue
    C. Red salmon color
    D. Hypopigmented and hyperpigmented brown spots on torso
    E. Itching.

40. Match the systemic treatment of choice for each of the following severe skin diseases:

    1. Lichen planus
    2. Plaque psoriasis
    3. Pityriasis rubra pilaris
    4. Dermatitis herpetiformis
    5. Discoid lupus erythematosus.

    A. Isotretinoin
    B. Prednisone
    C. Dapsone
    D. Chloroquine
    E. Methotrexate.

Choose the ONE BEST answer for the following question.

41. Cutaneous findings in pityriasis rubra pilaris include

    A. Keratoderma
    B. Islands of normal skin
    C. Follicular keratoses on fingers
    D. Ectropion
    E. All of the above.

Decide whether each of the following questions is TRUE or FALSE. Any combination of answers from all true to all false may occur.

42. Regarding the histopathologic findings of PRP,

    A. Microabscesses are common
    B. Perifollicular inflammation is seen
    C. Acanthosis is a feature
    D. Typical features include psoriasiform epidermal hyperplasia with laminated hyperkeratosis and scattered parakeratotic nuclei
    E. It closely resembles psoriasis.

43. Regarding the classic adult type of PRP,

    A. Onset in upper portion of body
    B. Never disappears
    C. Has no nail changes
    D. Is the most common type
    E. Is triggered by the sun.

44. Follicular hyperkeratoses on the elbows and knees can be found in

    A. Keratosis pilaris
    B. Darier's disease
    C. Pityriasis rubra pilaris
    D. Psoriasis
    E. Discoid lupus erythematosus.

45. Regarding high-dose vitamin A treatment for PRP,

    A. Pityriasis rubra pilaris is a vitamin A deficiency
    B. Pityriasis rubra pilaris patients have low vitamin A levels
    C. Vitamin A is effective because of its pharmacologic action
    D. To avoid the toxicity of vitamin A, isotretinoin and etretinate have been used
    E. One million units of vitamin A a day is an average dose.

Decide whether each of the following questions is TRUE or FALSE. Any combination of answers from all true to all false may occur.

46. Concerning the treatment of erythroderma,
    A. Systemic steroids are often used
    B. Topical steroids are of little value
    C. Topical antibiotics are often used
    D. Systemic antibiotics are of little value
    E. If known, treat the underlying cause.

47. Erythroderma in newborns and children differs from erythroderma in adults for which of the following reasons
    A. It comes on more quickly
    B. It can be due to candidiasis or staphylococcal disease
    C. It can be congenital
    D. It is easier to treat
    E. It does not usually accompany dermatopathic lymphadenitis.

48. Erythroderma has the following characteristics:
    A. The skin is lichenified
    B. The palms are always involved
    C. The skin may be scaly
    D. It is persistent
    E. Only the upper half of the body may be involved.

49. In dermatopathic lymphadenitis, the following are found on histologic examination:
    A. Large pale areas composed of reticular cells
    B. Destruction of normal lymph node architecture
    C. Presence of melanin
    D. Presence of lipid material
    E. Presence of Sternberg-Reed cells.

50. Dermatopathic lymphadenitis has the following clinical characteristics:
    A. Major involvement of the lymph nodes of the inguinal, axillary, and cervical areas
    B. Involvement of lymph nodes throughout the body
    C. Disappears over a number of months or years if the erythroderma disappears
    D. The lymph nodes are tender.

Choose the ONE BEST answer to each of the following questions.

51. All of the following are considered relatively common causes of erythroderma EXCEPT
    A. Atopic dermatitis
    B. Psoriasis
    C. Norwegian scabies
    D. Pemphigus foliaceus
    E. Drug reaction.

52. Systemic effects from erythroderma include all of the following EXCEPT
    A. Gynecomastia
    B. Disturbances in thermoregulation
    C. Impaired renal function
    D. Increased cardiac output
    E. Ankle edema.

53. The red man syndrome (l'homme rouge) has all of the following characteristics EXCEPT
    A. It is another name for exfoliative dermatitis of unknown etiology
    B. Keratoderma of the palms and soles is usually present
    C. The skin biopsy is diagnostic
    D. The disease lasts for years
    E. A few patients develop erythrodermatous mycosis fungoides.

For each numbered item in the following questions, choose the most likely associated lettered item. Each numbered item has only ONE answer. Within each group, each lettered item may be the answer to one, more than one, or none of the numbered items.

54. Match the most classic feature of pityriasis rubra pilaris with the five types listed.
    1. Classic adult   A. Most common type
    2. Atypical adult   B. Lasts 20 years
    3. Classic juvenile   C. Keratoses on elbows and knees
    4. Circumscribed juvenile D. Most often familial
    5. Atypical juvenile.   E. Onset by age of 2.

55. Match each of the following numbered items with the appropriate lettered item as the best clue to the cause of erythroderma.

1. Pityriasis rubra pilaris
2. Lichen planus
3. Atopic dermatitis
4. Eczematous dermatitis
5. Sezary's syndrome.

A. Results of skin biopsy
B. Stasis dermatitis
C. Family history of asthma and hay fever
D. Lesions on the buccal mucosae
E. Orangeish keratoderma
F. The enlarged lymph nodes can be seen.

56. Match the five following histologic findings with the most likely clinical condition.

    1. Corps ronds
    2. Cellules claires
    3. Nonspecific changes
    4. Abtropfung
    5. Spongiform micropustules in stratum malpighia.

    A. Erythroderma
    B. Compound nevi
    C. Psoriasis
    D. Darier's disease
    E. Epidermal melanocytes.

57. Match the eponyms with the appropriate disease.

    1. Darier's
    2. Wells'
    3. Bowen's
    4. Celsus'
    5. Vidal's.

    A. Lichen simplex chronicus
    B. Squamous cell carcinoma in situ
    C. Inflammatory ringworm of the scalp
    D. Eosinophilic cellulitis
    E. Keratosis follicularis.

Decide whether each of the following questions is TRUE or FALSE. Any combination of answers from all true to all false may occur.

58. The following conditions have occasionally been reported in patients with HIV infection:

    A. Hypopigmented and hyperpigmented spots on the torso ("raindrop pigmentation")
    B. Erythroderma
    C. Severe generalized cystic acne
    D. Pityriasis rubra pilaris
    E. Toxic epidermal necrolysis.

59. The following are characteristic of lichen simplex chronicus.

    1. Location on perianal skin and semimucosa
    2. A nonspecific histologic picture
    3. Hypopigmentation and atrophy centered about the pilosebaceous unit
    4. Koebnerization
    5. Isolated peripheral lichenified papules.

For the following questions, ONE or MORE of the following completions correctly finishes the incomplete statement. Choose

A. If only 1, 2, and 3 are correct
B. If only 1 and 3 are correct
C. If only 2 and 4 are correct
D. If only 4 is correct
E. If all are correct.

60. Lichen simplex chronicus is common in

    1. Patients with a history of hay fever and sensitivity to nickel
    2. Patients who are black
    3. Patients of Asian origin
    4. Patients who are white
    5. Patients with a history of extensive and long-standing eczema.

Choose the ONE BEST answer to each of the following questions.

61. Prurigo nodularis has the following histologic characteristics:

    A. Acanthosis
    B. May or may not show neural hyperplasia
    C. Mild upper dermal perivascular chronic inflammation
    D. Vascular hypoplasia.

62. All of the following statements are true of prurigo EXCEPT

    A. The lesions are itchy
    B. The lesions are grouped
    C. The lesions are traumatized
    D. Hypopigmentation and brown hyperpigmentation are commonly present
    E. The "tent" sign is negative.

63. All of the following statements are true of postherpetic neuralgia EXCEPT

    A. Amitriptyline can be used for control of pain
    B. Capsaicin is very frequently effective

C. The older the patient, the more likely the neuralgia

D. If the fifth cranial nerve root is involved, neuralgia is more common

E. The neuralgia tends to decrease with the passage of time.

Decide whether EACH of the following questions is TRUE or FALSE. Any combination of answers from all true to all false may occur.

64. Regarding the treatment of prurigo nodularis,
    A. Excising individual lesions is a reasonable treatment
    B. Systemic thalidomide may be helpful in severe cases
    C. Systemic prednisone is very effective
    D. In many patients, nothing seems to help
    E. Permanent occlusion where practicable is a useful treatment.

65. Regarding notalgia paresthetica,
    A. The differential diagnosis includes amyloidosis, lichen simplex chronicus, fixed drug eruption, and leprosy
    B. There are definite neurologic findings
    C. It may be associated with pudendal neuralgia
    D. It is more common in males
    E. It usually occurs on the inferomedial border of either scapula.

For each numbered item in the following questions, choose the most likely associated lettered item. Each numbered item has ONLY ONE answer. Within each group, each lettered item may be the answer to one, more than one, or none of the numbered items.

66. For each of the diseases, choose the most appropriate match.
    1. Also known as the trigeminal trophic skin syndrome
    2. Heel cracks with scarring
    3. Causalgia
    4. Commonly occur on the shin
    5. Commonly occur on pressure points.

    A. Reflex sympathetic dystrophy
    B. Neurotrophic ulcer
    C. Neuroanesthetic ulcers
    D. Ischemic ulcers
    E. Livedo with ulceration on the soles.

67. For each of the diseases, choose the most strongly suggestive finding.
    1. Trichotillomania
    2. Trichostasis spinulosa
    3. Alopecia areata
    4. Monilethrix
    5. Trichorrhexis invaginata.

    A. Exclamation point hairs
    B. Beaded hairs
    C. Multiple hairs in one follicle
    D. "Ball-in-socket" abnormality
    E. Absence of eyelashes.

For each of the following questions, the set of lettered items is accompanied by a list of numbered words or phrases. For each numbered word or phrase, choose

A. If the item is associated with A only
B. If the item is associated with B only
C. If the item is associated with both A and B
D. If the item is associated with neither A nor B.

68. For each of the statements below, choose whether it is characteristic of an ulcer, erosion, both, or neither.
    1. After healing, residual brown hyperpigmentation or hypopigmentation frequently occurs
    2. Is only caused by trauma
    3. Extends into the dermis
    4. Almost never scars
    5. Is the lesion normally seen in the mouth with primary herpes simplex.

    A. Ulcer
    B. Erosion
    C. Both
    D. Neither.

69. For each of the statements below, choose whether it is characteristic of a neurotic excoriation, dermatitis artefacta, both, or neither.
    1. The lesions of each disease in one patient are similar
    2. There is often an accentuation of the follicular orifices in the hypopigmented scar

    A. Neurotic excoriation
    B. Dermatitis artefacta
    C. Both
    D. Neither.

3. The condition is related to acne excoriée des jeune filles
4. The patient admits to picking and scratching easily
5. Oral pimozide is helpful.

A. Atopic dermatitis
B. Dermatitis artefacta
C. Acne vulgaris
D. Psoriasis
E. Urticaria.

Choose the ONE BEST answer to each of the following questions.

70. All of the following statements are true of parasitophobia EXCEPT
    A. It affects women over 40
    B. There are no primary skin lesions
    C. The patients often have scabies
    D. The patients have had repeated treatments by insecticides
    E. The patient cannot understand why there is no walking dandruff in the bits and pieces of lint, scabs, and skin that are brought in.

For the following questions, one or more of the following completions correctly finishes the incomplete statement. Choose

A. If only 1, 2, and 3 are correct
B. If only 1 and 3 are correct
C. If only 2 and 4 are correct
D. If only 4 is correct
E. If all are correct.

71. Skin lesions in mentally defective patients commonly include
    1. Those due to biting
    2. Those due to licking
    3. Those due to rubbing
    4. Those due to pulling
    5. Those due to sucking.

72. One or more of the following numbered words or phrases correctly finishes this statement: Vulvodynia can be associated with
    1. Vulvar dermatoses
    2. Cyclic vulvitis
    3. Papillomatosis
    4. Vestibulitis.

73. According to current beliefs, which of the following skin diseases are mainly or totally due to psychogenic abnormalities:

Decide whether EACH choice in the following questions is TRUE or FALSE. Any combination of answers from all true to all false may occur.

74. Regarding occupational hazards,
    A. Callosities occur on the medial aspect of the palm in carillonneurs
    B. Foreign body granulomata can occur in the finger web spaces of barbers
    C. Most cases of "white finger" are seen in chain saw operators
    D. "Hacksaw teeth" come from holding tacks in the teeth
    E. Lichenification and folliculitis can be seen under the chin of violinists.

75. Regarding vulvodynia,
    A. Itching is the predominant complaint
    B. Sexual inactivity is a direct result of symptoms
    C. It often follows an episode of acute inflammatory vulvitis
    D. The pain keeps the patient awake at night
    E. The pain disappears with topical application of the appropriate strength of topical corticosteroids.

76. Regarding glossodynia,
    A. The tongue is red and swollen
    B. It is common in women
    C. It is associated with a fissured or scrotal tongue
    D. It is common in the elderly
    E. It is associated with geographic tongue
    F. Orolingual paresthesias include glossodynia.

77. Regarding skin eruptions from psychotropic drugs,
    1. Pigmentation of the lid closure line is caused by chlorpromazine
    2. Lithium can cause a psoriatic keratoderma
    3. Sebum production increases when barbiturates are used

4. Cross-sensitivities frequently occur with carbamazepine, phenytoin, and the barbiturates

5. Phenytoin is a frequent cause of major erythema multiforme.

ANSWERS

1. B The amorphous protein that forms the matrix in which the tonofilaments are embedded is derived from keratohyaline granules. These granules appear first in the upper part of the spinous zone and become more prominent in the granular zone. They are the source of the protein profilaggrin that is degraded to filaggrin. On the other hand, keratinosomes, also known as lamellar bodies or Odland bodies, fuse with the plasma membrane and discharge their contents into the intercellular space. The contents consist of free sterol, polar lipids, and hydrolytic enzymes that contribute to the formation of a waterproof barrier. After their contents have been released, keratinosomes become organized into lamellae that constitute the structural basis for the barrier to epidermal permeability (Chapter 2).

2. D With a conventional microscope, the intercellular attachments, or bridges, can be seen between keratinocytes as spine-like processes (Chapter 2).

3. E The mean turnover of normal epidermis has been estimated to be 39 days, divided as follows: 13 days for the proliferative compartment (compared with 36 hours for psoriatic epidermis), 12 days for the differentiated compartment, and 14 days for the cornified layer. These times may vary according to cutaneous sites (Chapters 3 and 27).

4. A (T); B (F); C (T); D (T); E (T) It has been postulated that low intraepidermal levels of cAMP could lead to accelerated cell division, incomplete differentiation, and glycogen accumulation in the epidermis of psoriatic lesions (Chapters 3 and 27).

5. A (F); B (T); C (F); D (T); E (T) Fingernails show psoriatic changes more often than toenails. Pitting of the nail plate is the most common finding and is the result of focal involvement of that part of the nail matrix that gives rise to the superficial nail plate. A thick and onycholytic nail may contain *Candida albicans* or *Pseudomonas* organisms. However, the psoriatic nail seems peculiarly resistant to dermatophytes (Chapter 27).

6. A (T); B (T); C (T); D (F); E (F) Epidermal microabscesses composed of focal accumulations of neutrophils, microabscesses of Munro when they occur in the stratum corneum, and spongiform pustules of Kogoj when they are seen below it, are highly supportive of a diagnosis of psoriasis. They can nevertheless be seen in other conditions, such as seborrheic dermatitis, although serum is often present in the latter. In normal skin, mitoses are usually limited to a single layer of basal cells. In psoriasis, there are increased mitoses in multiple layers of basal cells. As a consequence of epidermal proliferation, the granular layer is either thin or absent, and on electron microscopy, tonofilament formation is seen to be reduced (Chapter 27).

7. E Sixty-three to 70% of patients with psoriatic arthritis have an asymmetric oligoarthritis affecting chiefly the hands and feet. Only 3% to 5% have distal interphalangeal arthritis (the "classic psoriatic arthritis"), 3% to 5% have arthritis mutilans, 5% to 7% have spondylitis, and 15% to 23% have rheumatoid arthritis–like involvement (Chapter 27).

8. B Antimalarials, beta-blockers, and lithium have been shown to exacerbate psoriasis in susceptible individuals. Alcohol in large quantities also seems to aggravate psoriasis. Withdrawal of systemic steroids may also provoke psoriasis (Chapter 27).

9. D The diagnostic features of psoriasis may not all be present at the same time, but they are useful in recognizing the numerous variants of psoriasis. The pale halo occasionally seen around psoriatic lesions is known as Woronoff's ring. The deep red color, silvery white scale, sharp borders, and symmetrical distribution are useful diagnostic features. Another helpful characteristic is the Auspitz sign, referring to fine bleeding points seen when the psoriatic scale is removed (Chapter 27).

10. E A number of papulosquamous conditions may at times be difficult to distinguish from psoriasis. These include seborrheic dermatitis, lichen planus, parapsoriasis, pityriasis rosea, and pityriasis rubra pilaris. Other conditions can also imitate some features of psoriasis. These include Reiter's disease, mycosis fungoides, psoriasiform tertiary syphilis, localized neurodermatitis, superficial fungal infections, and congenital ichthyosiform erythroderma (Chapter 27).

11. B Generalized pustular psoriasis of von Zumbusch is a rare and at times fatal form of acute psoriasis. The attacks are accompanied by high fever, leukocytosis, arthralgia, malaise, and other constitutional signs. The tongue and buccal mucosa may also be involved. The tongue often clinically resembles "geographic tongue." Hypocalcemia is frequent and may be a consequence of hypoalbuminemia. When it occurs in children, generalized pustular psoriasis has a better prognosis than the adult disease and is more likely to resolve spontaneously after a few weeks (Chapter 27).

12. E (Chapter 27).

13. i C; ii B; iii D; iv D; v A (Chapter 27).

14. i C; ii C; iii B; iv C; v C Retinoids and cyclosporine commonly cause an elevation of both cholesterol and triglycerides. This is especially important in long-term therapy because of the risk of accelerated atherosclerosis and cardiovascular disease. Headaches, often resistant to treatment with over-the-counter analgesics, are common in patients who take cyclosporine. They occur more commonly during the early weeks of therapy and tend to resolve spontaneously as treatment continues. Retinoids can also cause headaches that are likely due to increased intracranial pressure. Concomitant use of tetracyclines may increase this risk and should be avoided. Cyclosporine can induce both acute and chronic renal dysfunction, a primary concern in cyclosporine therapy. This is not the case with retinoids.

Transient elevations of serum hepatic transaminases are common with retinoids, although the risk of significant hepatotoxicity is low. With cyclosporine, there is a 50% incidence of hyperbilirubinemia. Other hepatic enzymes may also be abnormal. The risk of significant hepatotoxicity is also low. It is recommended that potentially hepatotoxic drugs be avoided during retinoid or cyclosporine therapy. Bone or muscle pains without objective evidence of abnormality and without sequelae is not uncommon with retinoids. With long-term therapy, the formation of spurs and calcification of interosseous membranes and tendons can occur. They are not usually symptomatic. Patients on cyclosporine may also complain of joint and muscle pain. Hyperuricemia is seen in as much as 15% of patients and there have been reports of gouty arthritis in these patients (Chapter 27).

15. i A; ii B; iii C; iv D; v C Conjunctivitis occurs in 20% to 50% of patients treated with retinoids. Staphylococcal superinfection may occur. There are two other ocular effects: (1) corneal erosions leading to opacities and (2) abnormalities of night vision. The corneal and conjunctival adverse effects are believed to be due to decreased tear formation and decreased lipid content of the tears. Blepharoconjunctivitis is not a regular occurence with methotrexate unless toxicity has occurred. Bone marrow toxicity is a major concern in patients who are on methotrexate. Leukopenia is the most frequent sign of marrow suppression. Thrombocytopenia usually occurs in conjunction with pancytopenia. Myelosuppression is not a regular feature of retinoid therapy. Both retinoids and methotrexate are teratogenic, but neither drug has been reported to cause malignancy. Mild alopecia has been reported with both drugs and is usually reversible after discontinuation (Chapter 27).

16. i A; ii C; iii A; iv C; v B Von Zumbusch's generalized pustular psoriasis and guttate psoriasis do not respond well to cyclosporine. Acrodermatitis continua of Hallopeau appears to respond well. Cyclosporine is particularly effective in erythrodermic psoriasis and severe plaque-type psoriasis. Retinoids are useful in all types of pustular psoriasis and in guttate psoriasis. Response of plaque-type psoriasis to retinoids is not usually satisfactory, although some patients do well (Chapter 27).

17. C Von Zumbusch's generalized pustular psoriasis seems to be resistant to cyclosporine. Some patients have shown a response, but only to very high doses. Localized pustular psoriasis responds better to cyclosporine. Etretinate has proven to be useful in both generalized and localized pustular psoriasis. Phototherapy in the form of the Goeckerman or Ingram regimen is contraindicated in generalized pustular psoriasis because of possible aggravation of the condition. PUVA, on the other hand, can initially be used with small doses and can be combined with etretinate therapy. Methotrexate is still considered the drug of choice for generalized pustular psoriasis or debilitating localized disease (Chapter 27).

18. E Risk factors for hyperlipidemia include all of the listed options and a family history of hyperlipidemia (Chapter 27).

19. E The presence of any of these factors to a significant degree should be considered when evaluating the need for a pre-methotrexate liver biopsy. The reader is referred to the revised methotrexate guidelines for use of methotrexate in psoriasis (Chapter 27).

20. A (T); B (F); C (T); D (F); E (T) There is mounting evidence that calcipotriol acts both by direct effects on the keratinocyte and by modulating the immune system. Calcipotriol has been shown to be a potent inhibitor of interleukin-1 and other cytokines. The best results are usually obtained after 6 to 8 weeks of application (Chapter 27).

21. D Etretinate is teratogenic and is therefore absolutely contraindicated in pregnancy. Severe skeletal malformations can occur, including failure of cranial fusion with meningomyelocele (Chapter 27).

22. D The risk of hyperlipidemia is the principal relative contraindication to etretinate use (Chapter 27).

23. E It is recommended that patients with hyperlipidemia increase active dynamic exercise during retinoid therapy. Patients with arthritis should be encouraged to swim, walk, or do other low impact exercise (Chapter 27).

24. E Etretinate has a long elimination time and has been detected in low concentrations in serum more than 2 years after discontinuation (Chapter 27).

25. C In about half the patients, the plaques of psoriasis increase in size between the second and fifth weeks of treatment with etretinate. After 1 month, thinning of the plaques is noted and scaling decreases. Within 3 to 4 months, the plaques clear, starting in the center of the lesions and progressing toward the edges (Chapter 27).

26. A During etretinate therapy, the nail becomes softer and thinner and the rate of growth increases (Chapter 27).

27. A Obesity is not a contraindication to methotrexate therapy. However, obese patients are at increased risk of liver toxicity. Other contraindications include liver chemistry abnormalities, liver cirrhosis, breast feeding, severe anemia, leukopenia or thrombocytopenia, excessive alcohol consumption, active infections, and an unreliable patient (Chapter 27).

28. B A liver biopsy is normally recommended after 1.5 g cumulative methotrexate dose, and at 1.0 to 1.5 g intervals thereafter. In a patient having prolonged significant liver test abnormalities or at least one risk factor for hepatotoxicity, a follow-up liver biopsy is recommended after a 1 g cumulative dose and repeated at 1 g intervals (Chapter 27).

29. D Beta-blockers do not interfere with the use of methotrexate but may aggravate psoriasis (Chapter 27).

30. B Methotrexate can produce abnormalities in spermatogenesis that are temporary and reversible when the drug is discontinued. Whether this results in fetal abnormalities is still unclear. When administered to women in the first trimester, it induces a high rate of spontaneous abortion. It is highly teratogenic, having a malformation rate of approximately 30%. In women, conception should be avoided for at least one ovulatory cycle after stopping the drug (Chapter 27).

31. C Phenytoin actually decreases cyclosporine blood levels and can result in poor therapeutic response. Other drugs that can increase cyclosporine blood levels are doxycycline, amphotericin B, cimetidine, the oral contraceptives, androgens, and danazol (Chapter 27).

32. B Cyclosporine is unique among immunosuppressive agents because it causes no significant degree of myelosuppression. There have been rare reports of normochromic normocytic anemia, thrombocytopenia, and leukopenia (Chapter 27).

33. E In Reiter's disease, recurrent attacks are the rule and may occur within months or may be delayed for decades. It may progress to chronic erosive arthritis of the lower limbs and sacroiliac joints (Chapter 28).

34. A *Chlamydia trachomatis* is the most important urogenital infective agent incriminated in Reiter's disease. It is also the most important factor in nongonococcal urethritis (Chapter 28).

35. A Keratoderma is more common on the soles of the feet than on the palms. Keratotic lesions are also quite common on the scalp; legs; and dorsal surfaces of the feet, hands, and fingers (Chapters 27, 30, and 175).

36. A (T); B (T); C (T); D (F); E (T) Because cyclosporine can significantly increase both systolic and diastolic pressures, it should be avoided in patients with uncontrolled hypertension. Cyclosporine is an immunosuppressive drug and is best avoided in combination with other immunosuppressive therapy such as ultraviolet B or PUVA. Patients with malignancies, serious infections, immunodeficiencies, drug or alcohol abuse, or abnormal renal function should not be given this drug (Chapter 27).

37. All true. The chart at the bottom of the page is a useful guide to the varieties of pityriasis rubra pilaris (PRP):

38. 1 B; 2 A; 3 C The white, flaky, laminated psoriatic scale is not present in PRP; the scale of PRP is fine and granular. Keratoderma may occur in psoriasis but is uncommon, whereas it is almost always present in PRP. The main location of seborrheic dermatitis is in the so-called seborrheic areas (Chapter 30).

39. 1 B; 2 C; 3 D; 4 E; 5 A The hypopigmented and hyperpigmented brown spots on the torso following long-term arsenic ingestion are called raindrop pigmentation. Multiple superficial multicentric basal cell carcinoma on the torso, as well as areas of Bowen's disease on nonexposed areas and multiple keratoses on the extremities are also found in this condition. Vohwinkel's disease is one of the familial keratodermas (Chapters 27, 30, 141, and 175).

40. 1 B; 2 E; 3 A; 4 C; 5 D (Chapters 20, 24, 27, and 30).

41. E Other important findings of PRP are the orangeish hue of the lesions and the widespread extent of the eruption (Chapter 30).

42. A (F); B (T); C (T); D (T); E (F) A biopsy generally is not needed to diagnose PRP—it can be diagnosed by the clinical findings. In the occasional case in which psoriasis or patch stage mycosis fungoides is considered, a biopsy may help exclude these last two diseases (Chapter 30).

43. A (T); B (F); C (F); D (T); E (F) An upper torso eruption suggesting an acute eczematous or seborrheic dermatitis is the common form of presentation of the classic adult type of PRP. In many cases, diagnosis is not possible at this early stage. In the classic adult type, which usually disappears in 2 to 3 years, patients' nails show subungual hyperkeratoses, thickening of the plate, distal yellow-brown discoloration, and splinter hemorrhages. Photosensitivity is not a precipitating feature of

TYPE	INCIDENCE (%)	CLEAR IN 3 YEARS (%)	CHARACTERISTICS
Adult			
Classic (I)	55	81	Acute onset; no precipitating pruritus; "classic" features
Atypical (II)	5	20	Long duration; alopecia; ichthyosiform scaling; eczematous areas
Juvenile			
Classic (III)	10	16	Onset before age of 2 yr; similar features to type 1
Circumscribed (IV)	25	32	Focal areas of erythema and hyperkeratosis; rarely progresses
Atypical (V)	5	0	Early onset and chronic course; predominantly hyperkeratosis; infrequent erythema; scleroderma-like changes on the palms and soles

From Cohen PR, Prystowsky JH. Pityriasis rubra pilaris: A review of diagnosis and treatment. J Am Acad Dermatol 1989; 20:801.

PRP but will make the eruption that is already present worse (Chapter 30).

44. A (F); B (F); C (T); D (F); E (F) Very few conditions apart from PRP cause an accentuation of the follicular orifices with some keratotic plugging. This finding also occurs on the dorsa of the fingers (Chapter 30).

45. A (F); B (F); C (T); D (T); E (F) The mechanism of action of vitamin A and the synthetic retinoids is not known. It is interesting that in phrynoderma there is dry, rough skin and follicular hyperkeratosis as well as night blindness, xerophthalmia, and keratomalacia (Chapter 27).

46. A (T); B (T); C (F); D (F); E (T) Almost all erythroderma for which no cause can be found requires systemic steroids. Systemic antibiotics are the preferred treatment for infection in patients with erythroderma. Remember that some erythrodermas, such as pityriasis rubra pilaris and Norwegian scabies, may require treatment specific for that disease (Chapter 31).

47. A (T); B (T); C (T); D (F); E (T) The staphylococcal scalded skin syndrome (SSSS) and toxic epidermal necrolysis are more common in newborns and children as a cause of erythroderma. They have a reasonably acute onset. It is not known why dermatopathic lymphadenitis is less common in newborn and childhood erythroderma (Chapters 31 and 106).

48. A (T); B (F); C (T); D (T); E (T) Although erythroderma commonly is universal, occasionally the palms, soles, and scalp may be spared. The synonym for *erythroderma* is *generalized exfoliative dermatitis*. Persistence is an important feature in the clinical concept of erythroderma (Chapter 31).

49. A (T); B (F); C (T); D (T); E (F) The preservation of the general architecture of the lymph node is an important factor in distinguishing dermatopathic lymphadenitis from malignant lymphomas. Sternberg-Reed cells are usually present in Hodgkin's disease (Chapter 31).

50. A (T); B (F); C (T); D (F); E (T) The painless lymphadenopathy that develops in patients with widespread or erythrodermic dermatoses involves mainly those lymph nodes in the axillae and inguinal and cervical areas. The internal lymph nodes are not involved. The enlarged lymph nodes can often be seen, particularly in the inguinal area (Chapter 31).

51. C Exact figures for the cause of erythroderma are difficult to obtain because up to 50% may have no clearly identifiable cause. Psoriasis, atopic dermatitis, generalized eczematous dermatitis, drug reactions, pityriasis rubra pilaris, and various reticuloses (either mycosis fungoides or systemic reticulosis) are not uncommon causes in reported series (Chapter 31).

52. C The most common systemic effects in erythroderma are disturbance of thermoregulation and ankle edema. The high-output cardiac failure, ankle edema, and gynecomastia are less common (Chapter 31).

53. C (Chapters 30 and 31).

54. 1 A; 2 B; 3 E; 4 C; 5 E See answer to Question 37 (Chapters 30 and 31).

55. 1 E; 2 D; 3 C; 4 B; 5 A It is not always possible to discover the cause of erythroderma. A common cause of eczematous erythroderma is the repeated application of one or more topical sensitizing agents to eczematous "stasis" dermatitis on the lower legs (Chapter 31).

56. 1 D; 2 E; 3 A; 4 B; 5 C

57. 1 E; 2 D; 3 B; 4 C; 5 A

58. A (F); B (T); C (T); D (T); E (F) (Chapters 30, 31, 49, 81, and 125).

59. 1 (T); 2 (T); 3 (F); 4 (F); 5 (T) Lichen simplex chronicus is common on the nape of the neck, upper inner thighs, perianally (involving the semimucosa but not the true mucosa), lateral aspects of legs, and forearms. It is to be distinguished from lichen sclerosus et atrophicus by the hypopigmentation and perifollicular atrophy that lichen sclerosus et atrophicus shows. Koebnerization occurs in psoriasis, lichen planus, and verruca plana. Lichenification seen in lichen simplex chronicus consists of a coalescence of nondescript excoriated and scaly lichenoid papules (Chapter 14).

60. A Lichen simplex chronicus is more common in those with Asian or African background. In a survey of 3700 patients with skin disease, 14.6% of the Asians and 2.2% of the whites had this disease. The exact relationship between atopic dermatitis and lichen simplex chronicus is not known. Certainly there is the strong clinical impression that those with atopic stigmata have a greater chance to develop lichen simplex chronicus (Chapter 14).

61. A Neural hyperplasia is not a diagnostic prerequisite in nodular prurigo, although in some patients it is a prominent histologic finding (Chapter 14).

62. B Examples of grouped lesions are those of herpes simplex or herpes zoster or of papular urticaria due to cat or dog flea bites. When you squeeze a dermatofibroma, the epidermis is puckered inwards because of the attachment of the dermal fibrous tissue to the epidermis. This does not occur in prurigo (Chapter 14).

63. B Capsaicin destroys sensory neurons containing the putative neurotransmitter substance P, which appears to be important in the transmission of pain. Fully controlled studies have indicated only a minor degree of benefit, if any (Chapter 14).

64. A (F); B (T); C (F); D (T); E (T) There is no effective therapy for many cases of prurigo nodularis. Intralesional corticosteroid will help individual lesions become less itchy and less thick, but the number of lesions and frequency of injection usually makes this method of treatment impractical. For severe cases, occlusion, PUVA, or even thalidomide may be worthy of a trial (Chapter 14).

65. A (T); B (F); C (F); D (F); E (T) The abnormal neurologic findings in notalgia paresthetica are minimal or nonexistent. Pudendal neuralgia is a neuropathic pain along the distribution of the pudendal nerve (Chapter 14).

66. 1 B; 2 E; 3 A; 4 D; 5 C Neurotrophic ulcer commonly follows section of the fifth cranial nerve to treat tic douloureux. Scarring and pain are common features of livedo with ulcerations on the heels. The hypertensive ischemic ulcer is common on the shin; the cause is not known. The neuroanesthetic ulcer is also called mal perforans (Chapter 89).

67. 1 E; 2 C; 3 A; 4 B; 5 D (Chapter 89).

68. 1 C; 2 D; 3 A; 4 B; 5 B An ulcer implies some underlying disease process; a wound results from external trauma. Erosions are most often caused by trauma (scratching, severe rubbing) but may also be caused by disease (candidiasis, primary syphilis). By definition, an ulcer scars because of destruction of a portion or all of the dermis. Ulcers of the oral mucosae are rarely seen except as a result of tuberculosis, deep fungi, cancers, or severe radiodermatitis; almost all lesions of the mouth commonly seen are erosions because they do not scar (Chapter 89).

69. 1 C; 2 A; 3 A; 4 A; 5 B *Neurotic excoriation* is the term given to superficial self-inflicted lesions consisting of circular or ovoid, whitish, slightly atrophic areas from 2 to 8 mm in diameter. Some are eroded and oozing; some show a fresh bloody crust; some show a dry, loosely attached crust; and some show an atrophic red area.

The lesions of dermatitis artefacta are deep, scarring lesions with bizarre shapes and are on easily accessible sites. The prominent follicular orifices in the white scars are commonly seen on the shoulder and back area in patients with neurotic excoriations. These patients also often freely admit they are itchy pickers and just cannot leave a scab or other skin abnormality alone. Pimozide is occasionally useful in dermatitis artefacta (Chapter 89).

70. C (Chapter 89).

71. E Self-inflicted disease of all sorts can frequently be seen as a result of the rhythmic destructive actions of these patients (Chapter 89).

72. E (Chapter 89).

73. B Although emotional factors may play a role in atopic dermatitis, acne vulgaris, psoriasis, and urticaria, they are not the main cause of these conditions (Chapter 89).

74. A (T); B (T); C (F); D (T); E (T) (Chapter 14).

75. A (F); B (T); C (T); D (F); E (F) Burning or pain are the most frequent complaint of patients with vulvodynia. The onset following an acute vulvovaginitis perhaps caused by *Candida* is often recorded. When the organism and inflammation has disappeared, the pain slowly takes over. Despite the discomfort from the pain, patients rarely state that it keeps them awake at night. The lack of response to any topical preparation is a feature of this condition. Usually the story is that many presumably bland and nonirritating topicals cause the condition to become worse (Chapter 89).

76. A (F); B (T); C (F); D (T); E (F); F (F) There are no abnormal findings on the tongue in glossodynia. At times the patient with glossodynia also complains of abnormal sensations on the lips and cheeks (Chapter 89).

77. 1 (T); 2 (T); 3 (F); 4 (T); 5 (T) The drugs that produce excessive seborrhea are those that produce extrapyramidal, Parkinson-like symptoms (Chapter 89).

Bibliography

Adam JE. Exfoliative dermatitis (erythroderma). Curr Probl Dermatol 1972; 4:1–23.

Borok M, Lowe NJ: Pityriasis rubra pilaris. Further observations of systemic retinoid therapy. Part 1. J Am Acad Dermatol 1990; 22:792–795.

Butterworth T, Strean LP. Behaviour disorders of interest to dermatologists. Arch Dermatol 1963; 88:859–867.

Cohen PR, Prystowsky JH. Pityriasis rubra pilaris: A review of diagnosis and treatment. J Am Acad Dermatol 1989; 20:801–807.

Danto, JL. Incidence of lichen simplex chronicus in Orientals and Caucasians. Can Med Assoc J 1956; 75:1029–1031.

Ellis CN, ed. Cyclosporine in Dermatology, Proceedings of a Symposium. J Am Acad Dermatol 1990; Volume 23, number 6, part 2, 1241–1334.

Ellis CN, Voorhees JJ. Etretinate therapy. J Am Acad Dermatol 1987; 16:270.

Fox RH, Shuster S, Williams R, et al. Cardiovascular, metabolic, and thermoregulatory disturbances in patients with erythrodermic skin diseases. Br Med J 1965; 1:619–622.

Fritsch PO. Retinoids in psoriasis and disorders of keratinisation. J Am Acad Dermatol 1992; 27:S11.

Griffiths WAD. Pityriasis rubra pilaris. Clin Exp Dermatol 1980; 5:105–112.

Jannigan CK, Gascon P, Schwartz RA, et al. Erythroderma as the initial presentation of the acquired immunodeficiency syndrome. Dermatologica 1991; 183:143–145.

Lim JT, Tham SN. Pityriasis rubra pilaris in Singapore. Clin Exp Dermatol 1991; 16:181–184.

Lindley RP, Payne CMER. Neural hyperplasia is not a diagnostic prerequisite in nodular prurigo. J Cutan Pathol 1989; 16:14–18.

Lyell A. Cutaneous artefactual disease. J Am Acad Dermatol 1979; 1:391–407.

Lynch PJ. Vulvodynia. J Reprod Med 1986; 31:773–779.

Martin AG, Weaver CC, Cockerell CJ, Berger TG. Pityriasis rubra pilaris in the setting of HIV infection: Clinical behaviour and association with explosive cystic acne. Br J Dermatol 1992; 126:617–620.

McKay M. Vulvodynia—a multifactorial clinical problem. Arch Dermatol 1989; 125:256–262.

Rebora A. Cyclosporin A in psoriasis. Clin Dermatol 1992; 9:516.

Roenigk HH Jr, Auerbach R, Maibach HI, et al. Methotrexate in psoriasis: Revised guidelines. J Am Acad Dermatol 1988; 19:145–157.

Ronchese F. Occupational Marks. New York: Grune & Stratton, 1948.

Shalita AR, Fritsch PO, eds. Retinoids: Present and Future, Proceedings of a Symposium. J Am Acad Dermatol 1992; Volume 27, number 6, part 2, S1–S46.

Thestrup-Pedersen K, Halkier-Sorensen L, Sogaard H, et al. The red man syndrome. Exfoliative dermatitis of unknown etiology: A description and follow-up of 38 patients. J Am Acad Dermatol 1988; 18:1307–1312.

Toole, JP. Mechanism of action of calcipotriol in the therapy of psoriasis. Can J Dermatol 1993; 5:385–388.

Woverton SE, Wilkin JK. Systemic Drugs for Skin Diseases. Philadelphia: WB Saunders Co., 1991.

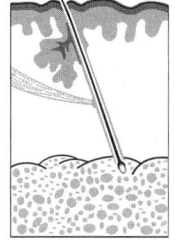

chapter 7

Diseases with Dermal Inflammation

MARK H. LOWITT

Choose the ONE BEST answer to each of the following questions.

1. A 36-year-old woman complains of a nonpruritic lesion of several weeks' duration that has expanded and slowly moved across her left shoulder. Physical examination reveals a polycyclic erythematous patch with a trailing scale. A potassium hydroxide preparation from the scale is negative. All of the following conditions may be associated with her condition EXCEPT
   A. Candidal infection
   B. Malignant neoplasm
   C. Dermatophytosis
   D. Urinary tract infection
   E. Drugs.

2. A 24-year-old man presents with fever; arthritis; chorea; pancarditis; and an erythematous, evanescent eruption. The most likely diagnosis for his skin condition is
   A. Erythema infectiosum
   B. Erythema annulare centrifugum
   C. Erythema marginatum
   D. Erythema chronicum migrans
   E. Erythema gyratum repens.

3. A 76-year-old man presents with a striking pattern of undulating wavy erythematous bands with the appearance of wood grain over the entire body. Which one of the following statements is TRUE?
   A. He is likely to have an associated leukocytosis
   B. This condition is always associated with an underlying malignancy
   C. The patient should be hospitalized for high-dose steroid therapy
   D. Treatment of an underlying malignancy may lead to resolution of the skin condition
   E. This condition may be triggered by severe tinea pedis.

4. Pustulation at the site of venipuncture occurs most commonly with
   A. Polyarteritis nodosum
   B. Erythema elevatum diutinum
   C. Behçet's syndrome
   D. Drug-induced leukocytoclastic vasculitis
   E. Sarcoidosis.

5. Idiopathic Sweet's syndrome is characterized by which of the following?
   A. Male predominance
   B. Frequent oral ulcerations

79

C. Peripheral lymphocytosis

D. Lack of response to systemic corticosteroids

E. Prior upper respiratory infection in 75% to 90%.

6. The malignancy most strongly associated with Sweet's syndrome is

   A. Acute myelogenous leukemia
   B. Acute lymphocytic leukemia
   C. Chronic myelogenous leukemia
   D. Chronic lymphocytic leukemia
   E. Hodgkin's lymphoma.

7. Which of the following is true regarding erythema dyschromicum perstans?

   A. It often is associated with high fever
   B. It is caused by a spirochete
   C. The blue-gray hue results from hemosiderin-laden macrophages in the epidermis
   D. The blue-gray hue results from melanin-laden macrophages in the epidermis
   E. It has no systemic manifestations.

8. All of the following statements regarding bromoderma are true EXCEPT

   A. Acneiform pustules are typical
   B. Plasma bromide levels parallel disease severity
   C. A follicular distribution is typical
   D. It may be mistaken for blastomycosis
   E. It may be mistaken for rosacea.

9. Which one of the following statements is TRUE regarding laboratory testing in sarcoidosis?

   A. A normal serum angiotensin–converting enzyme level rules out active sarcoidosis
   B. Hypocalcemia is frequently noted
   C. The Kveim reaction is positive if 10 mm induration occurs within 48 hours
   D. Serum globulins are often elevated
   E. Intradermal injections of mumps and *Candida* antigens yield positive reactions in 90% of patients with sarcoidosis.

10. In histologically differentiating sarcoidosis from lupus vulgaris, which one of the following statements is TRUE?

    A. The infiltrate is localized near the epidermis in lupus vulgaris and is more generalized in sarcoidosis
    B. A more marked lymphocytic infiltrate around the epithelioid cells is present in sarcoidosis
    C. Sarcoidal granulomas demonstrate more caseation than do those of lupus vulgaris
    D. Ulceration, acanthosis, and pseudoepitheliomatous hyperplasia are more frequently observed in sarcoidosis
    E. The two diseases are easily distinguished histologically.

11. Which of the following laboratory abnormalities is most likely to be associated with necrobiotic xanthogranuloma?

    A. Elevated glucose
    B. Elevated cholesterol
    C. Elevated triglycerides
    D. Elevated total protein
    E. Elevated calcium.

12. Which of the following lasers emits energy in the infrared range?

    A. Carbon dioxide
    B. Argon
    C. Q-switched ruby
    D. Pulsed dye
    E. Excimer.

13. Which one of the following statements is TRUE regarding sinus histiocytosis with massive lymphadenopathy?

    A. The histiocytes are S-100 positive
    B. Comma-shaped bodies are seen on electron microscopy
    C. Patients usually present in their sixth or seventh decade
    D. Eighty-five per cent of patients develop red-brown or yellow-brown papules or nodules
    E. Radiologic opacification of the maxillary sinuses is present in most cases.

14. If an individual urticarial wheal lasts more than 24 to 48 hours, histopathologic examination may be likely to reveal

    A. Atypical lymphocytes in the epidermis
    B. Vasculitis
    C. Heavy deposition of mucin (hyaluronic acid)
    D. "Coat-sleeving" of lymphocytes around superficial vessels
    E. Focal parakeratosis.

15. A 25-year-old woman develops hives within minutes of exposure to a medication. All of the following are likely to trigger direct, *non*immunologic mast cell degranulation EXCEPT

    A. Morphine
    B. *d*-Tubocurarine
    C. Polymyxin B
    D. Penicillin
    E. Acetylsalicylic acid.

16. Ultrastructural components of the mast cell include

    A. Large collections of immunoglobulin
    B. Fingerprint-like parallel filaments
    C. Chromogranin-positive granules
    D. Trilaminar elongate structures
    E. Absence of mitochondria.

17. The number of lobes in the nucleus of a typical eosinophil:

    A. One
    B. Two
    C. Three
    D. Four or more
    E. Eosinophil nuclei are not lobulated.

18. Which is the most common organ to produce clinical manifestations in the chronic, persistent type of sarcoidosis?

    A. Eye
    B. Lung
    C. Bone
    D. Salivary gland
    E. Nerve.

19. Which of the following is the most common cause of death from sarcoidosis?

    A. Sarcoidal glomerulonephritis
    B. Superimposed tuberculosis
    C. Cor pulmonale from pulmonary fibrosis
    D. Pulmonary hemorrhage
    E. Massive myocardial sarcoidal involvement.

20. Which one of the following statements regarding sarcoidosis is TRUE?

    A. Circulating levels of immunoglobulins are depressed
    B. Round cells at the periphery of granulomas are monocytes
    C. Phytohemagglutinin-stimulated transformation of lymphocytes is increased
    D. Touton giant cells predominate in the infiltrate
    E. The ratio of helper to suppressor T cells in the granulomas is lower than that found in the peripheral blood.

21. Which one of the following statements regarding necrobiosis lipoidica (NL) is TRUE?

    A. Between 60% and 70% of patients with NL have abnormal serum lipids
    B. Sixty-five per cent of patients with NL have diabetes
    C. Three per cent of diabetics develop NL
    D. Nondiabetic patients with NL are unlikely to have a family history of diabetes
    E. Twenty per cent of diabetics develop NL.

22. A patient presents with an indurated plaque on the scalp. Biopsy reveals granulomatous necrobiosis lipoidica. Which one of the following statements regarding this patient is TRUE?

    A. This patient is probably female
    B. This patient is probably a child
    C. This patient probably has diabetes
    D. This patient probably has an internal malignancy
    E. This patient probably has recently been bitten by a tick.

For the following questions, ONE or MORE of the completions correctly finishes the incomplete statement. Choose

   A. If only 1, 2, and 3 are correct
   B. If only 1 and 3 are correct
   C. If only 2 and 4 are correct
   D. If only 4 is correct
   E. If all are correct.

23. A patient with pyoderma gangrenosum has an increased probability of having which of the following conditions?

    1. Ulcerative colitis
    2. Monoclonal gammopathy
    3. Myelodysplastic syndrome
    4. Elevated serum bromide level.

24. Diagnostic criteria for Behçet's syndrome include

    1. Cutaneous vasculitis
    2. Synovitis

3. Genital ulcerations
4. Conjunctivitis.

25. Histologic features of leukocytoclastic vasculitis include
    1. Fibrinoid degeneration of the vascular wall
    2. Erythrocyte extravasation
    3. Endothelial swelling
    4. Karyorrhexis.

26. Features of the bowel-associated dermatitis–arthritis syndrome include
    1. Erythema nodosum
    2. Recurrent pustules on the arms and trunk
    3. Oral ulcerations
    4. Fever.

27. Types of granuloma annulare associated with diabetes mellitus include
    1. Perforating granuloma annulare
    2. Localized granuloma annulare
    3. Subcutaneous granuloma annulare
    4. Generalized granuloma annulare.

28. Which of the following extracutaneous sites may be involved in association with juvenile xanthogranuloma?
    1. Lung
    2. Meninges
    3. Pericardium
    4. Eye.

29. Clinical subsets of sarcoidosis include which of the following?
    1. Ichthyosiform
    2. Atrophic
    3. Subcutaneous
    4. Erythrodermic.

30. Subcutaneous nodules regularly occur in which of the following conditions?
    1. Rheumatoid arthritis
    2. Systemic lupus erythematosus
    3. Rheumatic fever
    4. Progressive systemic sclerosis.

Decide whether EACH of the following questions is TRUE or FALSE. Any combination of answers, from all true to all false, may occur.

Regarding leukocytoclastic vasculitis,

31. Medium-sized vessels in the skin are primarily involved.
32. Early lesions typically appear on the trunk.
33. Most cases are acute and self-limited.
34. Plasma cells are present in large numbers.

Concerning the histopathologic findings in granuloma annulare and necrobiosis lipoidica,

35. Mucin is more abundant in granuloma annulare.
36. Giant cells are more abundant in granuloma annulare.
37. Vascular changes are more pronounced in granuloma annulare.
38. More extensive lipid deposits are present in granuloma annulare.
39. Leukocytoclastic vasculitis is a common associated finding.

Regarding urticaria,

40. Chronic urticaria describes hives that have been recurring daily for 2 weeks or more.
41. Patients with aspirin-induced urticaria may experience cross-reactivity with tartrazine.
42. A definitive trigger can be identified in more than 75% of patients with chronic urticaria.

Regarding the granules of polymorphonuclear leukocytes,

43. Twenty per cent of granules are azurophilic.
44. Only azurophilic granules contain myeloperoxidase.
45. Only specific granules contain lysozyme.

In each of the following questions, a set of lettered headings accompanies a list of numbered words or phrases. For each numbered word or phrase, choose

  A. If the item is associated with A only.
  B. If the item is associated with B only.
  C. If the item is associated with both A and B.
  D. If the item is associated with neither A nor B.

For each of the following characteristics, choose whether it describes the hypereosinophilic syndrome, Well's syndrome, both, or neither.

46. Abnormal electrocardiogram   A. Hypereosinophilic syndrome

47. Peripheral eosinophilia
48. Flame figures.

A. Wells' syndrome
B. Wells' syndrome
C. Both
D. Neither.

For each of the following characteristics, choose whether it describes herpes gestationis, PUPPP, both, or neither.

49. Predilection for abdominal striae
50. Elevated 24-hour urinary chorionic gonadotropin
51. Recurrence with subsequent pregnancies
52. Complement-fixing IgA basement membrane zone antibody
53. Usually appears during the first trimester of pregnancy.

A. Herpes gestationis
B. PUPPP
C. Both
D. Neither.

For each of the following clinical findings, choose whether it describes Letterer-Siwe, Hand-Schüller-Christian, both, or neither.

54. Exophthalmos
55. May be clinically confused with seborrheic dermatitis or diaper dermatitis
56. Hoarseness, recurrent parotitis, papules along eyelid margins.

A. Letterer-Siwe
B. Hand-Schüller-Christian
C. Both
D. Neither.

For each of the following findings, choose whether it describes familial cold urticaria, essential acquired cold urticaria, both, or neither.

57. Lesions occur rapidly after cold exposure
58. Lesions are pruritic
59. Lesions last 48 hours.

A. Familial cold urticaria
B. Essential acquired cold urticaria
C. Both
D. Neither.

DISEASES WITH DERMAL INFLAMMATION 83

For each numbered item, choose the most likely associated lettered item. Each numbered item has ONLY ONE answer. Within each group, each lettered item may be the answer to one, more than one, or none of the numbered items.

Match each of the following histopathologic features with the appropriate lettered condition.

60. Pseudoepitheliomatous hyperplasia
61. Superficial zone of edema in papillary dermis
62. Doubly refractile lipid deposits
63. Prominent eosinophils.

A. Sweet's syndrome
B. Erythema elevatum diutinum
C. Granuloma faciale
D. Halogenoderma
E. Leukocytoclastic vasculitis.

Match each of the subsets of sarcoidosis with the appropriate eponym:

64. Lupus pernio
65. Fever, arthralgia, uveitis, hilar adenopathy, erythema nodosum
66. Subcutaneous sarcoid
67. Uveoparotid fever.

A. Darier-Roussy
B. Löfgren's
C. Heerfordt's
D. Osler's
E. Besnier's.

Match each of the following descriptions with the appropriate histopathologic finding:

68. Center stains brown-red and spikes stain blue with acid-hematoxylin
69. Round or oval with peripheral calcification
70. Formed from laminated residual bodies of lysosomes
71. Formed from collagen trapped between epithelioid cells during giant cell formation.

A. Schaumann's body
B. Farber's body
C. Birbeck's granule
D. Henderson-Patterson body
E. Asteroid body.

Match each of the following compounds with the foreign body granuloma it induces:

72. Mineral oil
73. Surgical gloves
74. Deodorant
75. Old fluorescent light bulbs.

A. Starch granuloma
B. Beryllium granuloma
C. Paraffinoma
D. Silica granuloma
E. Zirconium granuloma.

Match each of the following reactions with the tattoo pigment most likely to induce it:

76. Delayed hypersensitivity
77. Photosensitive reaction

A. Chrome green
B. Cinnabar red
C. India ink black
D. Cobalt blue
E. Cadmium yellow.

Match each of the following characteristics with the most closely associated histiocytic disease:

78. Usually occurs in childhood
79. Associated with mutilating arthritis
80. Usually accompanied by fever
81. Associated with internal malignancy in up to 25% of patients.

A. Progressive nodular histiocytoma
B. Generalized eruptive histiocytoma
C. Multicentric reticulohistiocytosis
D. Benign cephalic histiocytosis
E. Sinus histiocytosis with massive lymphadenopathy.

ANSWERS

1. D; **2.** C; **3.** D Erythema annulare centrifugum (EAC) is one of the gyrate erythemas, consisting of a slowly migrating, annular-polycyclic, erythematous, predominantly truncal eruption with a characteristic "trailing scale" (a line of scale that seems to follow the advancing rim of erythema). Although most cases remain unexplained, some have been linked with a variety of agents, including drugs, dermatophyte infection, candidal infection, blue cheese ingestion, and malignant neoplasms. There have been no reported associations with urinary tract infection.

The patient described in Question 2 exhibits several of the major criteria for acute rheumatic fever. The most characteristic skin manifestations of rheumatic fever include subcutaneous nodules and erythema marginatum—an erythematous, evanescent, rapidly moving annular or polycyclic eruption that characteristically appears and disappears over the course of hours. Erythema infectiosum (Fifth's disease) is a febrile exanthem of childhood. Erythema chronicum migrans typically accompanies early Lyme disease.

Erythema gyratum repens is another figurate erythema that demonstrates a striking widespread "woodgrain" pattern of erythema and scale. Many cases are associated with internal malignancy, particularly carcinoma of the breast, lung, and pharynx. Treatment of the underlying malignancy has been reported to cause resolution of the skin findings.

4. C Behçet's syndrome consists of a combination of the following findings: recurrent oral ulcerations, recurrent genital ulceration, uveitis, cutaneous vasculitis, synovitis, and meningoencephalitis. A sterile pustule at the site of saline injection (or needle prick) constitutes the "skin puncture" or "pathergy" test that is characteristic of this syndrome (Chapter 40).

5. E; **6.** A Sweet's syndrome (acute febrile neutrophilic dermatosis) constitutes a distinctive clinical entity in which large, rapidly growing, tender, pink pseudovesiculated plaques form on the upper body, commonly in conjunction with high fever and leukocytosis. Many cases are associated with underlying hematologic malignancy, particularly acute myelogenous leukemia. In idiopathic cases, a prior upper respiratory infection is frequently associated (Chapter 38).

7. E Erythema dyschromicum perstans, or ashy dermatosis, consists of gray-tan ashy patches that may have an indurated violaceous border. In the acute stage, a lichenoid dermatitis predominates. In the chronic stage, melanin-laden macrophages are present in the dermis. No systemic manifestations have been reported (Chapter 20).

8. B Bromoderma, an acneiform eruption resulting from ingestion of bromide-containing compounds often occurs in a follicular distribution. The clinical differential diagnosis includes acne, rosacea, and blastomycosis. Plasma bromide levels do not correlate with cutaneous disease activity (Chapter 49).

9. D Serum angiotensin–converting enzyme, although elevated in 60% of patients with sarcoidosis, is not sensitive enough to rule out the diagnosis. In sarcoidosis, activated pulmonary macrophages produce elevated amounts of dihydroxyvitamin D_3, leading to excessive intestinal calcium absorption and hypercalcemia. The Kveim test involves the intradermal injection of sarcoidal extract. The test becomes positive at 4 to 6 weeks. Hypergammaglobulinemia occurs in 50% of patients. Two thirds of patients with sarcoidosis are typically anergic (i.e., they do not manifest delayed-type hypersensitivity reactions to common antigens such as mumps or *Candida* organisms (Chapter 45).

10. A Histologically, the differences between sarcoidosis and lupus vulgaris (a variety of cutaneous tuberculosis) can be subtle. Several criteria can be used to differentiate the two conditions. In lupus vulgaris, the inflammatory infiltrate is typically localized close to the epidermis, whereas in sarcoidosis it is more generalized. Tuberculous infiltrates are generally heavy, but sarcoidal granulomas usually have a sparse infiltrate, resulting in "naked tubercles" (or granulomas without a surrounding rim of lymphocytes). Unlike tuberculoid granulomas, sarcoidal granulomas classically do not caseate. Ulceration, acanthosis, and pseudoepitheliomatous hyperplasia are more characteristic of lupus vulgaris (Chapter 45).

11. D Necrobiotic xanthogranuloma is a rare disorder, always associated with paraproteinemia and/or lymphoproliferative disease (Chapter 47).

12. A Most currently employed lasers emit light in the visible range with the exceptions of the carbon dioxide and the Nd:YAG lasers, which emit light in the infrared range, and the excimer lasers, which emit light in the ultraviolet range (Chapter 48).

LASER	WAVELENGTH
Excimer	248, 351 nm
Argon	488, 514 nm
Copper vapor	578 nm
Pulsed dye (vascular)	577, 585 nm
Pulsed dye (pigment)	510 nm
Q-switched ruby	694 nm
Nd:YAG	1060 nm
Carbon dioxide	10,600 nm

13. B Sinus histiocytosis with massive lymphadenopathy (Rosai-Dorfman syndrome) is a benign, self-limited condition defined by the proliferation of S-100 negative (non-Langerhans cell) histiocytes within lymph nodes that usually occurs in the first two decades of life. Cutaneous macules, papules, plaques, and nodules occur in only 10% of patients. Histologic examination of the cutaneous lesions reveals large collections of large pale histiocytes, sometimes aggregated in groups which resemble lymph node sinuses. Comma-shaped bodies are seen on electron microscopy. The maxillary sinuses are not involved (Chapter 154).

14. B Classic urticarial wheals are evanescent; individual lesions usually vanish after several hours. Biopsy should be considered for urticarial lesions persisting for more than 48 hours to rule out urticarial vasculitis. Lesions of urticarial vasculitis may itch or burn and may be associated with systemic lupus erythematosus, Sjögren's syndrome, and some infections. Systemic manifestations of vasculitis, including renal, gastrointestinal, respiratory, and central nervous system disease, have been reported in association with the skin lesions (Chapter 41).

15. D Mast cells may release histamine by immunologic or nonimmunologic means. An example of an immunologic trigger is seen in penicillin allergy, mediated by specific IgE molecules binding to mast cells, cross-linking and triggering mast cell degranulation. Several drugs, including morphine, d-tubocurarine, aspirin, nonsteroidal anti-inflammatory agents, and polymyxin B, can cause mast cells to degranulate directly in the absence of an immunologic trigger (Chapter 41).

16. B Ultrastructurally, mast cells contain fingerprint-like parallel filaments. Large collections of immunoglobulins are found in plasma cells. Chromogranin-positive structures are found in Merkel's cells. Trilaminar, elongate, tennis racquet–shaped structures (Birbeck's granules) are present in Langerhans cells. Mitochondria are present in all eukaryotic cells (Chapter 41).

17. B Eosinophil nuclei are typically bilobed (Chapter 35).

18. B; **19.** C Although all of the organs listed in Question 18 can be involved in chronic, persistent sarcoidosis, the lungs are the most likely organ to produce clinical symptoms. Fifty per cent of patients have symptomatic lung disease. The most common cause of death in sarcoidosis is cor pulmonale from extensive pulmonary fibrosis (Chapter 45).

20. B A variety of immunologic abnormalities occur in sarcoidosis. Humoral immunity alteration is manifested by high circulating levels of immunoglobulins. Cell-mediated immunity is likewise altered in several ways. Abnormal T-cell behavior is demonstrated by cutaneous anergy, an elevated helper:suppressor T-cell ratio within the lesions, and decreased transformation of lymphocytes in vitro with phytohemagglutinin. Langerhans giant cells are most abundant in the infiltrate. Although the small round cells at the periphery of sarcoidal granulomas were initially thought to be of lymphocytic origin, recent immunohistochemical staining has revealed that these cells contain lysosomal enzymes and thus actually are of monocyte origin (Chapter 45).

21. B Although necrobiosis lipoidica (NL) is not associated with any lipid abnormalities, it is strongly associated with diabetes mellitus. Sixty-five per cent of patients with NL have overt diabetes, an additional 15% have abnormal glucose tolerance, and 15% have positive family histories for glucose intolerance. Conversely, however, only 0.3% of diabetics develop NL (Chapter 47).

22. A Although classic necrobiosis lipoidica occurs most commonly on the anterior lower extremities, an atypical form of NL can manifest with sarcoid-like plaques on the head. This form of NL occurs most commonly in middle-aged nondiabetic women and demonstrates a histologically more granulomatous picture (Chapter 47).

23. A Pyoderma gangrenosum (PG) is a poorly understood inflammatory condition consisting of painful hemorrhagic nodules or pustules that progress into well-demarcated deep ulcers with characteristically overhanging, or "undermined," edges. Although idiopathic in 50% of patients, PG can be associated with a variety of underlying internal illnesses, including inflammatory bowel disease, rheumatoid and seronegative arthritis, monoclonal gammopathy, myeloid leukemia, multiple myeloma and other myelodysplastic syndromes, and collagen-vascular diseases, including lupus and Wegener's granulomatosis. Serum bromide levels are not elevated in association with PG (Chapter 39).

24. A Behçet's disease constitutes a systemic disease with prominent cutaneous and mucosal components. Its clinical diagnosis is defined by the presence of oral aphthous ulcers in association with at least two of the following: genital ulcerations, synovitis, cutaneous vasculitis, uveitis, or meningoencephalitis. The diagnosis of Behçet's disease can be made only after other collagen-vascular diseases have been excluded. Conjunctivitis, an important component of Reiter's syndrome, is *not* characteristically present in Behçet's disease (Chapter 40).

25. E The characteristic histologic findings in leukocytoclastic vasculitis include polymorphonuclear leukocytes invading the wall of cutaneous blood vessels (particularly venules), karyorrhexis (neutrophil fragmentation), fibrinoid degeneration of the vascular wall, endothelial swelling, erythrocyte extravasation, and fibrin thrombi within the vessel lumina. Leukocytoclastic vasculitis may occur in a wide range of inflammatory conditions, including collagen-vascular diseases (rheumatoid arthritis, systemic lupus), infections (bacterial and viral), drug reactions, and others (Henoch-Schönlein purpura, livedoid vasculitis, etc.) (Chapter 67).

26. C The bowel-associated dermatitis-arthritis syndrome is an episodic serum sickness–like reaction associated with crops of vesicopustules that occurs after ileojejunal bypass for morbid obesity or Billroth II gastroenterostomy. Fever, arthralgias, and malaise are common. The syndrome is thought to result from immune complexes formed in response to systemic absorption of peptidoglycans from overgrowing enteral bacteria (Chapter 38).

27. E The classic form of granuloma annulare (GA) manifests as annular, indurated, pinkish-yellow papules and plaques located on the distal dorsal extremities. Perforating, subcutaneous, and generalized forms of GA are also recognized. The generalized form, in which hundreds or thousands of 2 to 4 mm yellowish-pink papules are present on the trunk, is the only form of GA known to be associated with diabetes mellitus (Chapter 46).

28. E Juvenile xanthogranuloma is a benign aggregation of histiocytes with aggregation of lipid that typically occurs as a single yellowish papule in children. Ocular involvement is the most common extracutaneous manifestation. Lesions may also occur in the lungs, kidneys, pericardium, colon, ovaries, testes, meninges, and bones (Chapter 47).

29. E Skin lesions occur in 25% of patients with sarcoidosis. The cutaneous manifestations of sarcoidosis may vary widely in appearance. The most common skin lesions include indurated papules around the central face (lupus pernio), indurated plaques, and maculopapular eruptions. Other varieties of cutaneous sarcoidosis include ichthyosiform, atrophic, subcutaneous, erythrodermic, alopetic, and even verrucous lesions (Chapter 45).

30. E Rheumatoid nodules are firm, nontender, subcutaneous masses that occur at sites of trauma in 20% of patients with rheumatoid arthritis. Histologically, they fall into the necrobiotic category, resembling necrobiosis lipoidica and granuloma annulare. Subcutaneous nodules also occur in acute rheumatic fever. These lesions typically are found over bony prominences and are smaller and more transitory than the nodules of rheumatoid arthritis. Subcutaneous nodules in systemic lupus erythematosus are known as lupus profundus or lupus panniculitis. Subcutaneous inflammation may occur in both early morphea and progressive systemic sclerosis and may be referred to as morphea profunda (Chapter 47).

31. (F); 32. (F); 33. (T); 34. (F) Although all cutaneous blood vessels may be involved in leukocytoclastic vasculitis, the smaller, postcapillary vessels, particularly smaller venules, are primarily involved. Early lesions of leukocytoclastic vasculitis tend to occur on the lower extremities (as "palpable purpura"). In contrast with the skin lesions of the larger vessel vasculitides, the lesions of leukocytoclastic vasculitis tend to be more acute and self-limited (Chapter 67).

35. (T); 36. (F); 37. (F); 38. (F); 39. (F) Although their clinical appearances are distinctly different, necrobiosis lipoidica and granuloma annulare may frequently be difficult to distinguish histologically. Some of the histopathologic clues differentiating these conditions are as follows: mucin is more abundant in granuloma annulare; giant cells, vascular changes, and lipid deposits are more abundant in necrobiosis lipoidica (Chapters 46 and 47).

40. (F); 41. (T); 42. (F) Urticaria may be categorized as chronic when it has been present for more than 6 weeks. Patients with urticaria triggered by aspirin may also be sensitive to azo dyes (including tartrazine) and may have nasal polyps. Patients with asthma have an elevated incidence of aspirin intolerance (2% to 10% compared with 1% of the normal population). Cause of chronic urticaria can only rarely be identified (Chapter 41).

43. (T); 44. (T); 45. (F) Two major types of granules are present in polymorphonuclear leukocytes and are responsible for the killing and degradation of microorganisms, breakdown of collagen and other dermal components, and increasing vascular permeability. Azurophilic granules constitute 20% of all granules. They contain myeloperoxidase, acid hydrolases, neutral proteases, cationic proteins, and lysozyme. Specific granules (80%) are smaller and contain lysozyme, collagenase, alkaline phosphatase, and lactoferrin (Chapter 38).

46. A; 47. C; 48. B The hypereosinophilic syndrome is a severe disease, most commonly seen in men, with multiorgan system involvement and a high mortality rate if untreated. Peripheral blood eosinophilia and eosinophilic infiltration of internal organs occurs with involvement of the skin in 50% of patients. Cutaneous manifestations include papules, nodules, urticaria, angioedema, dermatographism, and, occasionally, mucosal ulcerations. Other organ systems involved may include the heart (with fibrosis, congestive heart failure, and abnor-

mal electrocardiogram), bone marrow, liver/spleen, lungs, and nervous system. Wells' syndrome, or eosinophilic cellulitis, is a more benign condition characterized by localized recurrent cellulitis-like swellings that spontaneously regress. Histopathologic examination reveals large collections of eosinophils associated with brightly eosinophilic amorphous material (flame figures), representing degenerated collagen and degranulated eosinophils. Peripheral eosinophilia may be present (Chapter 35).

49. B; **50.** D; **51.** A; **52.** D; **53.** D Pruritic urticarial papules and plaques of pregnancy (PUPPP) is a severely pruritic eruption typically occurring during the third trimester in primagravidas. The lesions have a predilection for the striae distensiae and are most frequently located on the abdomen and thighs. There is no reported associated fetal morbidity. Recurrence in subsequent pregnancies is unlikely. Herpes gestationis (HG) is also a pruritic dermatosis of pregnancy but is distinguished from PUPPP in several ways. It may occur at any point in pregnancy, with most cases appearing during the second trimester. The lesions are small vesicles or papulovesicles on an erythematous base. The abdomen is the most common site, but the eruption often extends to the extremities, chest, and back. Postpartum flares are frequent. Histology and direct immunofluorescence reveal a bullous pemphigoid–like pattern with linear C3 and IgG in the lamina lucida of the basement membrane zone. It is believed that the 180 kd bullous pemphigoid antigen may be identical to the antigen of HG. Circulating IgG directed against the basement membrane is measurable by indirect immunofluorescence in 25% of cases. Complement-fixing techniques increase this rate to 75%. Whether there is an increased risk of fetal morbidity in HG is the subject of considerable debate. Elevated urine chorionic gonadotropin levels have been reported in the papular dermatosis of pregnancy (of Spangler), a rare pruritic condition associated with a high incidence of fetal mortality (Chapter 37).

54. B; **55.** C; **56.** D Letterer-Siwe and Hand-Schüller-Christian diseases are both varieties in the spectrum of Langerhans cell histiocytoses (previously called histiocytosis X). Classically, Letterer-Siwe disease occurs in infants and manifests with erythematous papules and scaly nodules, frequently in the diaper area, trunk, or scalp, and may initially be confused with seborrheic dermatitis or candidiasis. Involvement of the liver, spleen, and other internal organs is typical, and the disease often takes an aggressive course. Hand-Schüller-Christian disease is classically characterized by the triad of exophthalmos, diabetes insipidus, and multiple lytic lesions in the skull. The constellation of hoarseness, parotitis, and eyelid papules is more typical for lipoid proteinosis (hyalinosis cutis et mucosae) (Chapter 155).

57. B; **58.** B; **59.** A Two major forms of cold urticaria are recognized. Essential acquired cold urticaria, which develops during adulthood, is the most common type. Associated hypotension and laryngeal edema are frequently associated findings. The lesions occur within minutes of exposure to cold, then resolve rapidly. Entire body cooling may be fatal. Familial cold urticaria, an extremely rare condition, may be distinguished from essential acquired cold urticaria in several ways. The onset is generally in infancy. The lesions classically occur some period of time following cold exposure and cause a burning sensation rather than itch and may last for more than 2 days. Chills, fever, and joint pains are often present as well (Chapter 41).

60. D; **61.** A; **62.** B; **63.** C All of the listed conditions involve dermal infiltrates by cells of granulocyte lineage. Halogenoderma (most importantly, bromoderma and iododerma) contain a dense infiltrate of neutrophils with nuclear dust, eosinophils, and extravasated erythrocytes. Later lesions include increasing numbers of lymphocytes and histiocytes. Epidermal changes are typically profound and include intraepidermal abscesses and pseudoepitheliomatous hyperplasia. Sweet's syndrome (acute febrile neutrophilic dermatosis) is characterized histologically by a dense perivascular infiltrate of neutrophils associated with prominent upper dermal edema. No vasculitis is seen. In contrast, erythema elevatum diutinum displays, in addition to a dense infiltrate of neutrophils, extensive vasculitis, granulation tissue, and fibrosis, as well as prominent extracellular lipid deposits, particularly cholesterol esters. The histology in granuloma faciale includes a dense infiltrate of eosinophils, with associated neutrophils, mononuclear cells, plasma cells, and mast cells. Vasculitis is observed (Chapter 38).

64. E; **65.** B; **66.** A; **67.** C Lupus pernio (of Besnier) describes the shiny smooth firm papules and plaques on the face and acral areas seen in sarcoidosis. Löfgren's syndrome is an acute variety of sarcoidosis that may manifest with hilar adenopathy, erythema nodosum, fever, arthralgia, and uveitis. It is more common among patients of Scandinavian descent. Sarcoidosis involving the subcutaneous tissues is referred to as Darier-Roussy sarcoid. Heerfordt's syndrome, or uveoparotid fever, is an unusual form of sarcoidosis that includes uveitis, parotid gland enlargement, and facial nerve palsy (Chapter 45).

68. E; **69.** A; **70.** A; **71.** E Giant cells in sarcoidosis may contain asteroid bodies or Schaumann's bodies. Asteroid bodies are stellate structures that stain best with phosphotungstic acid–hematoxylin. The centers stain brown-red, and the peripheral spikes stain blue. Asteroid bodies most likely arise from collagen that becomes trapped between epithelioid cells during granuloma formation. Asteroid bodies may be found in cat-scratch disease, tuberculosis, and a variety of other conditions. Schaumann's bodies are round or oval, calcified, and laminated. It appears that they develop from residual bodies of lysosomes. Farber's bodies are comma-shaped curvilinear bodies (lipid-containing vacuoles) found in lipogranulomatosis (Farber's disease). Henderson-Patterson bodies are large intracytoplasmic inclusion bodies, characteristic for molluscum contagiosum. Birbeck's granules are lamellar tennis racquet–shaped bodies present within Langerhans cells that are formed by invaginations of the cell membrane (Chapter 45).

72. C; **73.** A; **74.** E; **75.** B Introduction of a variety of exogenous substances into the skin may lead to a spectrum of granulomatous foreign body responses. Injection of oils (e.g., mineral oil) lead to the characteristic "Swiss cheese" appearance of paraffinoma, in which fibrotic strands of connective tissue surround large cavities containing oily material that stain positive with Oil Red O and Sudan IV. Starch granulomas occur when wounds are contaminated with powder from surgical gloves (containing cornstarch). Starch granules are found within giant cells and are PAS and methenamine silver–positive. The granules are also birefringent by polariscopic examination, displaying a Maltese cross–like pattern. Foreign body reactions to zirconium in underarm deodorants results from an allergic sensitization to zirconium. The histologic picture resembles that of sarcoidosis; spectrographic analysis may be needed to confirm the presence of zirconium. Old fluorescent light bulbs contained an interior beryllium coating. Traumatic injuries involving this glass led to lacerations with a necrotic appearance clinically and histologically. Silica granuloma results from the introduction of silica (from soil or glass) into the skin. Although the histologic pattern is similar to that of sarcoidosis, polarizable particles of differing sizes can be found within giant cells (Chapter 48).

76. B; **77.** E Granulomatous reactions to tattoos are not common. The most common dye causing a hypersensitivity reaction is cinnabar red, which contains mercuric sulfide. Other, less common, causes of hypersensitivity reactions are chrome green and cobalt blue. Photosensitivity reactions to tattoo pigments occur most frequently with cadmium yellow, which is occasionally also used to enhance the brightness of red tattoos (Chapter 48).

78. D; **79.** C; **80.** E; **81.** C The non-X (non-Langerhans cell) histiocytoses include a variety of conditions ranging from benign to fulminant and life-threatening. Benign cephalic histiocytosis is a benign proliferation of histiocytes containing comma-shaped bodies that occurs on the face in infants. The lesions resolve spontaneously. In multicentric reticulohistiocytosis, red-brown nodules appear on the hands and fingers, arms, scalp, face, neck, and mucous membranes. Polyarthritis and arthralgias are frequently present, and the arthritis may progress to the severely deforming arthritis mutilans. Multiple internal organs may likewise be involved. Spontaneous resolution and death have both been reported. In sinus histiocytosis with massive lymphadenopathy (Rosai-Dorfman syndrome) patients present with fever, massive adenopathy (usually cervical), leukocytosis, and an elevated sedimentation rate. Widespread yellow-brown papules and nodules occur in 10% of patients. Comma-shaped bodies are present on electron microscopic examination (Chapter 154).

Bibliography

Callen JP. Cutaneous vasculitis: relationship to systemic disease and therapy. Curr Probl Dermatol 1993; 5:45–80.
Cooper KD. Urticaria and angioedema: diagnosis and evaluation. J Am Acad Dermatol 1991; 25:166–174.
Duguid CM, Powell FC. Pyoderma gangrenosum. Clin Dermatol 1993; 11:129–133.
Goh CL. Eosinophilic cellulitis (Wells' syndrome). Int J Dermatol 1992; 31:429–430.
Hanno R, Saleeby ER, Krull EA. Disorders of pregnancy. Clin Dermatol 1994; Unit 29-1:1–15.
Lever WF, Schaumberg-Lever G. Histopathology of the Skin. Philadelphia: JB Lippincott, 1990.
Lowitt MH, Dover JS. Necrobiosis lipoidica. J Am Acad Dermatol 1991; 25:735–748.
Mehregan DR, Hall MJ, Gibson LE. Urticarial vasculitis: a histopathologic and clinical review of 72 cases. J Am Acad Dermatol 1992; 26:441–448.
Samtsov AV. Cutaneous sarcoidosis. Int J Dermatol 1992; 31:385–391.
Schwartz LB. Mast cells and their role in urticaria. J Am Acad Dermatol 1991; 25:190–203.
von den Driesch P. Sweet's syndrome (acute febrile neutrophilic dermatosis). J Am Acad Dermatol 1994; 31:535–556.

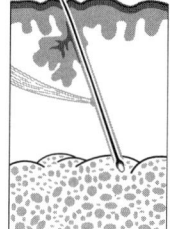

chapter 8

Follicular Inflammation and Inflammation of Cartilage

HEIDI ANN WALDORF

HAIR FOLLICLE AND APPENDAGEAL INFLAMMATORY DISEASES

For each of the following questions, decide whether EACH choice is TRUE or FALSE. Any combination of answers from all true to all false may occur.

1. Regarding sebaceous glands,
   A. Sebaceous glands are distributed over the entire surface of the body
   B. The density is highest on the face and scalp
   C. The largest sebaceous glands are found on the face
   D. In the pilosebaceous unit, sebaceous gland size varies directly with the size of the associated hair.

2. Regarding sebum,
   A. Secretion is holocrine
   B. Sebum production begins at puberty
   C. Sebum secretion is continuous
   D. Sebum lipids are derived predominantly from the circulation
   E. On the face, most surface lipid is derived from sebum.

3. To quantitate absolute sebum production,
   A. Apply cigarette paper to the skin for 3 hours followed by gravimetric analysis
   B. Apply cigarette paper to the skin for 12 hours followed by gravimetric analysis
   C. Apply bentonite gel (15% bentonite clay and 0.2% carboxymethylcellulose) for 3 hours followed by thin-layer chromatography
   D. Apply bentonite gel (15% bentonite clay and 0.2% carboxymethylcellulose) for 12 hours followed by thin-layer chromatography
   E. Apply an oil red O stain and visual image analysis.

4. Special characteristics of sebaceous gland fatty acids include
   A. The predominant chain length is 16 carbons
   B. Both odd- and even-numbered chain lengths occur
   C. Double bonds are most common between the sixth and seventh carbons in unsaturated acids ($\Delta 6$-unsaturated acids)
   D. Methyl-branching of saturated acids is relatively common.

5. Regarding the regulation of sebum production,
   A. Progesterone is inhibitory in physiologic doses
   B. The primary direct stimulatory effect is androgenic
   C. Sebaceous glands are unresponsive to neurotransmitters
   D. Exogenous estrogens can lower sebum secretion
   E. Pituitary hormones may exert a stimulatory effect.

6. Factors in the pathogenesis of acne include
   A. *Propionibacterium acnes*
   B. Free fatty acid formation
   C. Retention hyperkeratosis
   D. Diet
   E. Dihydrotestosterone.

7. Regarding comedonal acne,
   A. Comedonal acne is more frequent in younger patients
   B. Closed comedones are precursors of inflammatory acne
   C. Inflammatory acne is always preceded by comedonal acne
   D. Sebaceous gland enlargement is frequently seen in comedones
   E. The black color of open comedones is derived from oxidized lipid materials.

8. Appropriate therapy for comedonal acne may include
   A. Topical tretinoin
   B. Benzoyl peroxide
   C. Systemic tetracycline
   D. Comedone extraction
   E. Aggressive cleansing.

9. Regarding the mechanism of action of tetracycline and its derivatives, these drugs
   A. Suppress *P. acnes*
   B. Reduce sebum secretion
   C. Decrease the concentration of free fatty acids
   D. Suppress end-organ sensitivity of sebaceous glands to androgens
   E. Correct follicular keratinization.

10. An obese 16-year-old female presents with a 4-year history of progressively worsening acne unresponsive to several courses of systemic antibiotic treatment. On physical examination, she has ice-pick scarring of the cheeks, few closed comedones, and multiple inflammatory papules, cysts, and large nodules on the face and upper trunk. Important additional information to obtain from the history before prescribing therapy should include
    A. History of sexual activity
    B. Menstrual history
    C. Contact lens use
    D. Topical treatment regimen
    E. Family history of coronary artery disease.

11. Concerning the mechanism of action of oral isotretinoin in acne,
    A. Sebum suppression is noted within the first 2 weeks of treatment
    B. Sebum secretion is reduced indefinitely
    C. Isotretinoin is bactericidal to *P. acnes* in vitro
    D. The elimination of corneocyte debris is expedited
    E. Chemotaxis of neutrophils is inhibited in vitro.

12. Clinical side effects of isotretinoin therapy may include
    A. Cheilitis
    B. Diarrhea
    C. Pseudotumor cerebri
    D. Hair loss
    E. Cutaneous staphylococcal infections.

13. Regarding dermabrasion of acne scars,
    A. Postoperative erythema and telangiectases may last for months
    B. Dermabrasion is most effective if done within 4 weeks of the completion of isotretinoin therapy
    C. Dermabrasion is the therapy of choice for deep ice-pick scars
    D. History of recurrent cold sores is a contraindication to dermabrasion
    E. Patients who have undergone x-ray irradiation for severe acne are good candidates for dermabrasion.

14. Regarding steroid-acne,
    A. Histologically, hyperkeratinization is prominent
    B. Lesions are predominantly cystic

C. Lesions are predominantly comedonal

D. Scarring is unusual

E. Lesions often arise within 2 weeks of steroid use.

15. Characteristics of acne conglobata include:

    A. More males than females are affected

    B. Coagulase-positive staphylococci are frequently isolated from lesions

    C. Comedones are absent

    D. Systemic corticosteroids are often indicated

    E. The nodulocystic component subsides after adolescence.

16. Acne conglobata has been associated with

    A. Hidradenitis suppurativa

    B. Basal cell epithelioma

    C. Dissecting cellulitis of the scalp

    D. Pilonidal cysts

    E. Squamous cell carcinoma.

17. A 15-year-old boy presents with acute onset of painful, highly inflammatory nodules on the back and chest that ulcerate and form necrotic plaques. Supportive of a diagnosis of acne fulminans is (are)

    A. Polyarthralgia

    B. Leukocytosis

    C. Osteolytic bone lesions

    D. Polyporous comedones

    E. History of anabolic steroid use.

18. Effective in the therapy of nodulocystic acne is (are)

    A. Cryotherapy

    B. Systemic corticosteroids

    C. Intralesional corticosteroids

    D. Dapsone

    E. Isotretinoin.

19. A 13-year-old girl presents with mild papulopustular acne. Appropriate topical antibiotic(s) for her treatment regimen is (are)

    A. Gentamicin

    B. Clindamycin

    C. Erythromycin

    D. Mupirocin

    E. Minocycline.

20. A 25-year-old man presents with facial hypertrichosis, milia and bullae on the dorsum of his hands, and acneiform sinuses, nodules, and scars on his trunk and extremities. Exposure to which of the following could give rise to this constellation of findings?

    A. Polyhalogenated naphthalenes

    B. Potassium dichromate

    C. Polychlorinated dibenzodioxins

    D. Polymethyl methacrylate

    E. Pramoxine hydrochloride.

21. A 35-year-old woman presents complaining of recent development of acneiform papules and pustules on her upper trunk and, to a lesser extent, her face. A history of which of the following may be relevant?

    A. Seizure disorder

    B. Health food diet

    C. Asthma

    D. Hepatitis

    E. Depression.

22. Laser treatment of erythrotelangiectatic rosacea might involve the

    A. Pulsed-dye laser

    B. Carbon dioxide laser

    C. Q-switched ruby laser

    D. Argon laser

    E. Q-switched Nd:YAG laser.

23. Rosacea-related flushing may be aggravated by

    A. Caffeine

    B. Ultraviolet radiation

    C. Alcohol

    D. Isordil

    E. Clonidine.

24. Clinical expressions of rosacea may include

    A. Telangiectasia

    B. Comedones

    C. Pustules

    D. Edema

    E. Granuloma.

25. Ophthalmic manifestations of rosacea may include

    A. Blepharitis

    B. Conjunctivitis

C. Iritis

D. Keratitis

E. Blindness.

26. Which of the following oral contraceptive preparations is (are) likely to improve acne?

　A. Ethinyl estradiol (35 μg) with ethynodiol diacetate (1.0 μg)

　B. Ethinyl estradiol (50 μg) with ethynodiol diacetate (1.0 μg)

　C. Ethinyl estradiol (30 μg) with norgestrel (0.3 μg)

　D. Mestranol (100 μg) with ethynodiol diacetate (1.0 μg)

　E. Mestranol (100 μg) with norethynodrel (2.5 μg)

For each numbered item, choose the most likely associated lettered item. Each numbered item has ONLY ONE answer. Each lettered item may be the answer to one, more than one, or none of the numbered items.

For each of the following descriptions, choose the most appropriate lettered item.

27. Essential fatty acid
28. Marker for sebum
29. Marker for surface epidermal lipid
30. Circulating lipid incorporated into differentiated sebocytes
31. Implicated in follicular hyperkeratosis.

　A. Linoleic acid
　B. Δ 6-unsaturated acid
　C. Cholesterol
　D. Squalene
　E. None of the above.

For each of the systemic medications used to treat acne listed below, choose the side effect that has been most closely associated with its use.

32. Minocycline
33. Erythromycin
34. Estradiol
35. Dapsone
36. Clindamycin.

　A. Hemolytic anemia
　B. Pseudomembranous colitis
　C. Thromboembolism
　D. Mucosal pigmentation
　E. Cardiac arrhythmia.

For each of the acne variants listed below, choose the exposure with which it is most strongly linked.

37. Acne estivalis
38. Acne varioliformis
39. Acne keloidalis nuchae
40. Acne venenata
41. Acne fulminans.

　A. Coal tar
　B. Estrogen
　C. Ultraviolet radiation
　D. Anabolic steroids
　E. None of the above.

Match each of the following descriptions with the appropriate lettered item.

42. May decrease sebum secretion 30% to 50%
43. 5 α-Reductase inhibitor
44. Androgen receptor inhibitor
45. May produce gynecomastia in men
46. Directly inhibits conversion of testosterone to dihydrotestosterone.

　A. Cyproterone acetate
　B. Spironolactone
　C. Cimetidine
　D. A and B
　E. All of the above
　F. None of the above.

Match each of the following descriptions with the appropriate lettered item.

47. Grouped hyperkeratotic follicular papules on the neck and trunk
48. Atopic diathesis
49. Childhood onset typical
50. Follicular plugging.

　A. Keratosis pilaris
　B. Lichen spinulosus
　C. Lichen nitidus
　D. A and B
　E. B and C.

For each of the following causes of neonatal vesicles, choose the characteristic finding on cytologic examination of a smear made from a typical vesicle.

51. Erythema toxicum neonatorum
52. Transient neonatal pustular melanosis
53. Herpes simplex virus infection
54. Miliaria crystallina
55. Impetigo neonatorum.

　A. Neutrophils
　B. Eosinophils
　C. Bacteria
　D. Multinucleated giant cells
　E. None of the above.

Match each of the following disorders with the primary site of pathogenicity.

56. Hidradenitis suppurativa

　A. Sebaceous gland
　B. Apocrine gland

57. Acne conglobata
58. Miliaria pustulosa
59. Pseudofolliculitis barbae
60. Fox-Fordyce disease.

C. Eccrine gland
D. None of the above.

Match each of the following descriptions with the appropriate lettered item.

61. Comedones predominate
62. Affects women more frequently than men
63. May be associated with topical steroid abuse
64. Demodex folliculorum mites are the cause
65. First-line therapy includes topical tretinoin.

A. Acne rosacea
B. Perioral dermatitis
C. A and B
D. None of the above.

PERFORATING DISORDERS

For each of the following questions, decide whether EACH choice is TRUE or FALSE. Any combination of answers from all true to all false may occur.

66. A 15-year-old boy presents with an annular plaque on the nape of the neck. On closer examination, the plaque consists of a ring of erythematous, 2- to 3-mm papules, each with a tightly adherent keratotic plug. Biopsy reveals narrow channels filled with degenerated elastic fibers and keratotic debris. Which of the following statements regarding the appropriate workup and treatment of this patient are true and which are false?
    A. A potassium hydroxide (KOH) examination of a scraping from the lesions may be helpful before performing a biopsy
    B. Dermabrasion is the treatment of choice
    C. Histopathologic diagnosis is confirmed with acid orcein stain
    D. Glucose tolerance testing is critical
    E. The patient should be warned that widespread dissemination of lesions is likely.

67. A 2-year-old girl presents with a 3-week history of several 3- to 4-mm umbilicated keratotic papules in a linear array on the forearm. Biopsy reveals basophilic collagen and keratotic debris within a cup-shaped depression in the epidermis. Which of the following statements regarding the patient's disease are true and which are false?
    A. Hypertrophic scarring is likely
    B. Acid orcein or resorcin-fuchsin stains are helpful
    C. This disorder is often associated with Down syndrome
    D. Spontaneous resolution is the rule
    E. Glucose tolerance testing is critical.

For each numbered item choose the most likely associated lettered item. Each numbered item has ONLY ONE answer. Within each group, each lettered item may be the answer to one, more than one, or none of the numbered items.

Match each of the following histopathologic descriptions with the appropriate diagnosis.

68. Formation of hyperplastic elastic fibers in dermal papillae
69. Hyperkeratotic plug in hair follicle containing a curled-up hair
70. Calcified, short, elastic fibers in the reticular dermis
71. Trauma-induced subepidermal foci of necrobiotic basophilic collagen
72. Foci of dyskeratotic, rapidly proliferating cells in the epidermis.

A. Kyrle's disease
B. Perforating folliculitis
C. Elastosis perforans serpiginosa
D. Reactive perforating collagenosis
E. None of the above.

Match each of the following with the disease with which it is most closely associated.

73. Down syndrome
74. Chronic renal failure
75. Penicillamine
76. Arthopod bite
77. Osteogenesis imperfecta.

A. Acquired perforating disease
B. Elastosis perforans serpiginosa
C. Reactive perforating collagenosis.

INFLAMMATION OF CARTILAGE

For each of the following questions, a set of lettered headings is followed by a list of numbered words or phrases. For each numbered word or phrase, choose

- A. If the item is associated with A only
- B. If the item is associated with B only
- C. If the item is associated with both A and B
- D. If the item is associated with neither A nor B.

For each of the following characteristics, choose whether it describes chondrodermatitis nodularis helicis, relapsing polychondritis, both, or neither.

78. The ear lobe is typically uninvolved
79. Nasal chondritis is common
80. Immunity to type 2 collagen may play a pathogenic role
81. Elevation in erythrocyte sedimentation rate is common
82. Cartilage is frequently normal.

A. Chondrodermatitis nodularis helicis
B. Relapsing polychondritis
C. Both
D. Neither.

ANSWERS

HAIR FOLLICLE AND APPENDAGEAL INFLAMMATORY DISEASES

1. A (F); B (T); C (T); D (F) Sebaceous glands are located on all skin surfaces except the palms, soles, and dorsa of the feet. The density of sebaceous glands is highest on the face and scalp (400 to 900 glands/cm^2) and lowest on the extremities (0 to 100 glands/cm^2). In general, the size of a sebaceous gland varies inversely with the diameter of its associated hair. There are three types of pilosebaceous units. Sebaceous follicles are composed of a tiny vellus hair and large, multilobular sebaceous glands. These follicles are largest and most numerous on the face, but are also found on the ear lobes, neck, and upper trunk. The duct of a sebaceous follicle joins the hair follicle near the base. Sebaceous follicles are the critical structure in the development of acne. They are particularly susceptible because of their deep, wide follicular canal, small hair unit, and large sebaceous glands.

Like sebaceous follicles, the size of the sebaceous gland in vellus follicles is disproportionately large compared with the associated hair. However, as a result of duct insertion higher in the hair canal and a small follicular orifice, vellus follicles are not involved in acne. Vellus follicles are the most common type of pilosebaceous unit on the face.

The terminal follicles of the scalp and beard are the exception, containing a stiff, wide, long hair and a large sebaceous gland. The steady growth of the hair and wide diameter relative to the follicular lumen enables the canal to remain relatively free of corneocyte debris (Chapter 49).

2. A (T); B (F); C (T); D (F); E (T) Sebum secretion is holocrine. As the outer layer of undifferentiated sebocytes proliferate, they are forced to migrate centripetally. During this process, the cytoplasm fills with lipid-containing vacuoles, increasing cell volume more than 100-fold. The vacuoles enlarge and fuse with each other. Ultimately, the mature, lipid-laden sebocytes rupture, releasing lipid and the remnants of their organelles and cell membrane into the sebaceous duct. The process is continuous: it takes 2 to 3 weeks for an undifferentiated cell to reach the skin surface as sebum. Sebaceous glands are functional from their formation in the 13th to 15th gestational week. They reach peak activity during the third trimester under the influence of maternal and fetal androgens. This secretion accounts for the vernix caseosa, which is the white material that covers babies at birth. It contains fatty acids, squalene, and wax esters such as sebum and also sterol and sterol esters. The sebaceous glands remain active in the neonatal period, accounting for neonatal acne; however, shortly after birth, the glands involute as androgen levels decline (surface lipid reaches low levels at approximately 6 months). The glands redevelop between ages 7 and 8 at the time of adrenarche. They reach peak development and activity in the mid to late teens. Sebaceous glands synthesize the majority of their secreted lipids de novo. Endogenous lipids include a variety of unusual fatty acids characterized by odd and even chains (predominantly C14, C16, and C18), saturated and unsaturated acids, both with methyl-branching and Δ6-unsaturated acids. Cholesterol, linoleic acid, and Δ9-unsaturated fatty acids are not produced by differentiated sebocytes (although cholesterol and D9-fatty acids may be produced by undifferentiated cells) and may be taken up at cell division during formation of new cell membranes. Once differentiation occurs, no circulating lipid is incorporated into the cell. Evidence of their minor role is based on the proportional decrease in exogenous lipids compared with endogenous lipids with increasing sebaceous gland activity. In sebaceous gland–rich skin, greater than 95% of the surface lipid is derived from the sebaceous glands (Chapter 49).

3. A (F); B (T); C (F); D (T); E (F) Absorbent materials, including cigarette paper, bentonite clay, and absorbent tape, are used experimentally to collect skin lipids. The materials are then analyzed, using a gravimetric method (cigarette paper) or thin-layer chromatography (bentonite clay or absorbent tape). Because excretory ducts of sebaceous glands contain a significant amount of preformed sebum, the collection material must be left in place for 12 to 14 hours in order to deplete this reservoir and reach a constant rate of sebum absorption. A shorter collection time may be used for comparative purposes of sebum excretion.

Oil red O stains lipids orange to bright red on frozen or formalin-fixed tissue. It is useful to locate lipids in sebocytes in routine histologic sections. It is also used in rabbit ear comedogenicity tests: epidermal sheets from the ear canal can be stained with oil red O and studied with image analysis to determine the surface area covered with comedones (Chapter 49).

4. A (T); B (T); C (T); D (T) Sebaceous gland lipids include a variety of unusual fatty acids that differentiate them from lipids produced in other tissues. Although odd-chained fatty acids are uncommon elsewhere, sebaceous gland acids are characterized by both odd and even chains (predominantly C14, C16, and C18). The predominant double-bond site in the unsaturated fatty acids is between carbons 6 and 7 (Δ6-unsaturated) rather than the usual site between carbons 9 and 10 (Δ9-unsaturated). In the saturated fatty acids, a relatively high proportion of methyl-branching is found (Chapter 49).

5. A (F); B (T); C (T); D (T); E (T) The development and secretory activity of sebaceous glands is androgen-dependent. Levels of adrenal and gonadal androgens decline shortly after birth, increase in adolescence, and reach a peak in the mid to late teen years. Androgen levels are normally higher in men than women, declining after menopause in women and after the seventh decade of life in men. Exogenous administration of testosterone in children, eunuchs, or postmenopausal women increases sebum secretion. Orchiectomy reduces sebum production. The adrenal androgen, dehydroepiandrosterone, appears to be the critical sebogenic stimulus prepuberty. Postpuberty sebum production relies on testosterone.

Estrogen opposes the effect of androgens, apparently by inhibiting the uptake of testosterone and its conversion to dihydrotestosterone by the sebaceous glands. Progesterone in physiologic amounts has no effect on sebaceous glands. At supraphysiologic doses, progesterone may increase sebum production. Sebaceous glands, with the exception of the Meibomian glands, are not innervated and do not respond to exogenous neurotransmitters such as acetylcholine and norepinephrine. Pituitary hormones, such as growth hormone, melanocyte-stimulating hormone, and prolactin, have been shown to be sebogenic in animals and may act synergistically to optimize end-organ response to androgens. Indeed, untreated acromegalics have increased sebum production. Thyroid hormone and adrenal cortisol have also been implicated in the control of sebaceous gland function (Chapter 49).

6. A (T); B (T); C (T); D (F); E (T) Acne is a multifactorial disease. The primary alteration occurs in the pattern of keratinization in the sebaceous follicle in the lower portion of the infundibulum. Increased cohesion between corneocytes and an increased follicular epithelial cell turnover result in retarded desquamation, impaction at the follicular orifice, and microcomedone formation. Ultrastructurally, the corneocytes are notable for increased keratohyaline granules, decreased lamellar granules, and the intracellular formation of lipid granules. As retained cells block the follicular orifice, sebum and vellus hair fragments are trapped, and the anaerobic diphtheroid, *P. acnes,* proliferates. Sebum is comedogenic and proinflammatory. Microbial lipases, predominantly from *P. acnes,* convert sebaceous triglycerides into free fatty acids, which are chemotactic for neutrophils. *P. acnes* may also secrete chemotactic factors and activate complement pathways. As the inflammatory response ensues, neutrophils ingest *P. acnes.* Hydrolytic enzymes are released that produce follicular epithelial damage and rupture. Sebaceous follicles are particularly susceptible to this process. Patients with acne tend to have larger sebaceous glands and produce more sebum. Although plasma levels of testosterone are normal in most acne patients, there is a marked increased conversion of testosterone to dihydrotestosterone in the skin of both men and women with acne. Androgens stimulate sebaceous glands to produce sebum. Although total fasting decreases sebum production, there is no evidence that diet influences acne (Chapter 49).

7. A (T); B (T); C (F); D (T); E (F) Comedonal acne is often the first expression of adrenarche in prepubertal children. Closed comedones (whiteheads) either gradually enlarge into open comedones (blackheads) or rupture and incite an inflammatory response. Open comedones may remain stable for years or may form secondary comedones (cysts, fistulated comedones, draining sinus) through recurrent focal rupture, abscess formation, and re-encapsulation. As comedones enlarge, the sebaceous glands gradually regress, and the ducts are integrated into the comedone wall. Inflammatory acne lesions frequently arise from microcomedones before true comedones are clinically apparent. The dark cap of open comedones consists of giant melanosomes transferred into the extruded corneocytes from the cells of the apical infundibulum and interfollicular epidermis. Closed comedones and the lower portion of open comedones are nonpigmented (Chapter 49).

8. A (T); B (T); C (F); D (T); E (F) Comedonal acne is best managed with topical tretinoin because of its keratolytic effect. The primary effect of benzoyl peroxide is antibiotic; however, it also has a mild comedolytic effect. Salicylic acid, α-hydroxy acid, and azelaic acid may also act as comedolytics. The adjuvant use of a comedone extractor facilitates clearing.

Vigorous cleansing, including the use of abrasive cleansers, is not useful in acne because the site of primary obstruction is the infrainfundibulum, not the orifice, of the follicle. Indeed, excessive scrubbing can increase inflammation. Oral antibiotics, such as tetracycline and erythromycin, are most useful for inflammatory, not comedonal, acne (Chapter 49).

9. A (T); B (F); C (T); D (F); E (F) Like erythromycin, tetracycline is bacteriostatic, not bactericidal, to *P. acnes*. In high doses, systemic tetracycline reduces the population of *P. acnes* up to 50%. Perhaps more important to its therapeutic role, tetracycline has anti-inflammatory activity by reducing the concentration of free fatty acids and other proinflammatory products of the bacteria. Topical antibiotics have a similar mechanism; however, they are limited by cutaneous absorption. Systemic doxycycline and minocycline are more lipophilic and therefore have better penetration into the sebaceous follicle. Tetracyclines have no effect on sebum production, androgen sensitivity, or follicular keratinization (Chapter 49).

10. A (T); B (T); C (T); D (T); E (T) The described patient has severe, recalcitrant, scarring acne and will likely require oral isotretinoin. Because isotretinoin is teratogenic, it is critical prior to treatment to establish the sexual history and history of contraceptive use of any female patient of childbearing years. Effective contraception must be in use for at least 1 month and a negative serum pregnancy test or a negative urine pregnancy test with a sensitivity of at least 50 mU/ml must be obtained within 1 week prior to beginning therapy. The most common side effect of isotretinoin use is dryness of the skin and mucous membranes. Thus topical astringents and keratolytics should be discontinued. Contact lens use may also have to be discontinued during therapy because of discomfort or blepharoconjunctivitis. Isotretinoin may also induce an elevation of triglycerides and a decline in high-density lipoproteins. Patients with a strong family history of coronary artery disease or hyperlipidemia, but who are unaffected themselves, may be given isotretinoin with close follow-up. Women with recalcitrant acne associated with hirsutism, obesity, or menstrual abnormalities may have increased androgen levels. Endocrine evaluation for polycystic ovary disease or tumors of the ovaries or adrenal glands should be instigated if suggested by the history and physical examination. Laboratory studies should include total testosterone, free testosterone, and dihydroepiandrosterone sulfate (Chapter 49).

11. A (T); B (F); C (F); D (T); E (T) Oral isotretinoin causes a rapid, dose-dependent suppression of sebum secretion that reaches almost 90% after 3 months of therapy at a dose of 1.0 mg/kg body weight. Despite the profound inhibition during therapy, sebum production gradually returns to pretreatment levels 10 to 12 months after discontinuance of therapy in the majority of patients. Isotretinoin does not kill bacteria directly. Rather, the reduction in *P. acnes* as well as gram-negative organisms noted is explained by the reduction of intrafollicular lipids necessary for bacterial growth. Although the precise mechanism is unknown, isotretinoin improves corneocyte turnover and dehiscence. In vitro, serum from patients on isotretinoin inhibits neutrophil chemotaxis. In vivo, an anti-inflammatory effect is evidenced clinically by the reduction of edema, erythema, and inflammatory lesions (Chapter 49).

12. A (T); B (F); C (T); D (T); E (T) Almost all patients treated with isotretinoin complain of cheilitis. Other common symptoms related to skin and mucous membrane dryness include xerosis, epistaxis, conjunctivitis, and pruritus. Less common side effects include hair thinning, headache, pyogenic granuloma formation, and bone and joint pain. Disseminated interstitial skeletal hyperostosis is a rare radiologic finding and is generally asymptomatic. Pseudotumor cerebri, or benign intracranial hypertension, may be dose-dependent and should be ruled out in a patient complaining of unusual neurologic symptoms. The risk of pseudotumor cerebri increases if tetracycline and isotretinoin are used in combination. Isotretinoin may promote colonization and impetiginization with *Staphylococcus aureus* (Chapter 49).

13. A (T); B (F); C (F); D (F); E (F) Common complications of dermabrasion include hyper- and hypopigmentation, milia, keloids, persistent erythema, and telangiectasia. Atypical keloid formation has been reported in patients undergoing dermabrasion within 6 months of isotretinoin therapy. Dermabrasion can eliminate shallow, well-demarcated acne scars, including shallow ice-pick scars and can soften the edges of rolling scars. Dermabrasion alone will not improve and may worsen the appearance of deep, ice-pick type of scars. These scars require a tissue replacement technique, such as scar revision excision, punch elevation, or punch grafting, prior to dermabrasion. An active herpes simplex infection is a contraindication to dermabrasion. Patients with a history suggestive of herpes simplex infection, but without active lesions, should be placed on oral acyclovir prophylactically for several days before dermabrasion and until the skin has re-epithelialized. Chronic radiodermatitis, which may be seen in patients who have undergone x-ray therapy for facial acne, is usually a relative contraindication to dermabrasion (Chapter 49).

14. A (F); B (F); C (F); D (T); E (T) Steroid acne may arise within 2 weeks of systemic steroid use or after prolonged topical steroid use. Steroid-induced acne differs from acne vulgaris in distribution and lesion morphology. The lesions are predominantly monomorphic papules and pustules concentrated on the upper trunk with lesser involvement of the face. Histology reveals a focal folliculitis without prominent hyperkeratosis (Chapter 49).

15. A (T); B (T); C (F); D (T); E (F) Acne conglobata is most commonly seen in men with onset in adolescence. Although comedones, papules, and pustules are present, nodules and cysts predominate with formation of abscesses, sinus tracts, and scars. The inflammatory lesions are tender and often have foul-smelling drainage. Cultures of purulent drainage often reveal coagulase-positive staphylococci in addition to resident coagulase-negative staphylococci and anaerobic diphtheroids. Polyporous comedones are characteristic in long-standing acne conglobata secondary to scarring. Systemic corticosteroids are often required concomitant to isotretinoin in order to avoid a severe flare during the first weeks of therapy. Without treatment, the disease tends to run a recalcitrant, chronic course (Chapter 49).

16. A (T); B (F); C (T); D (T); E (T) The follicular occlusion tetrad refers to hidradenitis suppurativa, acne conglobata, dissecting cellulitis of the scalp, and pilonidal cyst formation. These diseases are characterized by chronic follicular inflammation with sinus tract formation. Well-differentiated squamous cell carcinoma has been reported arising in lesions of acne conglobata and hidradenitis suppurativa. There is no association with basal cell carcinoma (Chapters 49 and 50).

17. A (T); B (T); C (T); D (F); E (T) Acne fulminans describes the abrupt development over days to weeks of ulcerative nodulocystic acne lesions on the trunk of teenage males. The onset of acne is associated with fever, arthritis, arthralgias, and myalgias. Associated physical findings include joint swelling and splenomegaly. Laboratory work-up may reveal leukocytosis, elevated erythrocyte sedimentation rate, and proteinuria. Osteolytic lesions may be seen on x-ray in areas of tenderness. Iatrogenically induced androgen excess with testosterone therapy or anabolic steroids can trigger acne fulminans or acne conglobata. Polyporous or fistulated comedones are not seen in acne fulminans. These lesions develop over years as the result of recurrent rupture and re-encapsulation and are typical of acne conglobata (Chapter 49).

18. A (T); B (T); C (T); D (T); E (T) Systemic antibiotics are the mainstay of inflammatory acne treatment. When acne is recalcitrant to antibiotics, isotretinoin is the treatment of choice in patients without contraindications (see answer to Question 10). Systemic glucocorticoids have an adjunctive role as an anti-inflammatory agent at the start of isotretinoin therapy or as a sebosuppressant in combination with estrogens. Intralesional injection of a glucocorticosteroid can markedly shrink nodules and cysts. Local cryotherapy is used less commonly but can shrink deep nodules. Dapsone in doses of 50 to 200 mg/day may be used for severe nodulocystic acne if isotretinoin is contraindicated (Chapter 49).

19. A (F); B (T); C (T); D (F); E (F) Topical formulations of erythromycin, clindamycin, tetracycline, and benzoyl peroxide have antibacterial action in acne (see answer to Question 9). Minocycline is not available in topical form. Mupirocin is indicated for localized staphylococcal infections, but does not play a primary role in acne therapy (Chapter 49).

20. A (T); B (F); C (F); D (F); E (F) The constellation of symptoms described suggests the diagnosis of chloracne. Chloracne is induced by contact with halogenated hydrocarbons, including polyhalogenated naphthalenes, polyhalogenated biphenyls, polyhalogenated dibenzofurons, dioxins, azobenzenes, and azoxybenzenes. Initial exposure causes an acute chemical burn. Within weeks, pustules, nodules, and secondary comedones develop. Long-term inflammation results in massive scarring. Severe exposure may be complicated by liver disease, including porphyria cutanea tarda, as suggested by the hypertrichosis, vesicles, and milia in this patient. The pulmonary and central nervous system may also be affected.

Potassium dichromate is present in tanned leathers and may cause an allergic or irritant contact dermatitis. Polymethyl methacrylate is an acrylate polymer used in synthetic resins and is a common contact sensitizer. Pramoxine hydrochloride is a topical anesthetic (Chapter 49).

21. A (T); B (T); C (T); D (T); E (T) Phenytoin, lithium carbonate, prednisone, and isoniazid, used for seizure disorder, depression, asthma, and hepatitis, respectively, have all been reported to induce acneiform lesions. A health food diet is of interest if the patient ingests large quantities of kelp, high in iodine, or some vitamins, including B_1 or D. The acne lesions in these cases are generally monomorphic papulopustules on the upper trunk with relative sparing of the face (Chapter 49).

22. A (T); B (F); C (F); D (T); E (F) Patients with erythrotelangiectatic rosacea complain of prominent facial telangiectases and persistent erythema without a significant inflammatory component. These patients may benefit from laser therapy of telangiectases. Of the lasers listed, only the pulsed-dye and argon lasers are appropriate therapies for telangiectases. The carbon dioxide laser has been used to excise the hypertrophic tissue of rhinophyma, a complication of advanced rosacea. Q-switched ruby and Q-switched Nd:YAG lasers are effective in the removal of tattoos and do not play a role in the therapy for rosacea (Chapter 51).

23. A (F); B (T); C (T); D (T); E (F) Contrary to folklore, the cause of flushing following ingestion of hot coffee or tea is not the caffeine but the heat. Susceptible individuals challenged with hot and cold coffee, hot water, and caffeine only flush with the hot liquids. Ultraviolet radiation as well as extremes of temperature induce flushing. Alcoholic beverages and spicy foods aggravate flushing, perhaps by stimulating the release of neurotransmitters. Vasodilatory drugs, including nitrites and calcium channel blockers, worsen flushing in affected individuals. Clonidine, an α_2-adrenergic agonist, has been used to suppress flushing reactions (Chapter 51).

24. A (T); B (F); C (T); D (T); E (T) The earliest signs of rosacea are facial telangiectases and persistent erythema of the central face and, less often, the neck and upper chest. Most patients ultimately develop inflammatory follicular papules and pustules. Comedones, if present, are not a primary manifestation of rosacea but a result of other factors such as sun exposure (Favre-Racouchot disease). In a small proportion of patients, inflammation progresses, producing large nodules, edema, and tissue hyperplasia. A rare persistent nonpitting edema of the central face and forehead, similar to that reported in acne patients, has also been reported. Another variant, granulomatous rosacea, is characterized by multiple brown-red infiltrative papules and nodules. Biopsy reveals noncaseating granulomas (Chapter 51).

25. A (T); B (T); C (T); D (T); E (T) In a cooperative isotretinoin trial for rosacea, more than half of the patients were found to have some ophthalmic involvement, most commonly blepharitis and conjunctivitis. Other manifestations include iritis, iridocyclitis, hypopyon iritis, and keratitis. Rosacea keratitis can result in corneal opacities and blindness. Although ophthalmic complications are independent of the inflammatory component of cutaneous rosacea, the development of severe ocular rosacea has been correlated with the severity of flushing reactions (Chapter 51).

26. A (F); B (T); C (F); D (T); E (T) Oral contraceptives may be helpful in acne because of the estrogenic suppression of sebum production. Responsive patients may notice a decrease in skin oiliness after 3 or 4 months with a subsequent reduction of new acne lesions. Ethinyl estradiol and mestranol are the estrogens commonly used in oral contraceptive preparations. Combination pills containing less than 50 µg of ethinyl estradiol or mestranol have minimal effect on acne. Progestins may exert both androgenic and estrogenic effects. Ethynodiol diacetate and norethynodrel exert predominantly estrogenic effects. Oral contraceptives containing relatively androgenic progestins, such as norgestrel, may aggravate acne in susceptible women (Chapter 49).

27. A; 28. D; 29. C; 30. E; 31. A Linoleic acid is not produced by differentiated sebocytes and is therefore an essential fatty acid. (Δ9-Unsaturated fatty acids are also not produced by differentiated sebocytes but may be produced by undifferentiated cells.) It has been proposed that a relative deficiency of linoleic acid in the follicular epithelium, as is seen with dilution by increased endogenous fatty acid production during puberty, may cause comedogenesis by promoting hyperkeratinization and a reduced barrier to transepidermal water loss.

Circulating lipids, including cholesterol and linoleic acid, may be taken up at cell division during formation of new cell membranes. Once differentiation occurs, no circulating lipid is incorporated into the cell. A variety of unusual fatty acids, including Δ6-unsaturated acids are produced by sebaceous glands.

Fifty-seven percent of sebum and 65% of surface epidermal lipids are composed of triglycerides, diglycerides, and free fatty acids. Only sebum contains wax esters (26%) and squalene (12%). Conversely, surface epidermal lipids contain significant percentages of cholesterol (20%) and cholesterol esters (15%), which are found in only small quantities in sebum (about 5% combined) (Chapter 49).

32. D Patients on minocycline should be monitored for the development of blue-black discoloration, representing chelated iron, particularly of the gums, teeth, inflamed acne lesions, and scars. Pigmented post acne osteoma cutis and generalized blue-gray pigmentation have also been reported after minocycline use. Minocycline-induced pigmentation usually fades after discontinuation of therapy (Chapter 49).

33. E Ventricular arrhythmias, including torsades de pointes, have been reported in patients taking erythromycin concurrently with terfenadine.

34. C Exogenous estrogen use has been associated with the development of thrombotic diatheses, including thrombophlebitis, pulmonary embolism, and cerebrovascular accident. Estrogens should be avoided in acne patients with a history of hypercoagulability or thrombotic events (Chapter 49).

35. A Dapsone can produce a severe hemolytic anemia, particularly in patients with a deficiency of glucose-6-phosphate-dehydrogenase. Agranulocytosis and methemoglobinemia may also occur. Patients should be monitored closely (Chapter 49).

36. B Systemic clindamycin is now rarely used for acne because of the potential for severe pseudomembranous colitis. Use should be avoided in patients with a past medical history of gastrointestinal disease, particularly colitis. Topical clindamycin has not been associated with pseudomembranous colitis in healthy individuals. Its use in patients with a history of inflammatory bowel disease is controversial (Chapter 49).

37. C Acne estivalis, or Mallorca acne, is a rare form of acne consisting of monomorphic, firm, red, dome-shaped papules concentrated on the shoulders, arms, neck, and chest. Lesions develop abruptly in the spring, peak in the summer, and resolve without scarring in the fall. A similar eruption has been described in patients receiving ultraviolet A radiation, with and without psoralens (Chapter 49).

38. E Acne varioliformis, or acne necrotica, consists of recurrent umbilicated follicular papulopustules, alone or in clusters, on the scalp and temples that crust within days and leave depressed scars. *Staphylococcus aureus* and *P. acnes* are often isolated. The etiology is unclear (Chapter 49).

39. E Acne keloidalis nuchae is a chronic folliculitis and perifolliculitis of the terminal hair follicles of the nape of the neck that results in hypertrophic scarring and keloid formation. It may be complicated by bacterial superinfection (Chapter 49).

40. A Acne venenata is induced by contact with acnegenic compounds. In this category are acne cosmetica and the occupational acnes, including exposures to coal tar derivatives, insoluble cutting oils, petroleum oils, and chlorinated hydrocarbons (Chapter 49).

41. D Acne fulminans is a rarely seen, acute, ulcerative, nodulocystic acne associated with fever and systemic complaints. Onset has been associated with anabolic steroid abuse in bodybuilders and high-dose testosterone therapy for giantism. Cases have also been reported associated with isotretinoin therapy (see answer to Question 19) (Chapter 49).

42. D; 43. F; 44. D; 45. E; 46. F Cyproterone acetate and spironolactone are androgen receptor inhibitors used in acne therapy that act at the level of the sebaceous gland to reduce sebum secretion. The sebum excretion rate must be decreased by at least 40% to 50% to affect the course of acne. Cimetidine, a histamine receptor antagonist, is weakly androgenic and has not been shown to significantly affect sebum secretion. The enzyme 5α-reductase converts testosterone to dihydrotestosterone. It is unclear if finasteride, a 5α-reductase inhibitor used to treat benign prostatic hypertrophy, has any effect on sebum secretion or acne. The major side effect of antiandrogens in men is feminization (Chapter 49).

47. B; 48. A; 49. D; 50. D Lichen spinulosus is characterized by the occurrence of crops of nonpruritic, hyperkeratotic, spiny follicular papules grouped into indi-

vidual or polycyclic patches on the neck, trunk, and extensor surfaces of the extremities. The keratotic follicular papules of keratosis pilaris are distributed diffusely over the lateral upper arms, anterior thighs, and, less commonly, the cheeks and buttocks. Keratosis pilaris is closely associated with atopic dermatitis and ichthyosis vulgaris. Lichen nitidus is a disorder of asymptomatic, flesh-colored pinpoint papules found on the penis, arms, and abdomen. Keratosis pilaris and lichen spinulosus arise most commonly in childhood. Lichen nitidus has no age predisposition. Histologic examination of keratosis pilaris and lichen spinulosus lesions reveals a dilated follicle with a cornified plug and a coiled hair. Lichen nitidus is not a primary follicular disease (Chapter 54).

51. B Erythema toxicum neonatorum is a benign, self-limiting disorder of unknown cause. It consists of blotchy erythematous macules with a central vesicle or pustule that appear during the first few days of life. Biopsy reveals a perifollicular accumulation of eosinophils. Wright's stain of vesicle fluid is significant for the presence of eosinophils with relatively few neutrophils (Chapter 82).

52. A Transient neonatal pustular melanosis presents at birth as vesicles and pustules that rupture leaving a hyperpigmented macule with a collarette of scale. Histologic examination of a fresh lesion reveals a neutrophilic intraepidermal vesicle. In contrast to erythema toxicum, cytologic examination of vesicle fluid with Wright's stain reveals neutrophils, cellular debris, and only rarely, eosinophils. The disorder occurs primarily in black newborns, its cause is unknown, and it follows a self-limited course (Chapter 82).

53. D Neonatal herpes is transmitted from the maternal genital tract during vaginal delivery or is acquired shortly after birth. Grouped vesicles on an erythematous base are noted up to 3 weeks after exposure. Vesicles may also be noted at birth after intrauterine exposure to herpes, usually when the mother experienced primary herpes simplex infection during pregnancy. Diagnosis may be made by finding multinucleated giant cells on Wright's stained smear of the vesicle base, by culture, or by immunofluorescent identification of herpes antigen on a smear or tissue specimen. Early diagnosis and treatment of neonatal herpes are essential to avoid serious central nervous system complications or death. Exposure to herpes in utero has also been associated with congenital anomalies, including microcephaly, microphthalmos, chorioretinitis, and intracerebral calcification (Chapter 121).

54. E Miliaria crystallina appears as superficial, clear, noninflammatory pinpoint vesicles and represents obstruction of the eccrine sweat duct. The inflammatory papulovesicles and pustules of miliaria rubra result from the leakage of retained sweat into surrounding tissues. Miliaria are particularly common in the neonatal period because of the relative immaturity of the eccrine ducts (Chapter 82).

55. C Impetigo neonatorum is a superficial bacterial infection that manifests as superficial vesicles, pustules, or bullae on an erythematous base. Although lesions often erode, the crust formation typical of childhood or adult impetigo is uncommon. The predominant pathogen is *Staphylococcus aureus,* which may be identified by culture or by Gram stain examination of vesicle fluid. Although neutrophils are also identified, diagnosis relies on identification of the organism (Chapter 105).

56. B; **57.** A; **58.** C; **59.** D; **60.** B Hidradenitis suppurativa presents as tender, inflammatory abscesses and draining sinuses in the apocrine gland–bearing skin. The primary defect is keratinaceous occlusion of the apocrine duct. As the process progresses, the apocrine, eccrine, and pilosebaceous units are destroyed by chronic inflammation, bacterial infection, and scarring. The primary defect in acne conglobata, the most severe expression of acne vulgaris, is an alteration of keratinization within the sebaceous follicle combined with excessive sebum production. Miliaria pustulosa are pustules formed by the leakage of retained sweat into tissue surrounding plugged eccrine ducts. Pseudofolliculitis barbae appears as inflammatory follicles in the beard area, particularly in black men. The primary defect is not in the sebaceous gland but in the vicinity of the follicle as a foreign body reaction to ingrown hairs. Fox-Fordyce disease is a chronic pruritic papular eruption of apocrine areas and represents keratinous plugging of the apocrine duct with subsequent rupture. This disorder should be distinguished from Fordyce's spots, sebaceous glands of the lip and buccal mucosa (Chapters 49, 51, 53, and 82).

61. D; **62.** C; **63.** C; **64.** D; **65.** D Both acne rosacea and perioral dermatitis are inflammatory acneiform eruptions. Primary comedones are notably absent. Although its most severe manifestations are usually seen in men, rosacea is most common in postmenopausal women. Perioral dermatitis is classically seen in women of childbearing age. Although both disorders may initially improve with topical steroids, with chronic use patients develop follicular papulopustules and, ultimately, atrophy and telangiectases. An initial flare after withdrawal of steroids should be expected, but the conditions subsequently improve. Demodex follicularum mites are common skin saprophytes. Although it has been hypothesized that excessive demodex colonization could be responsible for both disorders, no difference between these patients and normal controls have been found. Because these are inflammatory disorders, antibiotics, particularly systemic tetracyclines, not comedolytics like tretinoin, are the treatment of choice (Chapters 51 and 52).

PERFORATING DISORDERS

66. A (T); B (F); C (T); D (F); E (F) The clinical and histologic description of this patient is most consistent with elastosis perforans serpiginosa (EPS). EPS usually manifests in the second decade of life as circinate arrays of umbilicated erythematous papules with a central keratotic plug. Lesions are most common on the posterior and lateral neck and are often symmetrically distributed. In EPS there is an increase in the number and size of elastic fibers in the upper dermis, particularly in the dermal papillae. The epidermis envelops the hyperplastic elastic fibers to form narrow, winding channels. In the channels, the elastic fibers degenerate and then are extruded with basophilic debris as a keratotic plug. In the uppermost portion of the canal, the elastic fibers lose their ability to react with elastic tissue stains, such as acid orcein, resorcin-fuchsin, or Verhoeff-van Gieson. A scraping of a lesion stained with KOH will rule out tinea corporis and may reveal elastic fibers. Attempts to remove plaques of EPS with dermabrasion or electrocautery often result in keloid formation. Success has been achieved with cryosurgical ablation, perhaps because of accelerated elimination of the hyperplastic elastic fibers by blister formation. EPS has not been associated with diabetes mellitus; therefore, glucose tolerance testing is not necessary on the basis of this diagnosis alone. Although disseminated EPS has been reported, in most cases EPS remains localized (Chapter 42).

67. A (F); B (T); C (F); D (T); E (F) In reactive perforating collagenosis (RPC), pinhead-sized keratotic papules are first noted in infancy or early childhood at sites of minor trauma such as scratch marks or insect bites. Lesions grow to as much as 10 mm over 3 to 4 weeks and develop a central umbilication filled with an adherent keratotic plug. These papules spontaneously resolve, leaving a minor scar. Treatment of early lesions with topical tretinoin may limit the overall number of lesions. Superficial trauma induces subepidermal foci of collagen degeneration. This necrobiotic collagen is then extruded through the epidermis. Once the altered collagen is eliminated, the epidermis regenerates and closes the perforation. Unlike EPS, on elastic tissue stain there is no increase in elastic fibers in the upper dermis, and elastic fibers are notably absent in the perforating canal. Although RPC had been reported in association with chronic renal failure and diabetes in adults, these cases have now been reclassified as acquired perforating dermatosis. Classic childhood RPC has not been associated with other disorders (Chapter 42).

68. C See answer to Question 66.

69. B The inflammation and degeneration in perforating folliculitis is focused at sites where hairs have perforated the follicular infundibulum. Local collagen and elastic fibers are degenerated and eliminated through the hair follicle to form keratotic plugs (Chapter 42).

70. E This histopathology describes perforating calcific elastosis. Short, thick, curled, calcified elastic fibers in the reticular dermis are expelled through the epidermis in a wide channel or through a tunnel ending in a keratin-filled crater (Chapter 42).

71. D See answer to Question 67.

72. A In Kyrle's disease, abnormal epidermal keratinization characterized by rapid proliferation and the formation of dyskeratotic foci leads to the formation of parakeratotic columns that extend deeper into the epidermis and ultimately into the dermis. Perforation of the dermis results in a granulomatous reaction. Proliferating epidermal cells surround this granulomatous focus and force it upward to be eliminated as basophilic debris within the keratotic plug (Chapter 42).

73. B; **74.** A; **75.** B; **76.** C; **77.** B Three major groups of patients with elastosis perforans serpiginosa (EPS) have been distinguished. An idiopathic form of EPS may occur without underlying disease. Reactive EPS is seen in patients with Down syndrome or with certain heritable connective tissue disorders, including Ehlers-Danlos syndrome type 4, osteogenesis imperfecta, Marfan's syndrome, Rothmund-Thomson syndrome, scleroderma, and acrogeria. Penicillamine-induced EPS has been reported in several patients undergoing treatment for Wilson's disease and cystinuria. Classic childhood reactive perforating collagenosis (RPC) is believed to be a familial disorder. Both autosomal dominant and autosomal recessive patterns of inheritance have been suggested. Although an acquired form of RPC had been reported in adults, these cases are now generally classified as acquired perforating disease.

Acquired perforating disease describes a group of eruptions associated most commonly with diabetes and chronic renal failure. This category includes some cases previously diagnosed as Kyrle's disease, perforating folliculitis, and reactive perforating collagenosis. Cases have also been associated with chronic liver failure and malignancies. Patients present with multiple, pruritic, umbilicated keratotic papules on the extensor surfaces of the extremities and, less commonly, on the trunk, neck, face, and scalp. Plaque formation and a prurigo-like appearance are induced with chronic rubbing. Histologic findings in these cases have included combined transepidermal elimination of both collagen and elastic fibers (Chapter 42).

INFLAMMATION OF CARTILAGE

78. C; **79.** B; **80.** B; **81.** B; **82.** A Relapsing polychondritis is a rare disease involving recurrent episodes of inflammation and subsequent destruction of cartilaginous tissues throughout the body. Manifestation is often with unilateral or bilateral auricular chondritis characterized by erythema, warmth, swelling, and tenderness of the cartilaginous portion of the external ear. Other manifestations include nonerosive seronegative inflammatory polyarthritis, nasal chondritis, ocular inflammation, respiratory chondritis (which may lead to airway collapse or obstruction and death), and audiovestibular damage. Cardiovascular complications include systemic vasculitis and ruptured aneurysms. Histology of the auricular and nasal chondritis is significant for a loss of the normal basophilia of cartilage with a perichondrial inflammatory infiltrate. End-stage disease is characterized by fibrotic replacement of cartilage. Laboratory work-up reveals an elevated erythrocyte sedimentation rate with or without leukocytosis and anemia. Circulating antibodies to type 2 collagen are detected in one third of patients.

Treatment consists of immunosuppressive and anti-inflammatory agents, including systemic corticosteroids, dapsone, and indomethacin.

Chondrodermatitis nodularis helicis is a benign disorder typically characterized by a single, small, intensely painful, round-to-oval nodule on the free border of the helix of the ear. It is thought to be initiated by minor trauma with subsequent dermal inflammation, edema, and necrosis. Histologic examination reveals a circumscribed area of epidermal hyperplasia covered by a hyperkeratotic or parakeratotic cap. The surrounding dermis is marked by edema, fibrinoid degeneration, collagen necrolysis, granulation tissue, and a moderately dense, diffuse infiltrate of lymphocytes and histiocytes. The perichondrium is thickened. Cartilage may show calcification and ossification but is usually normal. Treatment consists of high-potency topical corticosteroids, intralesional injections of corticosteroids, carbon dioxide laser, or excision (Chapters 55 and 56).

Bibliography

HAIR FOLLICLE AND APPENDAGEAL INFLAMMATORY DISEASES

Arndt KA, Rand RE. Follicular syndromes with inflammation and atrophy. In: Fitzpatrick TB, Eisen AZ, Wolff K, et al., eds. Dermatology in General Medicine, New York: McGraw Hill, 1993: 766–770.

Downing DT, Stewart ME, Wertz PW, Strauss JS. Lipids of the epidermis and the sebaceous glands. In: Fitzpatrick TB, Eisen AZ, Wolff K, et al., eds. Dermatology in General Medicine, New York: McGraw Hill, 1993:210–221.

Drake LA, Ceilley RI, Cornelison RL, et al. Guidelines for care of acne vulgaris. J Am Acad Dermatol 1990; 22:676–680.

Hurwitz S. Clinical Pediatric Dermatology. A Textbook of Skin Disorders of Childhood and Adolescence. Philadelphia: WB Saunders Co., 1993.

Lowe NJ, Behr KL, Fitzpatrick R, et al. Flash lamp–pulsed dye laser for rosacea-associated telangiectasia and erythema. J Dermatol Surg Oncol 1991; 17:522–525.

Plewig G, Kligman AM. Acne and Rosacea. New York: Springer-Verlag, 1993.

Pochi PE. Sebum: Its nature and physiologic responses. In: Moschella SL, Hurley HJ, eds. Dermatology. Philadelphia: WB Saunders Co., 1992:88–93.

Pochi PE. The pathogenesis and treatment of acne. Annu Rev Med 1990; 41:187–198.

Roenigk HH. Dermabrasion. In: Roenigk RK, Roenigk HH, eds. Dermatologic Surgery: Principles and Practice. New York: Marcel Dekker, 1989:959–978.

Shalita AR. Acne. In: Roenigk RK, Roenigk HH, eds. Dermatologic Surgery: Principles and Practice. New York: Marcel Dekker, 1989:749–752.

Stewart ME. Sebaceous gland lipids. Seminars in Dermatology. Philadelphia: WB Saunders Co., 1992:100–105.

Stegman SJ, Tromovitch TA, Glogau RG. Cosmetic Dermatologic Surgery. Chicago: Year Book Medical Publishers, 1990.

PERFORATING DISORDERS

Lever WF, Schaumberg-Lever G. Histopathology of the Skin. Philadelphia: JB Lippincott, 1990.

Patterson JW. The perforating disorders. J Am Acad Dermatol 1984; 10:561–581.

Patterson JW. Progress in the perforating dermatoses. Arch Dermatol 1989; 125:1121–1123.

Rapini RP, Hebert AA, Drucker CR. Acquired perforating dermatosis. Evidence for combined transepidermal elimination of both collagen and elastic fibers. Arch Dermatol 1989; 125:1074–1078.

Wolff-Schreiner E. Kyrle's disease and other perforating disorders. In: Fitzpatrick TB, Eisen AZ, Wolff K, et al., eds. Dermatology in General Medicine, New York: McGraw Hill, 1993:571–576.

Wolff-Schreiner E. Elastosis perforans serpiginosa and reactive perforating collagenosis. In: Fitzpatrick TB, Eisen AZ, Wolff K, et al., eds. Dermatology in General Medicine, New York: McGraw Hill, 1993:1280–1284.

INFLAMMATION OF CARTILAGE

Ceilley RI. The ear. In: Roenigk RK, Roenigk HH, eds. Dermatologic Surgery: Principles and Practice. New York: Marcel Dekker, 1989:357–381.

Coldiron BM. The surgical management of chondrodermatitis nodularis chronica helicis. J Dermatol Surg Oncol 1992; 18:640–641.

Katz SI. Relapsing polychondritis. In: Fitzpatrick TB, Eisen AZ, Wolff K, et al., eds. Dermatology in General Medicine. New York: McGraw Hill, 1993:2183–2185.

Taylor MB. Chondrodermatitis nodularis chronica helicis. Successful treatment with the carbon dioxide laser. J Dermatol Surg Oncol 1991; 17:862–864.

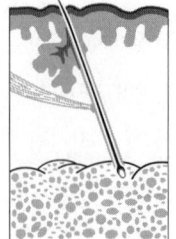

chapter 9

Vasculitis and Disorders of Vascular Reactivity

WARREN W. PIETTE, MICHELE HOLDER, and SUSAN M. MENARD

For the following questions, the set of lettered headings is followed by a list of numbered words or phrases. For each numbered word or phrase, choose

A. If the item is associated with A only
B. If the item is associated with B only
C. If the item is associated with both A and B
D. If the item is associated with neither A nor B.

For each of the following characteristics, choose whether it describes Henoch-Schönlein purpura, urticarial vasculitis, both, or neither.

1. IgA deposition often seen in cutaneous vessels
2. Lesions are often pruritic
3. Abnormal urinary sediment.

    A. Henoch-Schönlein purpura
    B. Urticarial vasculitis
    C. Both
    D. Neither.

For each of the following characteristics, choose whether it describes granuloma faciale, erythema elevatum diutinum, both, or neither.

4. Grenz zone typically seen
5. Vasculitis seen on histopathology

    A. Granuloma faciale
    B. Erythema elevatum diutinum
    C. Both
    D. Neither.

6. Has been associated with chronic infections and myeloproliferative diseases
7. Tendency toward spontaneous regression of cutaneous lesions
8. Extracellular cholesterolosis may be seen
9. Associated with systemic vasculitis
10. Most commonly seen in men
11. Lesions usually pruritic
12. Often see follicular prominence of clinical lesions
13. Systemic corticosteroid therapy is universally successful.

102

Choose the ONE BEST answer to each of the following questions.

14. Pustular vasculitis manifestations include all of the following EXCEPT
    A. Erythema nodosum–like lesions
    B. Coexistence of bowel-bypass syndrome
    C. Polyarthralgia
    D. IgA paraproteinemia
    E. Frequent recurrent pustular lesions on the arms and trunk.

15. Knowledge concerning antineutrophil cytoplasmic antibodies (ANCA) is expanding rapidly. Using ethanol-fixed granulocytes as substrate, c-ANCA staining is most often due to which antigen in neutrophils?
    A. Lactoferrin
    B. Myeloperoxidase
    C. Leukocyte elastase
    D. Proteinase 3
    E. None of the above.

16. The sensitivity of c-ANCA testing in Wegener's granulomatosis is approximately
    A. 80%
    B. 60%
    C. 40%
    D. 20%
    E. Less than 20%.

For the following questions, decide whether EACH choice is TRUE or FALSE. Any combination of answers from all true to all false may occur.

17. Perinuclear ANCA staining is found in 50% or greater of patients with
    A. Idiopathic crescentic glomerulonephritis
    B. Wegener's granulomatosis
    C. Polyangiitis overlap syndrome
    D. Microscopic polyarteritis
    E. Churg-Strauss syndrome.

18. Henoch-Schönlein purpura is the most common form of systemic vasculitis in children. The second most common form of pediatric vasculitis is Kawasaki disease. A firm diagnosis of Kawasaki disease requires five of six recognized criteria to be present. Decide whether EACH of the following are part of the six criteria.
    A. Fever persisting for five days or more
    B. Thrombocytosis
    C. Changes in peripheral extremities
    D. Polymorphous exanthema
    E. Bilateral conjunctival injection.

19. Which changes in the peripheral extremities or the lips and oral cavities are important when considering a diagnosis of Kawasaki disease?
    A. Erythema of palms and soles
    B. Indurative edema of hands or feet
    C. Strawberry tongue
    D. Lip erythema
    E. Diffuse injection of oral and pharyngeal mucosa.

20. Current recommended therapy for Kawasaki syndrome includes
    A. High-dose prednisone
    B. Aspirin
    C. Intravenous gamma globulin
    D. Dapsone
    E. Colchicine.

Choose the ONE BEST answer to the following question.

21. Which of the following is most true concerning the epidemiology of Kawasaki disease?
    A. Occurs more often in girls
    B. Recurrences are common
    C. Eighty per cent of cases occur before the age of 5 years
    D. It is rare before the age of 2 years
    E. There is no racial predilection.

For the following questions ONE or MORE of the following completions may correctly finish the incomplete statements; choose
   A. If only 1, 2, and 3 are correct
   B. If only 1 and 3 are correct
   C. If only 2 and 4 are correct
   D. If only 4 is correct
   E. If all are correct.

22. The skin lesions in giant cell arteritis
    1. Classically reveal erythema, heat, swelling, and tenderness of involved superficial vessels

2. Often reveal tender nodules anywhere on the scalp
3. May reveal tender nodules in involved temporal arteries
4. Often present as scalp necrosis in severe cases.

23. Laboratory findings that are supportive of but not necessary for diagnosis of giant cell arteritis include
   1. Elevated erythrocyte sedimentation rate
   2. Normochromic anemia
   3. Thrombocytosis
   4. Elevated serum alkaline phosphatase.

For the following questions decide whether EACH choice is TRUE or FALSE. Any combination of answers from all true to all false may occur.

24. Regarding giant cell arteritis,
   A. More frequently affects men than women
   B. Virtually unseen in patients less than 50 years old
   C. Often associated with polymyalgia rheumatica
   D. Constitutional symptoms are rare
   E. Usually manifests with clinically apparent temporal artery involvement.

25. Regarding the arteritis seen in giant cell arteritis,
   A. Involves numerous different arteries, quite commonly the renal and pulmonary arteries
   B. Leads to absent pulses in about 65% of affected superficial vessels
   C. Is most frequently noted in occipital arteries, which are superficial and easily visible
   D. When it involves temporal arteries, the patient or the spouse often notices a bulging, worm-like appearance of temporal vessels
   E. Clinical evidence of arteritis is patchy and usually unilateral
   F. May involve clinically normal-appearing vessels.

26. Compared with autoimmune-related antibodies, infection-related antiphospholipid antibodies are more likely to
   A. Be IgM
   B. Bind with low avidity to phospholipid
   C. Have anticoagulant activity in vitro
   D. Be associated with thrombotic complications
   E. Require a cofactor.

27. Likely mechanisms of antiphospholipid antibodies in promoting thrombosis include
   A. Inhibition of protein C-protein S-thrombomodulin pathway
   B. Induction of immune complex vasculitis
   C. Enhancement or induction of platelet aggregation
   D. Effects on endothelial cell function
   E. Stimulation of prostacyclin release.

28. The following are associated with the clinical findings of antiphospholipid antibody syndrome.
   A. Livedo reticularis
   B. Pulmonary hypertension
   C. Libman-Sacks endocarditis
   D. Glomerulonephritis
   E. Habitual abortion.

Choose the ONE BEST answer to each of the following questions.

29. Of the following cutaneous findings associated with the antiphospholipid (APS) antibody syndrome, which is the most common?
   A. Skin infarction
   B. Atrophie blanche
   C. Subungual splinter hemorrhages
   D. Superficial thrombophlebitis
   E. Livedo reticularis.

30. Tests for antiphospholipid antibodies include all of the following EXCEPT
   A. False-positive VDRL
   B. Prolongation of activated partial thromboplastin test (aPTT)
   C. Prolonged viper venom time
   D. Platelet neutralization procedure
   E. Positive antinuclear antibody (ANCA).

For each numbered item, choose the most likely associated lettered item. Each numbered item has ONLY ONE answer. Each lettered item may be the answer to one, more than one, or none of the numbered items.

Noninflammatory occlusion of the cutaneous microvasculature can be seen in a variety of syndromes, and involves many different mechanisms. Match the diseases that can produce such vascular occlusion with the most likely mechanism.

31. Coumadin necrosis
32. Heparin necrosis
33. Cryoglobulins
34. Ecthyma gangrenosum
35. Neonatal purpura fulminans
36. Atherosclerotic plaques.

A. Platelet plugs
B. Protein gel formation
C. Organisms growing in or around vessels
D. Protein-C alterations
E. Embolization.

For the following questions, decide whether each choice is TRUE or FALSE. Any combination of answers from all true to all false may occur.

37. Regarding atrophie blanche,
    A. Recurrent ulcerations heal with a reticular pattern
    B. Exacerbation is often seasonal
    C. Dermatopathology shows hyalin thrombi without vasculitis
    D. Ulcers are often painless
    E. Treatment options include aspirin, ethylestranol, or dipyridamole.

Choose the ONE BEST answer to the following question.

38. The most common cause of death in malignant atrophic papulosis (Degos' disease) is
    A. Cerebral infarction
    B. Renal insufficiency
    C. Myocardial disease
    D. Peritonitis
    E. Cutaneous ulcers with sepsis.

For the following question, ONE or MORE of the following completions correctly finishes the incomplete statement; choose

A. If only 1, 2, and 3 are correct
B. If only 1 and 3 are correct
C. If only 2 and 4 are correct
D. If only 4 is correct
E. If all are correct.

39. Regarding erythromelalgia
    1. Paroxysms may be brought on by exposure to cold
    2. It may lead to painful acrocyanosis and peripheral gangrene
    3. It most frequently affects hands
    4. It is often seen as a secondary phenomenon in association with polycythemia vera.

For the following questions, decide whether EACH choice is TRUE or FALSE. Any combination of answers from all true to all false may occur.

40. Regarding erythromelalgia,
    A. Relief of symptoms for up to 3 days by a single low dose of aspirin may be used as a diagnostic criterion
    B. Calcium channel blockers are effective therapy
    C. Phlebotomy is effective therapy in some cases
    D. Indocin and aspirin are interchangeable therapies with identical results
    E. Sympathectomy may be necessary in severe cases.

41. Regarding the cutaneous manifestations of carcinoid syndrome,
    A. Flushing
    B. Hyperkeratosis with dry scaling and gray-black pigmentation on the lower legs, forearms, trunk
    C. Nailfold telangiectasias
    D. Tender, firm nodules
    E. Scleroderma-like lesions on lower extremities.

For the following questions, the set of lettered headings accompanies a list of numbered words or phrases. For each numbered word or phrase, choose

A. If the item is associated with A only
B. If the item is associated with B only
C. If the item is associated with both A and B
D. If the item is associated with neither A nor B.

For each of the following findings, choose whether it describes the carcinoid syndrome, mastocytosis, both, or neither.

42. Bronchospasm, flushing, hypotension, diarrhea may occur
43. Diagnosis is confirmed by documenting increased levels of urinary 5-hydroxyindoleacetic acid

A. Carcinoid syndrome
B. Mastocytosis
C. Both
D. Neither.

44. Typically, paroxysms of flushing of the face and trunk last 10 to 30 minutes

45. Occurrence of flushing confirms presence of hepatic metastases

46. Antihistamines may be effective symptomatic treatment.

For the following question, decide whether EACH choice is TRUE or FALSE. Any combination of answers from all true to all false may occur.

47. Flushing is

    A. Commonly seen in pheochromocytoma

    B. Unlike most other types of flushing, menopausal flushing does not have any known precipitants

    C. Menopausal flushing seems to be caused by direct action on vascular smooth muscle

    D. Commonly caused by monosodium glutamate

    E. May be caused by eggplant ingestion.

In the following questions, ONE or MORE of the following completions correctly finishes the incomplete statement; choose

   A. If only 1, 2, and 3 are correct
   B. If only 1 and 3 are correct
   C. If only 2 and 4 are correct
   D. If only 4 is correct
   E. If all are correct.

48. Regarding (primary) Raynaud's disease,

    1. Diagnosis should be made no less than 5 years after symptoms have been present without findings of any associated diseases

    2. It is usually asymmetrical

    3. There is a high risk of developing gangrene

    4. It is most common in young women.

49. Occupational risks for Raynaud's phenomenon include

    1. Pneumatic percussion drill operation

    2. Typing

    3. Chain saw operation

    4. Vinyl chloride exposure.

50. Treatments that effectively relieve symptoms in many cases of Raynaud's include

    1. Nifedipine

    2. Discontinuation of smoking

    3. Surgical sympathectomy

    4. Propranolol.

Choose the ONE BEST answer for each of the following questions.

51. Concerning Raynaud's syndrome

    A. The classic triad is sequential phases of rubor, pallor, cyanosis

    B. All three color phases in the triad are required for diagnosis

    C. In men it tends to manifest at an older age and to be more often associated with malignancy than in women

    D. When secondary to vascular occlusive disease it is often asymmetrical, involving few digits

    E. It occurs with equal frequency in men and women.

52. Precipitants of Raynaud's phenomenon include all EXCEPT

    A. Emotional stress

    B. Piano playing

    C. Bleomycin injection

    D. Ergotamine ingestion

    E. Aspirin ingestion.

53. Proposed pathophysiologic mechanisms for Raynaud's syndrome include all EXCEPT

    A. Local vascular hypersensitivity to the cold

    B. Cryoprecipitable proteins

    C. Impaired cyclooxygenase activity

    D. Vascular hypersensitivity to serotonin

    E. Circulating immune complexes.

54. The condition most commonly associated with Raynaud's phenomenon is

    A. Systemic lupus erythematosus

    B. Rheumatoid arthritis

    C. Cryoproteinemia

    D. Scleroderma

    E. Thoracic outlet syndrome.

55. Predictors of future diagnosis of an associated disorder in apparent idiopathic Raynaud's include

    A. Female sex

    B. Aged less than 20 years

C. Nailfold capillary abnormalities

D. Anemia

E. Positive antinuclear antibodies

F. Basilar fibrosis on chest radiograph.

For the following questions decide whether EACH choice is TRUE or FALSE. Any combination of answers from all true to all false may occur.

56. Chronic lymphedema is
    A. Usually easily managed with leg elevation and diuretics
    B. Predominantly pitting
    C. May be primary or secondary
    D. May be a complication of malignancy
    E. May be complicated by malignancy.

57. The Stewart-Treves syndrome
    A. Follows an indolent course
    B. Is seen exclusively after radical mastectomy
    C. Skin lesions are pink, scaling macules
    D. One subset consists of distant recurrences of breast carcinoma
    E. Develops, on average, 9.5 years after mastectomy.

Choose the ONE BEST answer to the following question.

58. Of Milroy's disease, all are true EXCEPT
    A. Lymphedema is present at birth
    B. More common in males
    C. Inheritance is autosomal dominant
    D. May be unilateral or bilateral
    E. Develops secondary to hypoplastic distal lymphatics.

For the following questions, decide whether EACH choice is TRUE or FALSE. Any combination of answers from all true to all false may occur.

59. With respect to telangiectasias,
    A. Papular telangiectasias are frequently a part of a genetic syndrome such as Rendu-Osler-Weber disease
    B. Hemorrhagic telangiectasias can be effectively treated with tetracycline
    C. The gravid uterus is responsible for the development of telangiectasias during pregnancy
    D. Telangiectasias on the legs arise primarily from arterioles; those on the face arise from venules
    E. Telangiectasias often recur after treatment with dermabrasion.

60. The following are side effects of sclerotherapy with hypertonic saline:
    A. Burning at site of injection
    B. Skin necrosis
    C. Telangiectatic matting
    D. Hyperpigmentation
    E. Muscle cramps.

61. According to its proponents, post-sclerotic compression is helpful because the pressure:
    A. Helps seal vascular lumina
    B. Decreases the likelihood of recanalization
    C. Minimizes postinflammatory hyperpigmentation
    D. Minimizes thromboses.

Choose the ONE BEST answer to each of the following questions.

62. Which one of the following sclerosing agents has the highest incidence of allergic reaction?
    A. Hypertonic saline
    B. Polidocanol
    C. Tetracycline
    D. Sodium tetradecyl sulfate.

63. The major risk factor for lower extremity ulceration is
    A. Chronic edema
    B. Venous insufficiency
    C. Diabetes
    D. Obesity
    E. Trauma.

For the following questions, decide whether EACH choice is TRUE or FALSE. Any combination of answers from all true to all false may occur.

64. With regard to pressure ulceration,

    A. Deep tissue necrosis and volume loss are often disproportionately larger than the overlying skin injury

    B. Compression forces are not distributed equally over the total body surface area, making areas overlying bony prominences more susceptible to ulceration

    C. Muscle fibers are more resistant to degenerative changes from pressure than the overlying skin

    D. Clinically, the ulcers have violaceous, rolled borders that are ill-defined and show satellite violaceous papules at the border

    E. Pressure ulcer pathogenesis includes interstitial pressure exceeding venous capillary pressure, resulting in increased total tissue pressure, edema, and cell autolysis.

65. Regarding the diabetic foot ulcer,

    A. *Pseudomonas* is the most commonly isolated bacteria

    B. Ulcers are frequently located on the metatarsal fat pad

    C. Autonomic dysfunction leads to shunting of blood to muscle and subcutaneous tissue and away from the skin

    D. Atherosclerosis is the primary cause of ischemia

    E. Patients often present with hypoglycemia.

For the following questions, the set of lettered headings accompanies a list of numbered words or phrases. For each numbered word or phrase, choose

   A. If the item is associated with A only
   B. If the item is associated with B only
   C. If the item is associated with both A and B
   D. If the item is associated with neither A nor B.

For each of the following characteristics choose whether it describes venous ulcers, arterial ulcers, both, or neither.

66. Most commonly located on the lateral surface of the leg

67. Increased levels of protein C, D-dimer, and fibrin degradation products

    A. Venous ulcers
    B. Arterial ulcers
    C. Both
    D. Neither.

68. Ulcers are deep, indolent, and dry

69. Pain increases as leg is elevated.

Choose the ONE BEST answer to each of the following questions.

70. Advantages of occlusive dressings include of all the following EXCEPT

    A. Decrease wound tenderness
    B. Decrease voltage gradient between wound base and lateral wound margin
    C. Foster normal bacterial microflora
    D. Prevent crust and desiccation.

71. When measured at the level of the ankle, compression stockings should exert a resting pressure of at least how many mm Hg?

    A. 0 to 10 mm Hg
    B. 10 to 20 mm Hg
    C. 20 to 30 mm Hg
    D. 30 to 40 mm Hg
    E. 40 to 50 mm Hg.

72. All of the following drugs have an inhibitory effect on wound healing EXCEPT

    A. Anticoagulants
    B. Aspirin
    C. Diphenylhydantoin
    D. Phenylbutazone
    E. Colchicine.

73. When sutures are removed after 2 weeks, the wound has what percentage of its original strength?

    A. 5%
    B. 10%
    C. 15%
    D. 20%
    E. 25%.

74. What type of collagen is found in greater abundance during the substrate and proliferative phases of wound healing compared with normal skin?

    A. type I
    B. type II
    C. type III
    D. type IV

For the following questions, decide whether EACH choice is TRUE or FALSE. Any combination of answers from all true to all false may occur.

75. Regarding the substrate phase of wound healing,
    A. Polymorphonuclear (PMN) leukocytes stimulate fibroplasia
    B. Lymphocytes secrete fibrinolytic enzymes that aid in breaking down and remodeling the fibrin scaffolding
    C. Platelets release proteolytic enzymes responsible for the initiation of the alternate complement pathway
    D. Fibrin scaffolding provides temporary stability to the wound, hemostasis, and a framework over which macrophages and epithelial cells can migrate
    E. Macrophage inhibition factor and macrophage activation factor are released from lymphocytes.

76. Regarding fibronectin in wound healing,
    A. Promotes phagocytosis of denatured collagen
    B. Produced by keratinocytes
    C. Degraded by keratinocytes
    D. Necessary for adhesion of fibroblasts to fibrin
    E. A constituent of the fibrin clot.

77. Regarding wound contraction,
    A. Contraction begins 1 month after healing
    B. Contraction rate is independent of wound size
    C. Contraction rate is independent of wound shape
    D. Contraction is due to the contractile forces of the myofibroblast.

78. With regard to epidermal allografts,
    A. Newborn foreskin is often used as a donor allograft
    B. After grafting, pain relief at ulcer site is seen within 24 hours
    C. Human leukocyte antigen matching is required
    D. There is no risk of infection transmission
    E. Grafts become adherent within 3 weeks and develop complete basal lamina.

For the following questions, the set of lettered headings accompanies a list of numbered words or phrases. For each numbered word or phrase, choose

A. If the item is associated with A only
B. If the item is associated with B only
C. If the item is associated with both A and B
D. If the item is associated with neither A nor B.

For each of the following findings decide whether it describes PMN, macrophage, both, or neither.

79. Stimulates fibroplasia
80. Releases proteinases and collagenases
81. Plays no regulatory role in subsequent phases of wound healing
82. Can tolerate an environment with low oxygen tension.

A. PMN
B. Macrophage
C. Both
D. Neither.

For each numbered item, choose the one most likely associated lettered item from those provided. Each numbered item has ONLY ONE answer. Each lettered item may be the answer to one, more than one, or none of the numbered items.

83. Produced by keratinocytes, endothelial cells, and mature leukocytes; acts as an autocrine hormone, resulting in up-regulation of proliferation
84. Precursor is membrane-bound and produced by keratinocytes; it phosphorylates proteins in cells, leading to activation of cellular DNA
85. Promotes angiogenesis and the production of 1,25 dihydroxyvitamin D, assisting in keratinocyte differentiation
86. Stored as a precursor in keratinocytes and released after epidermal damage; causes skin inflammation, fever, malaise

A. Epidermal growth factor
B. Granulocyte-macrophage colony–stimulating factor
C. Interleukin 1
D. Interleukin 2
E. Interleukin 6
F. Tumor necrosis factor alpha
G. None of the above.

87. Produced by lymphoid cells and keratinocytes; stimulates B- & T-cell blastogenesis and differentiation

88. Secreted by activated T cells following antigen stimulation; main function is to regulate expression of class I and class II major histocompatibility complex.

ANSWERS

1. A; **2.** D; **3.** C Henoch-Schönlein purpura is also known as anaphylactoid purpura or purpura urticans. The syndrome includes purpura, nephritis, arthritis, and gastrointestinal involvement (abdominal pain, melena, or hematochezia). The lower extremities and buttocks are the most common sites of skin lesions. Renal involvement frequently occurs and manifests as hematuria, proteinuria, hypertension, or impaired function. Immunopathology often shows IgA deposition in cutaneous vessels.

Urticarial vasculitis is distinguished from urticaria by lesions that persist longer than 24 hours and that are burning or painful instead of pruritic. Lesions often resolve with purpura. Patients may have glomerulonephritis, hypocomplementemia, or pulmonary disease. Histopathologically, the lesions show leukocytoclastic vasculitis with fibrinoid necrosis (Chapter 67).

4. C; **5.** C; **6.** B; **7.** B; **8.** B; **9.** D; **10.** A; **11.** D; **12.** A; **13.** D Granuloma faciale presents with single or multiple soft, violaceous to red-brown papules and nodules, often smooth-surfaced, but with follicular prominence, most commonly on the faces of men. Rarely, burning, stinging, tenderness, and pruritus are associated. Lesions may be seen on the trunk. Lesions seldom spontaneously remit and are extremely resistant to medical therapy. Varying degrees of success have been achieved with dapsone, psoralen plus ultraviolet A (PUVA), and clofazamine. Surgical therapies are often required: simple excision, treatment with cryotherapy, argon and carbon dioxide lasers, or dermabrasion. The characteristic histology of granuloma faciale involves a dense, perivascular, mixed infiltrate of neutrophils and eosinophils separated by a Grenz zone from the epidermis and adnexal structures. Vasculitis with fibrinoid necrosis is usually seen. This infiltrate evolves to a more mononuclear cell predominant infiltrate only when the lesions are treated or regressing. The cause is unknown.

Erythema elevatum diutinum is a chronic skin-limited vasculitis, occurring with equal frequency in men and women. Violaceous, deep red or brown papules and plaques occur over extensor joints of the extremities, buttocks, and ear pinnae and may become yellowish in their chronic stages. Although usually asymptomatic, they may have a burning quality or be painful. Histologically, early lesions are characterized by a small-vessel leukocytoclastic vasculitis and a dense upper and mid dermal neutrophilic infiltrate sparing the Grenz zone. In later lesions, the infiltrate is partially replaced by granulation tissue, fibrosis, and sometimes by deposition of extracellular lipid material ("extracellular cholesterolosis"). The most common disorders associated with erythema elevatum diutinum are hematologic diseases, especially an IgA monoclonal gammopathy, but chronic infections (HIV, hepatitis B, and tuberculosis) have also been associated. Dramatic response to dapsone is seen in most cases, but lesions usually recur with cessation of therapy. Spontaneous resolution of lesions does occur, and the disease itself often remits within 5 to 10 years (Chapter 60).

14. D Pustular vasculitis is frequently associated with fever, polyarteritis, and myalgias. It is seen in Behçet's disease, bowel bypass, and inflammatory bowel disease, manifesting clinically as erythematous plaques (as seen in Sweet's syndrome), erythema nodosum–like and pyoderma gangrenosum–like lesions, and most commonly as pustules. The pustules are commonly seen on the arms and trunk, last 2 to 3 days, and are often recurrent. Systemic symptoms include fever, polyarthritis, and myalgias (Chapters 38 and 40).

15. D c-ANCA staining in ethanol-fixed granulocytes is almost always due to anti–proteinase 3, a component of primary (azurophilic) granules in granulocytes. Leukocyte elastase and myeloperoxidase are also contained in primary neutrophil granules, whereas lactoferrin is a component of secondary granules. All of these antigens reside in the cytoplasm, but in ethanol-fixed neutrophils, the positively charged lactoferrin, elastase, and myeloperoxidase molecules are apparently able to migrate to the highly negatively charged perinuclear membrane, causing a perinuclear (p-ANCA) staining pattern. A third staining pattern has been identified in patients with autoimmune liver diseases, ulcerative colitis (occasionally Crohn's disease), and rheumatoid arthritis, which produces both a perinuclear and diffuse cytoplasmic staining pattern. Termed u-ANCA by some (u for ulcerative colitis), the antigens responsible for this staining pattern have not been identified (Chapters 38 and 59).

16. A c-ANCA staining, although not completely specific for Wegener's granulomatosis (WG), is highly suggestive of Wegener's or a Wegener-like disease and is present in roughly 80% of patients with WG. Extended WG (the triad of granulomatous inflammation of the respiratory tract, systemic vasculitis, and necrotizing crescentic glomerulonephritis) is c-ANCA–positive in more than 90% of patients. In limited WG (without renal involvement), c-ANCAs are detected in 67% to 86% of patients. Taken together, these two groups of active-disease WG patients are positive 81% of the time. c-ANCA staining is also positive in roughly 50% of patients with pauci-immune glomerulonephritis and systemic small-vessel vasculitis but without granulomatous inflammation of the respiratory tract. This group is often termed microscopic polyarteritis and shows many clinical features of classic WG (Chapters 38 and 59).

17. A (T); B (F); C (F); D (T); E (T) p-ANCA staining is seen in 50% of patients with microscopic polyarteritis syndrome, in 70% of patients with idiopathic crescentic glomerulonephritis, and with Churg-Strauss syndrome. Less than 20% of patients with Wegener's granulomatosis or the polyangiitis overlap syndrome are p-ANCA–positive. Overlapping features of extended WG, classic polyarteritis nodosa, and Churg-Strauss syndromes may be seen in individual patients, and such variations of classic disease presentation have been called the polyangiitis overlap syndrome (Chapter 59).

18. A (T); B (F); C (T); D (T); E (T) Thrombocytosis, although often present and supportive of the diagnosis, is not a diagnostic criterion for Kawasaki disease. The remaining two diagnostic criteria are acute nonpurulent cervical lymphadenopathy and changes in the lips and oral cavity. If coronary artery aneurysms are visualized on two-dimensional echocardiography, only four of the six diagnostic criteria are required.

19. A–E (T) The induration of hands and feet occurs acutely; the additional membranous desquamation is a convalescent finding.

20. A (F); B (T); C (T); D (F); E (F) The most important complication of Kawasaki disease is coronary artery injury, which can result in long-term sequelae of impaired coronary distensibility, coronary artery stenosis, and myocardial infarction. The most effective therapy for preventing these complications includes aspirin and intravenous gamma globulin used in combination (Chapter 13).

21. C Kawasaki disease occurs somewhat more often in boys and usually manifests before the age of 2 years in both sexes. Recurrences are rare. Although there does appear to be a racial predilection, it may have a geographic basis. The annual attack rate for Kawasaki disease in Japan is 67 per 100,000 children under 5 years old, while the comparable attack rate in the United States is only 6 to 9 per 100,000 under 5 years old. This results in about 2000 cases per year in the United States (Chapter 13).

22. A Skin lesions are not common in giant cell arteritis. Scalp arteries are frequently involved, even with frank occlusion. Tender scalp nodules are one of the most frequently encountered skin findings and are often first noted by patients. Because of the extensive anastomoses of the scalp's blood supply, necrosis is unusual (Chapter 57).

23. E Elevated IgG levels also support the diagnosis but are not diagnostic. A positive temporal artery biopsy confirms, but is not necessary for, the diagnosis. Unfortunately, there are no established clinical criteria for diagnosis. Confirmation of diagnosis is desirable before committing a patient to the side effects of treatment with long-term, high-dose steroids (Chapter 57).

24. A (F); B (T); C (T); D (F); E (F) Giant cell arteritis involves women three times as frequently as men and is seldom seen in patients less than 50 years old. It is associated with polymyalgia rheumatica (in about 50%), which may develop before, during, or after the clinical presentation of arteritis. The relationship between the two entities is unclear. Systemic findings are common, including malaise, weight loss, anorexia, night sweats, fever, and depression. These are often the initial and sometimes the only findings and may suggest a diagnosis of infection or malignancy. A minority of patients present with temporal artery involvement (Chapter 57).

25. A (F); B (F); C (F); D (T); E (F); F (T) The severity of arteritis in giant cell arteritis may vary greatly. At the mild end of the spectrum is pain, swelling, and erythema; at the severe end is total arterial occlusion with ischemia and necrosis. Commonly involved are the superficial temporal, ophthalmic, maxillary, posterior auricular, occipital, facial, aortic, and coronary arteries. Pulmonary and renal artery involvement is rare. Clinical signs of inflammation are most frequently noted in temporal, not occipital, arteries. Patients often notice the increased size of temporal vessels. Arterial involvement is patchy. Although usually bilateral, this may be temporally dyssynchronous or unequal in severity. The strength of the temporal pulse on a single examination is not very helpful, but serial examinations revealing decreasing pulses can be a most helpful diagnostic finding. Only rarely are superficial pulses entirely absent as a result of giant cell arteritis (Chapter 57).

26. A (T); B (T); C (F); D (F); E (F) In contrast to infection-related antibodies, autoimmune antiphospholipid (APS) antibodies are more likely to be IgG, to bind with high avidity, to frequently have anticoagulant activity measured by prolongation of the activated partial thromboplastin time (aPTT), to be present in sustained high titer, and to require a cofactor for binding. This cofactor is now known to be β_2-glycoprotein I (Chapter 63).

27. A (T); B (F); C (T); D (T); E (F) A, C, and D are the three most commonly implicated mechanisms for thrombus induction by APS antibodies. There is little evidence to support immune-complex formation as part of this syndrome. Rather than stimulating prostacyclin release, inhibition of endothelial cell production of prostacyclin is thought to be an important mechanism for thrombus in some patients. It is likely that mechanisms for thrombus formation vary from patient to patient, based on the precise antigenic specificity of individual antiphospholipid antibodies (Chapter 63).

28. A (T); B (T); C (T); D (F); E (T) APS antibody syndrome is defined as yielding an elevated titer of lupus anticoagulant or anticardiolipin antibody with a history of vascular occlusive events, thrombocytopenia, or recurrent fetal loss. The thrombotic events can manifest in any organ, causing myocardial infarction (MI), pulmonary hypertension, stroke, or glomerular thrombi, leading to renal insufficiency and hypertension. Glomerulonephritis is not commonly seen. Cardiac manifestations include not only MI but also valvular heart disease, intracardiac clot, and Libman-Sacks endocarditis (sterile valvular vegetations) (Chapter 63).

29. E Livedo reticularis is the most commonly reported finding in these patients. In addition to the other features listed, Sneddon's syndrome (idiopathic livedo reticularis with cerebrovascular accidents), deep thrombophlebitis, and fulminant disseminated gangrene syndrome have also been reported (Chapter 13).

30. E The false-positive Venereal Disease Research Laboratory (VDRL) is often seen in patients with APS antibody syndrome. However, a false-positive VDRL can occur in patients with lupus and other connective tissue diseases. Likewise, the aPTT is subject to both false-positive and false-negative results. The aPTT prolongation usually does not correct with a 1:1 mix with normal plasma. APS antibodies also frequently prolong the Russell's viper venom time. Platelet phospholipid frequently corrects the aPTT prolongation, suggesting the APS. A positive ANCA is not seen in patients with APS antibody syndrome (Chapter 13).

31. D; **32.** A; **33.** B; **34.** C; **35.** D; **36.** E

37. A (T); B (T); C (T); D (F); E (T) Atrophie blanche may manifest as painful petechial lesions or purpuric papules that evolve into ulcerations, leaving atrophic, depressed scars, occasionally in a reticulate pattern. Livedo reticularis is often associated with the lesions. Some patients may experience a seasonal variation in disease activity. Dermatopathology shows extravasated red blood cells (RBCs), and dermal vessels occluded with hyalin thrombi. A perivascular infiltrate is often seen, but usually there is no vasculitis. Agents used in treatment inhibit platelet aggregation, e.g., acetylsalicylic acid (ASA) and dipyridamole, or increase endogenous fibrinolytic activity–ethylestranol (Chapter 63).

38. D Peritonitis due to perforation, usually of the small intestine, is the most common cause of death in malignant atrophic papulosis. Surgical specimens, autopsy findings, and, most recently, endoscopy show similar white lesions with telangiectatic rims in the gastrointestinal tract, anywhere from the oral cavity to the anus (Chapter 63).

39. C Erythromelalgia is a condition characterized by erythema, burning, pain, and paresthesias of acral lower and, less commonly, upper extremities. Paroxysms are brought on by exposure to warm temperatures, exercise, and dependency of the limb. Cooling or resting the limb provides relief. In severe cases, erythromelalgia may lead to painful acrocyanosis and peripheral gangrene. The disease may be primary or secondary, the most common associated disease being polycythemia vera. Other associations include primary thrombocythemia, hypertension, diabetes mellitus, systemic lupus erythematosus, and peripheral vascular disease (Chapter 61).

40. A (T); B (F); C (T); D (F); E (F) The pathogenesis of erythromelalgia is poorly understood. Platelet-derived prostaglandins seem to be involved. Therapeutic response to aspirin is so characteristic that it can be of diagnostic use. Aspirin, which irreversibly inhibits cyclooxygenase (such as indomethacin) provides relief for less than 24 hours. Calcium channel blockers may exacerbate or induce erythromelalgia. Phlebotomy can be effective therapy in patients with underlying polycythemia vera or thrombocythemia. Other effective treatments have included epinephrine, methysergide, lumbar ganglionectomy, and nitroglycerin ointment. Sympathectomy is not effective treatment (Chapter 61).

41. A (T); B (T); C (F); D (T); E (T) Carcinoid tumors secrete large amounts of serotonin, diverting as much as 60% of the body's tryptophan supply to its production. Both niacin and serotonin are synthesized from tryptophan. When food intake is poor, niacin deficiency can result, with the characteristic pellagra rash on sun-exposed skin (described in B). Telangiectasias may develop on the cheeks, nose, and forehead after several years of constant facial erythema, resulting from recurrent flushing attacks. Rarely, carcinoid produces cutaneous metastases, which are seen as tender, firm nodules. Scleroderma-like lesions can also be seen, especially on lower extremities (Chapter 61).

42. C; **43.** A; **44.** B; **45.** D; **46.** C Carcinoid is a tumor of chromaffin cells arising in the terminal ileum, other gastrointestinal (GI) locations, the lungs, and in ovarian and testicular teratomas. The tumor secretes kinins, serotonin, prostaglandins, histamine, and substance P, which induce bronchial constriction, gastrointestinal hypermobility, cardiac disease, and flushing. Serotonin seems to cause most of the symptoms. Flushing from gastric carcinoid can be blocked by a combination of H_1 and H_2 blockers, implicating histamine; it often occurs after meals. Since vasoactive substances produced by carcinoid tumors are degraded by the liver, hepatic metastases must be present before *gastric* carcinoid can produce flushing. Because venous drainage of bronchial or ovarian carcinoid bypasses the liver to reach the skin, flushing may occur in the absence of hepatic metastases. Flushing due to carcinoid typically lasts 1 to 2 minutes, and when severe, it can cause hypotension and shock. Diagnosis can be made by demonstrating increased levels of 24-hour urine 5-hydroxyindoleacetic acid.

Systemic mastocytosis involves mast cell proliferation in extracutaneous organs, most notably the GI tract and bone. GI manifestations are due to high circulating histamine levels and include nausea, vomiting, abdominal pain, GI hemorrhage, diarrhea, and steatorrhea. Pruritus and flushing are seen in about 30% of patients. Flushing episodes can be brought on by exercise, hot baths, emotional stress, and mast cell–degranulating drugs, such as aspirin and codeine. Systemic symptoms include pruritus, headache, bronchospasm, flushing, hypotension, tachycardia, dyspnea, syncope, and occasionally even death. Diagnosis is based on increased 24 hour urine histamine and its metabolite, 1-methyl-4-imidazoleacetic acid. Treatment includes antihistamines, disodium cromoglycate, and even aspirin (surprising, given aspirin's ability to induce symptoms) (Chapter 61).

47. A (F); B (F); C (F); D (F); E (T) Flushing is rare in pheochromocytoma, although a warm sensation may follow paroxysms of sweating and hypertension. Menopausal flushing is often brought on by hot beverages, physical exertion, and emotional upsets. It is characterized by its association with drenching perspiration. This implies an autonomic nerve–mediated (rather than direct vascular muscle) mechanism with concomitant effects on eccrine sweat glands. True monosodium glutamate flushing reactions are quite rare; most flushing from Chinese food is due to other ingredients. Tomatoes, spinach, eggplant, cheeses, red wine, chicken liver, and beefsteak are all high in histamine and can cause flushing (Chapter 61).

48. D Classic description and current teaching are that the diagnosis of Raynaud's disease (as a primary entity) should be made no less than 2 years after symptoms have been present without findings of underlying or associated diseases. If associated conditions exist, the term *Raynaud's phenomenon* is used. Some have found that longer periods of time may elapse before underlying connective tissue diseases are diagnosed. Therefore, many feel Raynaud's syndrome, which avoids prematurely making the distinction between Raynaud's as a phenomenon and as an idiopathic disease, is a more appropriate name. Classically, Raynaud's disease refers to a cold- or emotion-induced, usually bilaterally symmetrical, vasospastic phenomenon often involving multiple digits; it is associated with little or no gangrene (Chapter 62).

49. E Certain vibratory and traumatic activities can induce Raynaud's phenomenon, seemingly by direct arterial injury. Pneumatic drill, chain saw, and grinding and polishing wheel operation are the three most common occupations causing vibration-associated Raynaud's syndrome. The prevalence is 40% to 90% among chain saw operators. Exposure to vinyl chloride polymerization is another known occupational risk factor for Raynaud's (Chapter 62).

50. C Effective conservative therapy includes wearing gloves, avoidance of the cold, cessation of smoking, and avoidance of other known precipitants. Nifedipine is the most effective of medical therapies. Other calcium channel blockers, ketanserin (a serotonin-receptor blocker), prazosin, and prostaglandins are also considered first-line drugs. Less effective drug therapy includes methyldopa, reserpine, griseofulvin, and topical nitroglycerin application. Cervical sympathectomy is initially effective, but long-term follow-up reveals high relapse rates, especially in patients with underlying connective tissue disorders. (This suggests that increased sympathetic vasomotor activity alone does not cause symptoms.) Plasmapheresis has been effective in some instances. Beta-blocking agents, such as propranolol, can cause Raynaud's (Chapter 62).

51. D The classic triphasic color changes of Raynaud's are pallor, cyanosis, and rubor, resulting from initial vasoconstriction, tissue hypoxemia, and vasodilatory reperfusion. Numbness, tingling, and burning may accompany these phases. Only two thirds of patients experience all three phases. It usually manifests at an older age in men, and there is a higher risk of underlying vascular occlusive disease, such as arteriosclerosis or thromboangiitis obliterans. In contrast to Raynaud's disease, Raynaud's phenomenon tends to asymmetrically involve fewer digits. Sixty per cent to 90% of patients with Raynaud's syndrome are female (Chapter 62).

52. E In addition to the classically described precipitants of Raynaud's (direct cold exposure and emotional stress) there are numerous categories of other inciting agents and events. Drugs known to bring on symptoms include ergot compounds, methysergide, β-adrenergic blockers, sympathomimetic drugs, oral contraceptives, and cytotoxic drugs. Local trauma, such as piano playing, can also incite symptoms (Chapter 62).

53. C The pathogenesis of Raynaud's phenomenon is poorly understood. Raynaud's original hypothesis involved increased sympathetic vasomotor activity. The recurrence of symptoms despite sympathectomy has shed doubt on this hypothesis. All causes listed except impaired cyclooxygenase breakdown are proposed mechanisms. Enhanced platelet aggregation and activation, heightened blood viscosity, decreased blood fibrinolytic activity, imbalanced vasoactive prostaglandins, and reduced deformability of red blood cells have also been proposed. It is possible that numerous mechanisms exist for what is likely a heterogeneous syndrome (Chapter 62).

54. D All are associated with Raynaud's phenomenon. Scleroderma is the most common association. An incomplete list of associations would also include a variety of other connective tissue disorders, obstructive arterial diseases, neurovascular compression syndromes, hematologic abnormalities, occupational causes, numerous drugs, and neoplasia (Chapter 62).

55. C; E; F Other statistically significant predictors have included sclerodactyly, acro-osteolysis, subcutaneous calcification (seen on x-ray films of the hands), and digital pitted scars. The most frequent diagnosis is connective tissue disorder, especially scleroderma (Chapters 62 and 98).

56. A (F); B (F); C (T); D (T); E (T) Chronic lymphedema is classified as primary or secondary. Primary causes include congenital lymphedema and Milroy's disease. Secondary causes include inflammatory (venous stasis, infection, filariasis) and noninflammatory (postmastectomy, secondary to obstruction caused by malignancy). Although it may initially be pitting, it often becomes nonpitting. It responds poorly to therapy with leg elevation and diuretics. Postmastectomy lymphedema may be complicated by angiosarcoma or lymphoma (Chapter 64).

57. A (F); B (F); C (F); D (F); E (T) Stewart-Treves syndrome is the rare occurrence of angiosarcoma or lymphangiosarcoma in the face of chronic lymphedema. This is classically seen after radical mastectomy for breast carcinoma but is also described in lymphedema from other causes. It is rapidly fatal. Cutaneous lesions include ecchymoses, nodules, and bullae. Immunohistochemical studies have shown these tumors to be of endothelial origin and not recurrences of breast carcinoma. Development of angiosarcoma averages 9.5 years after lymphedema develops post mastectomy and 20 years after manifestation of lymphedema from other causes (Chapter 64).

58. A (T); B (F); C (T); D (T); E (T) Milroy's disease is congenital, painless lymphedema of one or both lower extremities. It is autosomal dominant and is more frequently seen in females. Often pitting, it results from hypoplastic distal lymphatics, usually only affecting feet, ankles, and lower legs. It often predisposes to recurrent β-hemolytic streptococcal infections (Chapter 64).

59. A (T); B (F); C (F); D (F); E (T) Telangiectasia can be divided into four different categories based on their clinical appearance: (1) sinus, or simple (linear); (2) arborizing; (3) spider, or star; (4) punctiform (papular). Papular telangiectasias are associated with genetic syndromes and collagen vascular diseases. Spider telangiectasias arise from arterioles in contrast to the blue linear or anastomosing telangiectasias commonly seen on the lower extremity, which arise from venules. Multiple causes have been proposed, but a common link to development of all telangiectasias is the release of vasoactive substances. Anoxia, infections, hormones, and physical factors may stimulate release of vasoactive substances. Telangiectasias of the legs develop in pregnancy in the first trimester, before the size of the uterus could compress the pelvic vasculature. Therefore, hormonal changes during pregnancy are thought to be responsible. Treatment options for telangiectasia include electrosurgery, laser, dermabrasion, medications, or sclerotherapy. Dermabrasion can be associated with recurrence. Hereditary hemorrhagic telangiectasia can be treated with estrogens. Generalized essential telangiectasia sometimes responds to tetracyclines (Chapter 66).

60. A–E (T) All sclerosing agents cause some discomfort on injection; skin necrosis may occur with all agents if the sclerosing agent extravasates. Hypertonic saline may produce necrosis without obvious extravasation. Extravasation of RBCs causes post-sclerotic hyperpigmentation. This side effect may be minimized by clearing the vessel of blood with the air-bolus technique. Muscle cramps may occur at the site of injection. Telangiectatic matting, blush areas, or collateralization usually occur on the thighs and are peripheral to and smaller than the area originally treated. Resolution often occurs spontaneously over 1 year, but 10% of patients require retreatment. Resistance to treatment is common and these mats may be permanent (Chapter 66).

61. A–D (T) Post-sclerotic compression helps seal the vascular lumina, minimizing the risk of thrombosis and subsequent hyperpigmentation. It also decreases the likelihood of recanalization. Prolonged compression cannot be applied to facial vessels, and thus these areas are more likely to develop necrosis and pigmentary changes (Chapter 66).

62. D Sodium tetradecyl sulfate has the highest incidence of allergic reactions of those sclerosing agents listed. Sodium morrhuate, an FDA-approved agent, has caused allergic reactions and even anaphylaxis because of protein contaminates. It is rarely used as a sclerosing agent (Chapter 66).

63. B Venous insufficiency. Venous hypertension results when a diseased venous system or faulty calf musculature prevents the predicted fall in pressure with ambulation. The venous system has one-way valves that direct blood only when there is a pressure differential between the deep and superficial venous systems. Venous insufficiency may be the result of dysfunction, neuropathies, or inflammatory diseases, leading to pump failure. Edema usually occurs secondary to venous insufficiency and leads to skin changes, increasing the risk of ulceration. Neuropathies (including diabetic neuropathy), obesity, and trauma may contribute to ulcer formation (Chapters 65 and 66).

64. A (T); B (T); C (F); D (F); E (T) Pressure ulcers have undermined edges, are punched-out in appearance, and are often draining. They are characterized by deep tissue necrosis that is often much greater in extent than the overlying skin defect. Muscle fibers are more sensitive to pressure than the skin. Compression forces are not uniform over the body; bony prominences of the sacrum, greater trochanter, ischial tuberosity of the calcaneus, and lateral malleolus are most affected (pressures as high as 2600 mm Hg). Decubitus ulcers result from a rise in tissue pressure, increased capillary filtration pressure, edema, and cell autolysis. Ischemic injury due to persistently occluded vessels further contributes to endothelial damage and an altered state of fibrinolysis.

Pyoderma gangrenosum ulcers are characterized by violaceous, rolled, boggy borders that are ill-defined and often show satellite violaceous papules at their border (Chapter 65).

65. A (F); B (T); C (F); D (T); E (F) Diabetics with foot ulcers often present with hyperglycemia and difficulty controlling their blood sugars. Examination shows ulcers commonly located on the metatarsal pad, heel, or on the hallux. Diabetics have a triad of motor, sensory, and autonomic nerve dysfunction. Motor dysfunction causes muscle atrophy with increase in extensor function that results in a claw-like deformity. More pressure is thus placed over the metatarsal pad in a patient who cannot sense the excessive pressure. Autonomic nerve dysfunction leads to decreased sweating and callus formation; skin becomes more susceptible to minor trauma. Autonomic nerve failure also leads to shunting of blood flow to the skin and away from muscle and subcutaneous tissue. Infection perpetuates ulcers once they have developed. Hyperglycemia impairs neutrophil function. *Staphylococcus aureus* is the bacteria most commonly isolated. Atherosclerosis further impedes wound healing by causing ischemia and poor nutrient delivery (Chapter 65).

66. B; **67.** A; **68.** D; **69.** B Arterial ulcers are typically located on the lateral aspect of the calf and ankle. An initial painful red plaque breaks down to form a superficial ulcer with minimal granulation tissue. Patients often have signs and symptoms of atherosclerosis-dependent rubor, claudication, coolness of the lower extremity, and pain with leg elevation. The pathogenesis of these ulcers may be related to increased vascular resistance without the compensatory relaxation that would normally occur distal to an arterial occlusion.

Venous ulcers are usually located over the medial aspect of the leg and are usually not very painful. Pain may be accentuated by a dependent position. Skin surrounding the ulcers shows signs of chronic stasis dermatitis and edema. Leakage of fibrogen into the dermis eventually forms a pericapillary cuff. This cuff may contribute to local anoxia. Patients have increased levels of protein C, fibrin-related antigen, and D-dimer, suggesting increased fibrin formation and breakdown.

Ulcers due to vasculopathies of morphea or scleroderma tend to be deep, indolent, and dry (Chapter 65).

70. B Occlusive dressings prevent crust formation and desiccation, thus enhancing the rate of epithelial migration. They also provide an environment with enhanced growth factors. Gradients of soluble ions are responsible for most of the electrical charge gradient, and as the wound dries out, the solute phase is lost as is the gradient. Epidermal migration may be influenced by electric fields within the wound. Bacteria thrive in a moist environment, but there has not been a problem with wound infection with the use of occlusive dressings. Wounds with large numbers of normal bacterial flora heal rapidly and without problems (Chapter 65).

71. C Compression stockings should be professionally fitted in the early morning when edema is minimal. A gradient pressure should be achieved, lower at the knee and at least 20 to 30 mm Hg at the level of the ankle. Occlusive arterial disease is not an absolute contraindication to compression stockings, but caution should be used and ankle systolic pressures evaluated (Chapter 65).

72. C Diphenylhydantoin may enhance rates of healing by inhibiting the secretion or synthesis of skin collagenase. It has been used to treat patients with recessive dystrophic epidermolysis bullosa. Anticoagulants may predispose patients to hematoma formation. Aspirin also has antiplatelet effects that can increase the likelihood of hematoma formation. Experimental animals have decreased tensile strength in healing wounds when given aspirin. Colchicine interferes with the microtubular system, preventing secretion of tropocollagen into the intercellular space. This drug may also stimulate collagenase. Phenylbutazone, a nonsteroidal anti-inflammatory drug, acts like aspirin to decrease tensile strength of wounds (Chapters 6 and 65).

73. A At 2 weeks after wounding, the wound has only 5% of its original strength, increasing to 40% at 1 month. A fully mature wound (by 18 months) has approximately 80% of normal strength (Chapter 6).

74. C During early phases of wound healing, type III collagen is produced in a collagen gel. Later, during the remodeling phase, type III is replaced by type I collagen and water and glycosaminoglycans are lost, leading to compression. The fibers therefore are closer together, aiding fiber cross-linking. Remodeling also includes realignment in which the fibers are reoriented parallel to the lines of tension.

Type II collagen is found in cartilage, and type IV collagen is found on the floor of the basement membrane zone (Chapter 6).

75. A (F); B (F); C (T); D (T); E (T) Wound healing can be divided temporally into three phases: substrate, proliferative, and remodeling. The substrate phase encompasses the first 3 to 4 days of healing, followed by 10 to 14 days of the proliferative phase. The remodeling phase lasts 6 to 12 months. The goal of the substrate phase is to prepare the defects for repair and to stabilize the wound. Initial hemostasis is achieved by vasoconstriction and platelet plugs. Activated thrombocytes release dense granules containing adenosine diphosphate and calcium important for fibrin formation. They release proteolytic enzymes, which are responsible for activation of the alternate complement pathway; C5a is a chemotactic factor for leukocytes. While polymorphonuclear leukocytes (PMNs) are the first participants in substrate phase inflammation, they do not stimulate fibroplasia. PMNs do assist with wound debridement and bacterial phagocytosis, and damaged PMNs release proteolytic, collagenolytic, and fibrinolytic enzymes. In the absence of wound infection, wounds heal normally in neutropenic animals. The neutrophil plays no regulatory role in subsequent phases of wound healing.

Macrophages in the wound are derived from blood monocytes. These cells can survive for long periods in the ulcer center, which is acid, anoxic, and avascular. Their presence is essential for normal wound healing. Macrophages release chemotactic and mitogenic factors that stimulate fibroplasia and angiogenesis as well as proteinases, elastases, and collagenases that further debride the wound.

The most important role of the lymphocytes is to secrete macrophage inhibition factor and macrophage activation factor. They do not directly assist with wound debridement by releasing fibrinolytic enzymes (Chapter 6).

76. A-E (T) Transforming growth factor B stimulates keratinocytes to produce fibronectin, which may promote macrophage phagocytosis of denatured collagen. Fibronectin is also found in the clot and acts as a stimulus for cell migration. Adhesion of fibroblasts to fibrin has been shown to require fibronectin. Keratinocyte migration is enhanced by fibronectin and, interestingly, the keratinocyte also degrades fibronectin, reconstitutes the fibronectin receptor, and produces more material for further attachment (Chapters 6 and 7).

77. A (F); B (T); C (F); D (T) Wound contraction begins 1 week after wounding. The contraction rate of 0.6 to 0.7 mm/day is independent of the size of the wound but dependent on the shape. Round wounds do not contract as completely or quickly as stellate or rectangular wounds. Fibroblasts are converted to myofibroblasts, which have prominent microtubules, providing the contractile force. Collagen, a rigid protein, does not contribute to wound contractivity (Chapters 6 and 7).

78. A (T); B (T); C (F); D (F); E (F) Epidermal allografts are often obtained from the foreskin of neonates. Studies have shown that young keratinocytes release growth factors that older keratinocytes do not. Thus, newborn cells are more responsive to growth stimulation by conditioned medium. Mothers are screened for risk factors for transmissible disease, and cultures are screened for bacterial or viral contamination. It was first thought that the original graft survived, but more recent studies have shown it is replaced by host keratinocytes. No human leukocyte antigen matching is performed. In contrast, cultured autografts become attached to the wound bed within 3 weeks and develop complete basal lamina. Graft sites are much less symptomatic within the first 24 hours after allografting (Chapter 65).

79. B; **80.** C; **81.** A; **82.** B (Chapter 7).

83. B; **84.** A; **85.** (F); **86.** C; **87.** E; **88.** G Epidermal growth factor (EGF) enhances proliferation of the keratinocytes and fibroblast by tyrosine kinase–induced phosphorylation of proteins, leading to activation of cellular DNA. EGF is produced by keratinocytes, and its precursor is membrane-bound.

Granulocyte-macrophage colony–stimulating factor is produced in basement membrane (BM) endothelial cells, keratinocytes, and leukocytes and is a potent factor for inducing growth and differentiation in the BM. Outside the marrow it acts as an autocrine hormone that stimulates proliferation.

Interleukin 1 (IL-1) is stored as a precursor in keratinocytes and is released after epidermal insult. Locally, IL-1 causes inflammation; systemically it causes fever, malaise, and elevation of C3 and acute-phase reactants. It also activates the liver to produce C3 and acute-phase reactants.

IL-2 (T-cell growth factor) is produced by lymphocytes. This cytokine stimulates natural killer cells, cytotonic T lymphocytes, and promotes B-cell production of antibodies. IL-2 stimulates T cells to produce gamma-interferon.

IL-6 is produced by lymphocytes and keratinocytes and stimulates B and T cells to blastogenesis and differentiation. IL-6 is also a pyrogen.

Tumor necrosis factor (TNF) is produced in the epidermis and can either stimulate or inhibit cell proliferation of epithelial and endothelial cells and fibroblasts. This factor plays an important role in maintenance of epidermal homeostasis, wound healing, and angiogenesis.

Interferon-γ is secreted by activated T cells. Its major function is in the regulation of class I and class II major histocompatibility antigens. It also down-regulates keratinocyte and endothelial cell proliferation as well as collagen synthesis by fibroblasts (Chapters 3 and 7).

Bibliography

Callen J. Current Problems in Dermatology 1993; 5:62–68.
Dibacco R, DeLeo V. Mastocytosis and the mast cell. J Am Acad Dermatol 1982; 7:709–722.
Dillon MJ. Systemic vasculitis. Clin Exp Rheumatol 1993; 11(Suppl 9):S19–S21.
Goldman M, Bennett R. Treatment of telangiectasia: A review. J Am Acad Dermatol 1987; 17:167–182.
Hammar H. Wound healing. Int J Dermatol 1993; 23:6–16.
Heller PE. Temperature-dependent skin disorders. J Am Acad Dermatol 1988; 18:1003–1019.
Jones JG. Clinical features of giant cell arteritis. In: Hazelman B, ed. Clin Rheumatol 1991; 5:413–430.
Kallenberg CGM, Mulder AHL, Tervaert JWC. Antineutrophil cytoplasmic antibodies: A still-growing class of autoantibodies in inflammatory disorders. Am J Med 1992; 93:675–682.
Klassen TP, Rowe PC, Gafni A. Economic evaluation of intravenous immune globulin therapy for Kawasaki syndrome. J Pediatr 1993; 122:538–542.
Kleinsmith DA. Raynaud's syndrome: An overview. Semin Dermatol 1985; 4:104–113.
Petri, M. Curr Prob Dermatol 1993; 4:173–201.
Piette WW. The differential diagnosis of purpura from a morphologic perspective. Adv Dermatol 1994; 9:3–24.
Piette WW. The antiphospholipid antibody syndrome. Curr Opin Dermatol 1994; 1:119–122.
Pollack S. Wound healing process. Clin Dermatol 1984; 2:8–16.
Yiannias J, El-Azhary RA, Gibson LE. Erythema elevatum diutinum: A clinical and histopathologic study of 13 patients. J Am Acad Dermatol 1992; 26:38–44.

chapter 10

Panniculitis, Fibrosing Disorders, and Atrophies

MICHAEL J. DANNENBERG, PHILLIP K. HALL,
GEORGIA A. KANNON, and JAMES W. PATTERSON

Choose the BEST answer to each of the following questions.

1. Partial lipodystrophy is associated with
   A. C1 esterase inhibitor
   B. C4 deficiency
   C. C1 deficiency
   D. C3 deficiency
   E. C567 abnormal function.

2. Weber-Christian panniculitis has been described in patients with which of the following disorders?
   A. Wilson's disease
   B. Chronic pancreatitis
   C. Gilbert's disease
   D. α_1-antitrypsin deficiency
   E. Crigler-Najjar syndrome.

3. You are asked to see a patient in the medical intensive care unit for atrophic, nonindurated, mildly erythematous patches on the right thigh and left upper arm who has been hospitalized with sepsis. The patient is reportedly febrile, with hypotension, and tachycardia, and has radiographic evidence of pneumonia. Abnormal laboratory values include serum bicarbonate, 15; pH, 7.14; sedimentation rate, 112; serum glucose, 892; serum osmolality, 360; serum amylase, 12; and lipase, normal. Results of coagulation studies and platelet count are normal. The most likely diagnosis is
   A. Pancreatic fat necrosis
   B. Cold panniculitis
   C. Localized lipodystrophy
   D. Lipogranulomatosis subcutanea of Rothmann-Makai
   E. Histiocytic cytophagic panniculitis.

4. All of the following may be associated with lobular panniculitis EXCEPT
   A. Lupus erythematosus
   B. Polyarteritis nodosa
   C. Sarcoidosis
   D. Post-steroid panniculitis
   E. Pancreatic fat necrosis.

5. A healthy-appearing 20-year-old male complains of deep nodules on his trunk and legs that are tender to the touch. He is otherwise healthy and has no history of fevers, chills, abdominal pain, weight

117

loss, or recent infections. The only laboratory abnormalities are an elevated sedimentation rate and mild leukocytosis. The most likely diagnosis is

A. Weber-Christian disease

B. Pancreatic fat necrosis

C. Bazin's disease

D. Histiocytic cytophagic panniculitis

E. Lipogranulomatosis subcutanea of Rothmann-Makai.

6. A 6-year-old girl developed firm, tender, itchy, red nodules on her trunk, extremities, and buttocks 1 month after she was discharged from the hospital. While hospitalized, she had been receiving intravenous methylprednisolone therapy for 7 days in addition to other drugs. You diagnose the condition as post-steroid panniculitis. Which of the following conditions is the most likely reason the patient was initially admitted to the hospital?

A. Tuberculosis

B. Leprosy

C. Rheumatic fever

D. Blastomycosis

E. Child abuse.

7. Erythema nodosum migrans is associated with all of the following EXCEPT

A. A history of streptococcal infections

B. A history of ulcerative colitis

C. Behçet's syndrome

D. A history of *Borrelia burgdorferi* infection

E. A history of oral bromide usage.

8. Which of the following is an example of septal panniculitis with vasculitis?

A. Erythema nodosum

B. Erythema induratum

C. Necrobiosis lipoidica

D. Superficial migratory thrombophlebitis

E. Eosinophilic fasciitis.

9. Systemic lobular panniculitis associated with a febrile course, hepatosplenomegaly, pancytopenia, liver function abnormalities, an unusual bleeding diathesis, and "bean bag" cells on histopathology would best characterize which of the following disorders?

A. Cytophagic histiocytic panniculitis

B. Weber-Christian disease

C. Sclerema neonatorum

D. Neonatal subcutaneous fat necrosis

E. Chronic lymphocytic leukemia.

10. A 22-year-old man presents with a painless subcutaneous tumor on the shaft of his penis that has been present for years. Histologic study of the mass after surgical removal reveals hyaline necrosis in the septa of the fat cells. An infiltrate of round cells, macrophages, and polymorphonuclear cells is seen. The collagen and fat are also altered. The most likely diagnosis is

A. Localized lipodystrophy

B. Zoon's balanitis

C. Sclerosing lipogranuloma

D. Post-steroid panniculitis

E. Lipoatrophia annularis.

11. Subcutaneous fat necrosis of the newborn is characterized by all of the following EXCEPT

A. Idiopathic hypercalcemia

B. Needle-shaped clefts within adipocytes

C. Calcification of subcutaneous nodules

D. Poor prognosis

E. Areas clear in a few months.

12. Sclerema neonatorum

A. Is thought to be linked to trauma or asphyxia at birth

B. May be linked to diabetes mellitus in the mother

C. Generally is associated with a poor prognosis

D. Is associated with a decreased saturated:unsaturated fatty acid ratio

E. Has no relation to perinatal hypothermia.

13. Partial lipodystrophy may be associated with all of the following EXCEPT

A. A positive family history

B. Abnormal complement profiles

C. Leprechaunism

D. Membranoproliferative glomerulonephritis

E. C3 nephritic factor.

14. The most common cause of pancreatic fat necrosis is

A. Chronic alcoholism

B. Pancreatic carcinoma

C. Traumatic pancreatitis

D. Oral contraceptives

E. Nonsteroidal anti-inflammatory drugs.

15. A 14-year-old boy presents with a complaint of unintentional weight loss. He states that his skin appears to be more wrinkled and "loose" and that he has started to grow hair between his scalp and eyebrows. On physical examination, he is seen to have acanthosis nigricans. He is also found to have hyperlipidemia and elevated serum glucose. This patient probably has

    A. Lipoatrophia annularis of Ferreira-Marques
    B. Total lipodystrophy
    C. Pancreatic carcinoma (acinar type)
    D. Diabetes mellitus
    E. Abdominal lipodystrophy.

16. **For each numbered item choose the most likely associated lettered item. Each numbered item has ONLY ONE answer.**

    1. Total lipodystrophy
    2. Lipoatrophia annularis
    3. Weber-Christian disease
    4. Cytophagic histiocytic panniculitis
    5. Factitial panniculitis
    6. Pancreatic fat necrosis
    7. Cold panniculitis
    8. Lipogranulomatosis subcutanea
    9. Erythema nodosum
    10. Erythema induratum
    11. Superficial migratory thrombophlebitis
    12. Partial lipodystrophy
    13. Lupus profundus
    14. Infectious panniculitis
    15. Post-steroid panniculitis
    16. Subcutaneous fat necrosis of newborn
    17. Sclerema neonatorum.

    A. Nodules may liquefy and calcify; may be related to trauma at birth
    B. Biopsy positive for infectious organism
    C. Associated with glomerulonephritis
    D. Tuberculoid granulomas are characteristic
    E. Localized form of lobular panniculitis
    F. Elevated serum lipase and amylase
    G. Unusual bleeding diathesis present
    H. Area of bracelet-shaped atrophy about limb
    I. Fatal in 70% of cases; hypothermic etiology proposed
    J. Ninety per cent with a history of rheumatic fever
    K. Hyalinization of lipocytes
    L. Associated with pancreatic and lung carcinoma
    M. Sarcoidosis
    N. May be seen in children eating popsicles
    O. Foreign material may be seen on polarization
    P. May be related to α_1-antitrypsin deficiency
    Q. Similar findings may be seen in leprechaunism.

Choose the ONE BEST answer to each of the following questions.

17. The pathology of all of the following conditions reveals a lobular panniculitis without vasculitis EXCEPT

    A. Cold-induced panniculitis
    B. Erythema induratum
    C. Pancreatic panniculitis
    D. Post-steroid panniculitis.

18. All of the following are symptoms of Lofgren's syndrome EXCEPT

    A. Parotiditis
    B. Erythema nodosum
    C. Hilar adenopathy
    D. Fever.

19. The most frequent infectious cause of erythema nodosum is:

    A. *Staphylococcus aureus*
    B. Group A streptococci
    C. Tuberculosis
    D. *Pseudomonas* organisms.

20. A 30-year-old white woman develops recurrent febrile episodes of crops of erythematous, tender, symmetrical, subcutaneous nodules on the thighs and legs. The nodules do not ulcerate and gradually involute over a few weeks, leaving hyperpigmented, atrophic scars. These episodes are accompanied by arthralgia, fatigue, and malaise. Skin biopsy reveals a lobular panniculitis without vasculitis, but with fat necrosis and an infiltrate of foamy histiocytes. Laboratory results reveal a

markedly elevated sedimentation rate. The most likely diagnosis is

A. Sarcoidosis

B. Erythema nodosum secondary to lupus

C. Weber-Christian disease

D. Lupus panniculitis.

21. A 3-day-old infant develops indurated, firm areas on the buttocks that rapidly evolve over the entire body surface, and the skin feels woody, waxy, hard, and cold. The disease continues to progress, and the infant dies 2 weeks later. The most likely diagnosis is:

A. Sclerema neonatorum

B. Infectious panniculitis with secondary sepsis

C. Subcutaneous fat necrosis of the newborn

D. Leukemia panniculitis.

22. A 1-week-old infant develops violaceous, firm nodules and plaques on his cheeks and buttocks. The overlying skin is woody and cannot be pinched. The child's birth was traumatic and prolonged. With development of the skin lesions, the child becomes irritable and will not eat resulting in failure to thrive. At day 14, he undergoes cardiac arrest, and is resuscitated. The most likely cause of this child's cardiac arrest is

A. Respiratory arrest

B. Sepsis

C. Hypercalcemia

D. Malnutrition.

23. Post-steroid panniculitis occurs most commonly in

A. Elderly women

B. Children

C. Black men

D. Black women.

24. Neonates are uniquely susceptible to cold-related injury and cold panniculitis for all of the following reasons EXCEPT

A. Newborn fat has higher melting and solidification points

B. Newborns have a lower ratio of saturated to unsaturated fat

C. Newborns have a higher ratio of body surface area to weight

D. Newborns have a higher ratio of saturated to unsaturated fat.

25. A 60-year-old white man presents with multiple, large, inflamed, ulcerated subcutaneous nodules and large ecchymoses on the arms and legs that have been present for 6 months. On physical examination, he is febrile (102° F) and has diffuse lymphadenopathy and hepatosplenomegaly. Laboratory results reveal pancytopenia with coagulopathy, and elevated liver function. Histologic analyses of skin biopsy reveals lobular panniculitis with an infiltrate composed of large bean bag cells with phagocytosis of lymphocytes, platelets, and red blood cells. These same large cells are found on analysis of lymph node and bone marrow biopsies. The most likely diagnosis is

A. Infectious panniculitis secondary to tuberculosis

B. Panniculitis secondary to leukemia

C. Sarcoidosis

D. Histiocytic cytophagic panniculitis.

26. The most characteristic pathologic feature of the panniculitis associated with renal failure is

A. Mural calcification of arterioles and fat

B. "Ghost-like" fat cells with lipid necrosis

C. Mucin deposition within fat lobules

D. Vasculitis of septal subcutaneous vessels with thrombosis and fibrin deposition.

27. A previously healthy 70-year-old black man developed nodular, indurated plaques on his right thigh shortly after falling down some steps. Histopathologic analyses of skin biopsy revealed an inflammatory infiltrate of lymphocytes, histiocytes, and plasma cells within the fascia and septae of subcutaneous fat as well as sclerosis of these areas. The most likely diagnosis is

A. Scleroderma panniculitis

B. Traumatic induced panniculitis

C. Eosinophilic fasciitis

D. Eosinophilia-myalgia syndrome

28. All of the following are features, histologically, of lupus profundus EXCEPT

A. Lobular panniculitis

B. Septal panniculitis with evidence of vasculitis

C. Necrobiotic changes with fibrinoid deposits in fat lobules

D. Mucin deposition.

29. A 40-year-old black woman presents with a 3-month history of anorexia, weight loss, and dys-

pepsia. On physical examination, she is seen to be icteric, and a right upper quadrant mass is palpated. Skin examination reveals multiple, tender, red nodules in a linear configuration on the left leg. The most likely cause of the skin lesions is

A. Polyarteritis nodosa

B. Erythema induratum

C. Panniculitis secondary to lymphoma

D. Trousseau's syndrome.

30. The most likely underlying malignancy in the patient in Question 29 is

A. Pancreatic carcinoma

B. Lymphoma of the small bowel

C. Hepatoma

D. Gastric carcinoma.

31. Other diseases associated with superficial migratory thrombophlebitis include all of the following EXCEPT

A. Infections

B. Varicosities

C. Behçet's syndrome

D. Pregnancy

E. All of the above.

32. A 50-year-old white woman, a heavy smoker, presents with nodules on the lower legs and dorsal surfaces of the feet. A few of the nodules are pulsatile. Surrounding the lesions are areas of purpura with an overall background of livedo reticularis. The fifth toe has a mottled violaceous hue with a small area of gangrene. Upon further questioning, the patient gives a history of melena. Histopathologic analysis of a skin biopsy reveals a septal panniculitis with vasculitis. The most likely diagnosis is

A. Superficial migratory thrombophlebitis

B. Polyarteritis nodosa

C. Henoch-Schönlein purpura

D. Buerger's disease.

33. The most frequently affected arteries in polyarteritis nodosa include all of the following EXCEPT

A. Skin

B. Gastrointestinal tract

C. Central nervous system

D. Kidney.

34. Rothmann-Makai syndrome is

A. A triad of panniculitis, eosinophilia, and weakness

B. Treated with potassium iodide

C. Associated with malignancies

D. A localized type of lobular panniculitis without systemic manifestations

E. A sign of tertiary syphilis.

35. Erythema nodosum may be caused by all of the following EXCEPT

A. Birth control pills

B. Penicillin

C. Tuberculosis

D. Sulfonamides

E. Sarcoidosis.

36. All of the following are true statements regarding calciphylaxis EXCEPT

A. Histologically, it shows lobular panniculitis and mural calcification of small arterioles in the deep dermis

B. It is usually seen in patients with renal failure

C. Clinically, it manifests with subcutaneous nodules that often ulcerate

D. Ectopic calcification frequently occurs in this disease

E. It is thought to be secondary to decreased calcium and phosphate removal during the process of dialysis.

37. Scarring is commonly found with which panniculitis?

A. Erythema induratum

B. Erythema nodosum

C. Subcutaneous fat necrosis

D. Post-steroid panniculitis

E. Cold panniculitis.

38. Which of the following panniculitides are associated with subcutaneous fat necrosis, arthritis, and serositis?

A. Erythema nodosum

B. Histiocytic cytophagic panniculitis

C. Weber-Christian disease

D. Erythema induratum

E. Panniculitis associated with pancreatic disease.

39. Which panniculitis is not limited to the skin and is a systemic disease?

   A. Erythema nodosum migrans
   B. Post-steroid panniculitis
   C. Morphea profundus
   D. Nodular vasculitis
   E. Periarteritis nodosa.

For the following questions, the set of lettered headings is followed by a list of numbered words or phrases. For each numbered word or phrase, choose

   A. If the item is associated with A only
   B. If the item is associated with B only
   C. If the item is associated with both A and B
   D. If the item is associated with neither A nor B.

For each of the following characteristics, choose whether it describes subcutaneous fat necrosis of the newborn, sclerema neonatorum, both, or neither.

40. Typically affects severely ill newborns
41. A lobular panniculitis without any concomitant vasculitis
42. Occurs exclusively in children born to primigravid mothers
43. Resolves spontaneously without treatment.

   A. Subcutaneous fat necrosis of the newborn
   B. Sclerema neonatorum
   C. Both
   D. Neither.

For each numbered item, choose the most likely associated lettered item. Each numbered item has ONLY ONE answer. Each lettered item may be the answer to one, more than one, or none of the numbered items.

Match each of the diseases listed to the most appropriate histologic description.

44. Lobular panniculitis, with degeneration of lipocytes and numerous macrophages within the infiltrate
45. "Swiss cheese" appearance
46. Subcutaneous hemorrhage is frequently seen secondary to vessel necrosis and the development of aneurysmal dilatations
47. Early lesions show a neutrophilic infiltrate in the septum, affecting small and often medium-sized vessels without leukocytoclasis
48. Microgranulomatous foci (of Miescher) with lymphocytes, histiocytes, and giant cells are a characteristic finding.

   A. Weber-Christian disease
   B. Erythema nodosum
   C. Chemical (oil) panniculitis
   D. Polyarteritis nodosa.

For each of the diseases listed, match the best clinical description.

49. Painless bluish-red nodules or ulceration, typically on the calves of females
50. Recurrent, tender nodules that frequently ulcerate in a patient with emphysema and cirrhosis
51. Livedo reticularis surrounding tender subcutaneous nodules or ulcers, typically on the lower extremities
52. Tender, erythematous plaques on the shins of a patient with sarcoidosis.

   A. Cutaneous polyarteritis nodosa
   B. Erythema induratum
   C. Erythema nodosum
   D. α_1-antitrypsin deficiency panniculitis
   E. Factitial panniculitis.

Match the following diseases with the characteristics listed.

53. L-tryptophan
54. May involve underlying bone (cortical hyperostosis)
55. Emaciated face and trunk, with apparent obesity of hips, buttocks, and legs
56. "Cigarette paper" skin

   A. Linear scleroderma
   B. Eosinophilic fasciitis
   C. Eosinophilia-myalgia syndrome
   D. Partial lipodystrophy
   E. Anetoderma.

57. Indurated, "bound-down" skin following exercise.

ANSWERS

1. D There are normal levels of C4, C1, C1 esterase inhibitor, and normal function of C567 in partial lipodystrophy. This disorder, also known as progressive lipoatrophy or Barraquer-Simons syndrome, is characterized by a progressive loss of subcutaneous fat, usually of the cephalothoracic, or classic, type. It usually occurs in children between the ages of 5 and 8, and girls outnumber boys by 4:1. The upper half of the body seems emaciated, the cheeks sink in, and the skin over the rest of the face is drawn like a death mask. Unlike those with the classic form of the disease, patients with disease of the lower trunk seem often to have a positive family history of acanthosis nigricans, diabetes, or hepatosplenomegaly.

Autografts of normal fat to atrophic sites undergo wasting. In a study of 21 patients with partial lipodystrophy, 17 had decreased C3 with normal C1 and C4, and 6 had nephritis. Two thirds of patients with classic partial lipodystrophy have a protein called C3 nephritic factor in their serum. This is an autoantibody against alternative pathway C3 convertase C3b, Bb. It increases the half-life of the convertase and prevents cleavage of C3b by C3b inactivator. This leads to the development of membranoproliferative glomerulonephritis in many of these patients (Chapter 71).

2. D Of all of the listed choices that can be associated with disease of the liver, only α_1-antitrypsin deficiency has been reported to be associated with Weber-Christian panniculitis. Many authors currently consider that Weber-Christian panniculitis is not a specific entity but one that can be associated with a number of causes, including trauma and connective tissue disease. α_1-Antitrypsin deficiency is widely regarded as one, maybe the most significant, cause of the Weber-Christian syndrome (Chapter 71).

3. C The preceding clinical scenario seems to indicate that the patient is in a hyperosmolar diabetic state and has septicemia, probably stemming from the pneumonia seen on chest x-ray. The diagnosis of pancreatic fat necrosis is unlikely, since the amylase and lipase are normal. Cold panniculitis is usually seen in areas exposed to cold, and tends to be bilateral in distribution (i.e., cheeks of children, thighs of horseback riders). Lipogranulomatosis subcutanea is thought to be an idiopathic, benign variant of Weber-Christian panniculitis. Histiocytic cytophagic panniculitis is a rare disorder characterized by widespread erythematous, painful, subcutaneous nodules, febrile illness, hepatosplenomegaly, pancytopenia, liver dysfunction, and even hemorrhagic diathesis. This patient's lipodystrophy is in areas where he most probably injects his insulin (Chapter 71).

4. B Polyarteritis nodosa is associated with a septal panniculitis (with vasculitis). All other disorders listed are associated with lobular panniculitis. Note the following classification of panniculitides:

Lobular panniculitis
  Without vasculitis
    Idiopathic lobular panniculitis (Weber-Christian)
    Lipogranulomatosis subcutanea (Rothmann-Makai)
    Cytophagic histiocytic panniculitis
    Physical panniculitis
      Cold-induced
      Traumatic
      Chemical-induced
      Factitial
    Neonatal panniculitis
      Sclerema neonatorum
      Subcutaneous fat necrosis
    Pancreatic panniculitis
    Post-steroid panniculitis
    Lobular panniculitis of systemic disease
      Lupus erythematosus
      Sarcoidosis
      Granuloma annulare
      Leukemia and lymphoma
      Infections
  With vasculitis
    Nodular vasculitis (erythema induratum, or "Bazin's disease")
Septal panniculitis
  Without vasculitis
    Erythema nodosum
    Scleroderma panniculitis
    Eosinophilic fasciitis
    Necrobiosis lipoidica diabeticorum
  With vasculitis
    Superficial migratory thrombophlebitis
    Polyarteritis nodosa
    Cutaneous polyarteritis nodosa (Chapters 58 and 68 to 71)

5. E The only disease in the preceding list that appears in otherwise healthy individuals is lipogranulomatosis subcutanea. As mentioned in the answer for Question 3, it is thought to be a benign variant of Weber-Christian disease by many, and patients generally tend to be healthy. They often have tender, spherical subcutaneous nodules on the legs and sometimes on the trunk and arms, which vary from 2 to 30 mm in diameter. The average number of nodules is 12. There are no systemic symptoms, and fever is absent. The lesions usually last 6 to 12 months (Chapter 71).

6. C Post-steroid panniculitis is characterized by firm, pruritic, tender, erythematous, subcutaneous nodules occurring on the buttocks, trunk, and extremities of children 1 to 30 days after cessation of oral prednisone therapy. About 90% of reported cases have been in children on prednisone for rheumatic carditis. Fever, joint pain, and heart failure all may be present. All reported patients have received at least 2000 mg of prednisone or its equivalent. Post-steroid panniculitis is usually transient and disappears spontaneously (Chapter 71).

7. D Erythema nodosum is associated with all of the above conditions except history of Lyme disease. It is an inflammatory condition that is caused by a delayed hypersensitivity reaction involving the large blood vessels of the fibrous septae of the subcutaneous tissue. Other conditions in which one may see erythema nodosum include tuberculosis, sarcoidosis, fungal infections, lymphogranuloma venereum, cat-scratch fever, leptospirosis, leukemias, drugs, inflammatory bowel diseases, infectious diseases of the bowel, such as *Yersinia enterocolitica* and *Campylobacter jejuni* infections, and drug injection. Erythema chronicum migrans is associated *with Borrelia burgdorferi* infection (Chapter 68).

8. D Of the previous choices, only superficial migratory thrombophlebitis represents a septal panniculitis with vasculitis. Erythema nodosum, eosinophilic fasciitis, and necrobiosis lipoidica are septal panniculitides without vasculitis. Erythema induratum is a lobular panniculitis with vasculitis (Chapter 68).

9. A First described in 1980, cytophagic histiocytic panniculitis is a disorder that is characterized by widespread, erythematous, painful subcutaneous nodules, that may occasionally become ecchymotic or hemorrhagic and break down to form crusted ulcerations. There is a progressive febrile illness, with hepatosplenomegaly, pancytopenia, and liver dysfunction, resulting from the proliferation of benign-appearing histiocytes with a marked phagocytic capacity. Histologically, there is infiltration of the lobules by histiocytes and inflammatory cells with fat necrosis and hemorrhage. The typical cell is a bean bag cell (a histiocyte stuffed with phagocytized RBCs, lymphocytes, neutrophils, and platelets). Patients usually die of acute hemorrhage after a long illness (Chapter 71).

10. C These are the classic clinical and histologic findings of sclerosing lipogranuloma. Localized lipodystrophy is typically seen 6 months to 2 years after initiation of insulin injections in diabetics. Zoon's balanitis, also known as benign plasma cell erythroplasia and balanoposthitis chronica circumscripta plasmacellularis, is a benign inflammatory lesion with a plasma cell infiltrate. Clinically, it is characterized by a persistent inflammation, which is usually sharply demarcated and usually occurs on the inner surface of the prepuce and glans penis. Post-steroid panniculitis is usually seen in children after steroid therapy for rheumatic fever. Lipoatrophia annularis of Ferreira-Marques is circumferential atrophy of the subcutaneous fat preceded by swelling, redness, scaling, and paresthesia about an extremity followed by loss of subcutaneous fat, so that there is a depressed, atrophic, bracelet-like constriction (Chapter 71).

11. D Subcutaneous fat necrosis in newborn or young infants is characterized by localized, firm, purple-red, subcutaneous nodules present on the cheeks, back, buttocks, and thighs. These nodules do not pit on firm pressure. Softening and absorption of the indurated areas begins in about the fifth week and is complete in a few months. The nodules may frequently liquefy and may develop calcification. The cause is unknown, but trauma at birth, asphyxia, hypothermia, and diabetes mellitus in the mother may be possible predisposing factors. Fatal, idiopathic hypercalcemia may be associated with this illness, but most cases are associated with a good prognosis (Chapter 69).

12. C This disease begins during the first few weeks of life in premature or debilitated infants, who usually have an associated severe disease such as sepsis, respiratory distress, diarrhea, congenital heart disease, or dehydration. There is symmetrical hardening of subcutaneous fat, usually of the buttocks, shoulders, calves, and cheeks. The skin of the palms, soles, and genitalia is spared. The course is rapidly progressive and is fatal. It is not specifically associated with maternal diabetes mellitus. A substantial increase in the saturated to unsaturated ratio of fatty acids of the subcutaneous triglycerides in affected infants has been reported. These factors may make the newborn more susceptible to cold injury and may be responsible for the dramatic physical changes (Chapter 69).

13. C All of the listed choices are associated with partial lipodystrophy except leprechaunism, which appears clinically similar to total lipodystrophy. These patients have decreased or absent subcutaneous fat in a generalized distribution, wrinkled loose skin, acanthosis nigricans, hypertrichosis, dysplastic nails, thick lips, and gingival hypertrophy. Separating them from total lipodystrophy are the presence of muscular wasting, retarded bone age, retarded growth, and early death. (Also see answer to Question 1.) (Chapter 71).

14. A Pancreatic panniculitis is associated with excessive circulating pancreatic enzymes such as trypsin, amylase, and lipase. The lesions usually begin on the legs as painless, elevated, subcutaneous nodules that may clinically resemble erythema nodosum, drug eruption, periarteritis nodosa, or embolic abscesses. The patients are extremely ill, with fever, vomiting, and abdominal distention. Fifty per cent of cases are caused by pancreatitis, most often (approximately 50%) the result of chronic alcoholism. Of the remaining cases, 30% are due to pancreatic carcinoma, most often acinar type rather than the more common adenocarcinoma; 15% of patients have pancreatic pseudocysts; and traumatic panniculitis is the cause in 5% (Chapter 71).

15. B This is the classic description of total lipodystrophy. Other features may include clitoral or penile enlargement early in life, hepatomegaly, dolicocephalic skulls, lipodystrophic facies, hirsutism, prominent teeth, and a small chin. Lipoatrophia annularis is characterized by circumferential atrophy of the subcutaneous fat preceded by swelling, redness, scaling, and paresthesia about an extremity followed by loss of subcutaneous fat so that there is division into two parts by a depressed atrophic, bracelet-like constriction. These features are not those seen in pancreatic necrosis (described in answer to Question 14). Patients with diabetes mellitus do not have these clinical abnormalities, rather they may have localized lipodystrophy secondary to insulin injection. Abdominal lipodystrophy is also known as "Lipodystrophia centrifugalis abdominalis infantalis." It is a disease of childhood. Ninety per cent of cases begin by the age of 5 years. It is characterized by depression of the abdominal wall (caused by loss of fat), which enlarges centrifugally for 3 to 8 years, in most cases. Histologically, most or all of the fat is lost, with minimal inflammatory infiltrate. By the age of 8 to 13 years, the progression stops, and within a year or two, normal contours are restored in almost all cases. All but one reported case have been in Asians (Chapter 71).

16. 1. Q; 2. H; 3. P; 4. G; 5. O; 6. F; 7. N; 8. E; 9. M; 10. D; 11. L; 12. C; 13. K; 14. B; 15. J; 16. A; 17. I

17. B Answers A, C, and D indicate types of lobular panniculitis not associated with vasculitis. Erythema induratum, or nodular vasculitis, causes lobular panniculitis with vasculitis of medium-sized vessels. It is classically associated with tuberculosis; histology also reveals caseating granulomas within fat lobules (Chapters 68 and 71).

18. A Lofgren's syndrome of sarcoidosis consists of the tetrad of fever, bilateral hilar adenopathy, arthralgias, and erythema nodosum. Parotiditis, although a symptom of sarcoidosis, is not a feature of Lofgren's syndrome, which is generally associated with a good prognosis. Patients usually have mild disease, do not develop lung disease, and spontaneous remission generally occurs with or without treatment (Chapter 45).

19. B Whereas many bacterial, viral, and fungal infections are known to be associated with erythema nodosum, β-hemolytic streptococcal infection is the most well-established cause. Streptococcal infection is also the most common causative agent in recurrent erythema nodosum, especially in children. Skin lesions usually develop within 3 weeks post infection, and ASO and Streptozyme titers are frequently elevated. Streptococcal skin tests are positive and can sometimes precipitate erythema nodosum lesions. Infectious diseases associated with erythema nodosum include tuberculosis, leprosy, and tularemia as well as those caused by *Yersinia* and *Mycoplasma* organisms (Chapter 68).

20. C Weber-Christian disease, otherwise known as idiopathic lobular panniculitis or relapsing febrile nonsuppurative panniculitis, is generally seen in women aged 30 to 60 years and classically manifests as recurrent episodes of fever and crops of tender, red subcutaneous nodules most commonly located on the legs. These lesions resolve with hyperpigmentation and atrophy. Visceral involvement may occur as well, and if extensive, can be lethal. The sedimentation rate is markedly elevated. An α_1-antitrypsin level must be checked, since these diseases can be virtually identical.

Biopsy reveals a lobular panniculitis, initially consisting of neutrophils and lymphocytes, later showing foamy histiocytes and eventually, fibrosis and scarring. Histology of sarcoid panniculitis is lobular, but one should see noncaseating granulomas. Erythema nodosum is a septal panniculitis, and lupus panniculitis shows a predominance of lymphocytes and hyalinization of the subcutis (Chapter 70).

21. A Sclerema neonatorum is a lobular panniculitis that occurs exclusively in neonates within the first few days of life, begins locally, but then becomes generalized. These infants have a poor prognosis, and the disease is generally fatal. Subcutaneous fat necrosis of the newborn remains localized and carries a good prognosis. Leukemia and infectious causes need to be ruled out, but are less likely (Chapter 69).

22. C The child most likely had subcutaneous fat necrosis of the newborn characterized by localized areas of fat necrosis developing during the first few weeks of life. Unlike those with sclerema neonatorum, these children are generally healthy, and the lesions resolve spontaneously over a few months with little or no scarring. Traumatic birth or hypothermia may be associated with the disease. Although prognosis is usually excellent, the disease is occasionally complicated by hypercalcemia manifested as anorexia, marasmus, irritability, and constipation, or death is caused by arrhythmia. Serial calcium levels should therefore be monitored (Chapter 69).

23. B All cases of post-steroid panniculitis, to date, have occurred in children. This rare disorder occurs in children within two weeks post oral or intravenous steroid withdrawal. Patients have usually received short courses of high-dose steroids, often complicated by substantial weight gain during the course of therapy. The etiology is unclear, but it has been proposed that the panniculitis occurs in areas that show greater fat accumulation followed by rapid removal of fat with steroid withdrawal, leading to necrosis of adipocytes. Lesions resolve spontaneously or with resumption of steroid therapy (Chapter 71).

24. B Neonates are highly susceptible to cold injury because they have high surface area to body weight ratios and high ratios of saturated to unsaturated fat, which gives them higher fat melting and solidification points (Chapter 69).

25. D Histiocytic cytophagic panniculitis is a lobular panniculitis characterized by an infiltrate of benign large histiocytic cells with secondary phagocytosis of other blood cells. These same cells called bean bag cells also infiltrate lymph nodes, bone marrow, liver, and spleen. The cutaneous lesions have a tendency to ulcerate and form ecchymoses. These patients may be extremely sick with pancytopenia and coagulopathy. There is no effective treatment for the disease, although some people have responded to multidrug chemotherapy. It was once thought to be uniformly fatal but spontaneous remissions do occur. It is unclear whether this is a benign histiocytic response or a malignant T-cell disorder (Chapter 71).

26. A Panniculitis of renal failure, also known as calciphylaxis, is thought to be caused largely by secondary hyperparathyroidism, resulting in ectopic calcification in subcutaneous tissue—a hallmark of the disease. Histology reveals mural calcification in small arterioles of the deep dermis and the lobular areas of subcutaneous tissue. Ghost-like fat cells are characteristic of panniculitis associated with pancreatic disease. Mucin deposition is seen with the disease but is not a characteristic feature. Vasculitis is not present in calciphylaxis (Chapter 71).

27. C Eosinophilic fasciitis results in an inflammatory reaction of the septal fat and fascia. It occurs more commonly in men and patients usually give a history of previous trauma. Lesions are most commonly located over an extremity. Traumatic panniculitis is a lobular panniculitis that does not involve fascia. Panniculitis of scleroderma and the eosinophilia-myalgia syndrome both cause a septal panniculitis. This man was also previously healthy with no history of scleroderma or L-tryptophan ingestion (Chapters 98 and 99).

28. B The panniculitis of lupus, or lupus profundus, is a lobular panniculitis without vasculitis. Mucin is often present, and there are necrobiotic changes with fibrinoid deposits in fat lobules, hyalinization of fat with separation of fat cells by homogeneous eosinophilic collagen (Chapters 24 and 71).

29. D Superficial migratory thrombophlebitis is a septal panniculitis with thrombosis of the superficial veins at the dermal-subcutaneous border. Nodules occurring in a linear distribution on the legs is characteristic of the disease. The disease may be associated with hypercoagulable states. When the hypercoagulable state is secondary to an underlying malignancy, it is known as Trousseau's syndrome (Chapters 68 and 71).

30. A Pancreatic cancer is the malignancy most commonly associated with Trousseau's syndrome. Whereas gastric carcinoma is commonly associated with the disease as well, the presentation of jaundice, weight loss, and a right upper quadrant mass are more suggestive of carcinoma involving the head of the pancreas. The most commonly associated cancers are those of the pancreas, stomach, colon, ovary, prostate, lung, and gallbladder (Chapter 71).

31. E All are correct. Superficial migratory thrombophlebitis most frequently occurs as a complication of varicose veins. It is also associated with primary hypercoagulable states, such as deficiencies of proteins C and S and antithrombin III, the lupus anticoagulant, Factor XII deficiency, and dysfibrinogenemias. Other disease states associated with the disease are Behçet's syndrome, infections, drug abuse, pregnancy, and malignancy (Trousseau's syndrome) (Chapter 71).

32. B Polyarteritis nodosa is a vasculitis of small to medium-sized arteries that may be systemic or may remain localized to the skin. Twenty per cent of patients with systemic disease have skin lesions. Cutaneous disease manifests with punched-out ulcers and subcutaneous nodules which may be pulsatile on the dorsal surfaces of legs and feet. Gangrene may be present as well as purpura. Often there is livedo associated with the lesions. Skin biopsy reveals a septal panniculitis with vasculitis. Henoch-Schönlein purpura (HSP) and Buerger's disease are not causes of panniculitis. HSP manifests with a lower extremity purpura without ulceration or gangrene and Buerger's disease should not involve the gastrointestinal (GI) tract (Chapter 58).

33. C Polyarteritis nodosa affects the arteries of many organ systems but tends to spare the lungs and central nervous system. This may be a helpful clue in differentiating the disease from other causes of vasculitis (Chapter 58).

34. D Rothmann-Makai syndrome is a rare variant of idiopathic lobular panniculitis (Weber-Christian disease). Weber-Christian disease is a cutaneous-systemic panniculitis that may carry significant morbidity and mortality. The Rothmann-Makai syndrome lacks the systemic involvement and is localized to the skin (Chapter 71).

35. B Erythema nodosum is thought to be a hypersensitivity response to a wide variety of antigens. Many of the accepted stimuli include streptococcal infections, sarcoidosis, tuberculosis, and drugs (sulfonamides, oral contraceptives, and bromides). Other less common causes are inflammatory bowel disease, lymphoma and leukemia, bacterial infections (*Yersinia enterocolitica, Mycoplasma pneumoniae,* leprosy, and others), fungal infections (dermatophytoses, histoplasmosis, coccidioidomycosis, and blastomycosis), and viral infections (hepatitis B, infectious mononucleosis, and others). Penicillin is not a widely accepted cause of erythema nodosum (Chapter 68).

36. E Calciphylaxis (calcifying panniculitis of renal failure) is a lobular panniculitis. It is presumed to be the result of a secondary hyperparathryoidism occurring in patients with renal failure. Ectopic calcifications occur following sensitization and elicitation phases, with a normal calcium-phosphate product. Calcification within the subcutaneous fat results in nodules that frequently ulcerate. Histologically, this is a lobular panniculitis without any evidence of vasculitis. Necrosis develops, possibly as a result of mural calcifications within arterioles in the deep dermis and in the subcutaneous fat. This disorder is treated with phosphate-binding antacids (Chapter 71).

37. A When scarring occurs, it generally occurs during the healing stage of the panniculitis. It may occur secondary to fat necrosis, or during the healing of an ulcer that occurs as part of the primary process. Several panniculitides characteristically do not result in scarring. These include cold panniculitis (although many of the other physical panniculitides do result in scarring), subcutaneous fat necrosis, sclerema neonatorum, post-steroid panniculitis, and erythema nodosum. The panniculitides associated with systemic diseases are variable with regard to scarring (Chapters 68 to 71).

38. E Pancreatitis and pancreatic tumors may both result in a diffuse panniculitis. In these patients, the pancreas releases both lipase and amylase. These enzymes are able to cause not only panniculitis, but pleuritis, pericarditis, peritonitis, and arthritis as well. Subcutaneous fat necrosis and pancreatic fat necrosis also may occur secondary to the pancreatic enzymes (Chapter 71).

39. E Periarteritis nodosa (polyarteritis nodosa [PAN]) is the best answer to this question. PAN is an immune complex–mediated disease affecting small and medium-sized arteries. Skin involvement occurs in roughly 25% to 50% of cases and consists of septal panniculitis with vasculitis. Arteries of the kidney, gastrointestinal tract, and mesentery are also commonly affected. This disease carried an extremely high mortality rate before the advent of corticosteroids.

Although erythema nodosum may be associated with fever and malaise, the lesions are limited to the skin. Post-steroid panniculitis is found in patients being weaned from systemic steroids and usually resolves spontaneously. Morphea profunda is the panniculitis that sometimes manifests in patients with an overlying patch of morphea. Nodular vasculitis (erythema induratum) is a lobular panniculitis with vasculitis that is typically limited to the legs and is often associated with mycobacterial infections (Chapters 58 and 68).

40. B; 41. C; 42. D; 43. A Subcutaneous fat necrosis and sclerema neonatorum are both panniculitides of newborns. Both histologically are lobular, without any concomitant vasculitis. The causes of these diseases are not clear; however, they have been hypothesized to represent cold-induced injury. Subcutaneous fat necrosis occurs in relatively healthy newborns in the first weeks of life. Clinically, the violaceous plaques remain localized to the trunk, proximal extremities, or the cheeks. It is a benign condition and generally resolves spontaneously.

Sclerema neonatorum generally occurs in the first days of life in severely ill newborns. It usually begins on the buttocks, and the confluent induration spreads rapidly to the trunk and legs. This disease carries a high mortality. Treatment is generally aimed at the child's underlying systemic disease (Chapter 69).

44. A; 45. C; 46. D; 47. B; 48. B Weber-Christian disease progresses through a macrophagic into a fibrotic stage. In the macrophagic stage, macrophages are the predominant cell type in the infiltrate. These are seen as foam cells, since they digest the degenerated lipocytes. During the fibrotic stage, the macrophages are replaced with lymphocytes and fibroblasts.

Erythema nodosum is a septal panniculitis that may spread to the lobules in the late stages. The infiltrate is predominantly neutrophilic early and becomes lymphocytic. Unlike PAN, leukocytoclasis is not a feature of erythema nodosum. A finding considered virtually pathognomonic is the microgranulomatous focus of Miescher.

Vegetable oil or other oils injected into the skin often cause a panniculitis. This is generally a lobular panniculitis without evidence of vasculitis. Oil-filled vacuoles resemble Swiss cheese.

Polyarteritis nodosa can affect small and medium-sized arteries of many different organs. In the skin, a leukocytoclastic vasculitis is found in small septal arteries. Thrombi form within the vessels, resulting in the formation of "nodose" aneurysmal dilatations, vessel necrosis, and hemorrhage (Chapter 71).

49. B; 50. D; 51. A; 52. C Unlike systemic polyarteritis nodosa, cutaneous PAN is a benign disease localized to the skin. The clinical appearance is similar to that of systemic PAN, that is, a livedo reticularis pattern surrounding tender, erythematous nodules that frequently ulcerate. The distribution is commonly on the lower legs. Spontaneous resolution may be seen without significant scarring if ulcerations were not present.

It was formerly believed that erythema induratum (nodular vasculitis) occurred as a hypersensitivity response to tuberculosis. It is now recognized that although many cases do occur as a result of mycobacterial infection, there are other causative factors involved as well. It manifests with chronic, tender, erythematous nodules. The lesions are typically found on the legs, commonly on the calf. Ulceration is not unusual; such lesions have a violaceous border. Scarring is noted upon healing.

Erythema nodosum manifests as erythematous-to-bluish tender plaques, usually on the shins of young women. It may acutely progress with fever, chills, and malaise. Arthralgias may persist for longer periods of time. Although the cause of this disease is not clear, it is thought to represent a hypersensitivity response to a wide variety of antigens.

α_1-Antitrypsin deficiency panniculitis has a distribution that differentiates it from other panniculitides. The trunk and proximal extremities are the most common locations for the recurrent, tender, erythematous nodules that mark this disease. Ulceration is the rule, not the exception. α_1-Antitrypsin deficiency affects other organs as well, including the lungs (emphysema), liver (cirrhosis), and blood vessels (vasculitis). This is also one of the causes of angioedema.

Factitial panniculitis results from injection of foreign material, usually by the patient. The materials injected vary widely from oils to organic materials (e.g., milk and feces) to acids or alkalis or even drugs (e.g., Demerol). The nodules that form soon undergo liquefaction, releasing an oily fluid. Bizarre shapes, patterns, or distribution of the lesions as well as atypical behavior on the part of the patient should suggest such a diagnosis (Chapters 58, 68, 69, and 71).

53. C; 54. A; 55. D; 56. E; 57. B Linear scleroderma is a disorder in which patients develop linear patches of indurated, bound-down skin. Children are affected more often than adults. It usually affects the lower extremities more frequently than the upper extremities. When linear scleroderma occurs over a joint, range of motion may become limited. Bone involvement (melorheostosis), a rare complication, is seen radiologically as linear cortical hyperostosis. Treatment of this disorder is difficult.

Eosinophilic fasciitis occurs most commonly in men, usually following excessive exercise. Clinically, it simulates scleroderma because the panniculus becomes inflamed and adheres to the fascia. It usually appears as a localized patch on an extremity, although it may become generalized. Eosinophilia is always present.

Eosinophilia-myalgia syndrome is a systemic illness in which sclerodermoid skin changes are associated with myopathy, pulmonary disease, and eosinophilia. The disease has been associated with the ingestion of L-tryptophan. It has actually been found that some generic lots of L-tryptophan have possessed a contaminant thought to be responsible for this syndrome. The eruption generally improves with systemic corticosteroid therapy as well as discontinuation of the L-tryptophan.

Partial lipodystrophy typically occurs in young patients, females outnumbering males. The etiology is unknown, although it is associated with a complement (C3) deficiency. The most common type is the cephalothoracic variant in which lipoatrophy begins on the face, and progresses through the trunk over a span of 2 to 3 years. It normally spares the hips, buttocks, and legs. Excess fat is often actually deposited in these regions. No treatment is available for these patients other than tissue augmentation.

Anetoderma (macular atrophy) is a disorder of unknown cause in which elastic fibers fragment within clearly localized lesions. The result is a 5- to 10-mm macule that has the texture of cigarette paper. Palpation of these macules provides the sensation of herniation through the dermis. The only significant histologic finding is a loss of normal elastic fibers (Chapters 98, 99, and 103).

Bibliography

Alegre VA, Winkelmann RK: Histocytic cytophagic panniculitis. J Am Acad Dermatol 1989; 20:177.

Beacham BE, et al.: Equestrian cold panniculitis in women. Arch Dermatol 1980; 116:1025.

Belongia EA, et al.: An investigation of the cause of the eosinophilia-myalgia syndrome associated with tryptophan use. N Engl J Med 1990; 323:357.

Diaz-Perez JL, et al.: Cutaneous periarteritis nodosa. Arch Dermatol 1980; 116:56.

Epstein EH, Oren ME: Popsicle panniculitis. N Engl J Med 1970; 282:966.

Hendrick SJ, et al.: Alpha-antitrypsin deficiency associated with panniculitis. J Am Acad Dermatol 1988; 18:684.

Horio T, et al.: Potassium iodide in erythema nodosum and other erythematous diseases. J Am Acad Dermatol 1983; 9:77.

Kellum RE, et al.: Sclerema neonatorum. Arch Dermatol 1968; 97:372.

Löfgren S: Erythema nodosum studies on etiology and pathogenesis in 185 adult cases. Acta Med Scand (suppl) 1946; 174:1.

MacDonald A, Feiwel M: A review of the concept of Weber-Christian panniculitis with a report of five cases. Br J Dermatol 1968; 80:355.

Montgomery H, et al.: Nodular vascular disease of the legs. JAMA 1945; 128:335.

Norwood-Galloway A, et al.: Subcutaneous fat necrosis of the newborn with hypercalcemia. J Am Acad Dermatol 1987; 16:435.

Patterson JW, et al.: Infection-induced panniculitis. J Cutan Pathol 1989; 16:183.

Peters SM, Daniel Su WP: Lupus erythematous panniculitis. Med Clin North Am 1989; 73:1113.

Potts DE, et al.: Syndrome of pancreatic disease, subcutaneous fat necrosis and polyserositis. Am J Med 1975; 58:417.

Rademaker M, et al.: Erythema induratum (Bazin's disease). J Am Acad Dermatol 1989; 21:740.

Richens G, et al.: Calcifying panniculitis associated with renal failure. J Am Acad Dermatol 1982; 6:537.

Samlaska CP, James WD: Superficial thrombophlebitis in primary hypercoagulable states. J Am Acad Dermatol 1990; 22:975.

Saxena AK, Nigam PK: Panniculitis following steroid therapy. Pediatr Dermatol 1988; 5:92.

Smith KC, et al.: Clinical and pathologic correlations in 96 patients with panniculitis. J Am Acad Dermatol 1989; 21:1192.

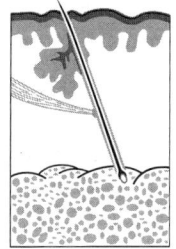

chapter 11

Drug Eruptions and Skin Manifestations of Immune Suppression

NEIL H. SHEAR, and RONALD PRUSSICK

DRUG ERUPTIONS

For the following questions decide whether EACH choice is TRUE or FALSE. Any combination of answers from all true to all false may occur.

Concerning toxic epidermal necrolysis (TEN),

1. TEN in children is usually secondary to a staphylococcal infection
2. The class of drugs most commonly implicated as the cause of TEN is sulfonamide antibiotics
3. The main difference between TEN and Stevens-Johnson syndrome is that patients with Stevens-Johnson syndrome have involvement of mucosal surfaces (e.g., eyes, nose, mouth, lips, genitalia)
4. TEN is best treated with systemic corticosteroids
5. The mortality rate in TEN is approximately 25%.

In the following question, ONE or MORE of the listed completions correctly finishes the incomplete statement; choose

A. If only 1, 2, and 3 are correct
B. If only 1 and 3 are correct
C. If only 2 and 4 are correct
D. If only 4 is correct
E. If all are correct.

6. A 50-year-old man presents with pharyngitis and receives ampicillin therapy. After 3 days he develops an eruption of erythema with scattered pinpoint pustules. This develops first on his face and intertriginous areas and then becomes disseminated over the back and upper legs. The patient has a temperature of 39° C and a peripheral neutrophil count of 7×10^9/L. He has no history of psoriasis.

   A skin biopsy reveals intraepidermal pustules with dermal edema and perivascular infiltrate of eosinophils. The differential diagnosis of this patient's eruption should include

   1. Acute febrile neutrophilic dermatosis
   2. Pustular psoriasis
   3. Eosinophilic folliculitis
   4. Acute generalized exanthematous pustulosis.

For the following question choose the ONE BEST answer.

7. A 9-year-old boy with cerebral palsy develops a rash. He had been diagnosed with grand mal sei-

zures and started on oral phenobarbital 3 weeks prior to the onset of the rash.

Two days before developing the rash, he developed a fever and cervical lymphadenopathy. On examination his rash is erythematous, nonscaly and flat. It is widespread over his trunk, arms, face, and upper thighs. There is no mucosal involvement. Physical examination is otherwise unhelpful. Microscopic hematuria is noted on urinalysis. The most likely diagnosis is

A. Infectious mononucleosis
B. Anticonvulsant hypersensitivity syndrome
C. Goodpasture's syndrome
D. Rubeola
E. Juvenile rheumatoid arthritis.

Decide whether EACH choice in the following questions is TRUE or FALSE. Any combination of answers from all true to all false may occur.

For each of the following statements about the phenytoin hypersensitivity syndrome decide whether it is TRUE or FALSE.

8. Pneumonitis may be part of the reaction.
9. Hepatitis is present in approximately 50% of patients.
10. Neutropenia may be present.
11. Thyroid antibodies can develop.
12. Myocarditis may be present.

Choose the ONE BEST answer to the following question.

13. A 5-year-old girl develops an urticarial eruption on her trunk and legs. She has a temperature of 39° C and complains of sore knees and ankles. She had a history of pharyngitis and otitis media and has been taking cefaclor for 10 days. Her other problems have resolved, but the rash, fever, and joint pain are new. Her complete blood count, liver function tests, and urinalysis are normal. The most likely diagnosis is

A. Urticaria
B. Serum sickness
C. Serum sickness–like reaction
D. Urticarial vasculitis
E. Rheumatic fever.

For each of the following questions, the set of lettered headings accompanies a list of numbered words or phrases. For each numbered word or phrase, choose

A. If the item is associated with A only
B. If the item is associated with B only
C. If the item is associated with both A and B
D. If the item is associated with neither A nor B.

For each of the following characteristics, choose whether it describes serum sickness, serum sickness–like reaction, both, or neither.

14. Regarding serum sickness,

   i. Circulating immune complexes
   ii. Caused by cefaclor
   iii. Hematuria
   iv. Anti–thymocyte globulin induced
   v. Associated with fever and arthralgias.

   A. Serum sickness
   B. Serum sickness–like reaction
   C. Both
   D. Neither.

Choose the ONE BEST answer to the following question.

15. A 20-year-old man develops an exanthematous eruption after taking amoxicillin for 5 days. The initial indication was pharyngitis. Which of the following would be the most helpful test?

A. Amoxicillin epicutaneous (prick) skin test
B. Liver function tests
C. Urinalysis
D. Antistreptolysin O test
E. Monospot test.

In the following question, ONE or MORE of the following completions correctly finishes the incomplete statement; choose

A. If only 1, 2, and 3 are correct
B. If only 1 and 3 are correct
C. If only 2 and 4 are correct
D. If only 4 is correct
E. If all are correct.

16. Which of the following beta-blockers is associated with drug-induced antinuclear antibodies in more than 1% of cases?

   1. Metoprolol
   2. Labetalol
   3. Propranolol
   4. Acebutolol.

For the following questions decide whether EACH choice is TRUE or FALSE. Any combination of answers from all true to all false may occur.

Decide whether each of the following statements about drug-induced lupus is TRUE or FALSE.

17. Antinuclear antibodies are present.
18. Anti-DNA antibodies are present.
19. Cutaneous lupus erythematosus is common.
20. The clinical presentation may be photosensitivity.

For the following questions, ONE or MORE of the following completions correctly finishes the incomplete statement; choose

A. If only 1, 2, and 3 are correct
B. If only 1 and 3 are correct
C. If only 2 and 4 are correct
D. If only 4 is correct
E. If all are correct.

21. A common clinical presentation of fixed drug eruption includes
    1. Erosion of glans penis
    2. Single bulla
    3. Hyperpigmented patch
    4. Psoriasiform plaque.

22. Lithium carbonate therapy often results in worsening or newly developing
    1. Psoriasis
    2. Photosensitivity
    3. Acne
    4. Pruritus.

For each numbered item, choose the most likely associated lettered item from those provided. Each numbered item has ONLY ONE answer. Within the group, each lettered item may be the answer to one, more than one, or none of the numbered items. For each eruption listed below choose the most likely drug cause listed.

23. Pityriasis rosea–like eruption
24. Lichenoid eruption
25. Pigmentation of hard palate
26. Erythema nodosum
27. Photo-onycholysis.

A. Hydroxychloroquine
B. Oral contraceptive
C. Intramuscular gold
D. Erythromycin
E. Doxycycline.

For each numbered item, choose the most likely associated lettered item. Each numbered item has ONLY ONE answer. Within each group, each lettered item may be the answer to one, more than one, or none of the numbered items.

For each of the following characteristics, choose whether it describes 5-fluorouracil, hydroxyurea, suramin, mitomycin D, or none.

28. Contact-type dermatitis
29. Atrophic violaceous papular eruption
30. Acral erythema
31. Keratoacanthomas
32. Supravenous flagellate hyperpigmentation
33. Porokeratosis.

A. 5-Fluorouracil
B. Hydroxyurea
C. Suramin
D. Mitomycin D
E. None of the above.

For each of the following characteristics, choose whether it describes interferon-α, interleukin-2, granulocyte colony–stimulating factor, all, or none of them.

34. Exacerbation of psoriasis
35. Cutaneous necrosis at injection sites
36. Delayed cutaneous reactions to intravenous contrast material
37. Telogen effluvium
38. Leukocytoclastic vasculitis.

A. Interferon-α
B. Interleukin-2
C. Granulocyte colony–stimulating factor
D. All of the above
E. None of the above.

For the following questions, the set of lettered headings accompanies a list of numbered words or phrases. For each numbered word or phrase, choose

A. If the item is associated with A only
B. If the item is associated with B only
C. If the item is associated with both A and B
D. If the item is associated with neither A nor B.

For each drug or disease described, choose whether it is associated with wet type–flushing associated with eccrine sweating, dry type–flushing related to vasodilatation, both, or neither.

39. Tamoxifen
40. Doxorubicin
41. Radiographic contrast agents
42. Flutamide
43. Carcinoid tumors.

A. Wet type–flushing associated with eccrine sweating
B. Dry type–flushing related to vasodilatation
C. Both
D. Neither.

For the following questions, decide whether EACH choice is TRUE or FALSE.

Concerning adverse cutaneous reactions resulting from bleomycin,

44. Flagellate pattern of hyperpigmentation following dermographism
45. Sclerodermoid changes of the skin
46. Raynaud's phenomenon
47. Bullous pemphigoid
48. Sweet's-like syndrome.

Choose the ONE BEST answer for each of the following questions.

49. All the following statements about neutrophilic eccrine hidradenitis are true EXCEPT
    A. Clinically, one sees tender erythematous macules, papules, or plaques
    B. It has been seen in patients treated with cytarabine
    C. Histology demonstrates neutrophils primarily around eccrine ducts
    D. It most likely represents a toxic reaction from chemotherapy
    E. It has been reported in patients with leukemia.

50. Possible adverse cutaneous reactions to granulocyte colony–stimulating factor include all of the following EXCEPT
    A. Sweet's-like syndrome
    B. Exacerbation of pemphigus vulgaris
    C. Leukocytoclastic vasculitis
    D. Bullous pyoderma gangrenosum.

SKIN MANIFESTATIONS OF IMMUNE SUPPRESSION

Choose the ONE BEST answer to each of the following questions.

A 28-year-old woman who is an immunocompromised renal transplant recipient is on maintenance treatment with prednisone and cyclosporine.

1. The patient is at increased risk for the following diseases EXCEPT
    A. Squamous cell carcinoma on sun-exposed skin
    B. Reactivation of tuberculosis
    C. Hodgkin's lymphoma
    D. Anogenital cancer
    E. Kaposi's sarcoma.

2. The previously described patient may develop any of the following complications EXCEPT
    A. Condyloma acuminata with squamous neoplasia of the cervix
    B. Increased incidence of post-herpetic neuralgia
    C. Molluscum contagiosum
    D. Ecthyma gangrenosum resulting from *Nocardia* sepsis
    E. Interstitial pneumonitis from *Pneumocystis carinii*.

3. All the following statements about immunocompromised patients are true EXCEPT
    A. Patients are at an increased risk of developing malignant melanoma
    B. Corticosteroids enhance susceptibility to infection by impairing neutrophil chemotaxis, suppressing cell-mediated immunity, and impairing monocyte killing
    C. Reactivation of varicella-zoster virus is particularly frequent in Hodgkin's lymphoma patients
    D. Oral labial herpes simplex infection may spread locally, particularly to the esophagus or respiratory tract
    E. Forty to fifty per cent of renal transplant patients develop verrucae, some of which may undergo malignant transformation, particularly on non–sun-exposed areas.

For each numbered item, choose the most likely associated lettered item from those

provided. Each numbered item has ONLY ONE answer. Within each group, each lettered item may be the answer to one, more than one, or none of the numbered items.

4. Pityrosporum folliculitis
5. Gingival hyperplasia and hypertrichosis
6. Non-Hodgkin's lymphoma
7. Nephrotoxicity with hypertension
8. Myelosuppression.

A. Prednisone
B. Cyclosporine
C. Azathioprine
D. All of the above
E. None of the above.

Choose the ONE BEST answer to the following question.

9. Cutaneous findings in patients with congenital forms of hypogammaglobulinemia may include the following EXCEPT

   A. Furunculosis and impetigo, often around the body orifices
   B. Atopic-like eczematous eruption
   C. Lichenoid papules and plaques consisting of lymphohistiocytic infiltrates that respond to high-dose immune serum globulin
   D. Pyoderma gangrenosum
   E. A dermatomyositis-like disorder related to disseminated herpes virus infection.

For each numbered item, choose the most likely associated lettered item. Each numbered item has ONLY ONE answer. Within each group, each lettered item may be the answer to one, more than one, or none of the numbered items.

For each of the following skin and systemic manifestations, choose the most likely congenital immunodeficiency disorder:

10. Extensive pyoderma, commonly staphylococcal abscesses, often with co-existent periorificial dermatitis and atopic-like dermatitis; defective ability of phagocytic leukocytes to kill intracellular organisms by the generation of oxidative metabolites

11. Frequent infections of the skin and lungs; atopic-like dermatitis, impetigo, furunculosis, paronychia, "cold" abscesses, defective neutrophilic chemotaxis, increased serum levels of IgE

12. X-linked recessive inheritance with thrombocytopenia; atopic-like dermatitis with purpuric excoriated areas and, often, secondary bacterial infection and eczema herpeticum, molluscum contagiosum, and verruca plana

13. Autosomal recessive inheritance with multiple telangiectasias and progeric facies. Cutaneous pyoderma, recurrent bacterial and viral sinopulmonary infections, malignant lymphoreticular neoplasms

14. Autosomal recessive inheritance with pigment dilution, nystagmus, and photophobia. Bacterial infections of the skin and lungs, deep skin ulcers resembling pyoderma gangrenosum, a lymphoma-like stage that may be precipitated by viruses such as Epstein-Barr virus.

A. Wiscott-Aldrich syndrome
B. Ataxia-telangiectasia
C. Hyperimmuno-globulinemia-E syndrome
D. Chediak-Higashi syndrome
E. Chronic granulomatous disease.

Choose the ONE BEST answer to the following question.

15. All the following are useful markers of human immunodeficiency virus (HIV) disease progression EXCEPT

    A. p24 antigen
    B. CD4 lymphocyte count
    C. Serum and urinary neopterin levels

D. B-lymphocyte count

E. β_2-microglobulin levels.

For the following question decide whether EACH choice is TRUE or FALSE. Any combination of answers from all true to all false may occur.

16. Which of the following statements regarding the herpesvirus family of infections in HIV-infected individuals are TRUE and which, FALSE?

    A. Periorificial erosions may enlarge into persistent painful ulcers

    B. Chronic perianal ulcers may be associated with herpetic colitis and ulcers in the oropharynx, with herpetic esophagitis

    C. Acyclovir-resistant herpes simplex most commonly results from loss of synthesis of the viral thymidine kinase

    D. Varicella-zoster virus may result in persistent primary varicella, multidermatomal zoster or persistent hyperkeratotic plaques

    E. The outbreak of zoster usually correlates with an advanced degree of immunodeficiency

    F. Oral hairy leukoplakia correlates with a moderate to advanced degree of immunodeficiency.

For the following questions, the set of lettered headings accompanies a list of numbered words or phrases; for each numbered word or phrase, choose

  A. If the item is associated with A only
  B. If the item is associated with B only
  C. If the item is associated with both A and B
  D. If the item is associated with neither A nor B.

For each of the following characteristic findings in patients with AIDS, choose whether it is associated with mild-to-moderate degree of immunosuppression, moderate-to-severe, both, or neither.

17. Multidermatomal zoster
18. Oral hairy leukoplakia
19. Oropharyngeal candidiasis
20. Seborrheic dermatitis on the face
21. Multiple molluscum contagiosum on the face.

  A. Mild-to-moderate degree of immunosuppression
  B. Moderate-to-severe degree of immunosuppression
  C. Both
  D. Neither.

Decide whether EACH choice in the following question is TRUE or FALSE. Any combination of answers from all true to all false may occur.

22. Which of the following statements regarding patients having both syphilis and HIV disease are TRUE and which, FALSE?

    A. Patients infected with *Treponema pallidum* may have rapid progression to tertiary disease within weeks to months of diagnosis

    B. All HIV-infected patients with syphilis should have cerebrospinal fluid (CSF) examination regardless of the stage

    C. Diagnosis of syphilis may be complicated by false-negative serologic tests and atypical clinical presentations

    D. The usually painless chancre of primary syphilis may be painful

    E. Neurosyphilis should be considered in the differential diagnosis of neurologic disease in HIV disease.

Choose the ONE BEST answer to each of the following questions.

23. All the following are characteristics of cutaneous findings in HIV-infected individuals EXCEPT

    A. Mild pre-existing psoriasis may undergo severe exacerbation

    B. Severe psoriasis may develop spontaneously in an individual after HIV seroconversion

    C. The incidence of Reiter's syndrome is increased in HIV-infected patients

    D. Methotrexate is one of the treatments of choice for widespread plaque psoriasis, psoriatic arthritis, or Reiter's disease.

    E. Seborrheic dermatitis is histologically distinguishable from the non–AIDS-related form of the disease.

24. All the following are TRUE about HIV disease in children EXCEPT

    A. Vertical transmission accounts for the majority of cases

    B. Early in the disease, B-cell defects are more common than T-cell defects

    C. Children commonly present with opportunistic infections such as *Pneumocystis carinii*–induced pneumonia (PCP)

    D. Staphylococcal skin infections are seen early in the disease

E. Atopic dermatitis may be difficult to control with the usual treatment regimens.

In the following questions, for each numbered item, choose the most likely associated lettered item. Each numbered item has ONLY ONE answer. Within each group, each lettered item may be the answer to one, more than one, or none of the numbered items.

Match the following with the most likely causative drug used in the treatment of HIV disease:

25. Oral or genital ulcers
26. Nail hyperpigmentation
27. The most common agent to cause adverse drug reactions in HIV-infected individuals
28. Ulcerations at injection sites
29. Cyanosis.

A. Zidovudine (AZT)
B. Trimethoprim-sulfamethoxazole
C. Foscarnet
D. Dapsone
E. Pentamidine.

Choose the form of Kaposi's sarcoma that is best described by the associated clinical features:

30. Benign nodular disease, but sometimes aggressive and fatal within 5 to 8 years
31. Fulminant lymphadenopathic disease, typically fatal within 2 to 3 years
32. Lesions are first seen on the legs and feet with associated lymphedema
33. Oral Kaposi's sarcoma may be a marker for more advanced immunosuppression.

A. Classic Kaposi's sarcoma
B. African-endemic Kaposi's sarcoma in adults
C. African-endemic Kaposi's sarcoma in young children
D. Iatrogenic, immunosuppressive drug–associated Kaposi's sarcoma
E. AIDS-associated (epidemic) Kaposi's sarcoma.

Choose the ONE BEST answer to the following question.

34. All the following statements about Kaposi's sarcoma are true EXCEPT

A. Kaposi's sarcoma induced by immunosuppressive agents in organ transplant recipients may spontaneously remit after discontinuation of treatment
B. Large differences in risk of acquiring epidemic Kaposi's sarcoma exist between different HIV transmission groups such as homosexual men, hemophiliacs, or females infected through heterosexual contact
C. Classic Kaposi's sarcoma is not a significant cause of death in affected patients
D. Studies have shown both cytomegalovirus and human papillomavirus DNA in Kaposi's sarcoma cells in patients with epidemic Kaposi's sarcoma
E. Visceral lesions in epidemic Kaposi's sarcoma are most commonly seen in the bone marrow and brain.

ANSWERS

DRUG ERUPTIONS

1. (F); **2.** (T); **3.** (F); **4.** (F); **5.** (T) Historically, *toxic epidermal necrolysis* (TEN) was a term that was used for any skin eruption that caused the epidermis to appear to blister and give a "scalded skin" appearance. In the literature, the term is used to describe both drug-induced TEN and the staphylococcal "scalded skin" syndrome. Now it is known that these are two separate entities. The staphylococcal "scalded skin" syndrome is due to a toxin from staphylococcus phage, type 2. This eruption has a superficial split in the upper epidermis, whereas TEN is associated with full-thickness epidermal necrosis and a sparse mononuclear infiltrate in the dermis.

Toxic epidermal necrolysis is generally drug-induced and in all situations, a drug cause should be elucidated. The most common drugs associated with TEN are, in order, sulfonamide antibiotics, anticonvulsants (carbamazepine, phenobarbital, phenytoin, and valproic acid), anti-inflammatories (nonsteroidal anti-inflammatories—in particular, oxicam derivatives and allopurinol). The differentiation between erythema multiforme major, Stevens-Johnson syndrome, and TEN is not completely clear. However, a recent international collaborative study on severe skin reactions to drugs has suggested that *all* of these severe reactions have mucosal involvement. The most helpful differentiating feature among severe reactions is the percentage of body surface area detachment from epidermis. The worst of these is TEN, and it is associated with a mortality rate of approximately 25%.

The incidence of severe TEN is approximately 1:1 million population per year, and this applies to both children and adults. Similarly, mortality rates are even across age groups. The treatment of TEN is controversial, but many experts advise against systemic corticosteroids as they may worsen the condition. Corticosteroids are not widely accepted therapy for TEN. Patients should be treated symptomatically and as burn patients.

Other organ involvement, including neutropenia and pneumonitis, must be watched for carefully and may necessitate intervention. Similarly, evidence of infection should also be treated promptly (Chapter 81).

6. D Acute generalized exanthematous pustulosis (AGEP) is a recently described, drug-induced pustular eruption. The most common drugs causing this include antimicrobials (amoxicillin, ampicillin, vancomycin, imipenem, cefaclor) and carbamazepine, etc.

The eruption is characterized by a widespread exanthem with nonfollicular pustules that are 1 to 3 mm in diameter. The most surprising clinical presentation is the early onset, 1 to 3 days after drug exposure. Patients may have a neutrophilia, malaise, chills, and low-grade fevers. A spontaneous resolution of pustules occurs with extensive desquamation in less than 15 days after withdrawal of the drug. The reaction can be re-created with re-challenge.

The differential diagnosis includes many other pustular eruptions. However, the intraepidermal involvement would rule out acute febrile neutrophilic dermatosis. The eosinophils would rule out pustular psoriasis, and the eruption is nonfollicular, thereby ruling out eosinophilic folliculitis (Chapter 43).

7. B; 8. (T); 9. (T); 10. (T); 11. (T); 12. (T) The anticonvulsant hypersensitivity syndrome is the term used to describe a delayed onset reaction from the first exposure to either phenytoin, phenobarbital, or carbamazepine. The syndrome features are identical for the three anticonvulsants, and terms such as *phenytoin anticonvulsant syndrome* are no longer appropriate. Patients develop fever approximately 2 to 4 weeks after initiating therapy. This is followed by erythema and swelling of the face and a generalized exanthematous eruption. Occasionally, the eruption may have features of a severe skin reaction such as erythema multiforme major, Stevens-Johnson syndrome, or toxic epidermal necrolysis. Internal organ involvement is present in most cases, and the most common is a rise in liver function tests. Liver damage can be hepatic necrosis. Granulomatous hepatitis has also been described. The lungs may be involved, with pneumonitis; neutropenia is not uncommon; and some patients may develop an aplastic anemia. Antimicrosomal antibodies may develop in a few patients, and ultimately these patients may become hypothyroid, requiring thyroid supplementation. Carditis is unusual, but can occur, and some patients have had severe cardiac involvement. Subtler changes may show on echocardiography with four-chamber enlargement or inverted T waves on electrocardiogram. The basis of the reactions is a genetically inherited inability to detoxify reactive metabolites of the anticonvulsant. The exact nature of the metabolite is not known.

Infectious mononucleosis may be associated with a very faint rash; however, this is more apparent when patients infected with Epstein-Barr virus take amino penicillins. Rubeola or measles is not associated with microscopic hematuria, and the lack of eye or nose involvement would make this an unlikely diagnosis. The rash of juvenile rheumatoid arthritis can be exanthematous, but there is no other description in this patient of anything associated with juvenile rheumatoid arthritis. Goodpasture's syndrome is not associated with a rash (Chapter 43).

13. C; 14. i A; ii B; iii B; iv A; v C Serum sickness describes the classic type 3, immune complex–mediated syndrome following exposure to foreign proteins such as anti–thymocyte globulin (ATG). The reaction occurs 10 days after exposure and is characterized by fever, arthralgia, and arthritis and vasculitis of the skin and kidneys.

Serum sickness–like reactions occur 5 to 10 days after antibiotic therapy and are characterized by urticarial, nonvasculitic eruption with fever and arthralgia. Immune complexes, hematuria, and depressed complement are *not* features of the serum sickness–like reaction. The drug most often incriminated is cefaclor (Chapter 43).

15. E Skin testing is most helpful in determining the relationship between penicillin and urticarial reactions. However, testing for exanthematous eruptions is not as helpful. Amoxicillin is not well established for either prick testing (for IgE-mediated immediate reactions) or for delayed cell-mediated reactions. Clearly, this test would not be helpful in this patient. The patient does not have features of a systemic reaction; therefore, liver function tests and urinalysis are not of major interest or value. A positive Antistreptolysin O test would indicate if the patient had a previous streptococcal infection. However, the main concern is that the amoxicillin caused a reaction in a patient with infectious mononucleosis. Almost 100% of patients with infectious mononucleosis develop a rash during treatment with amino penicillins. It is important to determine if a patient with an exanthem has infectious mononucleosis. A positive monospot test would suggest that the patient could use amino penicillins in future, as well as other penicillins. Some patients may refuse to take amino penicillins again; however, the risk associated with using penicillin and its derivatives would be the same as the baseline risk in any individual. This is exceedingly helpful information to patients and their physicians in future drug management (Chapter 43).

16. C; 17. (T); 18. (F); 19. (F); 20. (T) Labetalol and acebutolol are well associated with antinuclear antibodies (ANAs) and drug-induced lupus erythematosus. Patients do not characteristically have major skin involvement; however, they may present with photosensitivity and recent onset photosensitivity should prompt a check of ANA, especially in patients who are on labetalol and acebutolol. Because beta-blockers are not commonly associated with drug-induced antinuclear antibodies, this is often missed.

Although patients may develop ANAs, often in a speckled pattern, anti-DNA antibodies are not usually present (Chapter 43).

21. A Fixed drug eruptions are well-circumscribed oval patches approximately 1 to 2 cm in diameter that react on each exposure to a specific drug. There is no known cause other than drugs for these reactions. The commonest drugs associated with fixed drug eruptions are sulfonamide antibiotics, phenobarbital, tetracyclines, and phenolphthalein (Ex-Lax).

A fixed drug eruption can manifest as a red patch and on each exposure becomes red and tender again after 3 to 5 days. Eventually, a brown, hyperpigmented patch results and may be the presenting complaint.

Some of these drugs will cause bullae to develop. The oval area is usually one large blister rather than multiple small blisters. Mucous membranes such as the lips, vulva, and penis are often involved. Patients may have numerous involved areas and on re-exposure may develop new ones (Chapter 43).

22. B Lithium carbonate therapy is often associated with psoriasis in adults and acne in teenagers. Because of the unique properties of the drug, it is often difficult to stop, and patients may need more intensive therapy. It can be difficult to control the skin disease, and this may become a dominant factor in the patient's well-being. Current alternatives for lithium carbonate and the treatment of psychiatric disorders include valproic acid and carbamazepine (Chapter 43).

23. C; 24. C; 25. A; 26. B; 27. E Intramuscular gold is associated with both pityriasis rosea–like and lichenoid eruptions. Biopsies of the former may show dermatitic changes or lichenoid changes, but the clinical appearance is quite constant. Patients can be restarted on the drug, but on low doses at first with a gradual increase to therapeutic doses. Oral gold is not associated with eruptions as frequently; however, it may not be as effective in control of arthritis.

Antimalarials such as hydroxychloroquine are often associated with pigmentation around the ankles and on the hard palate.

Erythema nodosum is not a common reaction to drugs; however, it has been associated with estrogen. Patients can develop this on any form of estrogen, and it may recur during pregnancy.

Photo-onycholysis requires a combination of both drug and ultraviolet exposure. Doxycycline (Vibromycin) is a notorious problem. This photosensitizing drug is sometimes used for prevention of infectious diarrhea when patients travel to tropical areas, and patients may not realize that they have nail damage because of an accompanying sunburn. This nail damage make take several months to manifest. The lifting of the nail at the proximal end parallels the cuticle, reflecting the external nature of the insult. This should spontaneously resolve.

Erythromycin is not often associated with rashes; however, there have been anecdotal reports of TEN (Chapter 43).

28. D; 29. B; 30. A; 31. C; 32. A; 33. C 5-Fluorouracil is an antimetabolite that results in a variety of cutaneous side effects, including alopecia, photosensitivity, hyperpigmentation, acral erythema, and an acute flare of actinic keratoses. One form of hyperpigmentation overlying arm veins is termed serpentine supravenous fluorouracil hyperpigmentation.

Hydroxyurea has been reported to cause a variety of adverse reactions to the skin, including alopecia, xerosis, hyperpigmentation of the skin and nails, and a violaceous papular eruption that often appears atrophic and is usually found on the dorsum of the hands with some lesions appearing on the face. Skin biopsies of these atrophic papules resemble atrophic lichen planus. It has been proposed that inhibition of DNA synthesis by hydroxyurea may result in slowing of epidermal turnover, resulting in a thinner epidermis and widening of the granular layer.

Mitomycin C is an alkylating agent instilled intravesically in the treatment of superficial bladder cancer. Cutaneous reactions are common, and one often sees a dermatitis predominantly on the hands, buttocks, and genitals that may infrequently become generalized. The pathogenesis is unknown, but an allergic contact dermatitis mechanism has been proposed.

Suramin is a polysulfonated naphthylurea that is undergoing clinical trials as an antitumor agent for a variety of malignancies, including metastatic prostate carcinoma. The drug has a unique ability to block the receptors of various tumor growth factors such as platelet-derived growth factor, fibroblast growth factor-β, and transforming growth factor-β. A variety of cutaneous reactions have been described, including an erythematous maculopapular eruption that often fades within 3 to 5 days despite continuation of treatment. As well, multiple eruptive keratoacanthomas, disseminated superficial actinic porokeratosis, and syringosquamous metaplasia have been described (Chapter 44).

34. D; 35. A; 36. B; 37. D; 38. C There are three main types of interferons: interferon-α, mainly produced by leukocytes; interferon-β, produced by fibroblasts and epithelial cells; and interferon-γ, produced by lymphocytes. Interferon-α and interferon-β act as negative growth regulators, whereas interferon-γ acts as an immunomodulator. Systemic side effects are common, including flu-like symptoms such as fever, chills, headache, fatigue, myalgia, and nausea. Local reactions to recombinant interferon-α include cutaneous necrosis at injection sites and atrophic plaques, which may be pruritic. In addition, interferon-α has been reported to result in exacerbation of psoriasis vulgaris and may also result in alopecia, which may be related to telogen effluvium or acceleration of male-pattern baldness.

Interleukin 2 is a cytokine that enhances the immune system and therefore has been used in clinical trials in the treatment of various neoplastic diseases. It causes multiple toxic or hypersensitivity reactions, including transient flushing, a persistent erythema or erythroderma, bullous drug eruptions, urticaria, delayed reactions to intravenous contrast media, erythema nodosum, telogen effluvium, and oral erosions. It has also been known to induce or exacerbate various skin diseases, including psoriasis, and a number of autoimmune bullous disorders, including pemphigus vulgaris and linear IgA disease.

Granulocyte colony–stimulating factor is a neutrophil-specific growth factor that has been used in clinical trials to lessen the degree and duration of neutropenia in patients undergoing chemotherapy. Localized reactions include erythematous plaques or bullous pyoderma gangrenosum. Generalized reactions include a Sweet's-like syndrome, leukocytoclastic vasculitis, widespread folliculitis, and exacerbation of psoriasis (Chapter 44).

39. A; **40.** B; **41.** A; **42.** A; **43.** A Flushing reactions can be categorized as either wet flushing, associated with eccrine sweating and mediated by autonomic nerves, or dry flushing, resulting from vasodilation. Cancer chemotherapeutic agents are usually associated with dry flushing and include doxorubicin, mithramycin, cisplatin, and dacarbazine. Wet flushing can be produced by antihormones such as tamoxifen or flutamide or by radiographic contrast media. Various tumors can cause flushing usually associated with eccrine sweating, such as carcinoid tumors and others such as adenocarcinoma of the prostate or pancreatic tumors, which secrete vasoactive substances (Chapter 43).

44. (T); **45.** (T); **46.** (T); **47.** (F); **48.** (F) Bleomycin is an antibiotic with antineoplastic properties that inhibits the incorporation of thymidine into DNA. A reticulated patchy hyperpigmentation, most commonly seen on the trunk, in some cases is preceded by dermographism. It is believed to occur only in certain patients. Histologic findings show a normal number of melanocytes and melanophages but increased melanin in the basal layer. The pathogenesis is unknown but probably represents a toxic reaction in the skin in areas of increased drug concentrations. Other cutaneous findings include sclerodermoid changes, widespread erythema, buccal ulceration, glossitis, and Raynaud's phenomenon (Chapter 44).

49. C Neutrophilic eccrine hidradenitis was first described in a leukemia patient treated with cytarabine. Since this time, there have been many case reports attributing this reaction to various chemotherapeutic agents, and it has been reported in patients with various types of malignancies. Clinically, one sees tender erythematous macules, papules, or plaques. The histology is diagnostic, primarily showing neutrophils around the eccrine gland with some evidence of cellular damage. Necrosis spares the straight dermal and epidermal eccrine ducts. The pathogenesis is unknown but is thought to most likely be a toxic reaction from the drug itself (Chapter 44).

50. B See answer to Question 34.

ANSWERS

SKIN MANIFESTATIONS OF IMMUNE SUPPRESSION

1. C; **2.** D; **3.** E; **4.** A; **5.** B; **6.** B; **7.** B; **8.** C Most organ transplant recipients are treated with both prednisone and cyclosporine. Major cutaneous side effects of prednisone include skin fragility, atrophy with purpura, steroid acne, pityrosporum folliculitis, and hirsutism. Cyclosporine has many effects on the immune system but most importantly it inhibits T-lymphocyte proliferation. Its major benefit has been an absence of myelosuppression, although nephrotoxicity with hypertension is commonly seen. The most common mucocutaneous side effects include hypertrichosis and gingival hyperplasia. There has been a reported increased rate of non-Hodgkin's lymphoma at high dosages.

Other immunosuppressive agents such as methotrexate, azathioprine, and cyclophosphamide all can result in bone marrow suppression.

Common bacterial skin infections caused by *Staphylococcus* or *Streptococcus* may progress to widespread cellulitis. Ecthyma gangrenosum resulting from *Pseudomonas* sepsis and exogenous inoculation of the skin with opportunistic organisms such as *Nocardia* and atypical mycobacteria may be seen. Endogenous infection to the skin may occur with *Mycobacterium tuberculosis*.

Fungal infections are often caused by opportunistic organisms such as *Aspergillus, Candida,* and *Cryptococcus* and occasionally by primary pathogens, including *Coccidioides* and *Histoplasma*.

Dermatophyte infections are seen in approximately 12% of renal transplant patients, and onychomycosis is common.

Molluscum contagiosum infections are found in greater numbers and are more resistant to treatment in immunocompromised patients. Human papillomavirus (HPV) infection is seen in close to 50% of immunosuppressed renal transplant patients. The HPV-2 and HPV-4 types are most commonly detected, but HPV-1 and HPV-3 types can be seen. HPV-5 in some patients may result in lesions resembling epidermodysplasia verruciformis. The warts may undergo malignant transformation to squamous cell carcinoma, especially in sun-exposed areas. There is increased risk of squamous neoplasia of the cervix arising from condyloma acuminatum, particularly from types HPV-16, -18, -31, and -33.

Herpes simplex and varicella-zoster infections may be associated with prolonged viral shedding, decreased healing time, and increased risk of viral dissemination. Herpes simplex may result in local spread, commonly to the esophagus or respiratory tract, or in persistent, painful ulceration. Disseminated herpes zoster is seen in approximately 15% of renal transplantations and in patients with Hodgkin's disease. There is also an increased risk of post-herpetic neuralgia.

There is a threefold increase in malignancy in organ transplantation patients. Squamous cell carcinoma of the skin is the most common malignancy and may be locally aggressive with an increased incidence of local metastases. These patients are all at increased risk for developing Kaposi's sarcoma, and several reports document an increased incidence of various malignancies, including non-Hodgkin's lymphoma and malignant melanoma. Cancer of the anus, perianal skin, or external genitalia is also increased, especially in those with a history of condyloma acuminatum (Chapter 125).

9. E Various forms of hypogammaglobulinemia exist, the most common being the X-linked congenital form. Recurrent otitis, bronchiectasis, pneumonitis, and sinusitis are the earliest infectious manifestations. Bacterial skin infections are common, and other cutaneous findings include an atopic-like eczematous eruption, which is often resistant to immunoglobulin therapy; exfoliative erythroderma; and pyoderma gangrenosum. Disseminated echovirus infection may result in meningoencephalitis and dermatomyositis-like skin eruption with associated muscle weakness. Lichenoid papules and plaques may be seen as an early manifestation of the disease, which on biopsy shows aggregates of histiocytes and lymphocytes in the dermis. These lesions respond to monthly infusion of high doses of immune serum globulin (Chapter 125).

10. E; 11. C; 12. A; 13. B; 14. D Wiscott-Aldrich syndrome is an X-linked recessive disorder in which a purpuric, exfoliative, atopic dermatitis-like eruption develops. Secondary bacterial infection of the skin as well as eczema herpeticum, molluscum contagiosum, and verruca plana are common. Many patients die in infancy from infection, hemorrhage, or lymphoreticular malignancy. Bone marrow transplantation is often the treatment of choice.

Ataxia-telangiectasia is an autosomal recessively inherited disease. Characteristic telangiectasias, progeric faces, and greying of the hair is seen. Recurrent bacterial and viral sinopulmonary infections are common. Other features include growth retardation, endocrine disorders, and malignant lymphoreticular neoplasms. Both humoral and cellular immune defects are seen, and spontaneous chromosomal abnormalities are common.

Hyperimmunoglobulinemia-E syndrome is characterized by atopic-like dermatitis, recurrent cutaneous and systemic pyogenic infections, markedly increased serum levels of IgE, peripheral eosinophilia, and in most patients, defective neutrophil chemotaxis. Superficial skin abscesses are common. In some patients abscesses may be "cold," in that they lack the clinical signs of warmth, tenderness, and erythema. Many patients present with bronchitis, pulmonary abscesses, empyema, and pneumatoceles. Subsets of this syndrome include Buckley's (coarse facial features) and Job's syndromes (red hair, atrophic nails, hyperextensible joints).

Chediak-Higashi syndrome is a rare autosomal recessive disorder characterized by partial oculocutaneous albinism with nystagmus and photophobia. Deep skin ulcers may resemble pyoderma gangrenosum. An "accelerated" lymphoma-like phase may be precipitated by viruses such as the Epstein-Barr virus. This is characterized by hepatosplenomegaly, lymphadenopathy, pancytopenia, and leukemia-like gingivitis. Giant lysosomal granules are seen in various cell types, including neutrophils, monocytes, and lymphocytes. Treatment of choice for these patients is bone marrow transplantation.

Chronic granulomatous disease (CGD) is inherited as an X-linked form in the majority of patients; however, both autosomal recessive and dominant cases have been reported. Most patients have a mild dermatitis of the face and scalp that frequently becomes infected and may evolve into granulomatous lesions. Additional mucocutaneous findings include ulcerative gingivostomatitis, pyodermas, and subcutaneous abscesses. Systemic involvement may include lymph nodes, liver, spleen, bone, and lungs. Patients with CGD have deficient phagocyte killing because of an abnormality involving the nicotinamide-adenine dinucleotide phosphate (NADPH) oxidase system that produces superoxide and other toxic oxygen metabolites. Therapy includes treatment of infections with antimicrobial agents and drainage of abscesses. The use of interferon-γ appears to be helpful for some patients (Chapter 125).

15. D Human immunodeficiency virus (HIV) is a lymphotrophic human retrovirus. Two HIV types have been identified: HIV-1, the cause of nearly all HIV infections in North America and Europe, and HIV-2, the infection detected predominantly in West Africa. HIV infection results in progressive immunodeficiency in most patients, leading to end-stage acquired immunodeficiency syndrome (AIDS). In early HIV infection, p24 antigen, an HIV core antigen, is present for a short time in the serum but clears with subsequent antibody production. Later in the course of HIV disease, serum HIV-p24 reappears as the level of antibody to HIV-1 p24 antigen decreases. The CD4 lymphocyte (T4 or T-helper cell) count is the most important known marker of disease progression. The absolute CD4 count is used as a guideline for therapeutic intervention with low-dose zidovudine (AZT) therapy. Serum and urine neopterin and serum β_2-microglobin have also been found to be helpful indirect markers of disease progression (Chapter 125).

16. A (T); B (T); C (T); D (T); E (F); F (T) The majority of herpetic infections in HIV disease are reactivation of the latent virus. The most common sites for outbreaks include perianal, genital, orofacial, and digital sites. With increased immunodeficiency, erosions may enlarge and deepen into painful ulcers with raised margins. Chronic perianal ulcers may be associated with herpetic colitis. Herpes simplex virus (HSV) infection in the HIV-infected patient may occur in the oropharynx and extend to the esophagus, resulting in herpetic esophagitis. Rarely, HSV infection can disseminate hematogenously to the liver, lungs, and brain. HSV infection responds to oral or intravenous acyclovir therapy. Acyclovir-resistant virus commonly results from the loss of synthesis of the viral enzyme thymidine kinase. In HIV disease, patients may develop persistent varicella or in childhood develop dermatomal zoster within weeks of primary infection. Cutaneous dissemination of varicella-zoster virus (VZV), persistent hyperkeratotic plaques, and chronic ecthymatous lesions have been reported. Zoster occurring in HIV-infected patients may be multidermatomal, possibly involving two noncontiguous dermatomes. Its course may be atypical, persisting chronically for months. Acyclovir is usually the treatment of choice for HIV-infected patients.

Epstein-Barr virus (EBV) has a tendency to infect cells of the B-cell lineage and some types of squamous epithelium. In HIV-infected individuals, EBV is associated with oral hairy leukoplakia (OHL), which is characterized by white verrucous plaques usually found on the inferolateral aspects of the tongue.

Cytomegalovirus (CMV) is another herpes virus and a common viral pathogen in patients with advanced HIV–induced immunodeficiency. CMV skin lesions are nonspecific, and widespread exanthems, skin ulcers, and leukocytoclastic vasculitis have been reported. Intravenous ganciclovir is usually the treatment of choice (Chapter 125).

17. A; **18.** B; **19.** B; **20.** C; **21.** B An outbreak of herpes zoster in HIV-infected patients usually correlates with a moderate degree of immunodeficiency and may even be the first presenting feature that will alert the physician to the possibility of HIV infection. The clinical appearance of zoster usually occurs earlier in the course of HIV-induced immunodeficiency than OHL and oropharyngeal candidiasis. The appearance of OHL correlates with moderately advanced immunodeficiency and increased probability of developing full-blown AIDS.

Molluscum contagiosum represents a poxvirus infection. There is a tendency to develop multiple, frequently treatment-resistant lesions as immunodeficiency progresses. Seborrheic dermatitis of the face can be seen early on in asymptomatic HIV disease as well as in more advanced stages of immunodeficiency (Chapter 125).

22. A–E (T) In the normal host, the progression of syphilis, a sexually transmitted disease caused by the spirochete *T. pallidum*, from primary to secondary to tertiary stages takes place over a period of months and usually years. In an HIV-infected patient, rapid progression to tertiary disease and/or increased severity of clinical manifestations may occur. Diagnosis of syphilis in HIV-infected patients may be complicated by false-negative serologic testing and atypical clinical presentations. The usual painless chancre of primary syphilis may become painful from secondary infection with *S. aureus*. It is currently recommended that CSF examination be performed in all patients coinfected with syphilis and HIV regardless of clinical stage of syphilis (Chapter 125).

23. D Mild pre-existing psoriasis may suddenly undergo exacerbation to guttate-like plaque or pustular psoriasis. More commonly, psoriasis may develop spontaneously after HIV seroconversion in an individual who has had no history of pre-existing disease. Often lesions respond to traditional topical therapy, including topical corticosteroids, anthralin, or tar. Controversy exists as to whether ultraviolet B or oral psoralen with ultraviolet A (PUVA) should be used because of their theoretical ability to decrease cutaneous immunity. The incidence of Reiter's syndrome is increased in HIV-infected patients compared with normal controls. In both widespread psoriasis and Reiter's syndrome, methotrexate and other immunosuppressives are contraindicated because of the potential for further immunosuppression. Etretinate has been found to be a useful agent in widespread psoriatic disease.

Seborrheic dermatitis is a common feature in HIV disease and has some unusual clinical characteristics, especially with more advanced immunodeficiency. These include more severe hyperkeratotic lesions and more generalized involvement. Histologically, the AIDS-related disease may show features not usually seen in ordinary seborrheic dermatitis such as necrosis of keratinocytes, lymphocytic exocytosis, plasma cell infiltration, and focal leukocytoclasis (Chapter 125).

24. C HIV disease in children has many distinguishing features from the adult form. The majority of cases are transmitted vertically from an infected mother. In contrast to adult patients, children suffer from B-cell defects early in the course of disease. They usually present with multiple bacterial infections such as impetigo, cellulitis, skin abscesses, otitis media, and pneumonia.

Polyclonal hypergammaglobulinemia is an early feature; however, with time these patients develop defects of their cell-mediated immune system with low CD4 counts. Unlike some groups of adults, it is unusual for children to develop Kaposi's sarcoma or *Pneumocystis carinii* pneumonia (PCP). Other cutaneous signs of HIV disease in children include difficult-to-treat seborrheic and atopic dermatitis, Norwegian scabies with involvement of the scalp, hypersensitivity vasculitis, and drug eruptions. Patients may fail to thrive and have nutritional deficiencies with corresponding cutaneous signs (Chapter 125).

25. C; **26.** A; **27.** B; **28.** E; **29.** D Zidovudine (AZT) is currently given to HIV-infected patients with absolute CD4 counts less than $500/mm^3$. The most common cutaneous reaction to AZT is hyperpigmentation of the nails, often with longitudinal streaks, but diffuse pigmentation and transverse bands may occur. Hyperpigmentation of the mucous membranes or the skin may also occur but does so rarely. Other cutaneous findings include periungual erythema, a dermatomyositis-like syndrome and reticulated erythematous patches. Trimethoprim-sulfamethoxazole is given for prophylaxis or treatment of PCP. This is the most common offending agent causing drug reactions in HIV-infected individuals. The exanthematous erythematous eruption associated with fever is usually seen 8 to 10 days after starting therapy and has an incidence almost 10-fold higher than seen in the general population. Pentamidine is also used for the treatment of PCP and there have been reports of ulceration at injection sites. Foscarnet is used for the treatment of cytomegalovirus (CMV) infections and acyclovir-resistant herpes infections. It has been reported to cause fixed drug eruptions developing into painful oral, genital, or buttocks ulcers. Cutaneous side-effects from dapsone include cyanosis or an erythematous morbilliform eruption (Chapter 125).

30. B; **31.** C; **32.** A; **33.** E; **34.** E Classic Kaposi's sarcoma (KS) is primarily a skin disease that most commonly affects elderly men of Mediterranean origin with a peak incidence in the sixth decade. Lesions are usually first seen on the feet and legs with eventual associated lymphedema. The course of KS is chronic and is unlikely to result in death, but internal involvement, especially of the gastrointestinal tract, can occur. There are two forms of African endemic KS; one form is seen in young adults with a benign nodular disease. A rare form exists in which patients have an aggressive disease with both mucocutaneous and visceral involvement that may be fatal within 5 to 8 years. The second group is seen in young children who have fulminant lymphadenopathic disease that disseminates to lymph nodes and visceral organs, often in the absence of skin lesions and is fatal within 2 to 3 years. The iatrogenic form has been reported for a number of immunosuppressive drugs. Spontaneous remissions have been reported with discontinuation of immunosuppressive treatment.

AIDS-associated (epidemic) KS has been reported predominantly in homosexual men; there is a decreased risk in other subgroups of patients. Its pathogenesis is unknown, although a possible relationship with another sexually transmitted cofactor has been hypothesized. Clinically, the lesions vary from faint red macular lesions to purple papules, nodules, or plaques. In AIDS-KS, oral lesions are the first manifestation of the disease in 22% of cases and are markers for advanced HIV infection. Visceral involvement is common in AIDS-KS, and there is predilection for the gastrointestinal tract and lungs (Chapter 125).

Bibliography

DRUG ERUPTIONS

Bronner AK, Hood AF. Cutaneous complications of chemotherapeutic agents. J Am Acad Dermatol 1983; 9:645–663.

Colver GB, Inglis JA, McVittie E, et al. Dermatitis due to intravesical mitomycin C: a delayed-type hypersensitivity reaction? Br J Dermatol 1990; 122:217–224.

Gaspari AA, Lotze MJ, Rosenberg SA, et al. Dermatologic changes associated with interleukin 2 administration. JAMA 1987; 258:1624–1629.

Hebert AA, Sigman ES, Levy ML. Serum sickness-like reactions from cefaclor in children. J Am Acad Dermatol 1991; 25:805–808.

O'Donnell BP, Dawson NA, Weiss RB, et al. Suramin-induced skin reactions. Arch Dermatol 1992; 128:75–79.

Prussick R, Knowles S, Shear NH. Cutaneous drug reactions. Curr Probl Dermatol March/April 1994; 6(3):83–122.

Roujeau JC, Bioulac-Sage P, Bourseau C et al. Acute generalized exanthematous pustulosis. Arch Dermatol 1991; 127:1333–1338.

Shear NH, Spielberg SP. Anticonvulsant hypersensitivity syndrome. J Clin Invest 88; 82:1826–1832.

Vega JM, Blanca M, Carmona MJ, et al. Delayed allergic reactions to beta-lactams. Allergy 1991; 46:154–157.

Wilkin JA. Flushing reactions in the cancer chemotherapy patient. Arch Dermatol 1992; 128:1387–1389.

SKIN MANIFESTATIONS OF IMMUNE SUPPRESSION

Abel EA. Cutaneous manifestations of immunosuppression in organ transplant recipients. J Am Acad Dermatol 1989; 21:167–179.

Bentur L, Shear NH, Roifman, CM. Cutaneous lymphohistiocytic infiltrates in patients with hypogammaglobulinemia. J Pediatr 1990; 116:68–72.

Cohen PR, Grossman ME. Clinical features of human immunodeficiency virus–associated disseminated herpes zoster virus infection—a review of the literature. Clin Exp Dermatol 1989; 14:273–276.

Dover JS, Johnson RA. Cutaneous manifestations of Human Immunodeficiency Virus infection. Arch Dermatol 1991; 127:1383–1391 and 1549–1558.

Peacocke M, Siminovitch KA. Wiskott-Aldridge syndrome: new molecular and biochemical insights. J Am Acad Dermatol 1992; 27:507–519.

Sadick NS, McNutt NS, Kaplan MH. Papulosquamous dermatoses of AIDS. J Am Acad Dermatol 1990; 22:1270–1277.

Tappero JW, Conant MA, Wolfe SF, Berger TG. Kaposi's sarcoma. J Am Acad Dermatol 1993; 28:371–395.

section three

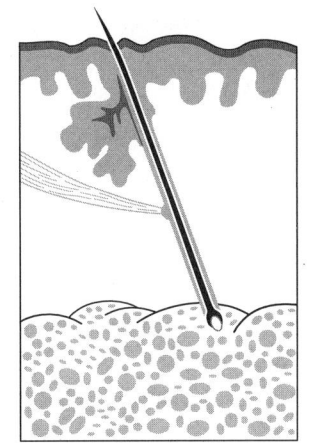

What Diseases Cause Blistering of the Skin?

chapter 12

Bullous Diseases

JO-DAVID FINE and ELIZABETH M. SPIERS

Choose the ONE BEST answer to the following question.

1. All of the following statements about the constituents of the dermoepidermal junction are correct EXCEPT

   A. Bullous pemphigoid antigen 1 (BPA-1) and $\alpha_6\beta_4$ integrin are associated with the hemidesmosome.

   B. Laminin is a glycosylated, cross-configured protein that is present within both the lamina lucida and the lamina densa.

   C. BPA-2 is a noncollagenous, hemidesmosome-associated protein.

   D. Heparin sulfate proteoglycan and chondroitin-6 sulfate proteoglycan are both present within the lamina densa of the dermoepidermal junction.

   E. Type IV collagen is the predominant collagen within the dermoepidermal junction and resides within the lamina densa.

For the following question, ONE or MORE of the following completions may correctly finish the incomplete statement; choose

   A. If only 1, 2, and 3 are correct
   B. If only 1 and 3 are correct
   C. If only 2 and 4 are correct
   D. If only 4 is correct
   E. If all are correct.

2. Altered expression of one or more of the following dermoepidermal junction antigens, as measured by diminished or absent monoclonal antibody staining, is observed in junctional epidermolysis bullosa (Herlitz variant) skin. This statement applies to

   A. Nicein (kalinin; epiligrin; GB3; BM-600)

   B. Laminin

   C. Uncein (19-DEJ-1)

   D. Chondroitin-6 sulfate proteoglycan

For the following questions decide whether each choice is TRUE or FALSE.

Regarding herpes gestations (HG)

3. HG usually has its onset in the second trimester of pregnancy.

4. HG typically flares just before, during, or immediately after the time of delivery.

5. Corticosteroid therapy may precipitate recurrent disease activity if given post partum.

6. HG is unassociated with any fetal morbidity or mortality.

7. The target antigen in HG is bullous pemphigoid antigen-1.

Regarding bullous pemphigoid (BP)

8. BP is an intraepidermal bullous disease characterized by the presence of tense, Nikolsky's sign–negative blisters.

9. Direct immunofluorescence of perilesional skin in BP typically is characterized by the presence of IgG and/or C3 in linear, homogeneous array along the dermoepidermal junction.

10. In BP, the most common autoantibody response is to BP antigen-2.

11. Autoantibody titers in BP correlate with the extent or severity of disease activity.

12. For each of the following statements regarding cicatricial pemphigoid (CP), decide whether it is TRUE or FALSE.

    A. The most common sites of blister formation in CP are the conjunctivae and the oral mucosa.

    B. Although it is a rare occurrence in CP, severe tracheolaryngeal involvement may occur.

    C. A variety of target antigens have been proposed in CP, including epiligrin.

    D. Circulating anti–skin basement membrane autoantibodies are observed in about 50% of CP patients.

    E. A rare variant of CP characterized by significant blistering of the face and head is referred to as Brunsting-Perry pemphigoid.

Regarding dermatitis herpetiformis (DH)

13. A characteristic histologic feature of DH is the presence of neutrophilic microabscesses within the upper papillary dermis.

14. DH patients may have associated gluten sensitivity.

15. Direct immunofluorescence of perilesional skin in DH reveals granular deposits of IgA within the upper papillary dermis.

16. Appropriate treatments for DH include dapsone, sulfapyridine, and a gluten-free diet.

17. Exogenous agents known to lead to flares in disease activity in DH include foods containing iodine and/or gluten and oral contraceptives.

In the following questions, a set of lettered headings accompanies a list of numbered words or phrases. For each numbered word or phrase choose

    A. If the item is associated with A only
    B. If the item is associated with B only
    C. If the item is associated with both A and B
    D. If the item is associated with neither A nor B

18. For each of the following characteristics, choose whether it describes pemphigus vulgaris, pemphigus foliaceus, both, or neither.

    1. Autoantibodies to desmoglein I
    2. Characterized by subepidermal blisters
    3. In vitro model is complement-independent
    4. Direct immunofluorescence of perilesional skin reveals IgG and/or complement bound to keratinocyte cell surfaces ("intercellular" pattern)
    5. Associated with thymoma and myasthenia gravis.

    A. Pemphigus vulgaris
    B. Pemphigus foliaceus
    C. Both
    D. Neither.

19. For each of the following characteristics, choose whether it describes dermatitis herpetiformis, linear IgA dermatosis, both, or neither.

    1. Associated with HLA-B8 and -DR3 haplotypes
    2. Direct immunofluorescence of perilesional skin reveals IgA in a continuous, homogeneous array along the dermoepidermal junction
    3. Small bowel biopsies reveal findings consistent with gluten-sensitive enteropathy
    4. Onset occurs only rarely in early childhood
    5. May be associated with autoimmune thyroid disease.

    A. Dermatitis herpetiformis
    B. Linear IgA dermatosis
    C. Both
    D. Neither.

For the following questions decide whether each choice is TRUE or FALSE.

Regarding epidermolysis bullosa acquisita (EBA)

20. EBA may clinically resemble bullous pemphigoid, cicatricial pemphigoid, dominant dystrophic epidermolysis bullosa, or porphyria cutanea tarda.

21. EBA is caused by autoimmunity to type VII collagen.

22. Autoantibodies to the EBA antigen bind to the epidermal portion of sodium chloride–separated normal human skin.
23. The presence of scarring and milia is more commonly observed in EBA than in bullous pemphigoid.
24. EBA usually is a self-limited disease that can be managed by conservative, topical approaches.

Regarding inherited epidermolysis bullosa (EB)

25. Patients with EB have pathophysiologically relevant anti–basement membrane autoantibodies within their sera.
26. All forms of EB are clinically apparent at or shortly after birth.
27. EB simplex is unassociated with an increased risk of infant mortality.
28. Major EB subtypes may be diagnosed by electron microscopy and/or specialized immunohistochemical techniques, using antibodies to specific skin basement membrane antigens
29. Junctional EB is associated with an increased risk of potentially fatal squamous cell carcinoma.
30. All forms of inherited EB are transmitted in either an autosomal dominant or an autosomal recessive manner.

For the following questions, decide whether EACH choice is TRUE or FALSE. Any combination of answers from all true to all false may occur.

31. Regarding recessive dystrophic EB (RDEB)
    A. More severe forms of RDEB may be associated with extracutaneous lymphoma.
    B. The mitis variant of generalized RDEB is characterized by the presence of short stature, marked multifactorial anemia, and severe mucous membrane involvement.
    C. Oral cavity findings in severe RDEB may include ankyloglossia, microstomia, widespread intraoral blisters and scars, and rampant caries.
    D. Clinical disease activity is usually more severe in dystrophic EB when the disease occurs in an autosomal dominant rather than an autosomal recessive manner.
    E. Type IV collagen is the target basement membrane protein in RDEB.

32. Regarding EB simplex (EBS)
    A. Scarring is not a feature of EBS.
    B. The Dowling-Meara variant of EBS is associated with an increased risk of infant mortality.
    C. All forms of EBS are transmitted in an autosomal dominant manner.
    D. Type VII collagen is the target protein in EBS.
    E. Blistering occurs within the epidermis in all forms of EBS.

33. Regarding junctional EB (JEB)
    A. Acute airway obstruction may be the cause of death during infancy in some patients with generalized JEB.
    B. Blisters occur with the lamina lucida in all forms of JEB.
    C. Laminin is believed to be the target protein in at least one known form of JEB.
    D. Exuberant granulation tissue is a pathognomonic feature in the Herlitz variant of generalized JEB.
    E. Mitten deformities are not a feature of JEB.

In the following question, a set of lettered headings accompanies a list of numbered words or phrases. For each numbered word or phrase choose

A. If the item is associated with A only
B. If the item is associated with B only
C. If the item is associated with both A and B
D. If the item is associated with neither A nor B.

34. For each of the following characteristics, choose whether it describes Cockayne-Touraine dominant dystrophic EB (DDEB), Pasini DDEB, both, or neither.

    1. Significant risk of tracheolaryngeal disease activity
    2. Albopapuloid lesions
    3. Absence of scarring and milia
    4. Nail dystrophy
    5. Predilection for localized cutaneous disease activity

    A. Cockayne-Touraine dominant dystrophic EB (DDEB)
    B. Pasini DDEB
    C. Both
    D. Neither.

For each numbered item, choose the most likely associated lettered item. Each numbered item has ONLY ONE answer. Within each group, each lettered item may be the answer to one, more than one, or none of the numbered items.

For each of the types of inherited epidermolysis bullosa (EB) listed below, choose the most characteristic associated ultrastructural feature in perilesional or lesional skin.

35. Intracytoplasmic stellate bodies within keratinocytes
36. Absent or rudimentary-appearing hemidesmosomes
37. Absent or rudimentary-appearing anchoring fibrils
38. Clumped tonofilaments within basilar keratinocytes
39. Cleavage within or at the level of the stratum granulosum

A. EB simplex herpetiformis (Dowling-Meara variant)
B. Recessive dystrophic EB, gravis (Hallopeau-Siemens variant)
C. Junctional EB, gravis (Herlitz variant)
D. Transient bullous dermolysis of the newborn
E. EB simplex superficialis.

For each of the autoantibodies listed below, choose the autoimmune bullous disease with which it is most strongly linked or in which it is most commonly found.

40. Anti–type VII collagen autoantibodies
41. Anti-gliadin and anti-reticulin autoantibodies
42. Anti–desmoglein I autoantibodies
43. Autoantibodies to bullous pemphigoid antigen-1
44. Autoantibodies to bullous pemphigoid antigen-2

A. Bullous pemphigoid
B. Dermatitis herpetiformis
C. Epidermolysis bullosa acquisita
D. Pemphigus foliaceus
E. Herpes gestationis.

Match each of the following bullous diseases with the most characteristic listed histologic or immunohistochemical finding.

45. Intracytoplasmic collections of type VII collagen within the epidermis
46. Eosinophils within the dermal infiltrate
47. Collections of polymorphonuclear leukocytes within the upper papillary dermis
48. Absence of visualizable type VII collagen along the dermoepidermal junction
49. Intraepidermal deposition of IgG and/or complement
50. Absence of type IV collagen along the dermoepidermal junction

A. Dermatitis herpetiformis
B. Recessive dystrophic epidermolysis bullosa, gravis (Hallopeau-Siemens)
C. Herpes gestationis
D. Transient bullous dermolysis of the newborn
E. None of the above.

For each of the basement membrane structures listed, choose the antigen with which it is most closely associated.

51. Uncein (19-DEJ-1)
52. Type VII collagen
53. Bullous pemphigoid antigen-1.

A. Anchoring fibril
B. Hemidesmosome
C. Anchoring filament
D. Lamina densa.

In each of the following questions, a set of lettered headings accompanies a list of numbered words or phrases. For each numbered word or phrase, choose

A. If the item is associated with A only
B. If the item is associated with B only
C. If the item is associated with both A and B
D. If the item is associated with neither A nor B.

54. For each of the following characteristics, choose whether it describes subcorneal pustular dermatosis, pustular psoriasis, both, or neither.

1. Dapsone is the treatment of choice
2. Psoriasiform dermatosis
3. Herpetiform grouping of lesions within flexural body sites

A. Subcorneal pustular dermatosis (Sneddon-Wilkinson disease)
B. Pustular psoriasis
C. Both
D. Neither

4. May rarely present as a life-threatening erythroderma associated with high fever and widespread pustulosis.

55. For each of the following characteristics choose whether it describes pemphigus vulgaris, transient acantholytic dermatosis, both, or neither.

    1. Intraepidermal cleavage with acantholysis
    2. May be associated with severe intraoral disease activity
    3. Autoantibodies to desmoglein I
    4. Autoantibodies to pemphigus vulgaris antigen
    5. Usually requires treatment with systemic corticosteroids, with or without the addition of a second immunosuppressant agent.

    A. Pemphigus vulgaris
    B. Transient acantholytic dermatosis
    C. Both
    D. Neither.

56. Altered expression of one or more of the following dermoepidermal junction antigens, as measured by diminished or absent monoclonal antibody staining, is observed in skin from patients with the Hallopeau-Siemens variant of recessive dystrophic EB:

    1. Chondroitin-6 sulfate proteoglycan
    2. Kalinin (nicein; epiligrin; GB3; BM-600)
    3. Type VII collagen
    4. Heparin sulfate proteoglycan.

    A. 1, 2, 3
    B. 2, 3
    C. 1, 3
    D. 4 only
    E. All of the above.

57. For each of the following statements regarding dermatitis herpetiformis and linear IgA dermatosis, decide whether it is TRUE or FALSE.

    A. Chronic bullous dermatosis of childhood is considered to be a subset of dermatitis herpetiformis.
    B. Dapsone is the treatment of choice for both dermatitis herpetiformis and linear IgA dermatosis.
    C. Both diseases are characterized by the presence of IgA in granular array along the dermoepidermal junction.
    D. Gluten-sensitive enteropathy is associated with both diseases.
    E. Dermatitis herpetiformis is usually a disease of the elderly.

In each of the following questions, a set of lettered headings accompanies a list of numbered words or phrases. For each numbered word or phrase, choose

    A. If the item is associated with A only
    B. If the item is associated with B only
    C. If the item is associated with both A and B
    D. If the item is associated with neither A nor B.

58. For each of the following statements, choose whether it describes bullous eruption of systemic lupus erythematosus, epidermolysis bullosa acquisita, both, or neither.

    1. Associated with HLA-DR2 haplotype
    2. Majority of patients with anti–basement membrane autoantibodies within their sera
    3. Associated with autoimmunity to type VII collagen
    4. Dapsone is the drug of choice
    5. Typically characterized by blister formation beneath the level of the lamina densa.

    A. Bullous eruption of systemic lupus erythematosus
    B. Epidermolysis bullosa acquisita
    C. Both
    D. Neither.

59. For each of the following characteristics, choose whether it describes bullous pemphigoid, pemphigus vulgaris, both, or neither.

    1. Blister formation is autoantibody-,

    A. Bullous pemphigoid
    B. Pemphigus vulgaris

complement-, and cell-dependent

2. Presence of IgG class autoantibodies within the skin

3. Autoantibody titers correlate with level of disease activity

4. Strongly associated with the presence of internal malignancy

5. May be associated with complement deposition within the skin.

C. Both
D. Neither.

Choose the ONE BEST answer to each of the following questions.

60. Eosinophilic spongiosis may be seen in which of the following conditions?

    A. Pemphigus vulgaris
    B. Herpes gestationis
    C. Bullous pemphigoid
    D. Arthropod bites
    E. All of the above.

61. Biopsies of transient acantholytic dermatosis may demonstrate all of the following EXCEPT

    A. Acantholysis
    B. Eosinophilic microabscesses
    C. Corps ronds
    D. Suprabasilar clefts
    E. Spongiosis.

In each of the following questions, a set of lettered headings accompanies a list of numbered words or phrases. For each numbered word or phrase, choose

A. If the item is associated with A only
B. If the item is associated with B only
C. If the item is associated with both A and B
D. If the item is associated with neither A nor B.

For each of the following histopathologic findings, choose whether it describes pemphigus vulgaris, paraneoplastic pemphigus, both, or neither.

62. Dyskeratotic keratinocytes
63. Acantholysis
64. Suprabasilar cleft formation
65. Vacuolar interface alteration.

A. Pemphigus vulgaris
B. Paraneoplastic pemphigus
C. Both
D. Neither.

For each of the following immunofluorescence findings, choose whether it describes pemphigus vulgaris, paraneoplastic pemphigus, both, or neither.

66. Intercellular IgG and complement by direct immunofluorescence
67. Basement membrane zone IgG and complement by direct immunofluorescence
68. Positive indirect immunofluorescence on rat bladder transitional epithelium
69. Negative indirect immunofluorescence studies.

A. Pemphigus vulgaris
B. Paraneoplastic pemphigus
C. Both
D. Neither.

For the following questions, ONE or MORE of the completions correctly finishes the incomplete statement; choose

A. If only 1, 2, and 3 are correct
B. If only 1 and 3 are correct
C. If only 2 and 4 are correct
D. If only 4 is correct
E. If all are correct.

70. The histologic differential diagnosis of a subcorneal blister includes

    1. Pemphigus foliaceus
    2. Impetigo
    3. Subcorneal pustular dermatosis
    4. Pustular psoriasis.

71. Histologic features of bullous pemphigoid may include

    1. Subepidermal blisters
    2. Neutrophil-rich inflammatory infiltrates
    3. Eosinophil-rich inflammatory infiltrates
    4. Paucity of inflammation.

72. The histologic differential diagnosis of bullous pemphigoid may include
    1. Epidermolysis bullosa acquisita
    2. Dermatitis herpetiformis
    3. Herpes gestationis
    4. Pemphigus vulgaris.

73. Herpes gestationis differs from bullous pemphigoid histologically by
    1. The presence of a subepidermal blister
    2. Eosinophils in the inflammatory infiltrate
    3. Eosinophilic spongiosis in some cases
    4. Vacuolar interface changes with necrotic keratinocytes

74. Cell-poor subepidermal blisters may be seen in which of the following conditions?
    1. Porphyria cutanea tarda
    2. Epidermolysis bullosa acquisita
    3. Bullosis diabeticorum
    4. Epidermolysis bullosa, simplex type.

75. Aggregates of neutrophils in dermal papillae are most typical of which of the following conditions?
    1. Subcorneal pustular dermatosis
    2. Bullous eruption of systemic lupus erythematosus
    3. Pemphigus vulgaris
    4. Dermatitis herpetiformis.

76. Neutrophils arranged in a band-like fashion along the dermoepidermal junction may be seen in which of the following conditions?
    1. Epidermolysis bullosa acquisita
    2. Dermatitis herpetiformis
    3. Bullous eruption of systemic lupus erythematosus
    4. Linear IgA bullous dermatosis.

Choose the ONE BEST answer to the following question.

77. All of the following are true regarding the histology of cicatricial pemphigoid EXCEPT
    A. Blisters are subepidermal.
    B. The inflammatory infiltrate is often mixed.
    C. Plasma cells may be observed.
    D. Fibroplasia and scarring may be present in the dermis.
    E. It is readily distinguishable from bullous pemphigoid.

In each of the following questions, a set of lettered headings accompanies a list of numbered words or phrases. For each numbered word or phrase, choose

    A. If the item is associated with A only
    B. If the item is associated with B only
    C. If the item is associated with both A and B
    D. If the item is associated with neither A nor B.

For each of the following histologic findings, choose whether it describes pemphigus vulgaris, pemphigus vegetans, both, or neither.

78. Acanthosis   A. Pemphigus vulgaris
79. Acantholysis   B. Pemphigus vegetans
80. Intraepidermal eosinophilic abscesses   C. Both
                        D. Neither.
81. Suprabasilar clefting

For each numbered item, choose the associated site of cleavage (lettered items) for the blistering diseases listed. Each numbered item has ONLY ONE correct answer.

Within each group, each lettered item may be the answer to one, more than one, or none of the numbered items.

82. Epidermolysis bullosa simplex, Weber-Cockayne variant
83. Epidermolysis bullosa simplex superficialis
84. Transient bullous dermolysis of the newborn
85. Bullous pemphigoid
86. Pemphigus erythematosus.

A. Subcorneal
B. Within basilar keratinocytes
C. Intra-lamina lucida
D. Sub–lamina densa.

Choose the ONE BEST answer to each of the following questions.

87. Regarding routine histology in the diagnosis of blistering diseases, all of the following are correct EXCEPT
    A. Nonspecific features may be present.
    B. A definitive diagnosis can always be rendered.
    C. Re-epithelialization of blisters may alter or mask the actual site of cleavage.

D. Technical problems, such as shearing of the blister roof, may occur.

E. Inflammatory infiltrates can change with age of lesion and secondary factors.

88. The biopsy technique that provides the most optimal specimen for histologic examination of a blistering disease is

A. Punch biopsy

B. Shave biopsy

C. Curette biopsy

D. Excisional biopsy

E. Either punch or excisional biopsy.

ANSWERS

1. C In contrast to BPA-1, which is a noncollagenous protein, BPA-2 contains two collagenous domains. Although it may be considered to be hemidesmosome-associated, BPA-2 presumably resides within the lamina lucida, whereas BPA-1 has been localized to the intracytoplasmic side of the hemidesmosome (Chapter 72).

2. B Uncein is undetectable along the dermoepidermal junction in 100% of cases of junctional epidermolysis bullosa (JEB), regardless of the subtype. With few exceptions, nicein is undetectable in Herlitz variant JEB skin specimens, whereas approximately 60% of non-Herlitz JEB specimens appear to have normal staining with the anti-nicein antibody, GB3. In contrast, laminin, type IV collagen, heparin sulfate proteoglycan, and chondroitin-6 sulfate proteoglycan all appear to be normally expressed, based on indirect immunofluorescence studies with antibodies specific for each.

3. (T); **4.** (T); **5.** (F); **6.** (F); **7.** (F) Herpes gestationis (HG) typically develops in the second trimester of pregnancy, as opposed to pruritic urticarial papules and plaques of pregnancy (PUPPP), which occurs usually during the last part of the third trimester. Flares in HG disease activity typically occur around the time of parturition. In the absence of medical intervention, there is an increased risk of prematurity or fetal death. Oral contraceptives, not corticosteroids, are known to precipitate recurrences in disease activity and therefore are considered to be contraindicated in patients with histories of previous HG. It is now known that bullous pemphigoid antigen-2 (BPA-2) is the target of autoimmunity in HG.

8. (F); **9** (T); **10.** (F); **11.** (F) Bullous pemphigoid (BP) is a subepidermal bullous disease. Like all other subepidermal blistering diseases, with the exception of dystrophic epidermolysis bullosa and epidermolysis bullosa acquisita, perilesional skin in BP is Nikolsky's sign–negative. Most positive BP antisera react against BPA-1. No correlation exists between the titer of BP autoantibody present in a patient's serum and the extent or severity of disease activity (Chapter 75).

12. A. (T); B. (T); C. (T); D. (F); E. (T) The most common sites of disease activity in cicatricial pemphigoid (CP) are the conjunctivae and the oral mucosa. Eye involvement, which is almost always bilateral, may range from mild conjunctival injection to active conjunctival vesiculation and scarring. Drying of the corneas may occur as a result of the inability of patients to fully close their eyes because of the development of symblepharons; if unchecked, corneal scarring and blindness may eventually ensue. The most common site of oral involvement is the gingivae. Although seen in some other autoimmune processes, including pemphigus vulgaris and lichen planus, the earliest hallmark of CP within the oral cavity is the presence of desquamative gingivitis. Autoimmunity to one of several different-sized basement membrane antigens has been reported in limited numbers of patients with CP. To date, the only well-characterized autoantigen is epiligrin (kalinin; nicein; GB3; BM-600), although only a few CP patients' sera have been shown to have autoreactivity against purified epiligrin. Anti–basement membrane autoantibodies are seen in only about 10% of CP patients' sera, and when present, are usually noted to be of only minimally measurable titer. Brunsting-Perry pemphigoid is considered by many to be a variant of CP, although others classify it as a scarring variant of bullous pemphigoid (Chapter 76).

13. (T); **14.** (T); **15.** (T); **16.** (T); **17.** (F) Most patients with dermatitis herpetiformis (DH) experience rapid exacerbation of their disease activity following ingestion of gluten. Smaller numbers of patients may complain of increased itching and/or vesiculation following meals rich in iodine, most notably shellfish. Whereas rare women may experience flares in their DH during or shortly before each menstrual cycle, the use of oral contraceptives is not known to be an exacerbator of disease activity in DH (Chapter 79).

18. 1. B; 2. D; 3. A; 4. C; 5. A Pemphigus vulgaris and pemphigus foliaceus have autoantibody responses against the pemphigus vulgaris antigen and desmoglein I, respectively. Both are intraepidermal blistering diseases. No adequate in vitro model of pemphigus foliaceus exists. In contrast, incubation of normal human skin explants in tissue culture with purified pemphigus vulgaris autoantibodies, in the absence of exogenous complement, results in autoantibody binding and lower intraepidermal cleft formation within skin identical to that occurring in vivo in patients with active pemphigus vulgaris. Pemphigus vulgaris has rarely been associated with the presence of thymoma and myasthenia gravis (Chapter 74).

19. 1. A; 2. B; 3. A; 4. A; 5. A The preceding HLA haplotypes are seen in DH patients, whereas they are characteristically absent in adults with linear IgA dermatosis. The most typical direct immunofluorescence finding in DH is the presence of granular deposits of IgA within the papillary dermis. Although usually these deposits are focal and are associated with neutrophilic microabscesses, they may rarely be present in linear but granular array along the dermoepidermal junction. This can be contrasted to linear IgA dermatosis, in which continous, homogeneous deposition of IgA can be observed along the dermoepidermal junction. Most DH patients who have undergone small-bowel biopsy have been found to have histologic features of gluten-sensitive enteropathy (i.e., celiac sprue–like), although most patients with DH admit to little or no gastrointestinal symptomatology. DH is usually a disease of young adults but may occur at any age. In contrast, one major subset of linear IgA dermatosis, also referred to as chronic bullous dermatosis of children, is a pediatric disease with onset usually during the preschool years. A minority of DH patients may have antithyroid autoantibodies within their sera; some may experience signs and symptoms of either hyperthyroidism or hypothyroidism (Chapters 79 and 80).

20. (T); **21.** (T); **22.** (F); **23.** (T); **24.** (F) Epidermolysis bullosa acquisita (EBA) may have many different presentations, although patients most commonly present with a generalized subepidermal blistering disease associated with fragile skin, atrophic scar formation, milia, and postinflammatory pigmentary changes. Anti–basement membrane autoantibodies directed against epitomes on the type VII collagen molecule are seen in the sera of the majority of EBA patients. These autoantibodies characteristically bind exclusively to the dermal portion of 1.0 M sodium chloride–split normal human skin. Although milia and scarring may be seen in essentially any subepidermal autoimmune bullous disease, they are commonly observed in EBA and porphyria cutanea tarda. Most patients with EBA have a generalized skin disease that requires aggressive medical therapy with combinations of systemic immunosuppressant drugs. Despite the latter interventions, however, many EBA patients eventually die either as a direct result of their disease or as a consequence of the potentially severe sequelae of chronic immunosuppressant therapy (Chapter 78).

25. (F); **26.** (F); **27.** (F); **28.** (T); **29.** (F); **30.** (F) None of the forms of inherited EB is associated with the presence of significant titers of circulating anti–basement membrane autoantibodies. This is physiologically reasonable, since inherited EB is not a disease of autoimmunity. Although patients with the most severe forms of inherited EB do have clinically detectable disease activity at or shortly after birth, some milder forms (e.g., localized EB simplex and EB progressiva) may have onset of blistering delayed until mid or late childhood. In contrast to most other EB simplex subsets, two generalized types, EB simplex herpetiformis (Dowling-Meara variant) and a type of autosomal recessive EB simplex associated with congenital neuromuscular diseases may be accompanied by an increased risk of death during early infancy. One form of inherited EB, the Mendes da Costa variant of EB simplex, is transmitted in an X-linked recessive manner. As suggested above, inherited EB is best confirmed and subclassified by the concurrent evaluation of skin biopsy samples with transmission electron microscopy and with an indirect immunofluorescence technique ("antigenic mapping") employing polyclonal and monoclonal antibodies to selected skin basement membrane proteins. Potentially life-threatening squamous cell carcinomas frequently arise in patients with severe, generalized recessive dystrophic EB and occasionally also occur in dominant dystrophic EB. Only one case of squamous cell carcinoma has been reported to date in junctional EB; in the absence of additional cases, the latter occurrence should not be interpreted to suggest an increased risk of this particular skin tumor in junctional EB patients (Chapter 73).

31. A. (F); B. (F); C. (T); D. (F); E. (F) Lymphoma is unassociated with any form of inherited EB. The features described under "B" are those of the gravis form of RDEB (referred to as the Hallopeau-Siemens variant). Significant extracutaneous involvement is only rarely observed in the mitis form of RDEB. As in the case of other genetic diseases, clinical findings are usually much worse in autosomal recessive than in autosomal dominant forms of dystrophic EB. Type VII collagen is the basement membrane protein involved in the pathogenesis of blister formation in RDEB. No reported abnormalities in the structure or expression of type IV collagen have been reported in any form of inherited EB, although autoimmunity to an epitope of type IV collagen is believed to be the immunologic target of injury in Goodpasture's syndrome (Chapter 73).

32. A. (F); B. (T); C. (F); D. (F); E. (T) All forms of EB simplex (EBS) are characterized by intraepidermal blister formation. With the sole exception of EBS superficialis, a rare variant defined by the presence of blistering at the level of the stratum granulosum, all other forms of EBS are associated with cleavage within the level of the basilar keratinocyte. Rare forms of EBS may be transmitted in an autosomal recessive or X-linked recessive manner. Keratins appear to be the targets of genetic mutation in all forms of EBS (Chapter 73).

33. A. (T); B. (T); C. (F); D. (T); E. (F) All forms of junctional EB (JEB) are characterized by the presence of blistering within the lamina lucida. The two proteins believed to be involved in the pathogenesis of blistering in JEB, nicein (kalinin; epiligrin; GB3; BM-600) and uncein (19-DEJ-1) are both anchoring filament–associated. Although mitten deformities are a classic feature of the Hallopeau-Siemens variant of severe, generalized recessive dystrophic EB, a rare subset of JEB, referred to as cicatricial JEB, has been reported to have mitten deformities that are phenotypically identical to those observed in severe recessive dystrophic EB (Chapter 73).

34. 1. D; 2. B; 3. D; 4. C; 5. D Tracheolaryngeal involvement is a feature of junctional EB, not dominant dystrophic EB (DDEB). Both major forms of generalized DDEB, Pasini and Cockayne-Touraine variants, are associated with cutaneous scarring, milia, and nail dystrophy. The presence of albopapuloid lesions explicitly defines the Pasini variant; no other differences exist between the Pasini and Cockayne-Touraine subsets of generalized DDEB (Chapter 73).

35. D; **36.** C; **37.** B; **38.** A; **39.** E (Chapter 73).

40. C; **41.** B; **42.** D; **43.** A; **44.** E (Chapters 75 to 79).

45. D; **46.** C; **47.** A; **48.** B; **49.** E (Chapters 73, 77, and 79).

50. E; **51.** C; **52.** A; **53.** B (Chapter 72).

54. 1. A; 2. C; 3. A; 4. B Both subcorneal pustular dermatosis and pustular psoriasis are classified among the psoriasiform dermatoses. Subcorneal pustular dermatosis is characteristically associated with the presence of pustules and scale in herpetiform or arcuate array, especially within body folds. Pustular psoriasis may be localized or generalized. Rare pustular psoriasis patients, especially those recently treated with systemic corticosteroids, may present with an acute, life-threatening, generalized pustular eruption, named pustular psoriasis of von Zumbusch, which is characterized by the development of widespread pustulation, erythroderma, and high fever (Chapter 27).

55. 1. C; 2. A; 3. D; 4. A; 5. A The histological findings in transient acantholytic dermatosis (Grover's disease) may closely mimic those of pemphigus vulgaris, although the extent of skin cleavage in the former is usually very focal. Pemphigus vulgaris is commonly associated with intraoral erosions; at times, widespread incapacitating denudation of tissue may occur. Autoantibodies to desmoglein I are a feature of pemphigus foliaceus. The target of the autoimmune response in pemphigus vulgaris is an epidermal cadherin referred to as the pemphigus vulgaris antigen. Although localized pemphigus vulgaris does occur, most patients with pemphigus vulgaris have severe, generalized disease necessitating treatment with one or more systemic immunosuppressant drugs (Chapters 30 and 37).

56. C Type VII collagen is usually undetectable by conventional indirect immunofluorescence technique in perilesional skin specimens from patients with the Hallopeau-Siemens variant of generalized recessive dystrophic EB (RDEB). Similar findings have been observed with a monoclonal antibody to chondroitin-6 sulfate proteoglycan. In contrast, heparin sulfate proteoglycan is normally expressed in all forms of inherited EB. Altered expression of kalinin is a feature of some forms of junctional EB (Chapter 72).

57. A. (F); B. (T); C. (F); D. (F); E. (F) Chronic bullous dermatosis of childhood is one of two forms of linear IgA dermatosis. Whereas continuous, homogeneous, linear deposits of IgA are the hallmark of linear IgA dermatosis (both adult and childhood forms), granular IgA deposits are characteristic of dermatitis herpetiformis. All forms of IgA-mediated autoimmune bullous diseases appear to respond to treatment with dapsone, but only dermatitis herpetiformis patients benefit from a gluten-free diet, since it is the only autoimmune bullous disorder that is associated with histologic evidence of a gluten-sensitive enteropathy. Dermatitis herpetiformis is usually a disease of young adults, although all ages may be affected (Chapter 80).

58. 1. C; 2. B; 3. C; 4. A; 5. C Both bullous eruption of systemic lupus erythematosus (BESLE) and epidermolysis bullosa acquisita (EBA) are associated with the HLA-DR2 haplotype and with autoimmunity to type VII collagen and usually have blister formation beneath the level of the lamina densa. Dapsone may be extremely effective in the treatment of BESLE but is only rarely beneficial in EBA. Most patients with EBA have measurable anti–basement membrane autoantibodies within their sera, especially when 1.0 M sodium chloride–split skin is used as the tissue substrate, whereas only a minority of BESLE patients do (Chapters 24 and 78).

59. 1. A; 2. C; 3. B; 4. D; 5. C Both bullous pemphigoid and pemphigus vulgaris are associated with IgG deposits within the skin, and each may be accompanied by evidence of complement fixation within the same ultrastructural locations as tissue-bound IgG. The titers of circulating autoantibodies to the pemphigus vulgaris antigen, but not to the bullous pemphigoid antigen, correlate well with the extent and severity of disease activity. Neither of these diseases is a significant marker of internal malignancy, although it does occur in a rare, newly defined variant of pemphigus named pemphigus paraneoplastica. The in vitro model of bullous pemphigoid, referred to as the leukocyte attachment assay, is autoantibody-, complement-, and cell-dependent. In contrast, the presence of only pemphigus vulgaris autoantibodies is required to reproduce blister formation in organ culture in vitro (Chapters 74 and 75).

60. E Eosinophilic spongiosis is a histopathologic reaction pattern consisting of spongiosis of the epidermis with or without microvesiculation and accompanied by exocytosis of eosinophils. It can be seen in a number of different disorders, including autoimmune bullous diseases (such as pemphigus vulgaris, herpes gestationis, bullous pemphigoid), as well as incontinentia pigmenti, allergic contact dermatitis, and arthropod bite reactions. Additional histologic findings may provide a specific diagnosis. Early pemphigus may demonstrate focal areas of acantholysis, whereas the urticarial phase of bullous pemphigoid is characterized by dermal infiltration with eosinophils and vacuolar alteration of the dermoepidermal junction, leading to subepidermal blister formation. In cases of autoimmune bullous diseases, however, direct immunofluorescence must be relied on to accurately determine the diagnosis (Chapters 74, 75, and 77).

61. B Transient acantholytic dermatosis (Grover's disease) generally shows a combination of histologic patterns, often occurring in the same specimen. Acantholysis may be seen in a suprabasilar location as in pemphigus vulgaris, more superficially as in pemphigus foliaceus, and throughout the full thickness of the epidermis as in Hailey-Hailey disease. Darier's disease–like dyskeratosis with the formation of corps ronds and grains may be observed, as well as foci of spongiosis. These changes are characteristically focal in nature but otherwise may closely simulate the other disease entities. A history of pruritic papulovesicles helps support the diagnosis of transient acantholytic dermatosis. Direct and indirect immunofluorescence are characteristically negative in transient acantholytic dermatosis. Although the inflammatory infiltrate may be admixed with scattered eosinophils, eosinophilic abscesses in the epidermis are not seen in this condition, whereas they typically occur in pemphigus vegetans (Chapter 32).

62. B; **63.** C; **64.** C; **65.** B (Chapter 74).

66. C; **67.** B; **68.** B; **69.** D Paraneoplastic pemphigus, an autoimmune blistering disease associated with internal neoplasia, shares histologic features with both pemphigus vulgaris and erythema multiforme. Findings in common with pemphigus vulgaris include acantholysis and suprabasilar cleft formation. Similarities to erythema multiforme include the presence of dyskeratotic keratinocytes, vacuolar interface change, and lymphocytic exocytosis. The inflammatory infiltrate may also be lichenoid in character, simulating lichen planus.

Paraneoplastic pemphigus demonstrates basement membrane zone–bound IgG and complement, in addition to the intercellular deposits characteristic of pemphigus vulgaris on direct immunofluorescence. Indirect immunofluorescence is frequently positive in both diseases, but the choice of substrate may allow some distinction of the two entities. The use of rat bladder transitional epithelium for indirect studies has been shown to have a high degree of specificity for the diagnosis of paraneoplastic pemphigus. This test may be a reliable method for accurate diagnosis when evaluation by immunoprecipitation technique is not available (Chapter 74).

70. E A subcorneal separation may be seen in the superficial forms of pemphigus (pemphigus foliaceus, pemphigus erythematosus), subcorneal pustular dermatosis, bullous impetigo, pustular psoriasis, staphylococcal scalded skin syndrome, and candidiasis. In pemphigus, a few dyscohesive acantholytic cells may be seen in the blister cavity. Neutrophils are prominent in the blisters of subcorneal pustular dermatosis, pustular psoriasis, impetigo, and candidiasis. They may also be seen in pemphigus if there is trauma to the blister or secondary infection. Candidiasis shows fungal hyphae and spores within the stratum corneum with PAS (periodic acid–Schiff) staining. Spongiform pustules may be seen in pustular psoriasis. Subcorneal pustular dermatosis and impetigo are histologically indistinguishable. Gram's stain will show gram-positive cocci in impetigo (Chapters 25 and 30).

71. E (Chapter 23).

72. A (Chapter 75).

73. D Bullous pemphigoid clinically shows tense blisters that may arise on urticarial plaques or normal-appearing skin. The clinical presentation correlates well with the histopathologic findings. Blisters are subepidermal in location, and the inflammatory infiltrate is of variable intensity. Cell-poor blisters with a paucity of inflammation are seen in lesions located on normal-appearing skin. When urticarial lesions are noted, eosinophils generally are the predominant inflammatory cell in the blister cavity and papillary dermis, where they may align along the dermoepidermal junction and form focal collections. Occasionally, however, neutrophils may predominate and papillary dermal microabscesses may be seen. In these cases, differentiation from dermatitis herpetiformis requires immunofluorescence studies. Epidermolysis bullosa acquisita (EBA) shares clinical and histologic features with bullous pemphigoid, although lesions often develop at sites of trauma and heal with the formation of milia. The use of immunoelectron microscopy shows the immunoreactants to be present in the lamina lucida for pemphigoid and in a sublamina densa location for EBA. Incubation of skin with saline causes a split to occur within the lamina lucida that can also be used diagnostically. Direct immunofluorescence with saline-split perilesional skin shows IgG in the roof of the blister in bullous pemphigoid and in the floor of the blister in EBA. Herpes gestationis is also histologically almost identical to bullous pemphigoid. Necrotic basal keratinocytes are not found in pemphigoid, however. Pemphigus vulgaris is an intraepidermal blister formed by acantholysis and should not be considered in the differential diagnosis (Chapter 75).

74. A Blisters that occur in a subepidermal location and contain a paucity of acute inflammatory cells in the blister cavity and underlying dermis may be seen in bullous pemphigoid, epidermolysis bullosa acquisita, bullous diabeticorum, porphyria cutanea tarda and pseudoporphyrias, coma bullae, and the inherited forms of epidermolysis bullosa (junctional and dystrophic types). In porphyria cutanea tarda, the dermal papillae retain their undulating architecture along the floor of the blister, in a so-called festooning pattern. Papillary dermal vessels show a thickening of their walls with PAS-positive eosinophilic material consisting of reduplicated basement membranes. Bullous diabeticorum occurs on the lower legs of some patients with diabetes mellitus and histologically may show a proliferation of small capillaries in the upper dermis in addition to the blister. Coma bullae occur at sites of prolonged pressure, often in the setting of barbiturate overdose. The histopathologic hallmark of this subepidermal blistering disorder is necrosis of eccrine sweat ducts. The inherited forms of epidermolysis bullosa are characterized by skin fragility. Ultrastructurally, the split occurs within the lamina lucida of the basement membrane zone in the junctional types and in a sub–lamina densa location in the dystrophic types. This leads to a subepidermal location of the blisters by light microscopy. In the simplex type of EB, blistering occurs within the basal cell layer, resulting in an intraepidermal split (Chapters 73, 78, and 169).

75. C; 76. E Subepidermal vesicles and bullae associated with predominantly neutrophilic inflammatory infiltrates may include dermatitis herpetiformis, linear IgA bullous dermatosis, bullous eruption of systemic lupus erythematosus, and epidermolysis bullosa acquisita. Papillary dermal microabscesses (collections of neutrophils, nuclear dust, and fibrin) are the prototypic histologic finding in dermatitis herpetiformis, whereas neutrophils arranged in a band-like fashion along the dermoepidermal junction are more frequently seen in linear IgA bullous dermatosis. In addition, extensive basal layer vacuolization occurs more commonly in linear IgA bullous dermatosis than in dermatitis herpetiformis and therefore may provide a further clue to diagnosis. Bullous lupus erythematosus may demonstrate both microabscesses and linear neutrophil infiltrates histologically. Occasionally, an underlying leukocytoclastic vasculitis or adjacent vacuolar interface change may be observed in bullous lupus, however (Chapters 24, 74, 78, and 80).

77. E Biopsies of cicatricial pemphigoid demonstrate subepithelial separations accompanied by a mixed inflammatory infiltrate composed of lymphocytes, plasma cells, eosinophils, and neutrophils. Cicatricial pemphigoid may show lesser numbers of eosinophils and more neutrophils than bullous pemphigoid, but this is a variable finding. Fibrosis and scarring of the dermis may develop secondary to repeated episodes of blistering (Chapter 76).

78. B; 79. C; 80. B; 81. C Pemphigus is an autoimmune blistering eruption that develops by acantholysis and loss of desmosomal attachments between epithelial cells. Acantholysis occurs in a suprabasilar location, giving rise to the so-called "row of tombstones" effect as seen in pemphigus vulgaris, pemphigus vegetans, and the newly described paraneoplastic type of pemphigus. Acantholysis of the more superficial (subcorneal-subgranular) layers is characteristic of pemphigus foliaceus and pemphigus erythematosus. Additionally, marked acanthosis, papillomatosis, and hyperkeratosis are typical of pemphigus vegetans, in contrast to pemphigus vulgaris. Intraepidermal collections of eosinophils are also a distinctive histologic feature of pemphigus vegetans (Chapter 74).

82. B; 83. A; 84. D; 85. C; 86. A All forms of epidermolysis bullosa simplex have cleavage planes within the epidermis. The variant known as epidermolysis bullosa simplex superficialis is characterized by a subcorneal split similar to peeling skin syndrome, whereas the Weber-Cockayne type shows primarily intra–basilar keratinocyte damage. Transient bullous dermolysis of the newborn is a self-limited form of dystrophic epidermolysis bullosa with cleavage occurring beneath the lamina densa. In addition, characteristic intracytoplasmic, stellate-shaped inclusions of type VII collagen may be identified within basal keratinocytes in the latter disorder if affected skin is examined by immunoelectron microscopic technique. Pemphigus erythematosus is a form of superficial pemphigus and as such, blister formation occurs within the upper epidermis in a subcorneal location. Bullous pemphigoid demonstrates cleavage within the lamina lucida of the dermoepidermal junction (Chapters 73 to 75).

87. B In many instances, a biopsy of a blistering disorder sent for routine histology may lead to only a differential diagnosis rather than a definitive diagnosis. This is because different diseases may share overlapping histologic characteristics. Ideally, the patient's clinical features, immunofluorescence results, and possibly split-skin studies or electron microscopy, in addition to the findings of routine histology, should be considered in order to most reliably establish the diagnosis. In some very early lesions, nonspecific features such as eosinophilic spongiosis may occur. Older lesions may show secondary changes due to trauma or impetiginization, and the actual composition of the dermal inflammatory infiltrate may also vary over time. Technical difficulties may arise with shearing of the blister roof. Biopsies of subepidermal blistering conditions may sometimes show an apparent intraepidermal location caused by re-epithelialization (Chapter 72).

88. E Biopsies obtained by punch or excisional techniques are most likely to provide the most optimal specimens for the diagnosis of blistering diseases. Curettage tends to destroy architectural features, and shave biopsies may not provide adequate visualization of the dermoepidermal junction or the underlying dermal inflammatory infiltrate. Samples that include the entire blister or the edge of the blister with adjacent uninvolved skin are most helpful (Chapter 72).

Bibliography

Anhalt GJ. Pemphigus: Vulgaris, foliaceus, and paraneoplastic. In: Fine JD, ed. Bullous Diseases. New York: Igaku-Shoin, 1993: 52–74.

Briggaman RA, Gammon WR, Woodley DT. Epidermolysis bullosa acquisita. In: Wojnarowska F, Briggaman RA, eds. Management of Blistering Diseases. London: Chapman & Hall Medical, 1990: 127–138.

Charles-Holmes R, Black MM. Herpes gestationis. In: Wojnarowska F, Briggaman RA, eds. Management of Blistering Diseases. London: Chapman & Hall Medical, 1990:93–104.

Crotty C, Pittlekow M, Muller SA. Eosinophilic spongiosis: A clinicopathologic review of seventy-one cases. J Am Acad Dermatol 1983; 8:337–343.

Fine J-D, ed. Bullous Diseases. New York: Igaku-Shoin, 1993:218 pp.

Fine J-D. Cicatricial pemphigoid. In: Wojnarowska F, Briggaman RA, eds. Management of Blistering Diseases. London: Chapman & Hall Medical, 1990:83–92.

Fine J-D. Cicatricial and localized pemphigoid. In: Jordon RE, ed. Immunologic Diseases of the Skin. East Norwalk, CT: Appleton-Century-Crofts, 1991:303–313.

Fine J-D. Pathology and pathogenesis of epidermolysis bullosa. In: Carter DM, Lin AN, eds. Epidermolysis Bullosa, Basic and Clinical Aspects. Springer-Verlag, 1992:37–62.

Fine J-D. Inherited epidermolysis bullosa. In: Fine J-D, ed. Bullous Diseases. New York: Igaku-Shoin, 1993:135–162.

Fine J-D, Briggaman RA, Gammon WR. Laboratory approach to the evaluation of vesiculobullous disorders. In: Fine J-D, ed. Bullous Diseases. New York: Igaku-Shoin, 1993:1–22.

Gammon WR, Briggaman RA, Inman AO III, et al. Differentiating anti–sublamina densa anti-BMZ antibodies by indirect immunofluorescence on 1.0 M sodium chloride–separated skin. Invest Dermatol 1984; 82:139–144.

Gammon WR, Fine J-D, Briggaman RA. Autoimmunity to type VII collagen: Features and role in basement membrane injury. In: Fine J-D, ed. Bullous Diseases. New York: Igaku-Shoin, 1993:75–96.

Horn TD, Anhalt GJ. Histologic features of paraneoplastic pemphigus. Arch Dermatol 1992; 128:1091–1095.

Korman NJ. Bullous pemphigoid. In: Fine J-D, ed. Bullous Diseases. New York: Igaku-Shoin, 1993:25–51.

Liu AY, Valenzuela R, Helm TN, et al. Indirect immunofluorescence on rat bladder transitional epithelium: A test with high specificity for paraneoplastic pemphigus. J Am Acad Dermatol 1993; 28:696–699.

Marsden RA. Linear IgA disease of childhood (chronic bullous disease of childhood). In: Wojnarowska F, Briggaman RA, eds. Management of Blistering Diseases. London: Chapman & Hall Medical, 1990:119–126.

McCord ML, Hall RP. IgA-mediated autoimmune blistering diseases. In: Fine JD, ed. Bullous Diseases. New York: Igaku-Shoin, 1993:97–120.

Morrison LH. Vesiculobullous disorders of pregnancy: Herpes gestationis and pruritic urticarial papules and plaques of pregnancy. In: Fine J-D, ed. Bullous Diseases. New York: Igaku-Shoin, 1993:121–132.

Sontheimer RD, Fine J-D. Biology of the dermoepidermal interface and the pathophysiology of bullous pemphigoid, epidermolysis bullosa acquisita, and lupus erythematosus. In: Soter NA, Baden HP, eds. Pathophysiology of Dermatologic Diseases. New York: McGraw-Hill, 1991:303–325.

Stanley JR. Pemphigus and pemphigoid as paradigms of organ-specific, autoantibody-mediated diseases. J Clin Invest 1989; 83:1443–1448.

Stevens SR, Griffiths GEM, Anhalt GJ, et al. Paraneoplastic pemphigus presenting as a lichen planus pemphigoides–like eruption. Arch Dermatol 1993: 129:866–869.

Wojnarowska F. Linear IgA disease of adults. In: Wojnarowska F, Briggaman RA, eds. Management of Blistering Diseases. London: Chapman & Hall Medical, 1990:105–118.

Wojnarowska F, Briggaman RA, eds. Management of Blistering Diseases. London: Chapman & Hall Medical, 1990: 119–126.

section four

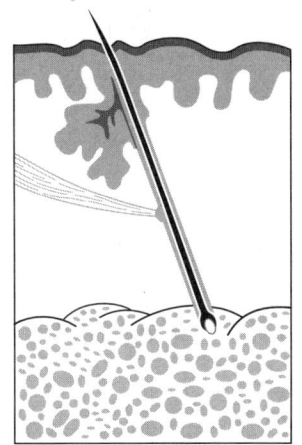

What Diseases Are Caused by Environmental Exposure or Physical Trauma?

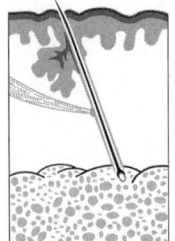

chapter 13

Photodermatoses

N. J. WAINWRIGHT, P. COLLINS, R. DAWE, and J. FERGUSON

Choose the ONE BEST answer to each of the following questions:

1. All of the following statements are true of polymorphic light eruption (PLE) EXCEPT
   A. It is more common in females
   B. Onset is usually within the first three decades
   C. An individual with PLE usually displays lesions of widely varying morphologies
   D. It may occur as an asymptomatic pruritus without a rash
   E. It may be clinically confused with solar urticaria.

2. Findings in PLE include all of the following EXCEPT
   A. A perivascular infiltrate of predominantly CD8-positive T cells within the first 48 hours of provocation
   B. Normal monochromator phototesting in the majority of cases
   C. It tends to clear in the winter months
   D. Some patients present with PLE having an erythema multiforme morphology
   E. A rise in prevalence of the condition on moving further from the equator.

3. All of the following statements are true of actinic prurigo EXCEPT
   A. The rash persists in the winter months
   B. There is a positive association with HLA-A2 and Cw4 antigens in the Native American sufferers
   C. The role of sunlight in the pathogenesis is readily apparent to all sufferers
   D. The distal nose is often affected
   E. Some ethnic groups may display associated conjunctivitis or pterygium formation.

4. A 56-year-old house painter reported itching and swelling of exposed skin and subsequently felt faint. The most helpful diagnostic test would be
   A. A hot bath
   B. Sunbed exposure
   C. Lupus serology
   D. Porphyrin profile
   E. Phototesting.

5. Erythematous facial plaques occur in all EXCEPT
   A. Lupus erythematosus
   B. Lymphocytoma cutis
   C. Jessner's lymphocytic infiltrate
   D. Amiodarone phototoxicity
   E. Polymorphic light eruption.

6. All the following have a vesicular phase EXCEPT
   A. Polymorphic light eruption
   B. Juvenile spring eruption
   C. Rothmund-Thomson syndrome

158

D. Actinic prurigo
   E. Hydroa vacciniforme.

7. A 96-hour phototest response on monochromator phototesting is a hallmark of
   A. Juvenile spring eruption
   B. Homozygous variegate porphyria
   C. Solar urticaria
   D. Hydroa vacciniforme
   E. Xeroderma pigmentosum.

8. Freckling is seen with all of the following EXCEPT
   A. Celtic phenotype
   B. Photochemotherapy
   C. Xeroderma pigmentosum
   D. Actinic reticuloid
   E. NAME syndrome.

9. On clinical examination, shaded sites include all of the following EXCEPT
   A. Retroauricular
   B. Submental
   C. Infranasal
   D. Periorbital
   E. Earlobe.

10. The following are therapeutic options for solar urticaria EXCEPT
    A. Terfenadine
    B. Photochemotherapy
    C. Phototherapy
    D. Thalidomide
    E. Plasmapheresis-plasma exchange.

11. All of the following statements about xeroderma pigmentosum are true EXCEPT
    A. Dry skin is a feature
    B. DNA excision repair is always defective
    C. Neurologic problems may be a feature
    D. Excessive exposed site freckling is a feature
    E. The underlying defect is in repair of DNA damage by environmental mutagens.

12. All the following are indicated in the management of xeroderma pigmentosum EXCEPT
    A. The patient must be advised not to smoke
    B. Routine chest radiographs at regular intervals to exclude early lung cancers
    C. Wearing of ultraviolet radiation (UVR) absorbing or –reflecting sunglasses
    D. Regular follow-up to detect skin cancers
    E. Physical therapies (speech therapy, occupational therapy, physiotherapy) for those with severe neurologic involvement.

For the following questions ONE or MORE of the following completions correctly finishes the incomplete statement.

A. If only 1, 2 and 3 are correct
B. If only 1 and 3 are correct
C. If only 2 and 4 are correct
D. If only 4 is correct
E. If all are correct.

13. In the treatment of polymorphic light eruption,
    1. Appropriate clothing and sunscreens are adequate measures in a minority
    2. An *Escherichia coli* filtrate has been recommended to be of prophylactic benefit
    3. The hardening effect of a course of UV desensitization is prolonged by diligent use of broad-spectrum sunblocks
    4. Psoralen plus ultraviolet A (PUVA) desensitization is likely to be beneficial even if the patient is found to be sensitive to UVA wavelengths on monochromator phototesting.

14. The following should generally be considered in the differential diagnosis of polymorphic light eruption:
    1. Lupus erythematosus
    2. Porphyria cutanea tarda
    3. Hydroa vacciniforme
    4. Xeroderma pigmentosum.

15. Which of the following statements is true of actinic prurigo?
    1. It may be difficult to distinguish from polymorphic light eruption
    2. On average, the age of onset is earlier than for polymorphic light eruption
    3. It is more common in females
    4. It may be complicated by glomerulonephritis.

16. The following are useful features in distinguishing between polymorphic light eruption and actinic prurigo:
    1. The seasonal variation in symptoms
    2. The presence of a lower lip cheilitis

3. The presence of scarring
4. Skin lesions with a vesicular morphology on presentation.

17. Histologic features of hydroa vacciniforme include
    1. Intraepidermal vesiculation
    2. Focal epidermal keratinocyte necrosis and spongiosis
    3. Mononuclear dermal infiltration
    4. Reticulate degeneration.

18. Appropriate therapeutic measures in hydroa vacciniforme include
    1. Reflectant sunscreen
    2. Absorbent sunscreen
    3. Protective clothing
    4. Thalidomide.

19. The following are appropriate investigations for the photosensitive patient:
    1. Lupus serology
    2. Plasma porphyrin fluorescent scan
    3. Provocation testing with ultraviolet (UV) A
    4. Monochromator phototesting.

20. Important questions to ask the patient with a photo-distributed eruption are
    1. Alcohol intake
    2. Presence of atopy
    3. Contact allergy history
    4. Recent drug therapy.

21. Causes of solar urticaria include
    1. Tar and pitch
    2. Erythropoietic protoporphyria
    3. Chlorpromazine
    4. Porphyria cutanea tarda.

22. Helpful therapeutic measures for solar urticaria include
    1. Sunlight avoidance
    2. Protective clothing
    3. Terfenadine
    4. Ranitidine.

23. Effects of UVB phototherapy include
    1. Three- to fivefold thickening of stratum corneum
    2. Increased melanin production
    3. Degradation of leukotriene B_4, a potent chemoattractant
    4. Increased *cis*-urocanic acid.

24. With regard to juvenile spring eruption,
    1. A change of hairstyle may help.
    2. It typically affects the helices of the ears
    3. It is a papulovesicular eruption
    4. The male:female incidence ratio is approximately equal

25. Abnormal photosensitivity can be a feature in
    1. Dermatomyositis
    2. Chloroquine treatment
    3. Antituberculous chemotherapy with isoniazid
    4. Dermatitis herpetiformis.

26. Photoaggravation is recognized in
    1. Lupoid sycosis
    2. Subacute cutaneous lupus erythematosus
    3. Lupus vulgaris
    4. Systemic lupus erythematosus.

Decide whether EACH of the following statements is TRUE or FALSE.

Concerning polymorphic light eruption (PLE),

27. The oral contraceptive pill tends to exacerbate episodes of the condition.
28. Symptoms usually start in the spring season.
29. The lesions of polymorphic light eruption heal with scarring in about 20% of patients.
30. It is provoked by a single irradiation with a solar simulator in the majority of persons.
31. It may be provoked by window glass–transmitted sunlight.
32. It may be precipitated by exposure to light emitted from a photocopier.
33. It may occur in individuals with skin types 3 and 4.
34. It may occur on areas covered by several layers of tightly woven cotton clothing.
35. It is a well-recognized consequence of long-term chlorpromazine therapy.
36. It may be the cause of photosensitive psoriasis.

Concerning actinic prurigo,

37. It is usually associated with contact allergy.
38. At presentation it may be difficult to distinguish from childhood eczema.
39. It tends to improve during early adulthood.
40. It displays pathognomonic histologic changes on biopsy of an established pruriginous lesion.
41. It is associated with an abnormal, delayed erythema action spectrum involving UVA wavelengths only.

Concerning the clinical features of hydroa vacciniforme,

42. It typically affects exposed and covered sites.
43. The reaction is maximal during sunshine months.
44. It never appears in winter.
45. A burning, stinging sensation is felt.
46. A reaction occurs within a few minutes of sunlight exposure.

In hydroa vacciniforme,

47. The reaction to sunlight gradually lessens and may cease.
48. Action spectrum studies are frequently normal.
49. Abnormal photosensitivity to UVA wavelengths is most frequently implicated.
50. Provocation testing with repeated UVA doses is a useful diagnostic test.
51. Histology is difficult to distinguish from other photodermatoses.

Idiopathic solar urticaria

52. Occurs more often in females.
53. Affects 0.1% of the population.
54. May occur with lymphocytoma cutis or PLE.
55. Is associated with atopy in a minority.
56. Typically affects teenagers.

In patients with solar urticaria,

57. Phototesting may be normal.
58. Phototesting most often reveals abnormal delayed erythemal response to UVA and visible wavebands.
59. The majority demonstrate improvement in phototest responses following treatment with H_1-receptor–blockers.
60. Sedating antihistamines are more effective than nonsedating types.
61. Resolves spontaneously as patients get older.

Patients with solar urticaria should

62. Try to desensitize themselves with natural sunlight.
63. Use a sunbed during winter months.
64. Have their porphyrin profile checked.
65. Have patch testing.
66. Consider purchasing protective film for car and house window glass.

Decide whether EACH of the following statements is TRUE or FALSE.

67. The following have been or are used in the therapy for polymorphic light eruption:
    A. Azathioprine
    B. Chloroquine
    C. UVB phototherapy
    D. Colchicine
    E. beta-Carotene.

68. The following circumstances would cast doubt on a diagnosis of polymorphic light eruption:
    A. Sparing of some maximally exposed sunlight areas
    B. Extensive covered site involvement
    C. Positive anti-Ro and/or anti-La antibodies
    D. Elliptical or linear scarring over the nose, cheeks, and forehead
    E. The absence of a positive family history.

69. The following are valuable in the therapy for actinic prurigo:
    A. 8-Methoxypsoralen (8-MOP) photochemotherapy
    B. UVB phototherapy

C. Reflectant sunscreens

D. Oral trioxsalen in the sunshine season

E. Oral indomethacin during exacerbations of the condition.

70. Regarding actinic prurigo,
    A. It is particularly common amongst Native Americans in North America but rarely seen among those in South America
    B. Covered site involvement is present in up to 50% of patients
    C. A positive family history is elicited more often than in polymorphic light eruption
    D. Hardened sites such as the face are usually spared by the rash
    E. Monochromator phototesting is required to distinguish it from polymorphic light eruption in some cases.

71. Regarding hydroa vacciniforme,
    A. It is more common in females
    B. It typically occurs in Amerindians
    C. It invariably begins in childhood
    D. It is frequently associated with atopy
    E. A familial tendency is present in many patients.

72. Features seen in hydroa vacciniforme include
    A. Photo-onycholysis
    B. Involvement of the eyes
    C. Papules on a background of edematous erythema
    D. Umbilicated vesicles that persist from days to weeks
    E. Characteristic varioliform scars.

73. The differential diagnosis of hydroa vacciniforme includes
    A. Juvenile spring eruption
    B. Hydroa estivale
    C. Rothmund-Thomson syndrome
    D. Erythropoietic protoporphyria
    E. Congenital erythropoietic porphyria.

74. Signs and symptoms of idiopathic solar urticaria include
    A. Pruritus
    B. Erythema, wheal and flare
    C. Wheals may appear only in fixed areas on exposed sites
    D. Resolution within an hour
    E. Marked cut-off at clothing-protected sites.

75. Regarding solar urticaria,
    A. Phototherapy or photochemotherapy may have to be done by exposing selected body areas
    B. Intradermal injection of photo-irradiated serum or plasma may help define patients responsive to plasma exchange
    C. Anaphylaxis may occur during plasmapheresis
    D. Response to plasma exchange is variable and thus should be restricted to severe, recalcitrant cases
    E. Repeat phototesting on antihistamines is useful to define improved tolerance to sunlight.

76. A 30-year-old woman who spent her childhood in Zambia but now lives in Scotland presents with a 3-year history of direct and window glass transmitted light having produced a rash of indurated erythematous plaques on photo-exposed sites except her face.
    A. She has solar urticaria
    B. Investigation should include sending blood to check antinuclear antibody (ANA)
    C. If the rash occurs in winter, this excludes polymorphic light eruption
    D. Phototesting may help in establishing the diagnosis
    E. Phototesting is likely to reveal abnormal photosensitivity.

77. A course of PUVA may be useful in the management of
    A. Idiopathic solar urticaria
    B. A patient with Cockayne's syndrome

C. Polymorphic light eruption
D. Photoaggravated psoriasis
E. Chronic discoid lupus erythematosus.

78. The following are clinical features of pellagra:
    A. Hallucinations
    B. Vaginitis
    C. Stomatitis
    D. Exposed-site dermatitis
    E. Weight loss.

79. Which of the following are true regarding xeroderma pigmentosum?
    A. Inheritance is autosomal dominant
    B. The same defect in DNA repair synthesis underlies all cases
    C. It is commoner in Japan than in the United States
    D. Abnormal photosensitivity may be a feature
    E. Internal neoplasms are a feature.

80. Decide whether each of the following statements concerning the patient with suspected photosensitivity is TRUE or FALSE.
    A. Histology is usually helpful
    B. Periorbital involvement points to genuine photosensitivity
    C. If covered sites are involved, an ultraviolet radiation–induced problem is excluded
    D. Monochromator phototesting is essential in all cases
    E. Facial sparing may be a feature in the patient with abnormal photosensitivity.

For the following questions the set of lettered headings accompanies a list of numbered words or phrases. For each numbered word or phrase, choose

A. If the item is associated with A only
B. If the item is associated with B only
C. If the item is associated with both A and B
D. If the item is associated with neither A nor B.

81. For each of the following characteristics, choose whether it describes polymorphic light eruption, lymphocytoma cutis, both, or neither.

    i. May appear as erythematous, papular lesions with a translucent component
    ii. May be exacerbated by sunlight
    iii. The predominant cells in the dermal infiltrate are B lymphocytes
    iv. Is commoner in males
    v. Is associated with malignant change.

    A. Polymorphic light eruption
    B. Lymphocytoma cutis
    C. Both
    D. Neither.

82. For each of the following statements, choose whether it describes polymorphic light eruption, porphyria cutanea tarda, both, or neither.

    i. May be precipitated by PUVA photochemotherapy
    ii. Commonly manifests as large blister formation on the hands
    iii. Is associated with an increased urinary excretion of the type 3 isomer of uroporphyrin
    iv. May manifest as hemorrhagic forms
    v. May be associated with pseudosclerodermatous changes in the skin.

    A. Polymorphic light eruption
    B. Porphyria cutanea tarda
    C. Both
    D. Neither.

83. For each of the following conditions, choose whether appropriate treatment includes beta-carotene, hydroxychloroquine, both, or neither.

    i. Polymorphic light eruption
    ii. Erythropoietic protoporphyria
    iii. Solar urticaria
    iv. Hydroa vacciniforme

    A. beta-Carotene
    B. Hydroxychloroquine
    C. Both
    D. Neither.

v. Frusemide photosensitivity.

84. For each of the following conditions, choose whether appropriate treatment includes UVB phototherapy, photochemotherapy, both, or neither.

i. Xeroderma pigmentosum variant
ii. Polymorphic light eruption
iii. Idiopathic solar urticaria
iv. Actinic prurigo
v. Pellagra.

A. UVB phototherapy
B. Photochemotherapy
C. Both
D. Neither.

85. Do the following statements about sunscreens apply to dibenzoylmethanes, benzophenones, both, or neither?

i. Offer significant protection against UVB wavelengths
ii. Offer significant protection against UVA wavelengths
iii. Offer significant protection against visible wavelengths
iv. Are associated with contact allergic dermatitis
v. Are associated with contact photoallergic dermatitis.

A. Dibenzoylmethanes
B. Benzophenones
C. Both
D. Neither.

86. For each of the following characteristics, choose whether it describes Bloom's syndrome, Rothmund-Thomson syndrome, both, or neither.

i. More common in females than males
ii. Cell mutation studies are abnormal
iii. Cutaneous squamous cell carcinomas not uncommonly occur during the second decade of life

A. Bloom's syndrome
B. Rothmund-Thomson syndrome
C. Both
D. Neither.

iv. Abnormal photosensitivity is not a feature
v. Poikiloderma is a *characteristic* feature.

87. For each of the following conditions, decide whether UVB desensitization, topical corticosteroids, both, or neither, may be useful treatment modalities.

i. Polymorphic light eruption
ii. Prurigo nodularis
iii. Idiopathic solar urticaria
iv. Actinic prurigo (hydroa estivale)
v. Hydroa vacciniforme.

A. UVB desensitization
B. Topical corticosteroids
C. Both
D. Neither.

For each numbered item, choose the most likely associated lettered item.

88. Actinic prurigo
89. Porphyria cutanea tarda
90. Pellagra
91. Nodular prurigo
92. Photosensitivity dermatitis/ actinic reticuloid syndrome (chronic actinic dermatitis).

A. Thalidomide
B. Chloroquine
C. Nicotinamide
D. All of the above
E. None of the above.

For each of the following, choose the single matching condition with which it has been described.

93. Hemolytic anemia
94. Erythropoietic protoporphyria
95. Atopy
96. Pseudoporphyria
97. Phytophotodermatitis.

A. Contact with giant hogweed
B. Congenital erythropoietic porphyria
C. Actinic prurigo
D. Solar urticaria
E. Naproxen.

ANSWERS

1. C Although a wide range of morphologies is seen in polymorphic light eruption, the eruption in an individual patient tends to be monomorphic. Rapid onset polymorphic light eruption (PLE) may be confused clinically with solar urticaria, and phototesting is required to confirm the diagnosis. Sunlight-induced asymptomatic pruritus without clinical signs is known as PLE sine eruptione (Chapter 86).

2. A Immunohistochemistry studies have shown an excess of CD4 T lymphocytes in PLE lesions up to 72 hours after irradiation with an excess of CD8 T cells thereafter (Chapter 86).

3. C The perennial nature of actinic prurigo means that some patients do not appreciate the central role of sunlight exposure in their condition. A positive association has been reported with HLA-A2 and Cw4 together with a negative association with the A3 antigen. Recent work has suggested that HLA-DR4 is a risk factor for actinic prurigo in British subjects. Late-onset actinic prurigo is associated with 30% to 40% of cases reported from Saskatchewan, Manitoba, and Mexico City, such that it is regarded as a particularly reliable sign of the disease, especially if seen in conjunction with distal nose involvement. These ethnic groups are also more likely to display conjunctivitis or pterygia formation (Chapter 86).

4. E The time course of the reaction will help define the diagnosis. This individual had idiopathic solar urticaria with obvious whealing at phototest sites to UVA and visible waveband on monochromator phototesting. Heat urticaria may be ruled out by provocation tests; see Question 76 (Chapter 86).

5. D Amiodarone phototoxicity induces a bronze pigmentation or slate-gray appearance; see Question 80 (Chapter 86).

6. C Rothmund-Thomson is a rare, autosomal recessive oculocutaneous syndrome affecting children, and 50% have abnormal photosensitivity. All have poikiloderma (telangiectasia, atrophy, and hypo- or hyperpigmentation) affecting face, upper limbs, and buttocks to a variable degree. Other common features include onset in infancy (93%), short stature (62%), absence or sparseness of hair (60%), family history (51%), and juvenile cataract (47%); see Question 14 (Chapter 175).

7. E Delayed maximal and persisting responses are characteristic of xeroderma pigmentosum. The phototest responses are maximal in the immediate phase, solar urticaria at 7 hours with the porphyrias, and at 24 hours with other photodermatoses listed (Chapter 168).

8. D Actinic reticuloid affects elderly males and is so named because it is induced by sunlight exposure, and the histology has some features of cutaneous lymphoma. Freckling is a common response in blue-eyed, fair-skinned subjects (skin type 1). PUVA "freckles" are lentigines associated with high, cumulative UVA doses and are best observed on the anterior thighs. NAME is the acronym given to a rare condition with nevi, bilateral atrial myomas, myxoid neurofibromata, and ephelides (freckles); see Questions 11 and 12 (Chapter 87).

9. E Clinical examination may help distinguish abnormal photosensitivity and airborne contact allergic dermatitis (no sparing of shaded sites); see question 80 (Chapters 86 and 87).

10. D Thalidomide may be used for patients with actinic prurigo; see Question 88. Terfenadine, an H_1 receptor antagonist is effective in controlling solar urticaria as adjunctive therapy to protective clothing and reflectant sunscreens. It is helpful to define the wavelengths that precipitate urticaria, because one can choose a suitable irradiation source—UVB or psoralen plus UVA—to desensitize the patients. Recalcitrant cases may be treated by plasmapheresis or plasma exchange, although the response is variable (Chapter 86).

11. B Xeroderma pigmentosum is a rare, inherited disease. DNA repair of UVR-induced damage is defective. It is thought that it is defective repair of DNA damage caused by ingested and other environmental mutagens that accounts for the occurrence of neurologic abnormalities in about 30% of cases. There is genetic heterogeneity among the DNA repair defects that are responsible for xeroderma pigmentosum (XP). Classic XP, in which the defect is in DNA excision repair, can be divided into several "complementation groups," which may also exhibit differing clinical features. In about 20% of XP patients, excision repair is normal and the defect is in another DNA repair process (postreplication repair); these cases are classed as XP variant.

The clinical presentation and course may vary from case to case, but characteristic features are dry skin (xeroderma) and abnormalities of pigmentation with excessive freckling and persistent hyperpigmented macules. Development of skin cancers from an early age is common (Chapter 168).

12. B In xeroderma pigmentosum, DNA repair after damage by environmental carcinogens, including tobacco smoke as well as UVR, is impaired. However, the greater risk of internal malignancy such as bronchogenic carcinoma does not justify deliberate exposure to x-rays. In fact, most patients with XP do not seem to be abnormally sensitive to therapeutic x-rays, but cultured cells from a few patients have been shown to be hypersensitive to x-rays, and it is wisest to reserve x-rays for times when there is a clear clinical indication (Chapter 168).

13. C Simple behavioral measures, clothing, and broad-spectrum sunscreen use are adequate for the majority of patients with PLE. *E. coli* filtrates have been recommended to be of prophylactic benefit, but controlled studies are required to support this claim. The hardening effect of UVB sensitization of course requires continued sun exposure if its benefit is to be prolonged after therapy. PUVA desensitization for PLE is often beneficial and is given on an incrementally increasing regimen based on the minimal phototoxic dose, which is established at the start of treatment. Narrowband UVB at 312 nm has also proved effective in desensitization (Chapters 85 and 86).

14. B The cutaneous lesions of lupus erythematosus may be clinically and histologically similar to chronic plaque-type PLE. Sunlight-provoked subacute cutaneous LE is associated with raised titers of anti-Ro or anti-La antibodies, a fact that is helpful in distinguishing it from PLE. Hydroa vacciniforme may be similar to PLE at an early stage, although the early age of onset and the development of characteristic vacciniforme scarring helps to distinguish the conditions (Chapters 24 and 86).

15. E Actinic prurigo usually arises in the first decade, whereas the onset of PLE occurs over the first three decades. Secondary infection of prurigo lesions with nephritogenic strains of *Streptococci* has been associated with epidemics of streptococcal glomerulonephritis (Chapter 86).

16. A Polymorphic light eruption tends to resolve in the winter months and is not associated with a lower lip cheilitis or the development of scarring, as with actinic prurigo, which is perennial in nature. Both may manifest with a vesicular eruption (Chapter 86).

17. E; **18.** A Reflectant sunscreens include titanium dioxide and zinc oxide. Absorbent sunscreens include para-aminobenzoic acid (PABA), PABA esters, cinnamaldehydes, benzophenones, and dibenzoylmethanes. Reflectant sunscreens are cosmetically less popular but provide better protection against longer UVA and visible wavelengths and result in much less contact and photocontact sensitization and contact urticaria (Chapter 85).

19. E; **20.** E Porphyria cutanea tarda is precipitated by alcohol. A personal history of atopy may be a feature in patients with actinic prurigo (40%) and polymorphic light eruption (20%). A history of contact allergy predates photosensitivity dermatitis/actinic reticuloid (PD/AR) syndrome in 40% of patients. Many drugs cause phototoxicity, and some photoallergy and abnormal photosensitivity may persist for several months after discontinuing the drug. Examples include quinine, thiazide diuretics, nonsteroidal anti-inflammatory drugs, quinolones, sulphonamides, tetracyclines, chlorpromazine and amiodarone (Chapter 169).

21. A; **22.** E The benefit of different H_1 receptor antagonists (e.g., terfenadine, cetirizine, optimine, astemizole) may be defined by repeating monochromator phototesting on the drug. Adding an H_2 receptor antagonist such as cimetidine or ranitidine increases the minimal urticarial dose in some patients (Chapter 86).

23. E Thickening of the stratum corneum and acanthosis of the epidermis is clinically demonstrated both by the fact that vitiligo patients develop high minimal erythema dose on the palms and soles and by the development of tolerance after increasing exposure to UVB phototherapy. Melanin is also induced and effectively absorbs UVB, ultraviolet (UV) A, and shorter visible wavebands. It is difficult to define accurately the relationship of other factors to photoprotection, but some include an effect on prostaglandin synthesis, a decrease in antigen-presenting cells, photodegradation of chemoattractants, and increased *cis*-urocanic acid. In mice these responses include suppression of contact and delayed hypersensitivity, rejection of transplant tumors, and skin allografts (Chapter 83).

24. A; **25.** B Photosensitivity is not characteristic of dermatomyositis but has been described as a feature in some patients. Isoniazid binds to some members of the vitamin B_6 group and causes loss of pyridoxine in the urine. Pyridoxine is an important cofactor in tryptophan metabolism, and so isoniazid-induced pyridoxine deficiency can cause a photosensitivity similar to that in pellagra. Chloroquine may suppress abnormal photosensitivity in some of the photodermatoses, although not through a sunscreening action. Neither chloroquine nor dermatitis herpetiformis are described as causing abnormal photosensitivity.

26. C Photoaggravation has long been recognized as a problem in chronic discoid lupus erythematosus, subacute lupus erythematosus, and the cutaneous manifestations of systemic lupus erythematosus.

Cutaneous tuberculosis of the lupus vulgaris type is not known to be exacerbated by UV or visible light irradiation, and indeed Niels Finsen was awarded the Nobel Prize for Medicine in 1903 in recognition of his work on the treatment of this condition with artificial light produced by the carbon arc lamp. Lupoid sycosis is, as the name suggests, a scarring pyogenic infection of hair follicles and is not adversely influenced by light (Chapter 24).

27. (F); **28.** (T); **29.** (F); **30.** (F); **31.** (T) Polymorphic light eruption is rarely induced by standard single-dose monochromator or solar simulator phototesting, but repeated provocation testing on larger areas of skin with artificial UVA and UVB sources can induce the rash in up to 60% of cases. Window glass–transmitted sunlight contains UVA and visible wavelengths and is therefore capable of inducing polymorphic light eruption (PLE). The eruption heals without scarring. The oral contraceptive pill does not significantly influence PLE (Chapter 86).

32. (T); **33.** (T); **34.** (F); **35.** (F); **36.** (T) PLE may occur in people with high skin types and tends not to involve covered sites unless the clothing is light and open weave. UV radiation from sunbeds, photocopiers, and electric arc welding equipment can precipitate the condition. Chlorpromazine is well known as a cause of photosensitivity and subsequent pigmentation of the skin but is not a recognized cause of PLE. Photosensitive psoriasis may arise as a result of koebnerization of PLE in a psoriatic patient (Chapter 86).

37. (F); **38.** (T); **39.** (T); **40.** (F); **41.** (F) Contact allergy is a feature of PD/AR syndrome but not of actinic prurigo. An eczematous type of actinic prurigo is seen in some younger patients and often improves within the first decade; the more persistent plaque form predominates in older patients, but it too often improves in early adulthood. The histologic changes are nonspecific, and phototesting has revealed broad-spectrum abnormalities in both the UVA and UVB wavebands (Chapter 87).

42. (F); **43.** (T); **44.** (F); **45.** (T); **46.** (F); **47.** (T); **48.** (T); **49.** (T); **50.** (T); **51.** (F) The majority of hydroa vacciniforme cases resolve in late teenage years. Monochromator phototesting is normal in 60% of the authors' patients and is best demonstrated by repeat provocation testing with UVA for several days. The histology is distinctive unlike that of other photodermatoses, such as PLE and actinic prurigo, which may share similar histologic features (Chapter 86).

52. (T); **53.** (F); **54.** (T); **55.** (T); **56.** (F) The female to male ratio is 2:1; the majority are young adults. The precise prevalence is not recorded; however, it is a rare condition. Atopy is less frequent compared with other forms of urticaria (Chapter 86).

57. (F); **58.** (F); **59.** (T); **60.** (F); **61.** (F) In solar urticaria, abnormal phototesting is most frequently for UVA and visible wavebands but the responses are immediate, not delayed. Non-sedating antihistamine types (i.e., terfenadine) are frequently used. A comparative study has not been done (see Question 22) (Chapter 86).

62. (T); **63.** (F); **64.** (T); **65.** (F); **66.** (T) Natural sunlight desensitization may be effective for patients with mild abnormal photosensitivity. If urticaria develops on a large area of the body, patients may feel nauseated, become pale and hypotensive, and collapse. Solar urticaria may occur with erythropoietic protoporphyria. They have immediate, not delayed, hypersensitivity. Clear photoprotective film may protect from 290 to 400 nm and may be used on car window glass. Colored photoprotective film (290 to 460 nm) may be used on house window glass but is illegal on car windows because it restricts vision (Chapter 86).

67. A (T); B (T); C (T); D (F); E (T) Azathioprine can be useful in some patients with severe PLE, whereas chloroquine and beta-carotene have been tried although with dubious benefit. The antimalarials are associated with potential ocular toxicity; beta-carotene causes yellow discoloration of the skin known as carotenoderma; and azathioprine has significant immunosuppressive actions. UVB phototherapy, both broad- and narrow-band, as well as photochemotherapy are all valuable in the desensitization of PLE (Chapter 86).

68. A (F); B (T); C (T); D (T); E (F) The rash of PLE often spares perennially exposed sites such as the hands and face and appears on those sites revealed by summer apparel, such as the neck, forearms, and legs. This suggests that the perennially exposed sites have developed a degree of self-protection and thus are described as being ''hardened.'' A significant covered site involvement and a positive family history are uncommon in PLE but more common in actinic prurigo. The presence of anti-Ro and anti-La antibodies is suggestive of subacute cutaneous lupus erythematosus, whereas elliptical and linear scarring of exposed areas of the face is suggestive of erythropoietic protoporphyria (Chapter 86).

69. A (T); B (T); C (T); D (T); E (F) Oral trioxsalen in conjunction with natural sunlight has been used in the treatment of some Native American patients. Desensitization with UVB or PUVA can be helpful (Chapter 86).

70. A (F); B (T); C (T); D (F); E (F) Actinic prurigo is also commonly seen in South America, particularly Colombia, and Central America. The sparing of hardened sites such as the face and the back of the hands as seen in PLE is not a feature of actinic prurigo. PLE and actinic prurigo are usually diagnosed on clinical grounds and are not clearly distinguished by monochromator phototesting. Farr and Diffey have reported augmentation of UVA- and UVB-induced erythema by the topical application of indomethacin in actinic prurigo patients in contrast to the inhibition of UVB erythema in normal skin. Further validation of these findings is required, however (Chapter 86).

71. A (T); B (F); C (T); D (F); E (F)

72. A (T); B (T); C (T); D (T); E (T) Photo-onycholysis and eye involvement suggests the involvement of longer UVA wavelengths.

73. A (F); B (T); C (F); D (T); E (F) Hydroa estivale represents the vesicular form of actinic prurigo (Chapter 86).

74. A (T); B (T); C (T); D (T); E (T)

75. A (T); B (T); C (T); D (T); E (T) Many patients have abnormal photosensitivity to UVA wavebands, and so urticaria may be provoked using broad-band UVB (270 to 350 nm) or UVA (320 to 400 nm) sources. A new source, narrow-band UVB, offers an advantage because of its relatively monochromatic emission spectrum (312 ± 2 nm). It has been suggested that patients who develop a wheal and flare response to 0.1 ml intradermal serum (irradiated with causal wavelengths) may respond to plasma exchange therapy as compared with those who do *not* respond to the intradermal serum. Plasmapheresis has only been reported in six patients, and two developed anaphylaxis, possibly related to fluorescent lighting, during treatment (Chapters 83 and 86).

76. A (F); B (T); C (F); D (T); E (F) The differential diagnosis is mainly between PLE and idiopathic solar urticaria. Questioning should be directed toward discovering how long after sun exposure the rash starts and how long it persists if the patient then avoids further exposure. PLE, as the more common condition, is the more likely diagnosis; however, if the eruption is described as starting within a half-hour of sun exposure and clearing after only two hours this would point to solar urticaria as the diagnosis. PLE typically starts within several hours or days of exposure and persists for 1 to 2 weeks. It is usually confined to spring and summer but in severe cases can be perennial. Sparing of normally exposed sites, probably due to natural desensitization, may be a feature of both solar urticaria and PLE.

It is usually possible to make a diagnosis of PLE or solar urticaria on the history, but it is important to exclude an underlying photosensitivity due to lupus erythematosus (especially if PUVA or UVB desensitization is being considered), and so a blood sample should be analyzed to check for lupus. Phototesting is also a helpful investigation, although it is not always necessary. It can be valuable in differentiating between PLE and solar urticaria when the history is not clear and can also identify those cases in which these two conditions coexist (Chapter 86).

77. A (T); B (F); C (T); D (T); E (F) PUVA or UVB desensitization may be useful in the management of PLE and also in solar urticaria. In photoaggravated psoriasis, careful use of PUVA or UVB remains a valuable treatment (see also Answer 36). Phototherapy is contraindicated in lupus erythematosus and in the genophotodermatoses, including Cockayne's syndrome (Chapter 86).

78. A (T); B (T); C (T); D (T); E (T) Pellagra is a chronic wasting disease characterized by the "three Ds"—Dermatitis, Dementia, and Diarrhea. The dermatitis is symmetrical, bilateral, affects exposed sites, and is due to photosensitivity. The diarrhea is due to inflammation of gut mucosa, but there is widespread inflammation of mucosal surfaces including mucosa of vagina and mouth as well as of gut.

79. A (F); B (F); C (T); D (T); E (T) Xeroderma pigmentosus (XP) is usually inherited as autosomal recessive. In *classic* XP, which is divided into complementation groups A to G, the defect is in excision repair, whereas in *variant* XP the defect is in postreplication repair. Individuals usually have exaggerated and prolonged photosensitivity. Internal malignancy has been reported in XP, and incidence may be 10 to 20 times that in the population as a whole. This is probably related to the fact that DNA repair is defective throughout the body, and it is not only repair after UVR-induced damage that is affected (Chapter 168).

80. A (F); B (F); C (F); D (F); E (T) When a patient is referred with a possible photosensitivity disorder, the first thing to do is to take an appropriate history, which in most cases leads to the correct diagnosis. Physical examination is also helpful, especially in deciding whether or not an exposed site eruption is due to sunlight or to something else (such as an airborne contact allergen). Involvement of relatively shaded sites, including periorbital areas, is more suggestive of contact sensitivity than photosensitivity. However, covered site involvement does not exclude photosensitivity, and it should be borne in mind that UVA irradiation is transmitted through thin clothing. In some conditions, notably PLE, sparing of habitually exposed sites is not uncommon and is thought to result from a natural process akin to the artificially induced desensitization that plays a role in the treatment of some of these disorders.

Tests, including monochromator phototesting and histopathology, can be extremely important in the assessment of a patient presenting with a possible photodermatosis, but usually the likely diagnosis is determined on the basis of a comprehensive history and examination, and without these further investigation is futile (Chapter 86).

81. i C; ii C; iii B; iv D; v D Both PLE and lymphocytoma cutis may have an erythematous, translucent papular appearance, but the latter has a more chronic duration and can be distinguished by B-lymphocyte marker studies. Both conditions are benign and are commoner in females (Chapter 86).

82. i C; ii B; iii B; iv C; v B Repeated trauma and constant sun exposure may lead to pseudoscleroderma-tous change in porphyria cutanea tarda (PCT). PLE is not associated with any porphyrin abnormalities but, like PCT, can manifest in a hemorrhagic form (Chapter 169).

83. i D; ii A; iii D; iv A; v D **84.** i D; ii C; iii C; iv C; v D **85.** i B; ii C; iii D; iv C; v C Benzophenones protect up to 320 to 340 nm, dibenzoylmethanes for longer UVA wavelength. Reflectant sunscreens offer better screening but are less cosmetically acceptable (e.g., titanium dioxide). Although PABA has been associated with contact and photocontact sensitivity, alternative absorbants such as these are proving equally capable of sensitizing patients (Chapter 85).

86. i B; ii A; iii C; iv D; v B (Although poikiloderma *may* occur in Bloom's syndrome.).

87. i C; See Answer No. 13. ii B; Topical steroids are helpful in nodular prurigo, as is UVB phototherapy, but not as a desensitization course. iii A; Desensitization can help in solar urticaria, at least partially through induction of increased pigmentation and epidermal thickening resulting in reduced transmission of UVR. Antihistamines have a proven place in the management of solar urticaria, whereas topical steroids are unlikely to help much. iv C; v A; Treatment of hydroa vacciniforme involves advice about the condition, sunlight avoidance, sunscreen use, and when necessary, desensitization phototherapy (Chapter 86).

88. D; **89.** B; **90.** C; **91.** A; **92.** E Actinic prurigo has been treated successfully with thalidomide, but with the significant risks of peripheral neuropathy, teratogenicity, and nodular prurigo. Low-dose chloroquine increases the renal excretion of uroporphyrin, and nicotinamide was used in the treatment of pellagra; both agents have also been used with limited success in actinic prurigo. None of the agents are used in the treatment of photosensitivity dermatitis/actinic reticuloid syndrome in which management is largely dependent on avoidance of sunlight and relevant contact factors and suppression of the condition with topical steroids (Chapter 169).

93. B; **94.** D; **95.** C; **96.** E; **97.** A

Bibliography

Addo HA, Frain-Bell W. Actinic prurigo: A specific photodermatosis? Photodermatology 1984; 1:110–128.

Bickers DR, Demar LK, DeLeo V. Hydroa vacciniforme. Arch Dermatol 1978; 114:1193–1197.

Birt AR, Davis RA. Hereditary polymorphic light eruption of American Indians. Int J Dermatol 1975; 14:105–111.

Corbett MF, Hawk JLM, Hexheimer A, Magnus IA. Controlled therapeutic trials in polymorphic light eruption. Br J Dermatol 1982; 107:571–581.

Duschet P, Leyen P, Schwarz T, et al. Solar urticaria—effective treatment by plasmapheresis. Clin Exp Dermatol 1987; 12:185–188.

Farr PM, Diffey BL. Treatment of actinic prurigo with PUVA: Mechanism of action. Br J Dermatol 1989; 120:411–418.

Ferguson J. Idiopathic solar urticaria: Natural history and response to nonsedative antihistamine therapy. A study of 26 cases. Br J Dermatol 1988; 119(Suppl. 33): 16.

Fusaro RM, Johnson JA. Hereditary polymorphic light eruption in American Indians—photoprotection and prevention of streptococcal pyoderma and glomerulonephritis. JAMA 1980; 244:1456–1459.

Holzle E, Plewig G, Lehmann P. Photodermatoses—diagnostic procedures and their interpretation. Photodermatology 1987 4:109–114.

Lane PR, Hogan DJ, Martel MJ, et al. Actinic prurigo: Clinical features and prognosis. J Am Acad Dermatol 1992; 26:683–692.

Lovell CR, Hawk JLM, Kalman CD, et al. Thalidomide in actinic prurigo. Br J Dermatol 1983; 108:467–471.

Mathews-Roth MM. β-carotene therapy for erythropoietic protoporphyria and other photosensitivity diseases. Biochimie 1986; 68:875–884.

Morison WL, Momtaz K, Mosher DB, Parrish JA. UVB phototherapy in the prophylaxis of polymorphic light eruption. Br J Dermatol 1982; 106:231–233.

Murphy GM, Logan RA, Lavelle CR, et al. Prophylactic PUVA and UVB therapy in polymorphic light eruption—a controlled trial. Br J Dermatol 1987; 116:531–538.

Orr PH, Birt AR. Hereditary polymorphic light eruption in Canadian Inuit. Int J Dermatol 1984; 23:472–475.

Przybilla B, Heppeler M, Ruzicka T. Preventative effect of an *Escherichia coli*–filtrate (Colibiogen) in polymorphous light eruption. Br J Dermatol 1989; 121:229–233.

Ros A-M, Wennersten G. Photosensitive psoriasis—clinical findings and phototest results. Photodermatology 1986; 3:317–326.

Sonnex TS, Hawk JLM. Hydroa vacciniforme: A review of ten cases. Br J Dermatol 1988; 118:101–108.

Vennos EM, Collins M, James WD. Rothmund-Thomson syndrome: Review of the world literature. J Am Acad Dermatol 1992; 27:750–762.

section five

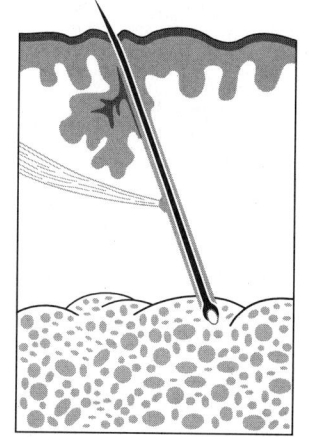

What Infections and Infestations Affect the Skin?

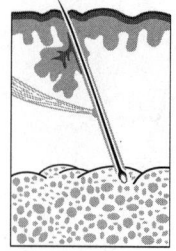

chapter 14

Bacterial and Rickettsial Infections

JAN V. HIRSCHMANN

For each numbered item in the following choose the most likely associated lettered item. Each numbered item has ONLY ONE answer. Within each group, each lettered item may be the answer to one, more than one, or none of the numbered items.

For each of the cutaneous infections listed, choose the responsible organism(s):

1. Nonbullous impetigo
2. Bullous impetigo
3. Blistering distal dactylitis
4. Ecthyma
5. Ecthyma gangrenosum
6. Erysipelas
7. Erysipeloid
8. Hot-tub folliculitis
9. Carbuncles
10. Scarlet fever.

A. *Staphylococcus aureus* only
B. *Streptococcus pyogenes* (group A streptococcus) only
C. Either *Staph. aureus* or *Strep. pyogenes*
D. *Pseudomonas aeruginosa*
E. *Erysipelothrix rhusiopathiae*.

For each of the sexually transmitted diseases, choose the responsible pathogen:

11. Lymphogranuloma venereum
12. Chancroid
13. Granuloma inguinale
14. Nongonococcal urethritis
15. Syphilis.

A. *Treponema pallidum*
B. *Calymmatobacterium granulomatis*
C. *Chlamydia trachomatis*
D. *Haemophilus ducreyi*
E. *Trichomonas vaginalis*.

Indicate the mode of spread of the following organisms to humans:

16. *Borrelia burgdorferi*
17. *Afipia felis*
18. *Rickettsia rickettsii*
19. *Vibrio vulnificus*
20. *Rickettsia akari*
21. *Ehrlichia canis*
22. *Rickettsia typhi*.

A. Tick
B. Mite
C. Flea
D. Water
E. Cat.

For the following questions, decide whether EACH statement is TRUE or FALSE.

23. Pitted keratolysis is caused by streptococci.
24. Trichomycosis axillaris is caused by gram-positive bacilli.
25. Although caused by corynebacteria, erythrasma responds to topical azoles such as miconazole or clotrimazole.
26. Axillary odor is related to the presence of coryneform bacteria.
27. Most cutaneous abscesses are caused by *Staphylococcus aureus*.
28. A risk of cutaneous infections caused by *Streptococcus pyogenes* (group A streptococcus) is acute rheumatic fever.
29. Early treatment of skin infections due to *Streptococcus pyogenes* clearly reduces the risk of acute post-streptococcal glomerulonephritis.
30. Needle aspiration of the leading edge of cellulitis usually yields a pathogen on culture.

31. The most common cause of cellulitis is probably *Staphylococcus aureus*.

32. In staphylococcal scalded skin syndrome, the skin separation is at the dermoepidermal junction.

33. Topical mupirocin (Bactroban) is as effective as oral erythromycin for treating most cases of non-bullous impetigo.

34. Unlike impetigo, ecthyma commonly heals with scarring.

35. *Streptococcus pyogenes* (group A streptococcus) is part of the normal cutaneous flora in about 20% of the general population.

36. One tablet (150 mg) of oral clindamycin per day markedly reduces the frequency of attacks in patients with recurrent staphylococcal skin infections.

37. The coral red appearance of erythrasma under Wood's light illumination is due to the production of porphyrins by the responsible corynebacteria.

For the following questions, choose the ONE BEST answer to each question.

38. The therapy of choice for *Nocardia asteroides* infections is
    A. Ciprofloxacin
    B. Streptomycin
    C. Penicillin
    D. Sulfamethoxazole-trimethoprim
    E. Cephalexin.

39. The therapy of choice for Rocky Mountain spotted fever is
    A. A third-generation cephalosporin
    B. Ampicillin
    C. Gentamicin
    D. Ciprofloxacin
    E. Tetracycline or doxycycline.

40. A 50-year-old man with alcoholic cirrhosis who lives in Florida develops fever, hypotension, and several hemorrhagic bullae on his legs 2 days after eating raw oysters. The most likely cause of his problem is
    A. *Pseudomonas aeruginosa*
    B. *Aeromonas hydrophila*
    C. *Vibrio vulnificus*
    D. *Escherichia coli*
    E. *Vibrio parahaemolyticus*.

41. A 20-year-old man working with goat hides in Iran develops an edematous, necrotic ulcer on his arm. The most likely responsible organism is
    A. *Bacillus anthracis*
    B. *Bacillus cereus*
    C. *Bartonella bacilliformis*
    D. *Erysipelothrix rhusiopathiae*
    E. *Corynebacterium diphtheriae*.

42. All the following cutaneous findings can occur with *Pseudomonas aeruginosa* bacteremia EXCEPT
    A. Subcutaneous nodules
    B. Hemorrhagic bullae
    C. Pink macules resembling "rose spots"
    D. Cellulitis
    E. Diffuse macular erythema.

43. Which of the following is responsible for at least some cases of cat-scratch fever?
    A. *Toxocara catis*
    B. *Afipia felis*
    C. *Nocardia caviae*
    D. *Coxiella burnetii*
    E. *Capnocytophaga canimorsus*.

44. Biopsies of skin lesions often reveal the responsible organism by the culture or special stains in all the following EXCEPT
    A. Toxic shock syndrome
    B. *Staphylococcus aureus* endocarditis
    C. Acute meningococcemia
    D. Typhoid fever
    E. Ecthyma gangrenosum.

45. A 40-year-old man who received a cardiac transplant 1 year ago develops several subcutaneous nodules on his lower extremities that yield pus on needle aspiration. A Gram stain demonstrates branching, beaded, gram-positive bacilli that are acid-fast on a modified acid-fast stain. The organism responsible is probably
    A. *Actinomyces israelii*
    B. *Mycobacterium tuberculosis*
    C. *Mycobacterium avium-intracellulare*
    D. *Propionibacterium acnes*
    E. *Nocardia asteroides*.

46. A 20-year-old woman develops tenosynovitis of her left wrist, myalgias, a mild fever, and scattered, painful lesions on her hands and feet. They are papular and pustular; one is a hemorrhagic bulla. A Gram stain of a pustule showed numerous neutrophils, but no organisms. The most likely cause is

    A. *Treponema pallidum*
    B. *Staphylococcus aureus*
    C. *Rickettsia akari*
    D. *Neisseria gonorrhoeae*
    E. *Salmonella typhi.*

47. A 29-year-old woman from India has had an eruption for about 2 years that consists of symmetrical, erythematous papules; pustules; and crusted ulcers located on her hands, feet, elbows, and knees. Numerous varioliform scars are present on the extremities. A skin biopsy shows a subacute lymphohistiocytic vasculitis with thrombosis and destruction of the small dermal vessels. The most likely diagnosis is

    A. Tuberculoid leprosy
    B. Chronic meningococcemia
    C. Papulonecrotic tuberculid
    D. Lupus vulgaris
    E. Typhoid fever.

48. A 73-year-old woman has had mild fever, anorexia, and weight loss for 2 months. She noticed a painful erythematous papule on the pulp of her right forefinger. The most likely diagnosis is

    A. Typhoid fever
    B. Subacute bacterial endocarditis
    C. Chronic meningococcemia
    D. Brill-Zinsser disease
    E. Tertiary syphilis.

49. A 40-year-old man, who is a butcher, noticed bright red, smooth, sharply demarcated plaques on the dorsum of his right hand, sparing the distal phalanges but involving the finger webs. They are painful and itchy. The most likely cause is

    A. *Staphylococcus aureus*
    B. *Bacillus anthracis*
    C. *Mycobacterium tuberculosis*
    D. *Erysipelothrix rhusiopathiae*
    E. *Treponema pallidum.*

50. A 45-year-old man has a nasal pack placed following nasal surgery. Two days later he develops fever, hypotension, watery diarrhea, myalgias, disorientation, and a diffuse macular blanching eruption on his trunk, abdomen, and extremities. The most likely diagnosis is

    A. Toxic shock syndrome
    B. Staphylococcal scalded skin syndrome
    C. Acute meningococcemia
    D. *Pseudomonas aeruginosa* bacteremia
    E. *Clostridium difficile* infection.

51. A 20-year-old woman who has recently traveled extensively throughout the world has had fever, headache, and myalgias for 1 week. She has had mild abdominal pain and constipation. Her temperature is 103° F, her heart rate 90, and blood pressure 120/80. Splenomegaly is present, as are several 1- to 4-mm erythematous macules on her chest and abdomen. Her chest radiograph is normal. The most likely infecting organism is

    A. *Shigella sonnei*
    B. *Rickettsia conorii*
    C. *Salmonella typhi*
    D. *Neisseria meningitidis*
    E. *Chlamydia psittaci.*

52. A 34-year-old man with acute leukemia undergoing chemotherapy becomes neutropenic. He develops fever of 104° F, hypotension, and a lesion in his right axilla that begins as an erythematous, edematous plaque, rapidly expands, and develops a hemorrhagic bulla in the center. The most likely organism responsible is

    A. *Staphylococcus aureus*
    B. *Salmonella typhi*
    C. *Streptococcus pyogenes*
    D. *Bacteroides fragilis*
    E. *Pseudomonas aeruginosa.*

53. A 38-year-old man with AIDS develops several dusky red, pedunculated nodules with adherent scale resembling pyogenic granulomas. Appropriate therapy is

    A. Liquid nitrogen cryotherapy
    B. Excision with electrodesiccation
    C. Oral erythromycin
    D. Oral cephalosporin
    E. Oral penicillin.

ONE or MORE of the completions for the following questions correctly finishes the incomplete statement; choose

A. If only 1, 2, and 3 are correct
B. If only 1 and 3 are correct
C. If only 2 and 4 are correct
D. If only 4 is correct
E. If all are correct.

54. Cutaneous findings of bacillary angiomatosis include
    1. Pyogenic granuloma-like lesions
    2. Subcutaneous nodules
    3. Indurated, hyperpigmented plaques
    4. Subcutaneous abscesses.

55. Toxic shock syndrome is associated with
    1. Fever
    2. Diffuse macular eruption
    3. Hypotension
    4. Desquamation, especially of palms and soles, 1 to 3 weeks after disease onset.

56. Penicillin is effective treatment for
    1. Typhoid fever
    2. Erysipeloid
    3. Rickettsialpox
    4. Erysipelas.

57. Prominent cutaneous findings in acute meningococcemia include
    1. Numerous pustules
    2. Involvement of the palms and soles
    3. Numerous vesicles and bullae
    4. Initial macular lesions evolving into petechiae and ecchymoses.

58. Cutaneous infections due to the following organisms can occur from water exposure:
    1. *Mycobacterium marinum*
    2. *Vibrio vulnificus*
    3. *Aeromonas hydrophila*
    4. *Pasteurella multocida.*

59. Effective therapy for erythema migrans includes:
    1. Amoxicillin
    2. Ciprofloxacin
    3. Doxycycline
    4. Rifampin.

60. Skin lesions that may be associated with *Mycobacterium tuberculosis* infections are
    1. Lupus vulgaris
    2. Erythema induratum
    3. Erythema nodosum
    4. Erythema marginatum.

61. The following is (are) characteristic of staphylococcal scalded skin syndrome:
    1. Most common in children over 6 years of age
    2. Usually fatal outcome
    3. In children is usually associated with intra-abdominal staphylococcal abscesses
    4. The Nikolsky sign is commonly present.

62. Secondary syphilis is associated with
    1. Condyloma lata
    2. Condyloma acuminata
    3. Mucous patches
    4. Gummas.

63. A false-positive treponemal test (FTA-ABS or MHA-TP) for syphilis may occur with
    1. Chancroid
    2. Lyme disease
    3. Chronic liver disease
    4. Systemic lupus erythematosus.

64. Similarities between the rashes of Rocky Mountain spotted fever and acute meningococcemia include
    1. Initially, blanching macules
    2. Initial appearance on wrists and ankles
    3. Petechial and purpuric lesions that may lead to cutaneous gangrene
    4. Involvement of palms and soles.

65. The following sexually transmitted organisms cause genital ulcers:
    1. *Treponema pallidum*
    2. *Haemophilus ducreyi*
    3. Herpes simplex
    4. *Calymmatobacterium granulomatis.*

66. The following is (are) characteristic of lupus vulgaris:
    1. Squamous cell carcinoma is a complication
    2. It may occur from primary inoculation of the skin with *Mycobacterium tuberculosis* (exogenous source)

3. It may occur from extension from a contiguous or distant focus of tuberculous infection (endogenous source)
4. Stains and cultures of skin biopsies are rarely positive for *M. tuberculosis*.

67. The following is (are) true about necrotizing fasciitis:
   1. *Staphylococcus aureus* is a common cause
   2. Antibiotic therapy without surgery is usually successful
   3. Pus is rarely present
   4. Gas formation may occur in affected tissue.

For the following questions, the set of lettered headings is followed by a list of numbered words or phrases. For each numbered word or phrase, choose

A. If the item is associated with A only.
B. If the item is associated with B only.
C. If the item is associated with both A and B.
D. If the item is associated with neither A nor B.

For each of the following, choose the type of effective therapy, whether doxycycline, penicillin, both, or neither.

68. Staphylococcal toxic shock syndrome
69. Primary syphilis
70. *Streptococcus viridans* endocarditis
71. Disseminated gonococcal infection
72. Lymphogranuloma venereum
73. Murine typhus.

A. Doxycycline is effective therapy
B. Penicillin is effective therapy
C. Both are effective therapy
D. Neither is effective therapy.

For each of the following characteristics, choose whether it describes tuberculoid leprosy, lepromatous leprosy, both, or neither.

74. Numerous organisms visible on skin biopsy
75. Leonine facies
76. Skin biopsy culture usually positive on Lowenstein-Jensen media
77. Strong cell-mediated immunity to *Mycobacterium leprae*

A. Tuberculoid leprosy
B. Lepromatous leprosy
C. Both
D. Neither.

78. Erythema nodosum leprosum is a complication
79. Dapsone alone is the recommended therapy
80. Few skin lesions.

ANSWERS

1. C; **2.** A; **3.** C; **4.** C In previous years nonbullous impetigo was thought to be caused primarily or exclusively by *Streptococcus pyogenes*. Although cultures often yielded *Staphylococcus aureus* as well, it was commonly considered a non–pathogenic colonizing organism. In recent years *Staph. aureus* has become the predominant isolate, usually in pure culture. When *Strep. pyogenes* is present, it is most often mixed with *Staph. aureus;* only occasionally is it the sole organism. Furthermore, trials of antibiotic therapy comparing agents effective against *Strep. pyogenes* alone versus those active against both *Strep. pyogenes* and *Staph. aureus* have demonstrated a higher cure rate for the latter, confirming the importance of *Staph. aureus* as a pathogen.

Bullous impetigo is exclusively due to *Staph. aureus* strains, usually group II, phage 71, capable of elaborating a toxin that causes cleavage in the epidermal layers. This is the same toxin that produces staphylococcal scalded skin syndrome when absorbed into the systemic circulation, usually from a mucosal surface, and causes widespread cutaneous damage. In bullous impetigo, the toxin exerts its effects only locally.

Blistering distal dactylitis is predominantly an infection of children and is usually due to *Strep. pyogenes*, but some cases have been caused by *Staph. aureus*. It is a superficial infection of the anterior fat pad of the distal portion of the fingers, or occasionally of the toes, causing a large blister on an erythematous base.

Ecthyma (Greek for pustule) is a deeper infection than impetigo, causing ulcerations surmounted by an adherent crust. The infection extends into the dermis and heals with scarring. The lower extremities are commonly affected, often in patients with poor hygiene. As is true of nonbullous impetigo, *Staph. aureus, Strep. pyogenes*, or both can produce this infection, and treatment should be with an agent effective against both organisms (Chapter 105).

5. D Ecthyma gangrenosum ("gangrenous pustule") is a manifestation of systemic infection with certain gram-negative bacilli, primarily *Pseudomonas aeruginosa*, although other organisms such as *Escherichia coli* or *Morganella morganii* have produced identical lesions. Patients are usually bacteremic, febrile, and often hypotensive. The lesions typically begin as erythematous plaques that rapidly enlarge and develop hemorrhagic bullae or gangrenous centers (Chapter 107).

6. B Erysipelas is a spreading erythematous infection of the epidermis and dermis. Although the term has been used in various ways, currently it typically refers to a streptococcal infection of the face (Chapter 105).

7. E Erysipeloid ("resembling erysipelas") is a cutaneous infection, usually of the hands, caused by *Erysipelothrix rhusiopathiae,* a gram-positive bacillus found in decayed animal products (Chapter 107).

8. D Hot-tub folliculitis is a superficial infection caused by *Pseudomonas aeruginosa* that has proliferated in inadequately disinfected hot water. Patients develop itchy, erythematous papules surrounding follicles in areas submerged during the patients' sojourn in the contaminated water (Chapter 107).

9. A Carbuncles are staphylococcal infections of the deeper portions of several adjacent follicles. They seem more common in diabetics and occur on the back of the neck, where they cause an inflammatory nodule with pus typically draining from several follicular orifices (Chapter 105).

10. B Scarlet fever is an infection, usually of the pharynx, by a lysogenic (virus-infected) strain of *Strep. pyogenes* that produces a toxin causing erythematous areas of the skin, changes in the papillae of the tongue, and desquamation of skin later in the course. The rash usually appears within 2 days after the throat becomes sore and involves the neck, upper chest, and back. It then spreads to the extremities, sparing the palms and soles. It consists of diffuse, blanching erythema with numerous 1- to 2-mm punctate papules that give the skin a "sandpaper" texture. The rash is accentuated in skinfolds, often producing Pastia's lines, linear streaks of petechiae from increased capillary fragility. The face is flushed except for circumoral pallor, and inside the mouth are petechiae on the soft palate and a thick, white covering of the tongue (white strawberry tongue) with patches of red, hypertrophied papillae. A few days later the coating disappears, leaving a red tongue (red strawberry or raspberry tongue). A few days after the rash appears, extensive desquamation occurs (Chapter 104).

11. C; **12.** D; **13.** B; **14.** C; **15.** A (Chapters 108 and 110).

16. A; **17.** E; **18.** A; **19.** D; **20.** B; **21.** A; **22.** C Tick-borne organisms include the cause of Lyme disease (*Borrelia burgdorferi*), Rocky Mountain spotted fever (*Rickettsia rickettsii*), and ehrlichiosis (*Ehrlichia canis*), a febrile disease occurring primarily in the southern United States that can sometimes cause a rash. *Afipia felis* is a cause of cat-scratch disease. The common house mouse is the reservoir for *Rickettsia akari,* transmitted to man by a mouse mite to cause rickettsialpox, a disease that occurs in crowded urban settings where mice are abundant. Rickettsialpox consists of fever, headache, myalgias, and an eruption of erythematous macules or papules with a central vesicle. *Rickettsia typhi* is the pathogen responsible for endemic (murine) typhus, transmitted to man from rats by rat fleas. It causes fever, headache, myalgias, and a macular eruption on the trunk and proximal extremities (Chapters 107, 109, 114, and 115).

23. (F) Pitted keratolysis may be caused by *Micrococcus sedentarius* or corynebacteria. It consists of small pitted erosions on the soles or, less commonly, the palms, especially in hot climates and in those wearing occlusive foot wear. It is often accompanied by pain, itching, and a pungent odor. Several therapies are effective, including topical azoles or topical erythromycin (Chapter 105).

24. (T) Although its name suggests a fungal infection (tricho*mycosis*), this disorder of the axillary hairs is produced by colonies of coryneform bacteria adherent to the hair shaft, creating yellowish-brown or black nodules. Treatment is shaving or a topical antibacterial agent such as clindamycin (Chapter 105).

25. (T) Erythrasma, which can cause toeweb erosions or scaly patches on the skin, is due to *Corynebacterium minutissimum*. Topical azoles are effective because they have some activity against gram-positive bacteria as well as fungi (Chapter 105).

26. (T) Adults, in general, tend to have an axillary flora in which either coryneform bacteria or gram-positive cocci predominate. The former create an impressive axillary odor, which can be reproduced by incubating apocrine sweat with the coryneform bacteria. Some axillary deodorants work, in part at least, by their ability to inhibit bacterial growth; neomycin, for example, is an extremely effective deodorant (Chapter 105).

27. (F) About 25% of cutaneous abscesses are due to *Staph. aureus,* usually in pure culture. It is the predominant isolate from breast abscesses in puerperal women and from hand and axillary abscesses. For most other sites, the infecting organisms have been a mixture of the local resident flora, sometimes combined with organisms from a nearby mucosal surface. Anaerobes are common in most abscesses (Chapter 105).

28. (F) Rheumatic fever, for unclear reasons, occurs only after streptococcal infection of the airway (predominantly pharyngitis). It has not followed streptococcal skin infections (Chapter 105).

29. (F) Acute post-streptococcal glomerulonephritis is a rare complication of streptococcal pyodermas and occurs only with certain "nephritogenic" strains. Often, kidney damage is already present when the patient seeks attention for the skin infection; furthermore, no study has conclusively demonstrated that early treatment reduces the risk (Chapter 105).

30. (F) Needle aspiration has a disappointing yield (about 5%) in most cases of cellulitis. Even skin biopsies are culture-positive in only about 20% (Chapter 105).

31. (F) When cultures of blood, skin biopsy, or needle aspiration are positive, the usual isolates are streptococci. Immunofluorescent techniques have commonly detected streptococcal antigens on skin biopsies, even when cultures are negative. These studies indicate that streptococci (group A and other types) are the most common cause of cellulitis (Chapter 105).

32. (F) The cleavage in staphylococcal scalded skin syndrome is in the epidermis, usually at the granular layer, an important distinction from toxic epidermal necrolysis, where the separation is at the dermoepidermal junction (Chapter 106).

33. (T) Several studies indicate that topical mupirocin is as effective as erythromycin. Other topical antibiotics are not as good. Mupirocin is an effective alternative to systemic therapy, unless the impetigo is widespread, when topical application may be impractical (Chapter 105).

34. (T) As indicated in the answer to Question 1, ecthyma is a deeper infection than impetigo, causes ulceration down to the dermis, and heals with scarring (Chapter 105).

35. (F) *Streptococcus pyogenes* does not survive on normal skin, presumably because it is inhibited by cutaneous fatty acids. *Staph. aureus,* however, does colonize the perineal area in about 10% to 20% of normal people and the anterior nares in 20% to 40% (Chapter 105).

36. (T) Many antibiotics are ineffectual in preventing recurrent furunculosis because they do not achieve adequate concentrations in the anterior nares, the probable reservoir of *Staph. aureus* in most patients with this problem. Clindamycin achieves high concentrations in the nasal secretions and has been effective in reducing the recurrence rates of furunculosis (Chapter 105).

37. (T) The simplest diagnostic evidence for erythrasma is the coral-red appearance with Wood's lamp illumination, which is produced by the porphyrins that the organisms excrete (Chapter 105).

38. D Sulfonamides remain the drug of choice for nocardial infections; most clinicians use the combination of sulfamethoxazole and trimethoprim, although it has not conclusively been demonstrated to be better than a sulfonamide alone (Chapter 113).

39. E None of the other agents listed is effective; an alternative to tetracycline or doxycycline is chloramphenicol (Chapter 114).

40. C *Vibrio vulnificus* is a gram-negative bacillus that lives in warm salt water. Exposure of open wounds to salt water can eventuate in a necrotizing cellulitis of the affected area. Skin lesions can also occur when patients develop bacteremia from ingesting inadequately cooked seafood. Many of the victims have alcoholic cirrhosis; probably the organisms enter the portal venous system from the gastrointestinal mucosa. Impaired hepatic phagocytosis or portal systemic shunts allow systemic bacteremia to occur. About 60% to 70% of those with bacteremia develop skin lesions, especially vesicles, bullae, erythematous swellings, and gangrene, typically on the lower extremities. The mortality rate is about 70% to 80% (Chapter 107).

41. A Anthrax typically occurs from local trauma, with inoculation of the spores of *Bacillus anthracis* into the skin from a contaminated animal product. Cases are rare in the United States, although the organism remains endemic in the soil of some Southern states. In recent years, disease has been frequent in Iran, Turkey, Greece, and southern Africa. The spores are ingested by herbivores, which usually die. Handling carcasses of infected livestock or their products, such as hides, hair, or bone meal, leads to infection in humans. After an incubation period of about 1 to 5 days, the skin lesion begins as a small, erythematous, and sometimes pruritic papule, typically on an exposed area such as the head, neck, and upper extremity. As the papule enlarges, vesicles form on its surface and nonpitting edema surrounds it. The center darkens first to brown, then black as an ulcer forms, which is then covered by a tough, black eschar. The encircling edema may become extensive, and regional lymph node enlargement, accompanied by pain and tenderness, is common. Gram stain and culture of the vesicular fluid or material obtained from the base of the eschar will usually demonstrate the organism, a gram-positive bacillus. Treatment is penicillin (Chapter 107).

42. E Cutaneous lesions occur in less than 5% of patients with *Pseudomonas aeruginosa* bacteremia, but all the forms listed except for E have been described (Chapter 107).

43. B Examining silver stains of tissue from patients with cat-scratch disease, researchers at the Armed Forces Institute of Pathology (AFIP) recognized gram-negative bacilli. An organism was isolated subsequently and named *Afipia* (in honor of the AFIP) *felis* (cat). Other investigations suggest that a rickettsia, *Rochalimaea,* may be a more common cause of cat-scratch disease (Chapter 115).

44. A In toxic shock syndrome, the cutaneous lesions occur from the action of a circulating toxin on the skin. *Staph. aureus* is usually present on a mucosal surface, not in the systemic circulation or the skin. In the other infections listed, circulating organisms lodge in the cutaneous vessels, causing vascular damage and often perivascular inflammation. Because live bacteria are present in the skin lesions, special stains and cultures commonly reveal the responsible organism (Chapters 106 and 107).

45. E *Nocardia asteroides,* a gram-positive branching rod that is partially acid-fast and lives in the soil, can cause cutaneous lesions in those with systemic infections. Most commonly, the victims have compromised cell-mediated immunity from an underlying disease or immunosuppressive therapy. The organism is inhaled into the lung and from that focus may spread via the systemic circulation to cause disease in distant sites, especially the brain or skin. Cutaneous lesions are usually cutaneous pustules or subcutaneous nodular abscesses (Chapter 113).

46. D Disseminated gonococcal infection typically causes myalgias, mild fever, suppurative arthritis, and tenosynovitis. About 50% to 75% of patients have skin lesions, which are typically few in number, distal, painful, and papular, pustular, or purpuric. Hemorrhagic bullae can occur. Commonly, the organism is present on a mucosal surface (pharynx, rectum, urethra, vagina) without causing local problems. Women are often menstruating or are pregnant, circumstances that change the

blood flow in the cervix and allow organisms to enter the systemic circulation. Blood cultures are positive in about one third to one half of patients (Chapters 107 and 110).

47. C Several forms of cutaneous tuberculosis exist. The description is classic for papulonecrotic tuberculid, which may be an immunologic reaction to infection elsewhere. Histology and cultures of skin biopsies rarely reveal the organism (Chapter 111).

48. B The lesion described is characteristic of Osler's node, a painful erythematous papule in the pulp of the fingers or toes. Although sometimes considered of immunologic origin due to deposition of immune complexes, Osler's nodes are probably septic emboli. Biopsies have often demonstrated the organisms on special stains or grown them on cultures (Chapter 107).

49. D The description is classic for erysipeloid, a cutaneous infection caused by *Erysipelothrix rhusiopathiae*, a gram-positive bacillus found in decayed animal products. It is an occupational hazard for fishermen, butchers, veterinarians, and farmers. After an incubation period of 1 to 7 days, the skin lesions described occur. A few patients have lymphangitis or systemic symptoms. The disease is usually self-limited, but resolution is hastened by treatment, and some patients develop systemic complications like endocarditis or septic arthritis. The organism is difficult to isolate from skin lesions, perhaps because it converts into a cell–wall deficient form that requires special culture techniques. Penicillin is the drug of choice, but the organism also appears susceptible to clindamycin, erythromycin, and cephalosporins (Chapter 107).

50. A Although many cases of toxic shock syndrome have involved females using tampons for menstruation, it has also occurred in other circumstances of mucosal colonization or deep infection with *Staph. aureus* strains producing the responsible toxins (Chapter 106).

51. C *Salmonella typhi*, an organism confined to humans and typically spread through contaminated food, is ingested into the gastrointestinal tract, from which it enters the blood stream. The early symptoms are headache, increasing fever, myalgias, and abdominal pain. Constipation, rather than diarrhea, is an early symptom. Splenomegaly and a heart rate lower than expected for the body temperature may be present. The skin lesions are "rose spots." Similar lesions can occur with *Pseudomonas aeruginosa* bacteremia or psittacosis, but the clinical presentation of a subacute disease is inconsistent with the former and the normal chest radiograph with the latter. Early in the disease, cultures of blood, bone marrow, and skin biopsies are commonly positive, stool cultures, negative. With time, the circulating organisms are phagocytized in the liver, excreted by the bile into the intestinal tract, and stool cultures become positive (Chapter 107).

52. E This is a characteristic setting and description of ecthyma gangrenosum, a skin lesion that occurs in a small minority of patients with *Pseudomonas aeruginosa* bacteremia. Needle aspiration of the lesion typically reveals the organism on Gram stain and culture. Skin biopsy discloses vascular damage with organisms causing destruction of the vessel wall and usually little inflammation (Chapter 107).

53. C The lesions are characteristic of bacillary angiomatosis, a disorder apparently caused by *Rochalimaea quintana* or *henselae,* rickettsia that may be transmitted by cats. Erythromycin is the drug of choice (Chapter 115).

54. A The main cutaneous forms of bacillary angiomatosis are the first three answers. These have been seen almost exclusively in patients with human immunodeficiency virus (HIV) infection (Chapter 115).

55. E These are among the defining criteria for toxic shock syndrome. Others include evidence of involvement of at least three of the following systems: gastrointestinal (vomiting or diarrhea), muscular (myalgia or elevated creatine phosphokinase levels), renal (elevated serum creatinine or urea nitrogen), hepatic (elevated bilirubin or aminotransferase), hematologic (thrombocytopenia), and central nervous system (disorientation or altered consciousness) (Chapter 106).

56. C (Chapters 105, 107, 114).

57. D (Chapter 107).

58. A *Mycobacterium marinum* causes "fish tank" granuloma; *Vibrio vulnificus,* found in salt water, causes cellulitis or necrotizing lesions during bacteremia; *Aeromonas hydrophila* is found in fresh or brackish water and can cause cellulitis in traumatized, contaminated skin. *Pasteurella multocida* is part of the oral flora of cats and dogs, causing cellulitis following bites or scratches from these animals (Chapters 107 and 111).

59. B Amoxicillin and doxycycline are equally effective in erythema migrans, the cutaneous manifestation of early infection with *Borrelia burgdorferi* (Lyme disease). Ciprofloxacin and rifampin are ineffective (Chapter 109).

60. A Erythema marginatum is a manifestation of acute rheumatic fever (Chapter 183).

61. D Most patients are under 5 years of age, the fatality rate is low, and the staphylococci are usually present on a mucosal surface (Chapter 106).

62. B Condylomata acuminata are genital warts; gummas are manifestations of tertiary syphilis (Chapters 108 and 123).

63. C Serologic tests for syphilis include treponemal (FTA-ABS, MHA-TP) or non-treponemal tests (e.g., VDRL, RPR). Chancroid and chronic liver disease can cause false-positive non-treponemal tests, but not false-positive treponemal tests (Chapter 108).

64. B The rash of Rocky Mountain spotted fever initially appears on the wrists and ankles and in acute meningococcemia on the trunk. Involvement of the palms and soles, characteristic of Rocky Mountain spotted fever, rarely, if ever, occurs with acute meningococcemia (Chapter 114).

65. E (Chapters 108, 110, and 121).

66. E Lupus vulgaris, a cutaneous manifestation of tuberculosis, may occur from primary inoculation of the skin by the organism or may spread from an endogenous site of infection. It typically occurs on the face, neck, or ears as red-brown plaques or nodules that can ulcerate and scar. Diascopy, pressure over the lesion with a magnifying lens, reveals "apple jelly" nodules. A rare complication is neoplastic change, usually into squamous cell carcinoma (Chapter 111).

67. D Necrotizing fasciitis is caused by *Streptococcus pyogenes* alone or more commonly by a mixture of aerobic and anaerobic organisms. Pus is usually present in the subcutaneous tissue, and surgery plus antibiotic therapy is necessary for cure. Gas formation from enteric gram-negative bacilli such as *Escherichia coli* or *Klebsiella* species or from anaerobes is common (Chapter 107).

68. D In addition to intravascular fluid, the management of toxic shock syndrome includes parenteral antimicrobial therapy against *Staph. aureus*. Because most isolates, even from outpatients, are penicillinase producers, penicillin is not satisfactory, and doxycycline is not a reliable agent against this pathogen either (Chapter 106).

69. C (Chapter 108).

70. B An important principle in the therapy for endocarditis is to employ antimicrobial therapy that kills the organism (bactericidal) rather than merely inhibits its growth (bacteriostatic). Doxycycline is bacteriostatic, penicillin is bactericidal against *Strep. viridans;* penicillin alone or combined with an aminoglycoside (streptomycin or gentamicin) remains the drug of choice for this infection (Chapter 107).

71. D Although both antibiotics were effective against *Neisseria gonorrhoeae* in the past, resistance against them is now common, and another antibiotic is required. Currently, ceftriaxone is the drug of choice (Chapter 110).

72. A (Chapter 110).

73. A (Chapter 114).

74. B; **75.** B; **76.** D; **77.** A; **78.** B; **79.** D; **80.** A The clinical manifestations of *Mycobacterium leprae,* an organism that has never been grown on artificial media, depend upon the host's cell-mediated immune response to this microbe. At one end of the spectrum are those with good immune response; clinically the number of skin lesions is small, and skin biopsies show few organisms and well-developed granulomas with mature epithelioid cells and Langerhans giant cells. These are features of tuberculoid leprosy. At the other extreme are those with poorly developed cell-mediated immunity; many skin lesions are present, extensive involvement can create a leonine facies, and skin biopsies show abundant bacilli, numerous macrophages, and no granulomas. These are features of lepromatous leprosy. Many patients have disease that lies between these two extremes. Erythema nodosum leprosum occurs in those with poor cell-mediated immunity; its manifestations may represent immune complex disease. It often occurs after therapy has begun and consists of crops of small pink nodules, frequently involving the face and extensor surfaces of the extremities. Fever, malaise, iritis, episcleritis, a chronic panniculitis, orchitis, bone pain, arthritis, and proteinuria are other findings. Because of the emergence of dapsone-resistant organisms, dapsone alone is not recommended for any form of the disease. For tuberculoid leprosy, dapsone plus rifampin is the regimen of choice; for lepromatous leprosy, dapsone, rifampin, and clofazimine are recommended (Chapter 112).

Bibliography

Beyt BE, Ortbals DW, Santa Cruz DJ, et al. Cutaneous mycobacteriosis: Analysis of 34 cases with a new classification of the disease. Medicine 1980; 60:95–109.

Cardullo AC, Silvers DN, Grossman ME. Janeway's lesions and Osler's nodes: A review of histopathologic findings. J Am Acad Dermatol 1990; 22:1088–1090.

Kingston ME, Mackey D. Skin clues in the diagnosis of life-threatening infections. Rev Infect Dis 1986; 8:1–11.

McCalmont C, Zanolli MD. Rickettsial diseases. Dermatol Clin 1989; 7:591–601.

Meyers WM, Marty AM. Current concepts in the pathogenesis of leprosy. Drugs 1991; 41:832–856.

Noble WC, ed. The Skin Microflora and Microbial Skin Disease. Cambridge, Engl: Cambridge University Press, 1992.

Resnick SD: Staphylococcal toxin–mediated syndromes in childhood. Semin Dermatol 1992; 11:11–18.

Spencer LV, Callen JP: Cutaneous manifestations of bacterial infections. Dermatol Clin 1989; 7:579–589.

chapter 15

Viral and Fungal Infections

TOBY A. MAURER

VIRAL INFECTIONS

Choose the ONE BEST answer to each of the following questions.

1. A 65-year-old man has herpes zoster involving his face. Ophthalmologic consultation should occur in which of the following situations?
   A. Lesions are seen on the tip and side of the nose
   B. Facial and auditory nerves are involved
   C. Supratrochlear and supraorbital nerves are involved
   D. Patient has Ramsay Hunt syndrome
   E. Maxillary branch of the fifth nerve is involved.

2. A 36-year-old man with AIDS develops a large, non-healing, perirectal ulcer caused by herpes simplex that is acyclovir-resistant. Which one of the following statements is true?
   A. The mechanism of resistance is due to altered viral DNA polymerase or altered thymidine kinase enzyme
   B. Mutant strains of thymidine kinase do not phosphorylate acyclovir into acyclovir triphosphate
   C. A reasonable alternative to acyclovir would be intravenous ganciclovir
   D. Resistance to HSV-1 has not been recognized
   E. The main side effects of foscarnet are hyperglycemia and anemia.

3. The following statement is true about molluscum contagiosum.
   A. The virus can be cultured on the chorioallantoic membrane of fertilized cells
   B. Genital lesions in children confirm sexual transmission of the virus
   C. Conjunctivitis and keratitis are complications of molluscum around the eyes
   D. Treatment in children is recommended because it will prevent recurrences
   E. Treatment in patients with AIDS is as effective as treatment is in the non-immunocompromised patient.

4. Which of the following is true of treatment for warts?
   A. Wart virus has been found in the plume of carbon dioxide lasers
   B. Radiation is one recommended treatment for warts
   C. Podophyllin is safe for use in pregnancy
   D. Dinitrochlorobenzene works by causing an irritant dermatitis, thereby destroying the cells infected with wart virus
   E. Areas that become acetowhite following 3% to 5% acetic acid soaks of the genitals need to be treated definitively.

5. Epstein-Barr virus is associated with all of the following EXCEPT
   A. A generalized erythematous maculopapular eruption 10 days after initiation of penicillins
   B. The Gianotti-Crosti syndrome
   C. Oral hairy leukoplakia
   D. Atypical lymphocytes in the peripheral blood
   E. Erythema infectiosum.

6. Which one of the following statements is true about varicella during pregnancy?
   A. Varicella infection has more severe consequences for the pregnant woman than for the non-pregnant woman.
   B. Consequences to a 1-month-old newborn exposed to varicella are worse than if that child had been exposed to varicella in utero 5 days prior to birth
   C. A newborn whose mother developed varicella one month prior to birth should receive varicella zoster immunoglobulins
   D. Children who develop herpes zoster prior to 1 year of age may have been exposed to varicella in utero
   E. Central nervous system sequelae are the most common complications of adult varicella.

Decide whether EACH of the following questions is TRUE or FALSE. Any combination of answers from all true to all false may occur.

The following diseases are associated with "blueberry muffin babies."

7. Cytomegalovirus
8. Rubella
9. Toxoplasmosis
10. Syphilis
11. Herpes simplex virus.

Regarding fifth disease,

12. Dermatitis starts after the fever resolves.
13. Aplastic crises can occur.
14. Fetal mortality most commonly occurs if the mother has been exposed to the virus in the third trimester of pregnancy.
15. The patient may have fever, pharyngitis, and headache.
16. The rash can be morbilliform, confluent, circinate, or annular.

Eczema herpeticum may be seen with the following disorders.

17. Darier-White disease
18. Atopic dermatitis
19. Pemphigus foliaceus
20. Mycosis fungoides
21. Congenital ichthyosiform erythroderma.

A 20-year-old woman presents to a dermatology clinic reporting that her brother has epidermodysplasia verruciformis. Regarding this disease,

22. The most common mode of inheritance is autosomal dominant.
23. Squamous cell cancers on the forehead, scalp, and hands are associated with the wart virus in this disease.
24. Trauma is associated with malignant transformation of warts.
25. Verruciform, exophytic warts are the most commonly noted warts in this disease.
26. Lymph node and visceral metastases are common.

In each of the following questions, a set of lettered headings accompanies a list of numbered words or phrases. For each numbered word or phrase, choose

A. If the item is associated with A only
B. If the item is associated with B only
C. If the item is associated with both A and B
D. If the item is associated with neither A nor B.

For each of the statements below, choose whether it is associated with herpangina, gingival stomatitis, both, or neither.

27. Associated with herpes simplex virus
28. Lesions on tongue and buccal mucosa
29. Associated with fever, inability to eat, drooling
30. Associated with Coxsackie virus.

A. Herpangina
B. Gingival stomatitis
C. Both
D. Neither.

For each of the statements below, choose whether it is associated with orf, milker's nodules, both, or neither.

31. Multiple lesions   A. Orf

32. Six clinical stages have been described
33. Treatment with tetracycline is recommended
34. Prevalent in spring when contact with newborn animals is made.

    B. Milker's nodules
    C. Both
    D. Neither.

For each of the statements below, choose whether it is associated with rubella, rubeola, both, or neither.

35. Rash clears rapidly by the end of the second or third day
36. Red pinhead-sized spots in mouth
37. Rash first noted on head
38. Associated with severe congenital defects when mother exposed to the virus late in the third trimester.

    A. Rubella
    B. Rubeola
    C. Both
    D. Neither.

For each numbered item, choose the most likely associated lettered item. Each numbered item has ONLY ONE answer. Within each group, each lettered item may be the answer to one, more than one, or none of the numbered items.

For each of the viruses listed below, choose the virus family with which it is most closely linked.

39. Molluscum contagiosum
40. Measles
41. Rubella
42. Varicella
43. Cytomegalovirus.

    A. Poxvirus
    B. Togavirus
    C. Paramyxovirus
    D. Herpesvirus.

FUNGAL INFECTIONS

Choose the ONE BEST answer to each of the following questions.

44. *Epidermophyton floccosum*
    A. Can cause tinea capitis
    B. Frequently affects the groin
    C. Has few macroconidia and numerous microconidia
    D. Produces light yellow to orange surface pigment in culture
    E. Has macroconidia that are thin-walled with pointed ends.

45. Which one of the following statements is true about chronic mucocutaneous candidiasis (CMC)?
    A. It is always an inherited disease
    B. When onset is in adulthood, there can be an association with thymoma and myasthenia gravis
    C. Nail involvement occurs in all types of CMC
    D. Immunologic defects are found in all patients with CMC.

46. Which one of the following statements is true regarding congenital candidiasis in a newborn?
    A. The newborn is at high risk of being immunocompromised, and a workup should be initiated
    B. The newborn should be treated with intravenous antifungals
    C. Morbidity and mortality has been noted in newborns with low birth weight and respiratory illness
    D. Lesions are commonly seen in the diaper area and perioraly in congenital candidiasis.

47. A patient with leukemia develops widespread lesions; the blood cultures are positive for *Candida albicans*. All the following are true EXCEPT
    A. *C. albicans* can activate C5a, inducing neutrophilic chemotaxis
    B. Lesions occasionally resemble ecthyma gangrenosum
    C. *C. albicans* should be cultured on Sabouraud's agar without antibiotics because antibiotics will inhibit its growth
    D. True hyphae can be seen in *Candida*

E. *C. albicans* is germ tube test–positive, sucrose assimilation–positive, and forms chlamydospores on cornmeal agar.

48. Which one of the following statements is true about mycetoma?
    A. Clinical triad includes draining sinuses, swelling, and sulfur granules
    B. The most common eumycotic mycetoma, *Pseudallescheria boydii*, is partially acid-fast
    C. Eumycotic mycetomas are not caused by true fungi
    D. The upper leg is the most common site of involvement
    E. Staphylococci and streptococci do not cause mycetomas.

Decide whether EACH of the following questions is TRUE or FALSE. Any combination of answers from all true to all false may occur.

Regarding Wood's lamp examination of hair dermatophytes,

49. *Microsporum canis* variant, *M. canis distortum*, fluoresces.
50. *Trichophyton schoenleinii* fluoresces.
51. *Microsporum fulvum* fluoresces.
52. *Trichophyton tonsurans* fluoresces.
53. *Microsporum ferugineum* fluoresces.

Regarding tinea capitis,

54. Black dot tinea is caused by *Trichophyton tonsurans* and *T. verrucosum*.
55. Black dot tinea is not inflammatory.
56. *Microsporum audouinii* is a common cause for tinea capitis in North America.
57. The most common cause of scutula is *Trichophyton schoenleinii*, associated with conditions of malnutrition and poverty.
58. Children with tinea capitis should be kept at home until the scalp is clear of lesions.

Regarding griseofulvin,

59. The cure rate of tinea anguium, or toenail onychomycosis is 50%.
60. Hematologic abnormalities from this drug have been reported; therefore, white blood cell counts should be checked routinely.
61. Griseofulvin's primary mechanism of action is known to be the inhibition of ergosterol synthesis.
62. Resistance of *Trichophyton rubrum* to the drug has not occurred.
63. Griseofulvin increases the anticoagulant effect of warfarin through induction of hepatic microsomal enzymes.

Concerning disseminated histoplasmosis,

64. It is commonly associated with neurologic disease.
65. Dermal macrophages are packed with yeast forms.
66. Liver disease is rare.
67. It is associated with Addison's disease.
68. Ulceration of the soft palate has been noted.

In each of the following questions, a set of lettered headings accompanies a list of numbered words or phrases. For each numbered word or phrase, choose

A. If the item is associated with A only
B. If the item is associated with B only
C. If the item is associated with both A and B
D. If the item is associated with neither A nor B.

For each of the statements below, choose whether it is associated with endothrix, ectothrix, both, or neither.

69. *Trichophyton tonsurans*
70. Fluoresce
71. Tend to be more chronic infections
72. The location of the hyphae are outside the hair.

A. Endothrix
B. Ectothrix
C. Both
D. Neither.

For each of the statements below, choose whether it is associated with black piedra, white piedra, both, or neither.

73. *Piedraia hortae*
74. *Phaeoannelomyces wernekii* (previously *Exophiala wernekii*)
75. Reported in the United States
76. Causes disseminated infection in the immunocompromised host.

A. Black piedra
B. White piedra
C. Both
D. Neither.

For each numbered item, choose the most likely associated lettered item. Each numbered item has ONLY ONE answer. Within each group, each lettered item may be the answer to one, more than one, or none of the numbered items.

For each of the types of onychomycosis in the following list, choose the characteristic with which it is most strongly linked.

77. Starts at the free edge of the nail
78. *Trichophyton mentagrophytes* is the most common organism
79. Does not occur on the fingernails
80. Often surrounded by paronychial infection.

A. Distal subungual onychomycosis
B. Proximal subungual onychomycosis
C. White superficial onychomycosis
D. *Candida* nails.

For each of the following mechanisms listed, choose the antifungal drug or drug class with which it is most strongly linked.

81. Inhibits squalene epoxidase
82. Absorbed through the blood–brain barrier
83. Causes gynecomastia by inhibiting testosterone
84. Fungistatic and fungicidal.

A. Fluconazole
B. Ketoconazole
C. Allylamines
D. Nystatin.

For each of the following histologic features listed, choose the deep fungal disease with which it is most strongly linked.

85. Budding yeast in chains with narrow intercellular connections
86. Medlar bodies in giant cells or free tissue
87. Asteroid bodies
88. Giant sporangium with sporangiospores
89. Spherules with endospores all at the same level of development.

A. Rhinosporidiosis
B. Lobomycosis
C. Chromoblastomycosis
D. Sporotrichosis
E. Coccidioidomycosis.

ANSWERS

1. A Ophthalmic zoster has a high complication rate. Nasociliary involvement provides varicella-zoster virus with direct access to intraocular structures. Nasociliary branch involvement is marked by lesions on the tip and/or side of the nose. The eye is usually spared when the supraorbital and supratrochlear nerves are involved. The Ramsay Hunt syndrome consists of facial palsy in combination with involvement of the facial and auditory nerves and does not involve the eye. The maxillary branch of the trigeminal branch is less frequently involved and is marked by lesions of the facial skin in that area and of the oral mucosa, again without affecting the eye (Chapter 121).

2. B Acyclovir is activated by viral thymidine kinase (TK) to produce acyclovir triphosphate, which inhibits viral DNA polymerase. In patients with AIDS who have acyclovir-resistant HSV (most often HSV2), the mechanism of resistance is due to TK-deficient mutants rather than to altered mutants seen in patients with leukemia or renal transplants. Ganciclovir does not treat acyclovir-resistant HSV because it is also TK-dependent. Foscarnet is the reasonable alternative. Its side effects are renal failure, hypocalcemia, seizures, and penile erosions (Chapter 121).

3. C Molluscum contagiosum is caused by a poxvirus that, unlike other poxviruses, cannot be cultured in tissue. Although genital lesions in adults are probably sexually transmitted, outbreaks in children have been reported among those attending swimming pools. Lesions around the eyes can be associated with conjunctivitis and keratitis. Treatment is often not necessary in children, since this is a self-limited disease, and treatment does not prevent recurrences. In immunocompromised patients, molluscum can be refractory to standard treatments such as cryotherapy, curettage, and application of cantharidin, podophyllin, or trichloroacetic acid (Chapter 122).

4. A Because human papillomavirus has been found in the plume from carbon dioxide laser ablation of warts, appropriate protection, including goggles, high-filtration masks, gown, and gloves should be worn during treatment. Radiation is not recommended in the treatment of warts because of the potential for malignant transformation. Podophyllin is contraindicated in pregnancy. Dinitrochlorobenzene causes an allergic contact dermatitis that stimulates local immunity. Not everything that becomes acetowhite is a wart, and treatment should not rest on this finding (Chapter 123).

5. E In patients with Epstein-Barr virus (EBV), a generalized erythematous rash may appear on the trunk and extremities about 10 days after certain penicillins are used. The most common penicillin to produce this eruption is ampicillin, although other penicillins have been implicated. EBV is the most commonly reported virus to be associated with the Gianotti-Crosti syndrome, which is a cutaneous reaction to viral infection. It is characterized by erythematous papules that involve the face, limbs, and buttocks. EBV DNA has been found in lesions of oral hairy leukoplakia. The finding of atypical lymphocytes in the peripheral blood is one of the diagnostic hallmarks of EBV (Chapter 121).

6. D The complications of varicella in pregnant women are no more serious than in non-pregnant women. The most severe complication period for the fetus is when the mother develops varicella between 5 days before birth and 2 days after birth. The varicella infection is likely to be disseminated, involving lungs, liver, and brain, with a mortality of about 30%. Varicella-zoster immunoglobulin should be given to a newborn whose mother develops varicella during this time period. Children who develop herpes zoster during the first year of life are not necessarily immunocompromised but probably were exposed to varicella in utero without further sequelae. In adults, the most common complication of varicella is pneumonia. Central nervous complications are quite rare (Chapter 121).

7. (T); **8.** (T); **9.** (T); **10.** (T); **11.** (T) "Blueberry muffin" lesions are dark-blue to violaceous macules or papules that manifest within the first 24 to 48 hours after birth. They are due to the persistence of blood-forming elements in the dermis and can be seen in viral diseases that have an effect on the vascular mesenchyme. They are seen in up to 31% of infants born with the TORCH (toxoplasmosis, syphilis, rubella, cytomegalovirus, herpes) syndrome (Chapter 124).

12. (F); **13.** (T); **14.** (F); **15.** (T); **16.** (T) Fifth disease (erythema infectiosum) is caused by parvovirus B19. It is characterized by reticulated lesions on the extremities and bright red cheeks that have the appearance of having been slapped. The rash can also be morbilliform, confluent, circinate, or annular and occurs during the illness (unlike the rash of human herpesvirus 6, which occurs after the fever drops). The symptoms of the illness include headache, coryza, low-grade fever, and arthralgias. Complications of the virus include aplastic crises, chronic B19 infection in immunocompromised patients, and hydrops fetalis in the fetus of a mother exposed to B19, particularly in the first half of the pregnancy (Chapter 124).

17. (T); **18.** (T); **19.** (T); **20.** (T); **21.** (T) Eczema herpeticum is a widespread infection of the skin with herpes simplex virus. It occurs in patients with chronic skin diseases and has been reported in all of the above conditions. It begins with clusters of umbilicated vesicles that spread widely over a 7- to 10-day course. Treatment with acyclovir is recommended. Because the vesicular lesions coalesce into large erosions, there may be secondary bacterial infection (Chapter 121).

22. (F); **23.** (T); **24.** (T); **25.** (F); **26.** (F) The most common mode of inheritance of epidermodysplasia verruciformis (EV) is autosomal recessive, although X-linked recessive inheritance has been reported. Malignant tumors associated most commonly with human papillomavirus types 5 and 8 develop in areas of sun exposure and trauma (forehead, scalp, and hands). The most common clinical presentation of warts in EV is flat warts. The squamous cell carcinomas associated with EV have not been associated with visceral involvement or lymph node metastases (Chapter 123).

27. B; **28.** B; **29.** B; **30.** A Herpangina is associated with group A Coxsackie viruses. It is characterized by gray-white papules and vesicles on the tonsillar fauces, uvula, and tonsils. In contrast, gingival stomatitis is associated with herpes simplex virus. Lesions occur on the lips, tongue, and buccal mucosa. Children are more severely ill with fever, dysphagia, bleeding gums, and fetid odor of the breath (Chapter 124).

31. C; **32.** C; **33.** D; **34.** A Orf and milker's nodules are caused by viruses in the poxvirus family. Orf is endemic among sheep, goats, and oxen and can be transmitted to humans who handle these animals. Orf is prevalent in the spring when newborn sheep, who have decreased immunity, are infected with the virus. Milker's nodules are seen in persons who handle meat from infected cattle or milk from infected cows. Both viruses usually cause single lesions, although multiple lesions have been reported. With both viruses, the disease advances through six stages. Both diseases are self-limited, not requiring antibiotics unless there is secondary infection (Chapter 122).

35. B; **36.** C; **37.** C; **38.** D The rash of rubella (German measles) disappears after the first 2 to 3 days in contrast to rubeola (measles), which persists for 5 to 6 days. Both rubella and rubeola can manifest with an enanthem of red, pin-sized spots on the soft palate. In rubeola, these spots coalesce to produce a reddened pharynx. Both rashes begin on the head—rubella on the face and rubeola behind the ears and on the forehead. The importance of rubella is that if the fetus is exposed to the virus in the first trimester before completion of organ development, there can be devastating effects (heart disease, mental retardation, nerve deafness, cataracts, and low birth weight (Chapter 124).

39. A; **40.** C; **41.** B; **42.** D; **43.** D The poxvirus family is associated with molluscum contagiosum, orf, variola, and milker's nodules. Rubella is caused by the togavirus. Mumps and measles are caused by paramyxoviruses. The herpesvirus family includes herpes simplex virus, herpes zoster virus, Epstein-Barr virus, cytomegalovirus, human herpesvirus 6 and B virus (herpesvirus simiae). Human herpesvirus 6 was recently shown to be the cause of roseola infantum, a disease seen mostly in children between the ages of 6 months and 2 years (Chapter 122).

44. B *Epidermophyton floccosum* never affects the scalp. It is, however, a common cause of tinea cruris. In culture, it is characterized by numerous, thick-walled, and club-shaped macroconidia without microconidia. In culture, the topography is flat with central folds, the texture is feathery with a slightly powdery center, the surface pigment is bright yellow to dull gray-green with occasional white cottony mutants, and the reverse pigment is yellow to brown (Chapter 118).

45. B Chronic mucocutaneous candidiasis (CMC) is a distinct syndrome in which persistent candidal infection usually involves the mouth, skin, and nails. Although most types of CMC involve the nails, chronic oral candidiasis involves only the mouth. There have been several distinct categories of CMC identified, using genetic and clinical criteria. Autosomal recessive CMC starts in the first decade of life and manifests with oral and nail-plate infections. Autosomal-dominant CMC also occurs in childhood but individuals with this may be more severely affected than those with the recessive variety. Diffuse CMC describes a group of severely affected children without evidence of genetic predisposition. CMC with polyendocrinopathy has an autosomal recessive inheritance pattern and manifests in childhood. However, the candidal infections can precede the endocrine disease by many years. Endocrine problems include hypoparathyroidism, hypoadrenocorticism, hypothyroidism, pernicious anemia, vitiligo, and ovarian dysfunction. Late-onset CMC (no evidence of genetic pattern) presents in adulthood and can be associated with thymoma, myasthenia gravis, esophagitis, aplastic anemia, neutropenia, and hypogammaglobulinemia. Although numerous immunologic defects have been described (primarily involving cell-mediated immunity), 25% to 30% of affected individuals have no detectable immunologic defect (Chapter 119).

46. C Congenital candidiasis manifests at birth or within the first 12 hours and is due to infection in utero. This is a diffuse process that spares the diaper and the perioral areas. The papulovesicular lesions that later desquamate and resolve spontaneously do not indicate dissemination from an immunocompromised state. Fatalities have been reported in newborns with low birth weight and respiratory illness (Chapter 119).

47. C *C. albicans* activates complement by the alternative pathway and induces neutrophilic chemotaxis. This may explain why leukopenia and neutrophilic tissue response can be seen in disseminated candidiasis. The characteristic skin lesions are erythematous papules and/or nodules located on the trunk and extremities. Ecthyma gangrenosum–like lesions have also been described. Pseudohyphae and true hyphae can be seen on histopathology. *C. albicans* can be differentiated from other *Candida* species by the fact that it is germ tube–positive, sucrose assimilation–positive, and can produce chlamydospores on cornmeal agar. *C. albicans* will grow on Sabouraud's agar with antibiotics, unlike *C. tropicalis* (Chapter 119).

48. A Mycetoma is a deforming infectious disease characteristically affecting the feet, although it occasionally affects the back, hands, and shoulders. The hallmark of the disease is swelling, draining sinus tracts, and sulfur granules in the pus from the sinuses. Many organisms can cause mycetoma: eumycotic organisms (true fungi), actinomycotic mycetomas (bacteria), staphylococci, and streptococci.

Pseudallescheria boydii is the most common eumycotic organism to cause mycetoma but it is not acid-fast. *Nocardia,* an actinomycotic mycetoma, is partially acid-fast (Chapters 113 and 120).

49. (T); **50.** (T); **51.** (F); **52.** (F); **53.** (T) When an ultraviolet lamp with a Wood's filter is shone on the hair, fluorescent and nonfluorescent types of dermatophyte infections can be separated and identified. Wood's lamp examination of *Microsporum audouinii, M. canis, M. canis distortum,* and *M. ferugineum* produces a bright green band of fluorescence in the hair. The fluorescence is thought to be caused by ptheridine, a substance produced by the interaction of the growing hair and fungus. *Trichophyton schoenleinii* also fluoresces a dull gray color. *T. tonsurans* typically does not fluoresce (Chapter 118).

54. (F); **55.** (F); **56.** (F); **57.** (T); **58.** (F) Black dot tinea is caused by *T. tonsurans* and *T. violaceum.* This type of tinea can have a variable manifestation; most often there is scaling with minimal hair loss and inflammation, but there can be pustular folliculitis or frank kerion formation. *M. audouinii* was once the most common cause of tinea capitis in North America. The epidemiology has changed recently; *T. tonsurans* now predominates as the most common cause of tinea capitis. Segregation of children with tinea capitis is not necessary once adequate treatment has been instituted.

Adherent yellowish crusts and scales known as scutula are seen in favus, a chronic infection of the scalp that begins in early life and extends into adulthood. It is seen predominantly in rural, poor areas where there are conditions of malnutrition. The most common dermatophyte producing favus is *T. schoenleinii,* although other organisms have also been implicated in this infection (Chapter 118).

59. (F); **60.** (T); **61.** (F); **62.** (F); **63.** (F) The cure rate for fingernails with griseofulvin is 57%; for toenails it is far less (approximately 17%). Although leukopenia has rarely been reported, it is recommended that complete blood counts be obtained at baseline, after 1 month, and then every 3 months in long-term therapy. The exact mechanism of griseofulvin's action is unknown, although it is thought to inhibit fungal RNA, DNA, microtubular assembly, and cell-wall synthesis. Griseofulvin inhibits and therefore decreases the effect of warfarin-type anticoagulants. *Trichophyton rubrum* has been found to be the most common isolate in griseofulvin-resistant dermatophyte infections (Chapter 118).

64. (F); **65.** (T); **66.** (F); **67.** (T); **68.** (T) Cutaneous involvement in disseminated histoplasmosis is unusual except in elderly and immunocompromised patients. The lesions can occur as multiple erythematous papules and plaques resembling a guttate psoriasis pattern. Disseminated histoplasmosis affects the liver most commonly (approximately 80% of patients have evidence of liver disease). Ulceration of the oropharynx and soft palate are described. Neurologic disease is rare. Overt Addison's disease can occur. Histologic examination of the specimen shows parasitized macrophages. Parasitized macrophages are also seen in leishmaniasis, rhinoscleroma and granuloma inguinale. Amphotericin B is the recommended therapeutic agent for disseminated histoplasmosis. In this progressive form of the disease, 80% of patients die within 1 year of the diagnosis without treatment (Chapter 120).

69. A; **70.** C; **71.** A; **72.** D Endothrix and ectothrix refer to the location of arthrospores in or around the hair in tinea capitis; they do not refer to the location of the hyphae. *Trichophyton tonsurans* is an endothrix infection that leaves the hair fragile and causes it to break at its weakest point. Clinically, this infection resembles a black dot, hence the name. Although the majority of ectothrix infections fluoresce, there is only one endothrix infection that fluoresces—*T. schoenleinii*. The three common endothrix infections are *T. tonsurans*, *T. verrucosum,* and *T. schoenleinii*. Hair appears to be most susceptible to ectothrix infections during anagen phase, whereas endothrix infections continue past the anagen phase of the hair cycle into telogen; therefore, endothrix infections tend to lead to more chronic infections (Chapter 118).

73. A; **74.** D; **75.** B; **76.** C Piedra is an infection of the hair shaft. Black piedra is caused by *Piedraia hortae*, and white piedra is caused by *Trichosporon beigelii*. *Phaeoannelomyces wernekii* (previously *Cladosporum wernekii*) is the cause of tinea nigra. Black piedra and white piedra are seen in South America and the Far East. White piedra has been reported in the southern United States, and travel abroad has not been thought to be the source of infection. Both species cause disseminated infections exclusively in immunocompromised hosts (Chapter 117).

77. A; **78.** C; **79.** C; **80.** D Distal subungual onychomycosis is the most common type of onychomycosis and is marked by a brownish-yellow discoloration of the free edge of the nail in distinction to proximal subungual onychomycosis, which starts as a whitish area on the proximal part of the nail plate and is the least common variety of onychomycosis. White superficial onychomycosis affects only the toenails, the most common organism being *Trichophyton mentagrophytes*. Any area of the nail can be affected in white superficial onychomycosis. In *Candida* onychomycosis, the entire nail plate is invaded by the organism, and often there is a surrounding paronychial infection (Chapter 118).

81. C; **82.** A; **83.** B; **84.** D The imidazoles, which include ketoconazole, fluconazole, and itraconazole, inhibit ergosterol synthesis by blocking C14 demethylation. This results in a decrease in ergosterol and accumulation of lanosterol. The newer class of antifungal agents, the allylamines, inhibit squalene epoxidase, an early enzyme in the ergosterol synthesis pathway. Fluconazole and ketoconazole are fungistatic but not fungicidal. The allylamines are both fungistatic and fungicidal. Whereas ketoconazole appears to decrease testosterone plasma concentrations, fluconazole does not have this effect. Fluconazole and itraconazole are absorbed through the blood–brain barrier, but ketoconazole is not absorbed (Chapter 118).

85. B; **86.** C; **87.** D; **88.** A; **89.** E Lobomycosis characteristically manifests with keloidal verrucous lesions. Histologically, there are yeast buds with narrow intercellular connections that resemble a chain of pearls. Chromoblastomycosis is characterized by dark "copper penny" bodies known as medlar bodies. Sporotrichosis demonstrates cigar-shaped yeast (few in number seen on biopsy). Occasionally, asteroid bodies can be noted, but these are not specific to sporotrichosis and can be seen in sarcoidosis. Rhinosporidiosis is marked by large sporangium (350 μmL) filled with sporangiospores. Coccidioidomycosis has a much smaller spherule (30 to 60 μmL), and endospores are all the same size (Chapter 120).

Bibliography

VIRAL INFECTIONS

Belshe RB, ed. Textbook of Human Virology, 2nd edition. St. Louis: Mosby–Year Book, 1991.

Beutner KR. Human papillomavirus infection. J Am Acad Dermatol 1989; 20:114–123.

Cobb MW. Human papillomavirus infection. J Am Acad Dermatol 1990; 22:547–566.

Committee of Infectious Disease of the American Academy of Pediatrics. Red Book of the American Academy of Pediatrics, 22nd ed. Elk Grove Village, IL. 1991.

Darby G et al. Altered substrate specificity of herpes simplex virus: Thymidine kinase confers acyclovir resistance. Nature 1981; 289:81.

Fields JP et al. Hand, foot, and mouth disease. Arch Dermatol 1969; 99:243.

Gershon AA: Chickenpox, measles, and mumps. In: Remington JS, Klein JO, eds. Infectious Diseases of the Fetus and Newborn Infant. 3rd edition. Philadelphia: WB Saunders Co., 1990:140.

Gershon AA et al. Varicella vaccine: The American experience. J Infect Dis 1992; 166:S63.

Greenspan D et al. Oral hairy leukoplakia:human immunodeficiency virus status and risk for development of AIDS. J Infect Dis 1987; 155:474.

Jablonska S, Orth G, eds. Warts/human papillomaviruses. Clin Dermatol 1985; 3:71.

Lesher JL. Cytomegalovirus and the skin. J Am Acad Dermatol 1988; 18:1333.

Liesegang TJ. Diagnosis and therapy of herpes zoster ophthalmicus. Ophthalmology 1991; 98:1216.

Lowe L et al. Gianotti-Crosti syndrome associated with Epstein-Barr virus infection. J Am Acad Dermatol 1989; 20:336.

Miederman JC et al. Infectious mononucleosis: Clinical manifestations in relation to EB virus antibodies. JAMA 1968; 203:205.

Ostrow RS, Manias D, et al. Epidermodysplasia verruciformis. Arch Dermatol 1987; 123:1511–1516.

Risks associated with human parvovirus B19 infection. MMWR 1989; 38:81.

Robbins FC. Measles: Clinical features. Am J Dis Child 1962; 103:266.

Safrin S et al. A controlled trial comparing foscarnet with vidarabine for acyclovir-resistant mucocutaneous herpes simplex in the acquired immunodeficiency syndrome. N Engl J Med 1991; 325:551.

Takahashi K et al: Human herpesvirus-6 and exanthem subitum. Lancet 1988; 1:1463.

Weller TH. Varicella–herpes zoster virus. In: Evans AS, ed. Viral Infections of Man, Epidemiology and Control. 3rd ed. New York: Plenum Press, 1989:659.

FUNGAL INFECTIONS

Balows A et al. Manual of Clinical Microbiology. 5th ed. Washington, DC: American Society for Microbiology, 1991.

Baron R. Onychia and paronychia of mycotic, microbial and parasitic origin. In: Pierre M, ed. The Nail. New York: Churchill Livingstone, 1981:39.

Binazzi M et al. Skin mycoses—geographic distribution and present-day pathomorphosis. Int J Dermatol 1983; 22:92.

Drugs for treatment of deep fungal infections. Med Lett Drugs Ther 1990; 32:50.

Grossman ME et al. Cutaneous manifestations of disseminated candidiasis. J Am Acad Dermatol 1980; 2:111.

Hay RJ. Chronic dermatophyte infections. I. Clinical and mycologic features. Br J Dermatol 1982; 106:1.
Hay RJ, Shennan G: Chronic dermatophyte infections. II. Antibody and cell-mediated immune responses. Br J Dermatol 1982; 106:191.
Hernandez AD. An approach to the diagnosis and therapy of dermatophytosis. Int J Dermatol 1980; 19:540.
Jorizzo JL. Chronic mucocutaneous candidiasis: An update. Arch Dermatol 1982; 118:963.
Millikan LE, Shrum JP: Antifungal agents. In: Wolverton S, Wilkin J, eds. Systemic Drugs for Skin Diseases. Philadelphia: WB Saunders Co., 1991:25.
Ray TL. Candidiasis. In: Stone J, ed. Dermatologic Immunology and Allergy. St. Louis: CV Mosby, 1985:511.
Rippon JW. Medical Mycology: The Pathogenic Fungi and the Pathogenic Actinomycetes. 3rd ed. Philadelphia: WB Saunders Co., 1988.
Wheat LJ. Diagnosis and management of histoplasmosis. Eur J Clin Microbiol Infect Dis 1989; 8:480.
Zaias N. Onychomycosis. Dermatol Clin 1985; 3:445.

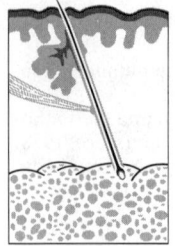

chapter 16

Zoonoses, Protozoal and Helminthic Infections, Bites and Stings

PETER G. EHRNSTROM, and STEVEN R. KOHN

In the following question, the set of lettered headings is followed by a list of numbered words or phrases. For each numbered word or phrase, choose

A. If the item is associated with A only
B. If the item is associated with B only
C. If the item is associated with both A and B
D. If the item is associated with neither A nor B.

1. Spiders from this genus live predominantly in webs
2. Black widow spider
3. Can cause systemic disease in humans
4. Reactions include viscerocutaneous and necrotic cutaneous forms
5. Brown recluse spider.

A. *Latrodectus*
B. *Loxosceles*
C. Both
D. Neither.

Choose the ONE BEST answer to each of the following questions.

6. Vector of cutaneous and visceral leishmaniasis:
    A. *Dermatobia hominis*
    B. Tsetse fly
    C. *Lutzomyia* species
    D. Deer fly (*Chrysops*)
    E. *Phlebotomus* species.

7. Vector of mucocutaneous leishmaniasis:
    A. *Dermatobia hominis*
    B. Tsetse fly
    C. *Lutzomyia* species
    D. Deer fly (*Chrysops*)
    E. *Phlebotomus* species.

8. A 23-year-old college student spent 6 months in Israel during the second semester of her senior college year. On returning, she had a scaly erythematous plaque on her right cheek which was diagnosed as psoriasis and treated with topical steroids. A second physician diagnosed a fungal infection and treated her with a topical antifungal agent. Throughout this 3-month period, the plaque continued to get larger and became slightly indurated. A hypodermic needle was inserted into the adjacent skin, and loosened debris and serum was aspirated. A positive result was obtained by incubation on Nicole-Novy-MacNeal medium. The diagnosis is
    A. Syphilis
    B. Yaws
    C. Leishmaniasis
    D. Pinta
    E. Lepromatous leprosy.

For each numbered item, choose the most likely associated lettered item. Each numbered item has ONLY ONE answer. Each lettered item may be the answer to one, more than one, or none of the numbered items.

9. *Leishmania braziliensis braziliensis*
10. *Leishmania mexicana*
11. *Leishmania tropica*
12. *Leishmania donovani.*

A. Kala azar
B. Mucocutaneous leishmaniasis
C. Cutaneous leishmaniasis.

Choose the ONE BEST answer to each of the following questions.

13. Transformation of the promastigote of *Leishmania* spp. into their amastigotic form takes place in the
    A. Human macrophage
    B. Fly-vector proboscis
    C. Human endothelial cells
    D. Fly-vector gut
    E. Human keratinocyte.

14. The main drug group used to treat leishmaniasis is
    A. Systemic imidazoles
    B. Topical imidazoles
    C. Aureal agents (gold)
    D. Antimonials
    E. Fluoroquinolones.

15. Eggs from this species are excreted in the urine of infected humans:
    A. *Schistosoma mansoni*
    B. *Schistosoma japonicum*
    C. *Wuchereria bancrofti*
    D. *Schistosoma haematobium*
    E. *Trypanosoma cruzi.*

For each numbered item, choose the most likely associated lettered item. Each numbered item has ONLY ONE answer. Each lettered item may be the answer to one, more than one, or none of the numbered items.

16. *Schistosoma haematobium*
17. *Schistosoma japonicum*
18. *Schistosoma mansoni.*

A. Prominent terminal spine
B. Prominent lateral spine
C. Vestigial spine.

Choose the ONE BEST answer to each of the following questions.

19. This is likely caused by an immune response to acute schistosomal infection:
    A. Oroya fever
    B. Dengue fever
    C. Katayama fever
    D. Mediterranean fever
    E. Tertian fever.

20. A 64-year-old man has returned from Costa Rica, where he spent 3 weeks in the jungle cataloguing bird species. He presents with seven painful, red, subcutaneous nodules on his back. Each of these nodules has a central punctum. Incision of one of these lesions reveals a live maggot. The diagnosis is
    A. Tumbu fly myiasis
    B. New World leishmaniasis
    C. Tungiasis
    D. Botfly myiasis
    E. Old World leishmaniasis.

21. The botfly is
    A. *Dermatobia hominis*
    B. *Latrodectus mactans*
    C. The tsetse fly
    D. The *Phlebotomus* sand fly
    E. *Simulium damnosum.*

For the following questions ONE or MORE of the following completions may correctly finish the incomplete statement; choose

A. If only 1, 2, and 3 are correct
B. If only 1 and 3 are correct
C. If only 2 and 4 are correct
D. If only 4 is correct
E. If all are correct.

22. Effective treatments for botfly myiasis include
    1. Excision
    2. Intralesional corticosteroids
    3. Oil occlusion
    4. Extracorporeal photopheresis.

23. It may cause cutaneous larva migrans:
    1. *Ancylostoma braziliense*
    2. *Dracunculus medinensis* (the Guinea worm)

3. *Bubostomum phlebotomum*

4. *Schistosoma mansoni.*

24. Effective treatments of cutaneous larva migrans include

    1. Oral beta-lactams
    2. Topical thiabendazole
    3. Ivermectin
    4. Oral thiabendazole.

25. Cutaneous manifestations of infection with *Onchocerca volvulus* may include

    1. Papular urticaria
    2. Lichenification
    3. Diffuse atrophy
    4. Widespread depigmentation.

26. Which of the following drugs is effective in treating onchocerciasis?

    1. Erythromycin
    2. Itraconazole
    3. Ethambutol
    4. Ivermectin.

Choose the ONE BEST answer to each of the following questions.

27. The head louse is a subspecies of

    A. *Phthirus pubis*
    B. *Pediculus humanus*
    C. *Rickettsia rickettsii*
    D. *Rochalimaea quintana*
    E. *Loxosceles rufescens*

28. Pruritic papules around the umbilicus, areolae, and penis suggest the diagnosis of

    A. Leishmaniasis
    B. Pityriasis rosea
    C. *Sarcoptes spp.* infection
    D. Botfly myiasis
    E. *Strongyloides spp.* infection.

29. A patient with a spinal injury at C4 develops 5-cm crusted plaques on the dorsa of his hands. Histologic examination shows numerous mites in the stratum corneum. The diagnosis is

    A. Infection by *Dracunculus medinensis*
    B. *Pityrosporon* folliculitis
    C. Erythema migrans
    D. Psoriasis vulgaris
    E. Norwegian scabies.

30. A patient presents with pruritic, erythematous macules and papules under the area covered by her bathing suit. She had been swimming in Long Island Sound the day before this visit. Samples of ocean water from the area show numerous 2- to 3-mm pink, round and oval, ciliated larvae which, in the laboratory, metamorphosed into the adult sea anemone *Edwardsiella lineata*. The most likely diagnosis in this patient is

    A. Seabather's eruption
    B. Contact dermatitis to laundry detergent
    C. Contact dermatitis to bathing suit material
    D. Swimmer's itch
    E. Clammer's itch.

31. All of the following statements regarding the most likely diagnosis in this patient are true EXCEPT

    A. This condition usually becomes chronic unless prompt treatment is administered
    B. Topical steroid preparations may offer symptomatic relief
    C. This condition can be prevented by rinsing with fresh water directly after swimming
    D. Distribution of the lesions on the skin is helpful in making the diagnosis
    E. *Edwardsiella spp.* have been implicated as causative agents in this eruption.

32. A 21-year-old woman student returns from a trip to Brazil complaining of a new painful lesion on the left sole. On examination, there is a 7-mm erythematous nodule with a central black punctum. Evacuation of the nodule reveals a 2-mm arthropod whose abdomen is swollen with eggs. The diagnosis is

    A. *Strongyloides stercoralis* infection
    B. Tropical leishmaniasis
    C. Tumbu fly myiasis
    D. Norwegian scabies
    E. Tungiasis.

For the following questions ONE or MORE of the following completions may correctly finish the incomplete statements; choose

A. If only 1, 2, and 3 are correct
B. If only 1 and 3 are correct

C. If only 2 and 4 are correct
D. If only 4 is correct
E. If all are correct.

33. Use of lindane in children is controversial. Which of the following is (are) contraindications to the use of lindane in children?
    1. Atopic dermatitis
    2. Congenital nevi
    3. Pityriasis rubra pilaris
    4. Plantar warts.

34. Chagas' disease may be transmitted
    1. Transplacentally
    2. Through blood transfusions
    3. Through donated organs
    4. By triatomine insects.

Choose the ONE BEST answer to each of the following questions.

35. The causative agent of Chagas' disease is
    A. *Dracunculus medinensis*
    B. *Trypanosoma cruzi*
    C. *Schistosoma hominis*
    D. *Strongyloides stercoralis*
    E. *Yersinia pestis*.

36. The main form of transmission of the etiologic organism of Chagas' disease to humans is through mucosal or parenteral contact with
    A. *Sarcoptes spp.* feces
    B. *Phlebotomus spp.* saliva
    C. *Phthirus spp.* saliva
    D. Reduviid bug feces
    E. *Simulium spp.* saliva.

37. The "Romaña sign" refers to
    A. Periumbilical purpura and unilateral inguinal lymphadenopathy
    B. Transient cranial nerve VII palsy
    C. Unilateral periorbital swelling, erythema, and preauricular lymphadenopathy
    D. Macroglossia and unilateral nasal mucosal edema
    E. Unilateral palpable perineural swellings.

For the following questions ONE or MORE of the following completions may correctly finish the incomplete statements; choose

A. If only 1, 2, and 3 are correct
B. If only 1 and 3 are correct
C. If only 2 and 4 are correct
D. If only 4 is correct
E. If all are correct.

38. Vector(s) of bancroftian filariasis is (are)
    1. *Culex*
    2. *Aedes*
    3. *Anopheles*
    4. *Latrodectus*.

39. Vector(s) of brugian filariasis is (are)
    1. *Aedes*
    2. *Mansonia*
    3. *Latrodectus*
    4. *Anopheles*.

Choose the ONE BEST answer to each of the following questions.

40. The microfilaria in *Wuchereria bancrofti* and *Brugia spp.* infections are found in the blood in greatest numbers
    A. Between 8 A.M. and 12 P.M.
    B. Between 12 P.M. and 5 P.M.
    C. Between 5 A.M. and 8 A.M.
    D. Between 9 P.M. and 2 A.M.
    E. During all daylight hours.

41. Calabar (transient subcutaneous) swellings are caused by
    A. *Loa loa*
    B. *Onchocerca volvulus*
    C. *Wuchereria bancrofti*
    D. *Brugia timori*
    E. *Enterobius vermicularis*.

42. A 60-year-old man born in Ecuador had been treated for 7 years for asthma with many courses of systemic corticosteroids. He was admitted to the hospital for respiratory distress, and intravenous methylprednisolone was started. Three days later, he had a respiratory arrest and was intubated. Two days after that, he was noted to have reticulated, periumbilical purpura which resembled many thumbprints on the abdomen. This eruption subse-

quently spread to his thighs and flanks. The most likely diagnosis is

A. Drug eruption to the methylprednisolone
B. Hyperinfection with *Strongyloides stercoralis*
C. Cutaneous *Mycobacterium avium-intracellulare* (MAI)
D. Giardiasis
E. Onchocerciasis.

ANSWERS

1. A; **2.** A; **3.** C; **4.** B; **5.** B Two types of spiders are of medical importance in North America—*Latrodectus* species (widow spiders) and *Loxosceles* species (recluse spiders).

The female black widow spider (*L. mactans*) bites humans. It spins a web, has a 1-cm diameter body, a 5-cm leg span, and has a red hour-glass mark on its abdomen. The bite may cause transient stinging, but severe local reactions are uncommon. The major effects are systemic, with diffuse central and peripheral nervous system excitation. Severe abdominal cramping, hypertension, nausea, vomiting, headache, and death due to cardiac and respiratory failure have all been reported.

Although *Loxosceles reclusa* (the brown recluse) is the most infamous of this genus, at least six species of *Loxosceles* spiders have been reported to cause human disease in North America. They are yellow to brown in color, approximately 10 to 15 mm in body size, have a classic violin or fiddle pattern on the dorsum of their cephalothorax, and do not spin webs. The bite of this spider may cause either necrotic cutaneous or viscerocutaneous disease. Locally, there may be extensive ischemic necrosis and secondary infection. Systemically, fevers, myalgias, disseminated intravascular coagulation, acute renal failure, and hemolysis may occur. Deaths from the bites of *Loxosceles* spiders have been reported and usually occur in children (Chapter 92).

6. E; **7.** C; **8.** C; **9.** B; **10.** C; **11.** C; **12.** A; **13.** A; **14.** D Leishmaniasis refers to different forms of disease caused in humans by *Leishmania* species. Cutaneous leishmaniasis is caused primarily by *L. tropica* (Old World leishmaniasis) and subspecies of *L. mexicana* (New World leishmaniasis). One subspecies of *L. braziliensis, L. braziliensis peruviana,* may also cause a form of cutaneous leishmaniasis called "uta." Mucocutaneous leishmaniasis, also called espundia, is caused primarily by *L. braziliensis braziliensis.* Visceral leishmaniasis (kala azar) is caused by *L. donovani.* The vector of the visceral and cutaneous forms of this disease is the phlebotomine sand fly, and mucocutaneous disease is transmitted to humans by way of *Lutzomyia* fly species.

The life cycle of *Leishmania* spp. begins as the infected sand fly bites the human. It deposits the promastigotes into the bite. These flagellate forms are quickly taken up by macrophages. Here the promastigote transforms into the amastigote. Lysis of the macrophage releases the amastigotes to other macrophages and also to either dermal cells or mucous membranes, depending on the type of disease. Finally, the amastigote is ingested by the sand fly again where it is retransformed to the promastigote.

Diagnosis is made by the identification of leptomonads by culture of material aspirated from perilesional skin incubated on Nicole-Novy-MacNeal medium at 22 to 35° C. The mainstay in treatment of leishmaniasis is antimonial agents (Chapter 92).

15. D; **16.** A; **17.** C; **18.** B; **19.** C Schistosomiasis is caused mainly by three *Schistosoma* species—*S. mansoni, S. japonicum,* and *S. haematobium.* Humans become infected after contact with water that contains the free-swimming, infective stage of the schistosome, called a cercaria. These cercariae penetrate intact skin. After 2 to 3 days there, the parasites migrate to the lungs and then through the portal vein to the intestines, bladder, or ureters, depending on the species. After another 4 to 9 weeks, the schistosomes begin to lay eggs that are then excreted back into water supplies in which they quickly become miracidia. The life cycle is completed in the soft tissues of snails in the water, where the miracidia mature into the free-swimming cercaria.

Acutely, patients may develop a strong immune response to the schistosomes. This response may include fever, chills, headache, angioedema, and diarrhea and is called Katayama fever. With *S. mansoni* and *S. japonicum,* the liver and mesentery are the primary sites of infection, as the eggs are shed through the feces. Individuals infected with *S. haematobium* shed eggs through the urine, since the bladder and ureters are the targets of this species.

Identification of the specific *Schistosoma* species can be made by examination of the morphology of the ova. *S. mansoni* eggs are oval, with dimensions of 114 to 175 microns in length and 45 to 68 microns in width. They have a prominent lateral spine. *S. haematobium* ova are approximately the same size but have prominent terminal spines. Finally, *S. japonicum* ova are slightly smaller and have only a vestigial spine (Chapter 127).

20. D; **21.** A; **22.** B *Dermatobia hominis,* the botfly, is found in the tropical regions of South, Central, and North America. The adult female botfly lays her eggs on the abdomens of other biting insects. They, in turn, deposit the eggs in the human host during the blood meal. These eggs hatch, and the maggot grows for 4 to 6 weeks in the dermis of the infected human, creating the botfly boil. Eventually, the maggot crawls out of the human host, pupates, and flies away.

Many methods have been proposed for extracting the maggot from the skin. Occlusion with oil, honey, chewing gum, and pork fat (among others) may cause the larva literally to come out for air. Simple surgical excision is also effective. There is no role for intralesional steroids or extracorporeal photopheresis (Chapter 92).

23. B Cutaneous larva migrans (creeping eruption, plumber's itch, duckhunter's itch) may be caused by many parasitic larvae. The characteristic feature of the lesion is its migratory nature as the larvae slowly move through the skin. Many hookworms such as *Ancylostoma braziliense, A. caninum, A. ceylonicum, Uncinaria stenocephala,* and *Bubostomum phlebotomum* may cause cutaneous larva migrans. *Strongyloides stercoralis* may cause a similar eruption called larva currens.

Dracunculus medinensis and *Schistosoma mansoni* do not cause cutaneous larva migrans (Chapter 127).

24. C; **25.** E; **26.** D Although the introduction of ivermectin as the primary treatment of onchocerciasis has made a significant impact on this disease, infection with *Onchocerca volvulus* remains a major health concern for much of the population of tropical Africa and Central and South America. Onchocerciasis continues to be a major cause of blindness, especially in Africa (river blindness). Cutaneous manifestations of infection with *O. volvulus* include granulomatous dermal nodules containing adult worms and microfilaria, papular urticaria, lichenification, atrophy, and depigmentation. Diagnosis is usually made by physical examination, but skin snippings can also show microfilaria under the microscope (Chapter 127).

27. B The head louse is a subspecies of *Pediculus humanus—P. humanus capitis* (Chapter 128).

28. C; **29.** E Probably because of their predilection for pilosebaceous follicles, *Sarcoptes scabiei*-infected lesions are common in the groin, around the umbilicus, and around the areolae. Crusted, or Norwegian, scabies refers to infection with this same organism but in much higher numbers. Often, patients who develop this form of the infection have a sensory loss, are demented, mentally retarded, or are immunosuppressed (Chapter 128).

30. A; **31.** A This is a classic description of seabather's eruption. For comparison, swimmer's itch or clammer's itch (cutaneous cercarial infection) lesions are found on uncovered skin. Both conditions are usually self-limited and may be prevented or diminished by prompt "rinsing off" after swimming (Chapter 90).

32. E *Tunga penetrans,* a sand flea, is the causative agent of tungiasis. Infection occurs when the impregnated female burrows her way into the foot pad of a large mammal, such as a human or pig. An inflammatory nodule with a central black punctum is the commonest cutaneous lesion. Removal is accomplished by curettage and cautery (Chapter 92).

33. B Use of lindane in the treatment of scabies in children has been associated with grand mal seizures as well as cases of aplastic anemia. Underlying skin conditions such as atopic dermatitis, psoriasis, and pityriasis rubra pilaris may increase the cutaneous absorption of lindane, thereby increasing toxicity (Chapter 128).

34. E; **35.** B; **36.** D; **37.** C Chagas' disease (American trypanosomiasis) is caused by *Trypanosoma cruzi.* This disease is endemic to Latin America and, since the 1970s, has been seen in increasing incidence in the United States (probably because of increased immigration from these areas). The protozoan parasite *T. cruzi* is passed to humans by mucosal contact with the feces of triatomine insects (reduviid bugs) that contain the infective organisms. Local amplification of these organisms gives way to their release into the circulation, where they may be ingested when the reduviid bug takes its meal from the infected human, thus completing the cycle. Transmission of *T. cruzi* has also been reported to occur through blood transfusions, transplacentally, and through donated organs.

Only one third of acutely infected individuals have clinical manifestations. Initially, there may be an intense local inflammatory reaction at the site of inoculation. An erythematous nodule called a chagoma appears within 1 to 3 weeks. There may also be a transient, generalized morbilliform or urticarial eruption at this point. If the site of initial infection is the conjunctiva, unilateral palpebral edema, painless conjunctivitis, and preauricular lymphadenopathy (Romaña's sign) may be present. Acute Chagas' disease is usually a mild illness, but the patient may go on to have chronic recurring disease; meningoencephalitis and severe heart disease, causing death, do occur, and the immunocompromised patient is at highest risk for these complications.

The best treatment for Chagas' disease is good prevention by the use of insecticides in homes in endemic areas, since there is no satisfactory pharmaceutical agent against the parasite once infection has occurred (Chapter 127).

38. A; **39.** C; **40.** D Filariasis refers to a group of diseases in humans caused by infestations with the nematodes in the superfamily Filarioides. The microfilaria are passed from the arthropod vectors into the next host during the arthropod's blood meal. *Culex, Aedes,* and *Anopheles* species are the vectors of *Wuchereria bancrofti,* and *Mansonia, Anopheles,* and *Coquillettidia* are vectors for *Brugia malayi* and *Brugia timori.* The microfilaria are found in the blood of infected individuals in greatest numbers between 9 P.M. and 2 A.M.—the best time to draw blood samples for diagnostic purposes (Chapter 127).

41. A Loiasis is caused by *Loa loa.* This organism may cause elephantiasis of extremities as a result of lymphatic occlusion and also may cause transient subcutaneous nodules called Calabar swellings (Chapter 127).

42. B The "thumbprint sign" has been described in patients with hyperinfection with *Strongyloides stercoralis.* All of the case reports have been of patients on ventilator assistance who have had a history of immunosuppression (usually with systemic corticosteroids). Skin biopsies of lesional skin in these patients show multiple larvae at all levels of the dermis and the subcutis (Chapter 127).

Bibliography

Bank DE, Grossman ME, Kohn SR, et al. The thumbprint sign: Rapid diagnosis of disseminated strongyloidiasis. J Am Acad Dermatol 1990; 2:324–326.

Champion RH, Burton JL, Ebling FJG, eds. Rook/Wilkinson/Ebling Textbook of Dermatology. 5th edition. Oxford: Blackwell Scientific Publications, 1992.

Ehrnstrom PG. Myiasis in a birdwatcher. Presented at Gross and Microscopic Symposium, American Academy of Dermatology 51st Annual Meeting, San Francisco, December 4–10, 1992.

Freudenthal AR, Joseph PR. Seabather's eruption. N Engl J Med 1993; 329:542–544.

Kirchoff LV. American trypanosomiasis (Chagas' disease)—a tropical disease now in the United States. N Engl J Med 1993; 392:639–644.

Wilson JD, Braunwald E, Isselbacher KJ, eds. Harrison's Principles of Internal Medicine. 12th edition. New York: McGraw-Hill, 1991.

section six

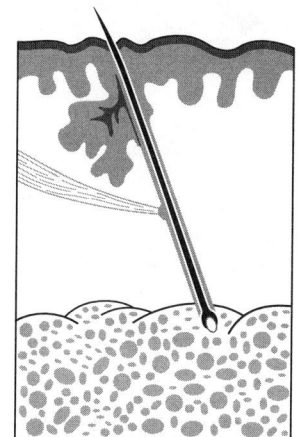

What Diseases Alter Skin Color, Hair, Nails, Sweat Glands, and Mucous Membranes?

chapter 17

Disorders of Pigmentation and Pigment Cell Biology

FRANK PINTO, and JEAN BOLOGNIA

ALBINISM AND OTHER DISORDERS OF HYPOPIGMENTATION

Choose the ONE BEST answer to each of the following questions:

1. Autoimmune endocrine disorders associated with vitiligo include all of the following EXCEPT

    A. Graves' disease

    B. Cushing's disease

    C. Hashimoto's thyroiditis

    D. Pernicious anemia

    E. Addison's disease.

2. In patients with vitiligo, which of the following areas would be LEAST likely to respond to psoralen plus UVA (PUVA) photochemotherapy?

    A. Fingers

    B. Face

    C. Trunk

    D. Elbow

    E. Dorsal hand.

3. A 40-year-old woman has depigmented patches on the upper back within which are perifollicular macules of normal pigmentation (Figure 17-1).* The underlying skin is indurated. This is most likely due to

    A. PUVA therapy

    B. Spontaneously repigmenting vitiligo

    C. Scleroderma

    D. Chemical leukoderma

    E. Melanoma-associated leukoderma.

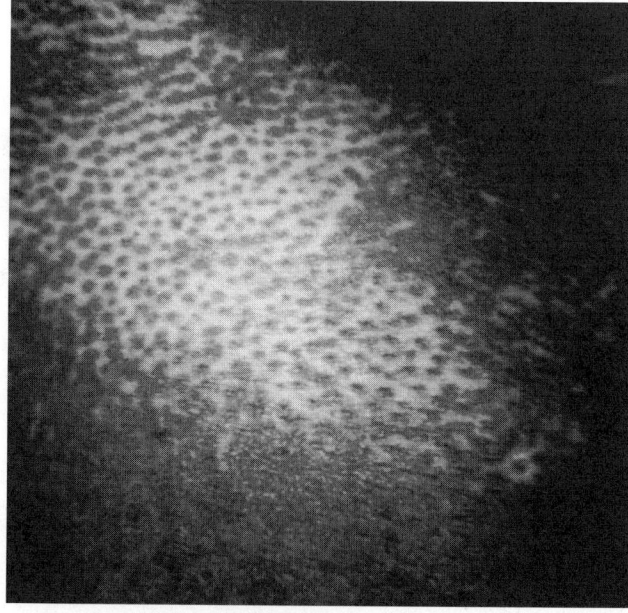

---

* From Yale Residents' Slide Collection.

4. A 60-year-old man has hypopigmented patches on the trunk. Skin biopsy shows an absence of melanocytes. The differential diagnosis includes all of the following EXCEPT
   A. Scleroderma
   B. Leukoderma associated with metastatic melanoma
   C. Piebaldism
   D. Tinea versicolor
   E. Vitiligo.

5. All of the following can cause chemical leukoderma EXCEPT
   A. Phenols
   B. Catechols
   C. Hydroquinones
   D. Mercaptoamines
   E. Aldehydes.

In the following questions, for each numbered item, choose the most likely associated lettered item. Each numbered item has ONLY ONE answer. Each lettered item may be the answer to one, more than one, or none of the numbered items.

6. Vitiligo
7. Piebaldism
8. Nevus depigmentosus
9. Ash-leaf spot of tuberous sclerosis
10. Hypomelanosis of Ito
11. Nevus anemicus.

A. Borders obscured by diascopy
B. Associated with chronic mucocutaneous candidiasis
C. Favors mid portions of extremities
D. Occurs in approximately 1 in 150 newborns
E. Associated with fibrous plaque on forehead
F. Associated with chromosomal mosaicism.

Choose the ONE BEST answer to each of the following questions:

12. Features of Waardenburg's syndrome include all of the following EXCEPT
    A. Dystopia canthorum
    B. Sensorineural hearing loss
    C. Fusion of medial eyebrows
    D. Uveitis
    E. Heterochrome irides.

13. The earliest manifestation of tuberous sclerosis is
    A. Adenoma sebaceum
    B. Connective tissue nevi
    C. Ash-leaf spots
    D. Lisch nodules
    E. Gingival fibromas.

14. The most common configuration for ash-leaf spots is
    A. Lance-ovate
    B. Polygonal
    C. Segmental
    D. Confetti-like
    E. Sworled.

15. Electron microscopic examination of ash-leaf spots reveals
    A. Absence of melanocytes
    B. Giant melanosomes
    C. Small, poorly melanized melanosomes
    D. Absence of melanosomes in keratinocytes
    E. Normal melanosomes.

16. A disorder that has an autosomal recessive inheritance pattern is
    A. Tuberous sclerosis
    B. Piebaldism
    C. Nevus depigmentosus
    D. Hypomelanosis of Ito
    E. Oculocutaneous albinism.

17. Cutaneous features of tuberous sclerosis include all of the following EXCEPT
    A. Sebaceous adenomas
    B. Facial angiofibromas
    C. Connective tissue nevi
    D. Periungual fibromas
    E. Poliosis.

In the following question, for each numbered item, choose the most likely associated lettered item. Each numbered item has ONLY ONE answer. Each lettered item may be the answer to one, more than one, or none of the numbered items.

18. Goltz' syndrome
19. Piebaldism

A. Autosomal dominant
B. Autosomal recessive

20. Nevus depigmentosus
21. Tuberous sclerosis
22. Most common form of ocular albinism.

C. X-linked dominant
D. X-linked recessive
E. No distinct inheritance pattern.

C. Schistosomiasis
D. Loiasis
E. Dracunculosis.

Choose the ONE BEST answer to each of the following questions:

23. Which of the following may manifest with hypopigmentation?
    A. Pityriasis lichenoides chronica
    B. Cutaneous T-cell lymphoma
    C. Sarcoidosis
    D. Lichen striatus
    E. All of the above.

24. Treatment options for patients with vitiligo include
    A. 20% monobenzyl ether of hydroquinone
    B. Psoralen plus UVA (PUVA) photochemotherapy
    C. Topical corticosteroids
    D. Autografts
    E. All of the above.

25. An 18-year-old Asian woman presents with headache, neck stiffness, dysacousis, and photophobia. She later develops depigmented areas of skin and hair. The most likely diagnosis is
    A. Waardenburg's syndrome
    B. Woolf's syndrome
    C. Vogt-Koyanagi-Harada syndrome
    D. Ziprkowski-Margolis syndrome
    E. Hermansky-Pudlak syndrome.

26. The differential diagnosis of hypopigmentation that follows Blaschko's lines includes all of the following EXCEPT
    A. Incontinentia pigmenti
    B. Goltz' syndrome
    C. Hypomelanosis of Ito
    D. Piebaldism
    E. Nevus depigmentosus.

27. Which of the following is characterized by skin depigmentation?
    A. Filariasis
    B. Onchocerciasis

In the following question, for each numbered item, choose the most likely associated lettered item. Each numbered item has ONLY ONE answer. Each lettered item may be the answer to one, more than one, or none of the numbered items.

28. Hermansky-Pudlak syndrome
29. Chédiak-Higashi syndrome
30. Griscelli's syndrome
31. Menkes' syndrome
32. Prader-Willi syndrome
33. Phenylketonuria.

A. Thrombocytopenia and silvery hair, but no macromelanosomes
B. Giant lysosomal granules in granulocytes
C. Interstitial lung fibrosis and absence of platelet-dense granules
D. Low serum ceruloplasmin
E. Eczematous dermatitis
F. Hypogonadism.

Choose the ONE BEST answer to each of the following questions:

34. Genetic studies in human piebaldism have shown
    A. Mutations in the *steel* locus
    B. Mutations of the tyrosinase gene
    C. Autosomal recessive inheritance
    D. Deletions in the *KIT* proto-oncogene
    E. Mosaicism.

35. The differential diagnosis of scalp poliosis includes all of the following EXCEPT
    A. Tuberous sclerosis
    B. Halo nevus
    C. Chédiak-Higashi syndrome
    D. Vogt-Koyanagi-Harada syndrome
    E. Waardenburg's syndrome.

In the following questions, decide whether EACH choice is TRUE or FALSE. Any combination of answers from all true to all false may occur.

36. Diagnostic criteria for the tuberous sclerosis complex include
    A. Calcified subependymal nodule

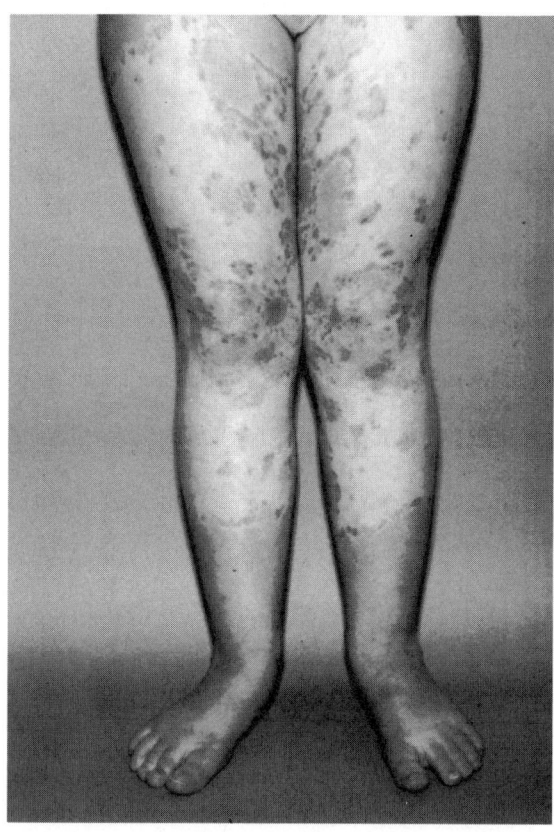

B. Renal angiomyolipoma
C. Pheochromocytoma
D. Cardiac rhabdomyoma
E. Acoustic schwannoma.

37. Findings that have been associated with the disorder seen in Figure 17–2* include
    A. Hirschsprung's disease
    B. Hyperthyroidism
    C. Upper limb defects
    D. Café au lait macules
    E. Deafness.

38. Associated findings in the Hermansky-Pudlak syndrome include
    A. Prolonged bleeding time
    B. Interstitial fibrosis seen on chest x-ray film
    C. Granulomatous colitis
    D. Thrombocytopenia
    E. Absence of granules in platelets.

---

*From Bolognia JL. Disorders of hypopigmentation. Current Concepts Skin Disorders, Winter 1992–1993; 13:11.

39. The differential diagnosis of multiple guttate hypomelanotic macules includes
    A. Tuberous sclerosis
    B. Darier's disease
    C. Pityriasis lichenoides chronica
    D. Side effect of PUVA therapy
    E. Lichen sclerosis et atrophicus.

40. In patients with leprosy lesions that frequently manifest with hypopigmentation include
    A. Tuberculoid leprosy
    B. Erythema nodosum leprosum
    C. Borderline lepromatous leprosy
    D. Lepromatous leprosy
    E. Indeterminant leprosy.

DISORDERS OF HYPERPIGMENTATION AND PIGMENT CELL BIOLOGY

Choose the ONE BEST answer to each of the following questions:

41. The key enzyme in the melanin biosynthetic pathway is tyrosinase. What metal does it require for its enzymatic activity?
    A. Iron
    B. Silver
    C. Gold
    D. Copper
    E. Arsenic.

42. The fact that tyrosinase depends on this metal for its activity explains the pigmentary findings in what disease?
    A. Hemochromatosis
    B. Argyria
    C. Chrysiasis
    D. Menkes' kinky hair syndrome
    E. Chronic arsenic intoxication.

In the following questions, for each numbered item, choose the most likely associated lettered item. Each numbered item has ONLY ONE answer. Within each group, each lettered item may be the answer to one, more than one, or none of the numbered items.

Ingestion of certain drugs can result in discoloration of the skin; the clinical findings are listed in questions 43 to 47, and the associated histologic findings are listed in questions 48 to 52.

43. Vitamin B$_{12}$
44. Chlorpromazine
45. Gold
46. Clofazimine
47. Silver.

A. Red-brown to dark brown hyperpigmentation; predilection for lesional skin
B. Slate-gray pigmentation
C. Blue-gray to brown discoloration, especially around the eyes
D. Tan or slate-gray pigmentation, especially in sun-exposed areas; phototoxicity plays a role
E. None of the above.

48. Trimethoprim-sulfamethoxazole
49. Minocycline
50. Amiodarone
51. Clofazimine
52. Silver.

A. Ceroid-lipofuscin deposits in macrophages
B. Granules that stain positive for iron distributed within macrophages
C. Granules in the basement membrane zone (BMZ) of sweat glands
D. Melanophages
E. None of the above.

For the following questions, a set of lettered items accompanies a list of numbered words or phrases. For each numbered word or phrase, choose

A. If the item is associated with A only
B. If the item is associated with B only
C. If the item is associated with both A and B
D. If the item is associated with neither A nor B.

For each of the following characteristics, choose whether it describes macular amyloidosis, notalgia paresthetica, both, or neither.

53.
i. Contains dermal deposits composed of immunoglobulin light chains
ii. Associated with pruritus
iii. Patients should be screened for autoimmune polyendocrinopathy, e.g., Addison's disease
iv. Contains dermal deposits of keratin proteins
v. Common location is the upper back.

A. Macular amyloidosis
B. Notalgia paresthetica
C. Both
D. Neither.

For each of the following characteristics, choose whether it describes linear and whorled nevoid hypermelanosis, incontinentia pigmenti, both, or neither.

54.
i. X-linked dominant
ii. Associated with ectodermal dysplasias (e.g., hair, nails)
iii. Streaks of hyperpigmentation along the lines of Blaschko
iv. Hyperpigmentation is due to increased melanin content of the basal layer
v. May be manifestation of chromosomal mosaicism.

A. Linear and whorled nevoid hypermelanosis
B. Incontinentia pigmenti
C. Both
D. Neither.

For each of the following characteristics, choose whether it describes Dowling-Degos disease, confluent and reticulated papillomatosis of Gougerot and Carteaud, both, or neither.

55.
i. Autosomal dominant inheritance pattern
ii. Associated with perioral scars
iii. Reticulated hyperpigmentation of the inframammary regions
iv. Women are more commonly affected
v. Biopsy specimens demonstrate changes similar to acanthosis nigricans.

A. Dowling-Degos disease
B. Confluent and reticulated papillomatosis of Gougerot and Carteaud
C. Both
D. Neither.

DISORDERS OF PIGMENTATION AND PIGMENT CELL BIOLOGY

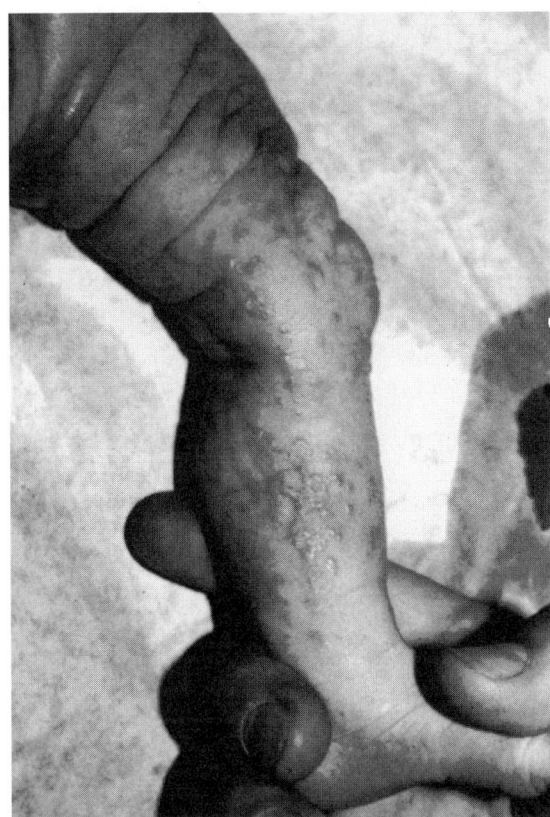

63. There are more stage IV melanosomes in tan-colored skin compared with black skin.
64. The keratinocytes in tan-colored skin are less efficient at engulfing melanosomes.
65. The turnover time of the epidermis is greater in black skin.

Decide whether EACH of the following statements regarding the clinical evaluation of melasma is TRUE or FALSE.

66. In a patient with melasma and skin type III, enhancement of the color contrast under Wood's lamp examination is a reflection of an increased number of melanophages in the dermis.
67. In a patient with melasma and skin type III, enhancement of the color contrast under Wood's lamp examination is a reflection of an increase in the melanin content of the epidermis.
68. In a patient with melasma and skin type III, no accentuation of color contrast is seen when there is an associated increase in the melanin content of the epidermis.
69. The most common form of melasma is mixed (epidermal and dermal).
70. The most common pattern for melasma is centrofacial.

Decide whether EACH of the following statements is TRUE or FALSE. Any combination of answers from all true to all false may occur.

Decide whether each of the following statements about the mother of the newborn in Figure 17–3* is true or false.

56. Her mouth should be examined to look for conical teeth.
57. It is likely that she had a papulovesicular eruption during the first trimester of pregnancy.
58. It is likely that she had a papulosquamous eruption during the first trimester of pregnancy.
59. A lacy pattern of hypopigmentation on her calves may be the only cutaneous finding.
60. A serum VDRL test should be done.

Decide whether EACH of the following statements regarding skin color differences is TRUE or FALSE.

61. The melanosomes in black skin are larger in size than in light tan skin.
62. The number of melanocytes/mm² is greater in black skin than in light tan skin.

Decide whether EACH of the following questions is TRUE or FALSE. Any combination of answers from all true to all false may occur.

71. Side effects of minocycline include the following:
    A. Diffuse blue-gray or muddy discoloration, especially of sun-exposed skin
    B. Gray or gray-green discoloration of permanent teeth in adults
    C. Blue to gray macules on the lower extremities
    D. Blue-black macules within scars or sites of inflammation
    E. Depigmentation of the hair.

72. Patients with erythema dyschromicum perstans can have
    A. A proliferation of melanocytes in the epidermis
    B. Unilateral distribution
    C. Lesions with an erythematous, raised border
    D. Slate-gray macules and patches on the head, neck, and upper torso
    E. Lesions that follow skin cleavage lines.

---
* From Yale Residents' Slide Collection.

73. Dyskeratosis congenita is characterized by reticulated hyperpigmentation and nail dystrophy as well as
    A. Epiphora
    B. Pancytopenia
    C. X-linked dominant inheritance
    D. Autosomal recessive inheritance
    E. Mucosal squamous cell carcinomas.

74. Pigmentary demarcation lines are seen
    A. In less than 30% of individuals with black skin
    B. Most commonly on the upper anterior arm and the midback
    C. In at least 60% of individuals with black skin
    D. Most commonly on the upper anterior arm and posteromedial portion of the leg
    E. Most commonly on the anterior abdomen.

In the following questions, ONE or MORE of the following completions correctly finishes the incomplete statement; choose

    A. If only 1, 2, and 3 are correct
    B. If only 1 and 3 are correct
    C. If only 2 and 4 are correct
    D. If only 4 is correct
    E. If all are correct.

75. Bilateral macular hyperpigmentation of the malar region is seen in
    1. Exogenous ochronosis
    2. Pigmented contact dermatitis
    3. Actinic lichen planus
    4. Melasma.

76. The following chemotherapeutic agents have been associated with hyperpigmentation (either diffuse or localized) of the skin:
    1. Busulfan
    2. Topical bis-chlorethyl-nitrosourea (BCNU)
    3. 5-Fluorouracil
    4. Bleomycin.

77. A young woman presents with diffuse hyperpigmentation and swelling of the distal extremities. What signs, symptoms, or tests would be useful in determining the underlying cause?
    1. Serum protein electrophoresis
    2. Insomnia
    3. Amenorrhea
    4. Mat telangiectasias.

ANSWERS

1. B Vitiligo is presumably an autoimmune disorder, and it is important to remember that it is associated with several autoimmune endocrine disorders, most commonly Graves' disease, Hashimoto's thyroiditis, and pernicious anemia. In children and adolescents, thyroid disease and polyglandular autoimmune syndromes are the most frequently observed associations. The latter includes hypoparathyroidism, chronic mucocutaneous candidiasis, and Addison's disease (Chapter 130).

2. A Significant (greater than 75%) repigmentation with PUVA therapy can be expected in the head and neck region and trunk of 40% to 60% of patients with vitiligo, especially those with more darkly pigmented skin. Repigmentation, however, can require 150 or more treatments, and some areas, such as the lips, fingertips, toes, palms, and soles, are particularly resistant to therapy (Chapter 130).

3. C; 4. D Vitiligo-like leukodermas can be seen in patients with scleroderma or melanoma. In scleroderma, the leukoderma is said to resemble "repigmenting vitiligo," with perifollicular pigmented macules within areas of amelanosis. This leukoderma tends to occur on extensor surfaces as well as the upper part of the trunk and can involve clinically normal skin. In contrast to idiopathic vitiligo, the depigmentation in patients with melanoma often begins on the trunk and spreads centrifugally. In two series of patients with metastatic melanoma, the presence of this leukoderma was associated with prolonged survival. The possibility exists that the destruction of normal melanocytes results from an immune response against malignant melanocytes and that this immune response retards melanoma growth (Chapter 130).

5. E The topical application of several compounds, including catechols, phenols, hydroquinone, and monobenzyl ether of hydroquinone, can result in a decrease or loss of cutaneous pigmentation. The chemical structure of these compounds is very similar to that of the melanin precursors, and their cytotoxic effects on pigment cells are also quite similar. Following early reports of monobenzyl ether of hydroquinone–induced leukoderma, it was used as a topical treatment for several disorders of hypermelanosis until it became clear that areas remote from the site could also undergo depigmentation, which was permanent in a significant number of patients. Today, the only clinical application for monobenzyl ether of hydroquinone is in the depigmentation of patients with widespread and unresponsive vitiligo. Hydroquinone can also cause destruction of melanocytes, but its effects are limited to the area of application, and the secondary hypopigmentation is usually neither complete nor irreversible, especially when low concentrations (2% to 3%) are employed (Chapter 130).

6. B; 7. C; 8. D; 9. E; 10. F; 11. A Vitiligo is associated with polyglandular autoimmune syndromes that include hypoparathyroidism, chronic mucocutaneous candidiasis, and Addison's disease (see Question 1). In addition to a white forelock, hypomelanotic areas in piebaldism are characteristically distributed over the forehead, neck, anterior trunk, flanks, and midportion of the extremities. Typically spared are the central back, shoulders, hips, hands, and feet. It is postulated that nevus depigmentosus results from a sporadic defect in embryonic development. Both sexes are equally affected, and there is no distinct pattern of inheritance. In tuberous sclerosis, a fibrous plaque may be seen on the forehead or scalp, and both fibrous plaque and shagreen patch are considered secondary clinical criteria for the diagnosis of this disorder. The fibrous plaque, like adenoma sebaceum, is an angiofibroma on histopathologic examination. In hypomelanosis of Ito, diploid/triploid mixoploidy and chromosomal mosaicism have been reported. One explanation for the association of chromosomal mosaicism with this pigmentary disorder that follows the lines of Blaschko is the proliferation and migration of two clones of primordial melanocytes with different pigment potential. Nevus anemicus is a localized area of vasoconstriction that is distinguished from nevus depigmentosus by having its borders obscured by diascopy (Chapter 130).

12. D Waardenburg's syndrome is an autosomal dominant disorder associated with a white forelock and skin lesions of piebaldism. It is characterized by the presence of lateral displacement of the inner canthi with normal interpupillary distance (dystopia canthorum), broad nasal root, hypertrichosis and fusion of the medial eyebrows, heterochromia of the irides, and congenital sensorineural hearing loss (Chapter 131).

13. C; 14. B; 15. C The earliest sign of tuberous sclerosis is the ash-leaf spot, which is present in at least 90% of patients with this disorder. These lesions are well-circumscribed macules or patches that have a partial rather than complete loss of pigmentation. In the majority of patients with tuberous sclerosis, ash-leaf spots are present at birth, but they may also appear in infancy or childhood. Once they appear, however, their size and shape remain stable. Most range in size from 1 to 3 cm. Although the lance-ovate configuration is considered characteristic, one study showed that only 18% of the lesions actually had this configuration, the polygonal form being the most common. Less commonly, ash-leaf spots manifest in a segmental distribution or as multiple "confetti-like" lesions ranging from 2 to 4 mm. They occur most commonly on the posterior trunk, where their long axes are oriented in a transverse direction; this is in contrast to the extremities, where the orientation of the lesions is cephalocaudal. Electron microscopic examination of ash-leaf spots has shown a normal number of melanocytes, a decreased number of melanosomes in melanocytes, and abnormally small melanosomes that are poorly melanized. The basic abnormality in ash-leaf spots appears to be an arrest in the maturation of melanosomes (Chapter 131).

16. E All forms of oculocutaneous albinism except one are inherited as autosomal recessive traits. Tuberous sclerosis is an autosomal dominant disorder, but in at least one half of the patients, it results from a spontaneous mutation. Piebaldism is also inherited in an autosomal dominant fashion with a high degree of penetrance. The majority of cases of hypomelanosis of Ito are sporadic, although there have been reports of autosomal dominant inheritance. There is no distinct inheritance pattern for nevus depigmentosus (Chapter 131).

17. A Cutaneous features of tuberous sclerosis other than ash-leaf spots include angiofibromas of the central face (adenoma sebaceum), which occur in over half of patients, and shagreen patches, which are connective tissue nevi; both lesions can begin to appear between the ages of 2 and 5 years. Periungual or subungual fibromas (Koenen's tumors) occur in 19% to 52% of cases, most commonly in females after puberty. They are seen most often on the toes and are associated with renal hamartomas. Fibromas also occur in the mouth as well as on the scalp, neck, and axilla. A fibrous plaque may be seen on the forehead or scalp. This lesion, like adenoma sebaceum, is an angiofibroma on histopathologic examination. In addition to the hypopigmented ash-leaf spots, poliosis of scalp hair, eyebrows, or eyelashes is also seen in patients with tuberous sclerosis as is circumscribed hypopigmentation of the iris or fundus (Chapter 131).

18. C; 19. A; 20. E; 21. A; 22. D Goltz' syndrome (focal dermal hypoplasia) presents with splashes and streaks of hypopigmentation in addition to defects of the musculoskeletal system, eyes, and teeth. Other cutaneous findings include linear areas of telangiectasis, hyperpigmentation, and dermal atrophy with fat herniation as well as periorificial papillomas, nail dystrophy, and focal alopecia. This disorder is thought to be inherited in an X-linked dominant fashion and is usually lethal in males. Piebaldism and tuberous sclerosis are both inherited in an autosomal dominant fashion but at least one half of tuberous sclerosis cases are the result of spontaneous mutation. The most common form of ocular albinism is the X-linked recessive Nettleship-Falls variant, which is characterized by macromelanosomes in the melanocytes and keratinocytes of the skin and in the pigment epithelium of the eye. A mild, generalized cutaneous pigmentary dilution is seen in some cases. There is no distinct inheritance pattern for nevus depigmentosus (Chapter 131).

23. E Pityriasis lichenoides chronica is characterized by multiple 3- to 7-mm papules that are red to red-brown in color. Macules of hypopigmentation that are of a similar size may be scattered among the inflammatory papules. The leukoderma may appear as the primary lesions heal, or it may appear de novo.

The diagnosis of hypopigmented cutaneous T-cell lymphoma (mycosis fungoides) is usually made histologically when atypical T lymphocytes are seen in the epidermis and dermis. By electron microscopy, degenerative changes in the melanocytes have been observed as has disordered melanogenesis with spherical melanosomes. Treatment with PUVA and topical alkylating agents has led to a reversal of the hypomelanosis.

The hypomelanosis occurring in patients with sarcoidosis can be seen in the form of nodules within areas of hypopigmentation or macular areas of hypopigmentation. Biopsy specimens of the infiltrated lesions have consistently revealed sarcoidal granulomas, whereas the majority but not all of the biopsy specimens from the macular areas have contained granulomas in the dermis.

Lichen striatus is an acquired inflammatory disorder that occurs most commonly in children ages 5 to 15. A linear array of flat-topped (lichenoid) papules that follows the lines of Blaschko appears, usually on an extremity. The color of the lesions ranges from pink to flesh-colored to tan (chapter 131).

24. E Treatment of vitiligo is somewhat limited for children less than 10 years of age. Low potency topical steroids may decrease the rate of spread of the lesions, and topical 8-methoxypsoralen plus UVA (PUVA) can be used in localized forms of the disease. In adolescents and adults, the most effective treatment is oral 8-methoxypsoralen plus UVA. Unfortunately, cosmetically significant repigmentation requires twice-a-week treatments for approximately 1 to 2 years. Autografts are particularly helpful in cases of segmental vitiligo, because this form of the disease is usually stable. In severe widespread vitiligo, depigmentation of the entire skin surface can be accomplished with topical monobenzyl ether of hydroquinone. The patient must be aware that depigmentation from this compound can occur in areas other than the sites of application and is often irreversible and that complete depigmentation can require up to 10 to 12 months of therapy (Chapter 130).

25. C Classic Vogt-Koyanagi syndrome consists of (1) vitiligo, (2) poliosis, (3) circumscribed alopecia, (4) acute nontraumatic anterior uveitis, (5) tinnitus, hearing loss, and dysacousis (ear discomfort from certain sounds). Harada's disease is characterized primarily by (1) posterior uveitis, (2) retinal detachment, and (3) aseptic meningitis. An overlap, however, frequently occurs, and they are routinely combined into one entity. Signs of meningeal irritation often precede the uveitis and dysacousis while depigmentation of the skin and hair frequently appears as a third phase of the disease. An increased incidence has been reported in patients with skin types 4 to 6 (Chapter 130).

26. D One explanation for a pigmentary pattern that follows Blaschko's lines is the migration of two different clones of cells with different pigmentary potential during embryogenesis. In the case of hypomelanosis of Ito, diploid/triploid mixoploidy and chromosomal mosaicism have been reported, whereas in X-linked dominant disorders such as incontinentia pigmenti and Goltz' syndrome, the presumed etiology is lyonization (random inactivation of the X chromosome). The differential diagnosis of hypomelanosis of Ito therefore includes those disorders with hypopigmentation that follow Blaschko's lines; these include the hypopigmented fourth stage of incontinentia pigmenti (see below), Goltz' syndrome (see the preceding), and the segmental and systematized form of nevus depigmentosus (Chapter 131).

27. B In patients with long-standing onchocerciasis, there can be areas of depigmentation in the pretibial region, the groin, and over bony prominences of the pelvic girdle. In advanced cases, the areas of involvement resemble "leopard skin." Preceding the leukoderma many patients have pruritus, excoriations, and lichenification (onchodermatitis) on the back, buttocks, and thighs. Additional stigmata of onchocerciasis include onchocercomas (nodules of adult worms), skin atrophy, adenolymphoceles ("hanging groin"), sclerosing lymphadenopathy of the groin and axilla, retinal degeneration, and punctate keratitis. All of these manifestations, including the dermatitis, are found more frequently in patients with the leukoderma (Chapters 127 and 131).

28. C; 29. B; 30. A; 31. D; 32. F; 33. E Patients with the Hermansky-Pudlak syndrome, a form of tyrosinase-positive albinism, have deposits of lipid and ceroid-like material in the macrophages of several organs (see Question 38). In the lung, these deposits can lead to interstitial fibrosis and restrictive pulmonary disease.

Patients with the Chédiak-Higashi syndrome have granulocytes with giant lysosomal granules that fail to discharge their contents into phagocytic vacuoles in a normal manner. This leads to recurrent sinopulmonary and cutaneous infections, usually secondary to *Staphylococcus aureus*. The abnormally large cytoplasmic granules, including lysosomes and melanosomes, are thought to be secondary to an ongoing fusion of organelles. The macromelanosomes in the melanocytes pass with difficulty to surrounding keratinocytes, and there is destruction of melanosomes within phagosomes in the melanocytes and keratinocytes of these patients. The combination of these events leads to a pigmentary dilution.

The differential diagnosis of Chédiak-Higashi syndrome includes the Griscelli syndrome, which is associated with (1) recurrent pyogenic infections, (2) immunodeficiency, (3) neutropenia, (4) thrombocytopenia, (5) hepatosplenomegaly, and (6) silvery gray hair, as well as areas of cutaneous hypopigmentation. The pigmentary changes seem to be secondary to a block in the transfer of melanosomes to keratinocytes, but there are no giant lysosomal or melanosomal granules in this disorder.

Other causes of generalized pigmentary dilution of the skin and hair include Menkes' kinky hair syndrome, Prader-Willi syndrome, and phenylketonuria (PKU), as well as homocystinuria, histidinemia, copper and selenium deficiencies, kwashiorkor, malabsorption secondary to chronic pancreatic disease, Angelman syndrome, Apert syndrome, the EEC (ectrodactyly, ectodermal dysplasia, and clefting) syndrome, and generalized vitiligo. Deletions in the region of the P gene on chromosome 15q have been identified in Prader-Willi syndrome and Angelman syndrome and therefore explain their overlap with type 2 (tyrosinase-positive) oculocutaneous albinism. Patients with Menkes' syndrome have low serum levels of ceruloplasmin as well as copper, the metal ion required for tyrosinase activity. In PKU, phenylalanine hydroxylase, which converts phenylalanine to tyrosine, is deficient, leading to an accumulation of the former metabolite. Possible explanations for the associated pigmentary dilution include a decrease in the amount of tyrosine available for melanin production, an inhibition of tyrosinase by phenylalanine, and the possibility that phenylalanine hydroxylase is involved in melanin biosynthesis. In the United States, however, it is unusual to see such patients because of mandatory screening for PKU in infants (Chapters 129 to 131).

34. D The *KIT* gene was first described as an oncogene in the feline sarcoma virus; it encodes for a cell-surface tyrosine kinase receptor. The ligand for this receptor is the *steel* factor, a protein encoded by the *steel* locus. The *steel* factor has several names that reflect its biologic properties; these include mast cell growth factor, stem cell growth factor, and melanocyte growth factor. In studies performed in human piebaldism, deletions in the *KIT* gene on chromosome 4q were observed as were at least nine different pathologic point mutations. To date, no mutations in the *steel* locus have been described in patients with piebaldism (Chapter 131).

35. C Poliosis, a localized area of white hair, is typically seen as a midfrontal white forelock in patients with piebaldism. In Waardenburg's syndrome, at least 17% of patients will have a white forelock and an estimated 12% of patients have skin lesions of piebaldism in addition to the white forelock. In addition to ash-leaf spots, poliosis of scalp hair, eyebrows, or eyelashes is seen in patients with tuberous sclerosis. In the classic form of the Vogt-Koyanagi-Harada syndrome, poliosis of the eyelashes, eyebrows, scalp, and body hair is seen in association with vitiligo. A halo nevus (leukoderma acquisitum centrifugum, or Sutton's nevus) of the scalp can also occur with poliosis. In Chédiak-Higashi syndrome, a form of oculocutaneous albinism, there is diffuse rather than localized pigmentary dilution of the scalp hair (Chapters 130 and 131).

36. A (T); B (T); C (F); D (T); E (F) Radiographic evidence of multiple calcified subependymal nodules protruding into a ventricle is a primary feature of the tuberous sclerosis complex. These lesions can be detected at an early stage by computed tomography or magnetic resonance imaging. Cardiac rhabdomyomata, a secondary feature, have been observed by echocardiography in 58% of children under 18 years of age with tuberous sclerosis and have been detected by ultrasound as early as 22 weeks of gestation. Another secondary feature is renal angiomyolipomas, which can also be detected by ultrasound. Acoustic schwannoma and pheochromocytoma are features of neurofibromatosis, another neurocutaneous disorder (Chapter 131).

37. A (T); B (F); C (T); D (T); E (T) Within the hypomelanotic areas seen in piebaldism, there are normally pigmented and hyperpigmented macules of varying size. Hyperpigmented macules that resemble café au lait macules can also be seen on normally pigmented skin; their presence does not require the diagnosis of a second genodermatosis. Piebaldism has been associated with Hirschsprung's disease, reflecting abnormal migration or differentiation of two neural crest–derived elements, melanocytes and myenteric ganglion cells. Congenital sensorineural hearing loss is seen in patients with piebaldism, particularly in those patients with Waardenburg's syndrome and Woolf's syndrome, the latter having been described in one Native American family. Because of the presence of deafness in patients with these two syndromes, individuals with piebaldism should routinely have auditory testing. Patients with Klein-Waardenburg syndrome have piebaldism in addition to congenital anomalies of the upper limbs (Chapter 131).

38. A (T); B (T); C (T); D (F); E (T) Patients with Hermansky-Pudlak syndrome, a form of oculocutaneous albinism, have a bleeding diathesis secondary to a platelet storage–pool defect. These platelets have decreased numbers of dense granules and decreased levels of substances normally stored within the granules, including serotonin and adenosine diphosphate. There are also deposits of lipid and ceroid-like material in the macrophages of the bone marrow, lymph nodes, liver, spleen, and lungs, the gastrointestinal mucosa, and renal tubular cells. In the lungs, these deposits can lead to interstitial fibrosis and restrictive pulmonary disease; in the gastrointestinal tract, they lead to granulomatous colitis (Chapter 131).

39. A (T); B (T); C (T); D (T); E (T) The most common shapes for the hypomelanotic macules seen in patients with tuberous sclerosis are polygonal, oval and ash-leaf, or lance-ovate. Less commonly, these lesions manifest in a segmental distribution or as multiple guttate "confetti-like" lesions 2 to 4 mm in size. Multiple hypomelanotic macules in a generalized distribution are also seen in pityriasis lichenoides chronica (PLC). In order to establish the clinical diagnosis of PLC, it is important to search for the characteristic red-brown, slightly scaly papules. Lichen sclerosis et atrophicus may manifest with white macules with associated epidermal atrophy and follicular plugging that demonstrate hydropic degeneration of the basal layer and homogenization of the papillary dermis on histologic examination. Punctate leukoderma can also be seen following psoralen plus ultraviolet A (PUVA) phototherapy and in patients with Darier's disease (Chapter 131).

40. A (T); B (F); C (F); D (F); E (T) Hypopigmentation is commonly observed in the tuberculoid and indeterminant forms of leprosy, while it is seen only rarely in the borderline lepromatous or lepromatous forms of the disease. Tuberculoid leprosy is characterized by a few asymmetrical patches of hypomelanosis that have associated anesthesia, anhidrosis, and alopecia. Enlargement of peripheral nerves is also seen in this form of the disease. In indeterminant leprosy, there are hypopigmented macules that are also hypoesthetic. In areas of involvement, the number of active melanocytes is usually decreased. Repigmentation follows treatment of the infection with dapsone (Chapters 112 and 131).

41. D; **42.** D In the melanin biosynthetic pathway, the enzyme tyrosinase catalyzes three reactions: (1) the oxidation of tyrosine to dihydroxyphenylalanine (DOPA); (2) the dehydrogenation of DOPA to dopaquinone; and (3) the conversion of 5,6-dihydroxyindole to melanochrome. Tyrosinase is a copper-dependent enzyme, which provides an explanation for the hypopigmentation of the hair that is seen in males with Menkes' kinky hair syndrome (it is an X-linked recessive disorder). In addition, streaks and sworls of hypopigmentation have been reported in female carriers of the disease, suggesting a mosaic state secondary to the Lyon phenomenon (random inactivation of the X chromosome). It has recently been shown that the genetic defect in this disease involves a copper transporting adenosine triphosphatase (Chapters 129 and 131).

43. E; **44.** D; **45.** C; **46.** A; **47.** B; **48.** D; **49.** B; **50.** A; **51.** A; **52.** C Vitamin B_{12} *deficiency*, as well as folate deficiency, is associated with diffuse hyperpigmentation, and the hyperpigmentation can be reversed by appropriate vitamin replacement. Chronic ingestion of chlorpromazine results in a diffuse tan or slate-gray color especially in sun-exposed skin. The pigmentation is thought to occur as a result of a phototoxic reaction and melanin–drug complexes in the lysosomes of dermal macrophages. Chrysiasis secondary to gold exposure is characterized by a blue-gray to brown pigmentation in sun-exposed areas; the periorbital region is a common site and often is the first site of involvement. Clofazimine is associated with a red-brown to dark brown discoloration of the skin, and in biopsy specimens of hyperpigmented skin, there are ceroid-lipofuscin deposits in dermal macrophages; similar deposits are seen in the gray-blue skin of patients treated with amiodarone. When patients with leprosy are treated with clofazimine, relative hyperpigmentation of lesions can be seen. Argyria is associated with a slate-gray discoloration of the skin, and, histologically, deposits of silver can be seen in the BMZ of the appendages and in association with elastic fibers. Trimethoprim-sulfamethoxazole is a common cause of fixed drug eruption. In the localized blue-black discolorations seen in patients taking minocycline, there are particles in dermal macrophages that stain positive for iron and probably also contain a metabolite of the drug complexed with protein (Chapter 132).

53. i D; ii C; iii D; iv A; v C Notalgia paresthetica and macular amyloidosis have several features in common—pruritus and macular hyperpigmentation, and the upper back is the most common location. In addition to hyperpigmentation, lesions of notalgia paresthetica may have erosions and hypopigmented scars secondary to scratching as well as decreased sensation to pinprick and temperature. One explanation given for the upper back location is the unique 90-degree path taken through the paraspinal muscles by the sensory fibers that innervate T2 to T6, which thereby increases the risk for damage to these nerves. Other names for notalgia paresthetica include *peculiar spotty pigmentation, hereditary localized pruritus,* and *puzzling posterior pigmented pruritic patches*. Macular amyloidosis can have a similar clinical appearance, but biopsy specimens demonstrate deposits of amyloid in the dermal papillae in addition to melanophages and changes secondary to rubbing (the latter two findings can be seen in notalgia paresthetica). It has been shown that the amyloid deposits in macular and lichen amyloidosis are composed of keratin proteins in contrast to the amyloid deposits in primary amyloidosis, which consist of immunoglobulin light chains.

The possibility that notalgia paresthetica and macular amyloidosis are related entities has been raised given the observation that repeated trauma or friction can lead to dermal deposition of degenerated keratin. More recently, there have been reports of the association of both notalgia paresthetica and lichen amyloidosis with the Sipple syndrome (multiple endocrine neoplasia type 2A characterized by an increased risk of medullary thyroid carcinoma, parathyroid hyperplasia, and pheochromocytoma) such that the skin lesions were considered a phenotypic marker. Cutaneous features of the autoimmune polyendocrinopathy syndromes include vitiligo, alopecia areata, and chronic mucocutaneous candidiasis (Chapters 130 and 132).

54. i B; ii B; iii C; iv A; v A Both linear and whorled nevoid hypermelanosis (LWNH) and incontinentia pigmenti (IP) can have reticulated hyperpigmentation as well as streaks and whorls of hyperpigmentation along the lines of Blaschko. LWNH usually appears by the age of 2 years, and biopsy specimens demonstrate an increase in the melanin content of the basal layer. Associated findings have been reported in a few patients and include atrial septal defect, dextrocardia, and chromosomal mosaicism. To date, all of the cases have been sporadic. In contrast, IP is inherited in an X-linked dominant fashion, which explains why the vast majority of individuals are female (the condition is usually lethal in hemizygous males). The third phase of IP is characterized by hyperpigmentation, whereas erythema and vesicles are seen in the first phase and verrucous lesions in the second phase. Histologically, numerous dermal melanophages ("incontinent pigment") are seen in the areas of hyperpigmentation and provide the basis for the name of this disease. Classically, the third phase of IP appears during the twelfth to twenty-sixth week of life, and when it follows phases I and II, the diagnosis is rather straightforward. However, there are a minority of cases in which the third phase is the initial phase and histologic examination of the skin is indicated to exclude LWNH. Additional clues to the diagnosis of IP include alopecia, dental anomalies, subungual tumors, and nail dystrophy as well as ocular and CNS abnormalities, e.g., retrolental fibroplasia, cataracts, and seizures. The remainder of the differential diagnosis of streaks of hyperpigmentation in an infant includes the early phase of an epidermal nevus (prior to the development of papillomatosis), chimerism, and Goltz' syndrome (Chapters 131 and 132).

55. i A; ii A; iii C; iv B; v B Both Dowling-Degos disease (DDD) and confluent and reticulated papillomatosis of Gougerot and Carteaud (CRP) are characterized by reticulated hyperpigmentation that coalesces centrally. In DDD, also known as reticulated pigmented anomaly of the flexures, the major sites of involvement are the axillae, inframammary regions, and groin. The pattern of inheritance is autosomal dominant, and the hyperpigmentation can be associated with pigmented follicular keratotic papules and pitted scars near the angles of the mouth. Histologically, there are thin interconnecting downgrowths of the epidermis that are heavily melanized. In CRP, the lesions usually involve the neck, inter- and inframammary areas, axillae, and midline of the back. The majority of lesions are elevated with associated scale; biopsy specimens demonstrate mild hyperkeratosis and papillomatosis. In some individuals, an increased number of *Pityrosporum* organisms has been observed in the stratum corneum; however, treatment with antifungals is not always successful in eradicating the disease (Chapter 132).

56. (T); **57.** (F); **58.** (F); **59.** (T); **60.** (F) The female child in this figure has incontinentia pigmenti (IP). The verrucous lesions (stage II) that have begun to form in several areas as well as the number of linear lesions are against the diagnosis of either herpes zoster or congenital syphilis. Patients with IP either represent a spontaneous mutation or they have inherited the disorder in an X-linked dominant fashion (from the mother in almost all cases). Adults with IP do not always know that they have the disease because the first two stages are transient (there are rare cases of persistent stage II), the hyperpigmentation associated with the third stage may fade, the cutaneous findings in the fourth stage can be subtle, and the associated nail, teeth, and hair abnormalities may be seen in other diseases or as isolated findings. The fourth stage of IP is characterized by lacy hypopigmentation primarily on the extremities. These areas may also be atrophic and lack hair; histologically, an absence of eccrine glands and pilosebaceous follicles has been described. Awareness of the fourth stage of IP is important because it may be the only cutaneous finding in an otherwise asymptomatic carrier. Associated ectodermal abnormalities in patients with IP include conical teeth, partial adontia, cicatricial alopecia, and nail dystrophy (Chapters 131 and 132).

61. (T); **62.** (F); **63.** (F); **64.** (F); **65.** (F) When black skin is compared with light tan skin, there are several differences. The melanosomes of black skin are larger in size, there are more stage IV (fully melanized) melanosomes in black skin, and the melanosomes are degraded more slowly in the keratinocytes of black skin. The latter characteristic is thought to be related to the observation that melanosomes are dispersed singly in the keratinocytes of black skin whereas melanosomes in the keratinocytes of lightly pigmented skin are aggregated into groups of two to three and bound by the membrane of a phagolysosome. There are no differences in the number of melanocytes/mm^2, the turnover time of the epidermis, or the ability of the keratinocytes to engulf the melanosomes (Chapter 129).

66. (F); **67.** (T); **68.** (F); **69.** (F); **70.** (T) Wood's lamp examination is an important component of the clinical evaluation of a patient with melasma. An increase in color contrast is seen when there is an increase in the melanin content of the basal and suprabasal layers of the epidermis (epidermal melasma). When there is an increase in the number of dermal melanophages (dermal melasma), no enhancement of the color contrast is seen under Wood's lamp examination. Epidermal melasma is more common than dermal melasma, and it is important to distinguish the two types because topical agents such as hydroquinone, tretinoin, and α-hydroxy acids are effective only in the epidermal form. A minority of patients have a mixed form of melasma in which some areas of hyperpigmentation are enhanced while other areas show no accentuation under Wood's lamp examination. Occasionally, in patients with skin types 5 and 6, lesions seen with visible light are no longer apparent under Wood's lamp illumination, and the histologic correlate is usually an increase in dermal pigment. The most common pattern of melasma is centrofacial (forehead, nose, cheeks, lateral aspects of the upper lip, and chin), whereas the malar and mandibular patterns are seen less often (Chapter 132).

71. A (T); B (T); C (T); D (T); E (F) There are several forms of minocycline-related hyperpigmentation, including circumscribed hyperpigmented macules (especially on the lower extremities) and dark blue–black macules that are localized to sites of cutaneous inflammation. The latter are seen most often in areas of acne scarring. Diffuse blue-gray to brown-gray discoloration of the skin has also been described with accentuation in sun-exposed areas and increased melanin in the epidermis and dermis. This is in contrast to the circumscribed forms of hyperpigmentation in which deposits stain positively for iron. Discoloration of permanent teeth secondary to minocycline is characteristically gray to gray-green in color and favors the incisors and premolar teeth. Additional side effects include pigmentation of the oral mucosa, nails, and sclerae; black staining of the thyroid gland; black galactorrhea; and green discoloration of bone. These side effects are not always dose-dependent and usually fade slowly after discontinuation of the minocycline. Depigmentation of the hair is seen in patients who have received antimalarials such as chloroquine (Chapter 132).

72. A (F); B (T); C (T); D (T); E (T) Erythema dyschromicum perstans is also known as ashy dermatosis; the latter name reflects the characteristic gray color of the lesions. The macules and patches are usually asymptomatic, but they may initially have an erythematous, slightly elevated border. The shape of the lesions is often oval or polycyclic and although the distribution is usually symmetrical, it can be unilateral. The upper half of the body is affected more often than the lower half, and, histologically, there is overlap with lichen planus, including hydropic degeneration, colloid bodies, and abundant dermal melanophages (incontinent pigment). Unfortunately, there is no effective treatment (Chapter 132).

73. A (T); B (T); C (F); D (F); E (T) Patients with dyskeratosis congenita (Zinsser-Cole-Engman syndrome) have reticulated hyperpigmentation that is usually most prominent on the trunk. Additional cutaneous findings (seen in ≥70% of patients) include nail dystrophy, skin atrophy, bullae, and hyperhidrosis and hyperkeratosis of the palms and soles. Leukokeratosis of the mucosal surfaces can be striking, and the development of squamous cell carcinomas is a serious problem in these patients. The inheritance pattern in dyskeratosis congenita is either X-linked recessive or autosomal dominant, and the majority of patients also have epiphora (excessive tearing secondary to lacrimal duct obstruction) and extensive caries or early dental loss. Abnormalities in the cellular immune system are associated with infections, including *Pneumocystis carinii*. During the second to third decades, the development of pancytopenia can lead to premature death (Chapter 132).

74. A (F); B (F); C (T); D (T); E (F) In one population survey from the United States, at least 75% of individuals with black skin had pigmentary demarcation lines. In general, these lines represent a sharp demarcation between outer more darkly pigmented skin and inner more lightly pigmented skin. The most common locations for these lines are (1) the upper anterior portion of the arm with extension onto the pectoral region (type A), (2) the posteromedial portion of the lower extremity (type B), and (3) the para- and presternal areas (type C). Type D (midback) and type E (extending from the mid third of the clavicle to the periareolar skin) pigmentary demarcation lines are seen infrequently (Chapter 132).

75. E Hyperpigmentation of the malar areas is seen in both the centrofacial and the malar patterns of melasma. Epidermal, dermal, and mixed forms of melasma can be seen in this location (see earlier). Exogenous ochronosis is characterized by darkening and coarsening of the skin in areas of application of hydroquinone. In addition, "caviar-like" papules can develop within these areas. The cheek is the most common location for exogenous ochronosis. Histologic examination of the skin confirms the diagnosis; yellow-brown, occasionally green, curled or banana-shaped fibers are seen in the dermis (similar to the histologic changes seen in alkaptonuria [ochronosis]). In cases of exogenous ochronosis reported in the United States, the strength of the hydroquinone has varied from 1% to 4%, and the duration of hydroquinone application has varied from 2 months to at least 3 years. Pigmented contact dermatitis can mimic melasma and most commonly affects the cheeks and/or forehead. It is associated with exposure to several chemicals, including lemon oil, benzyl salicylate, hydroxycitronella, geraniol, and the dyes D&C red 31 and yellow No. 11. Last, actinic lichen planus can also mimic melasma with brown to slate-gray patches on the face. However, a clue to the diagnosis is the presence of additional lesions in sun-exposed areas that are annular in shape or violaceous in color. A skin biopsy confirms the diagnosis because the histologic findings of lichen planus, including vacuolar degeneration and a band-like infiltrate of lymphocytes, is seen even in those cases that have only melasma-like lesions (Chapter 132).

76. E Bleomycin is a chemotherapeutic agent that is associated with flagellate linear hyperpigmentation (primarily of the upper trunk) and hyperpigmentation of extensor surfaces, especially the interphalangeal joints of the hands and feet. Topical BCNU and topical mechlorethamine (nitrogen mustard) can both cause the skin to become hyperpigmented. Histologically, an increase in the melanin content of the epidermis and an increase in the number of melanocytes is seen. 5-Fluorouracil can result in two types of hyperpigmentation: (1) diffuse with accentuation in sun-exposed areas and (2) serpiginous streaks that overlie superficial veins in which the drug was infused. Diffuse hyperpigmentation of the upper torso has been reported in patients treated with busulfan, whereas brown-black hyperpigmentation of the palmar-plantar surfaces has been observed in patients given doxorubicin (Chapter 132).

77. E The differential diagnosis in such a patient includes scleroderma, POEMS (*p*olyneuropathy, *o*rganomegaly, *e*ndocrinopathy, *M*-component protein [monoclonal gammopathy], and *s*kin changes) syndrome, eosinophilia-myalgia syndrome secondary to tryptophan ingestion, and less likely, toxic oil syndrome. The presence of mat telangiectasias, Raynaud's phenomenon, and digital ulcers would favor the diagnosis of scleroderma, whereas eosinophilia, myalgias, muscle weakness, polyneuropathy, and the history of a maculopapular eruption would raise the possibility of tryptophan ingestion. Of note, one of the ailments thought to respond to tryptophan was insomnia. In the POEMS syndrome, the most common endocrinopathies are impotence, gynecomastia, and amenorrhea, and cutaneous findings (in addition to hyperpigmentation and peripheral edema) include induration, hypertrichosis, hyperhidrosis, and multiple hemangiomas (Chapter 132).

Bibliography

Bologna JL, Pawelek JM. Biology of hypopigmentation. J Am Acad Dermatol 1988; 19:217–255.

Fulk CS. Primary disorders of hyperpigmentation. J Am Acad Dermatol 1984; 10:1–16.

Griffiths WAD. Reticulate pigmentary disorders—a review. Clin Exp Dermatol 1984; 9:439–450.

Lerner EA, Sober AJ. Chemical and pharmacologic agents which cause hyperpigmentation of the skin. In: Fitzpatrick TB, Wick MM, Toda K, eds. Brown Melanoderma. Biology and Disease of Epidermal Pigmentation. Tokyo: University of Tokyo Press, 1986:215–227.

Nordlund JJ, Ortonne J-P. Vitiligo and depigmentation. Curr Probl Dermatol 1992; 4:3–30.

Pinto FJ, Bologna JL. Disorders of hypopigmentation in children. Pediatr Clin North Am 1991; 991:1017.

Cutaneous Oral and Genital Diseases

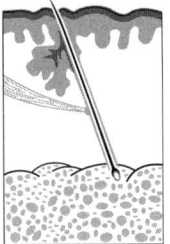

chapter 18, part I

Oral Diseases

JOHN SEXTON

Choose the ONE BEST answer to each of the following questions.

1. Which of the following anomalies are seen in Cowden's disease?
   A. Scrotal tongue
   B. Oral mucosal papillomatosis
   C. Lichenoid lesions of the gingiva
   D. Fibrocystic disease of the breast
   E. All of the above.

2. Aphthous ulcers occur
   A. On nonkeratinized mucosa
   B. Occasionally as part of multiple organ system disease
   C. As solitary ulcers
   D. As part of Behçet's syndrome
   E. All of the above.

3. Treatment of aphthous ulcers includes
   A. Topical and systemic steroids
   B. Colchicine
   C. Thalidomide
   D. Retinoids
   E. All of the above.

4. All of the following are true regarding aphthous stomatitis EXCEPT
   A. It may cause scarring
   B. It can last 2 to 4 weeks
   C. It has an undetermined cause
   D. It only occurs on keratinized mucosal surfaces
   E. It can be associated with trauma.

5. Which of the following is true of aphthous stomatitis?
   A. Is an infectious disease
   B. Recurrence is lessened by topical tetracycline
   C. Demonstrates diagnostic histopathology
   D. Shows a familial pattern
   E. Is worsened by smoking.

6. Aphthous-like ulceration is seen in all of the following EXCEPT
   A. Hypereosinophilic syndrome
   B. Chemotherapy mucositis
   C. Squamous cell carcinoma
   D. Chancre
   E. Sjögren's syndrome.

7. Geographic tongue
   A. May be associated with psoriasis
   B. Histologically, shows loss of filiform papillae
   C. May show microabscess formation
   D. May be symptomatic
   E. All of the above.

8. A mucocele
   A. May appear blue
   B. Is a true cyst
   C. Occurs most commonly on the upper lip
   D. Involves only the sublingual gland
   E. Is a common component of Sjögren's syndrome.

9. The oral epulis fissuratum is
   A. Premalignant
   B. Seen as a component of Melkersson-Rosenthal syndrome
   C. An inflammatory hyperplastic lesion
   D. A neurogenic lesion
   E. An acinic cell tumor.

10. A pathognomonic oral sign of Wegener's granulomatosis is
    A. Multiple, scarring aphthae
    B. Palatal tori
    C. Gingival fibromatosis
    D. Erythematous gingival enlargement with petechial hemorrhage
    E. Pseudomembranous palatopharyngitis.

11. Of the following oral lesions, the one that shows the greatest premalignant potential is
    A. Leukoplakia
    B. Erosive lichen planus
    C. Erythroplakia
    D. Sialometaplasia
    E. Discoid lupus erythematosus.

12. Malignant transformation of leukoplakia lesions occur most commonly when such lesions are found
    A. In the floor of the mouth (sublingually)
    B. On the buccal mucosa
    C. On the palatal mucosa
    D. On the lips
    E. In the mandibular or maxillary vestibules.

13. Necrotizing sialometaplasia
    A. May mimic mucoepidermoid carcinoma
    B. Heals in 6 to 12 weeks without recurrence
    C. Occurs primarily on the palate
    D. Is a benign, self-healing lesion
    E. All of the above.

14. Granular cell myoblastoma is an oral lesion seen most frequently on the
    A. Tongue
    B. Lips
    C. Soft palate
    D. Buccal mucosa
    E. Floor of the mouth.

15. A 30-year-old African-American patient shows grayish-white, somewhat folded and opalescent, buccal and labial mucosae. There is a history of smoking but no current tobacco abuse. The most likely diagnosis is
    A. Verrucous leukoplakia
    B. Oral submucous fibrosis
    C. Stomatitis nicotina
    D. Chronic trauma
    E. Leukoedema.

16. A recently diagnosed HIV-positive patient develops hairy leukoplakia on the tongue. This is
    A. A suggestion of recent infection
    B. A prognostic marker for the development of AIDS
    C. A finding consistent with HSV infection
    D. A manifestation of *Candida* infection
    E. Of no clinical significance.

17. A cutaneous fistula from an odontogenic source
    A. Is always associated with a painful tooth
    B. Responds to antibiotics
    C. Is a common presenting sign of dental sepsis
    D. Usually indicates actinomycosis
    E. None of the above.

18. Patients with ectodermal dysplasia have
    A. Oligodontia
    B. Anodontia
    C. Delayed eruption
    D. Abnormally shaped teeth
    E. All of the above.

19. The *overall* malignant transformation rate for oral leukoplakia is
    A. 30% to 60%

B. 10% to 15%
C. 3% to 6%
D. 0.5% to 2%
E. Unknown.

20. Among those patients referred for diagnosis and treatment of lichen planus, the type that is the most common is
    A. Erosive
    B. Bullous
    C. Reticular
    D. Atrophic
    E. Papular.

21. The hard palate of a 65-year-old pipe smoker appears white, rough, and nodular. The nodules exhibit central red spots. The diagnosis is
    A. Necrotizing sialometaplasia
    B. Nicotinic stomatitis
    C. Reactive papillary hyperplasia
    D. Erythroleukoplakia
    E. Verrucous carcinoma.

22. The most common of the vesiculobullous disorders manifesting oral lesions is
    A. Hereditary mucoepithelial dysplasia
    B. Pemphigoid
    C. Pemphigus
    D. Major aphthous stomatitis
    E. Erosive lichen planus.

In the following questions, ONE or MORE of the following completions correctly finishes the incomplete statement; choose

A. If only 1, 2, and 3 are correct.
B. If only 1 and 3 are correct.
C. If only 2 and 4 are correct.
D. If only 4 is correct.
E. If all are correct.

23. Benign mucous membrane pemphigoid
    1. Is seen more frequently in women
    2. Does not involve attached gingiva
    3. Infrequently demonstrates low titers of serum antibodies to basement membrane
    4. Shares the same target antigen as bullous pemphigoid.

24. Mucous membrane pemphigoid may
    1. Be precipitated by drug therapy
    2. Involve the vagina, respiratory tract or eye
    3. Be asymptomatic
    4. Be associated with glaucoma.

25. Which of the following are anatomic structures of the tongue surface?
    1. Foliate papillae
    2. Fungiform papillae
    3. Circumvallate papillae
    4. Filiform papillae.

26. Histologic characteristic(s) of lichen planus is (are)
    1. Hypergranulosis
    2. T-cell infiltrate
    3. Liquefaction degeneration of the basal cell layer
    4. Civatte and colloid bodies.

27. Eosinophilic ulcer of the oral mucosa
    1. Usually manifests on the lateral tongue
    2. Is usually solitary
    3. May manifest cellular atypia
    4. Is associated with multiple allergies.

28. Which of the following should be included in the differential diagnosis of a patient with desquamative gingivitis?
    1. Lichen planus
    2. Cicatricial pemphigoid
    3. Pemphigus
    4. Leukoedema.

For the following questions decide whether EACH choice is TRUE or FALSE.

Regarding cicatricial pemphigoid,

29. Rarely demonstrates circulating antibodies
30. Is similar in all respects to bullous pemphigoid
31. Involves the same antigens as bullous pemphigoid
32. Shows destruction of the basal lamina histologically.

Regarding verruciform xanthoma,

33. Is seldom seen as an oral lesion
34. Is easily confused with verrucous carcinoma
35. When manifested intraorally usually involves the gingiva or alveolar ridge

36. Shows extensive infiltration of xanthoma cells in the submucosal connective tissue.

In the following questions, ONE or MORE of the following completions correctly finishes the incomplete statement; choose

A. If only 1, 2, and 3 are correct.
B. If only 1 and 3 are correct.
C. If only 2 and 4 are correct.
D. If only 4 is correct.
E. If all are correct.

37. In Reiter's syndrome,
    1. Oral lesions are intensely painful
    2. Oral lesions last up to several weeks
    3. Mucosal lesions cause scarring
    4. Oromucosal lesions are psoriasiform and may initially manifest as a vesicle.

38. Necrotizing sialometaplasia histologically demonstrates which of the following?
    1. Necrosis of salivary gland lobules
    2. Pseudoepitheliomatous hyperplasia
    3. Squamous ductal metaplasia
    4. Epithelial dysplasia.

39. Cheilitis granulomatosa is characterized by
    1. An association with Crohn's disease
    2. Tender swelling
    3. Langhan's giant cells
    4. Caseating granulomas.

40. The most common oral mucosal manifestation(s) of chronic graft-versus-host disease is (are)
    1. Xerostomia secondary to minor salivary gland metaplasia
    2. Vesiculobullous erosions
    3. Erythema with atrophic and lichenoid changes
    4. Gingival hyperplasia.

41. Oral clinical findings in morphea include
    1. Fibrotic stricture of the attached gingiva, leading to periodontal disease
    2. Induration and atrophy of the muscles of the tongue, lips, and soft palate
    3. Tender, pale, and rigid oral mucosa
    4. Mucosal erosion.

42. A 25-year-old woman patient presents with keratotic and scaly lip lesions surrounded by a white, elevated zone. Her mucosal lesions are painful. This scenario is consistent with
    1. Discoid lupus erythematosus
    2. Dyskeratosis congenita
    3. Lichen planus
    4. Stomatitis areata (migratory stomatitis).

43. White sponge nevus is
    1. Identical to leukoedema
    2. Associated with palmoplantar hyperkeratosis
    3. Mildly dysplastic
    4. Inherited as an autosomal dominant trait.

44. Xerostomia can be induced by which of the following types of drugs?
    1. Antidepressants
    2. Antihypertensive drugs
    3. Beta-blockers
    4. Antiparkinsonian drugs.

45. Oral changes evident in dyskeratosis congenita include
    1. Childhood vesicular ulcerative lesions
    2. Mucosal atrophy
    3. Late onset dysplasia
    4. White, hyperkeratotic plaques.

46. Nevoid basal cell carcinoma syndrome predisposes to
    A. Multiple jaw cysts
    B. Osteomas of the mandible and maxilla
    C. Enamel hypoplasia
    D. Neurofibromas of the tongue
    E. None of the above.

ANSWERS

1. E Cowden's disease, also known as the multiple hamartoma and neoplasia syndrome, is a rare disease with an autosomal dominant inheritance pattern. Its major orofacial manifestations are multiple orocutaneous hamartomas. Orally, one finds papillomatous and lichenoid lesions of the gingiva and multiple small papules of the gingiva and palate, giving a cobblestone appearance. The tongue is scrotal with a pebbly surface. The oral mucosal papillomatosis is reported in more than 80% of cases. Onset of skin and mucosal lesions in Cowden's disease is not known, but patients become aware of lesions in the second to third decades. These lesions observed by the patient are often the first manifestation of the disease.

Histologic study of the oral lesions shows epithelial hyperplasia with acanthosis and parakeratosis. The facial skin lesions are histologically similar to trichilemmoma. Because patients with Cowden's disease are at risk for developing internal malignancy, especially of the breast and thyroid, careful monitoring of the patient and family members is important. Other hamartomas that occur with this disease include fibrocystic disease of the breast, thyroid adenomas, and ovarian cysts. Gastrointestinal and esophageal polyps are also features of the syndrome.

Treatment of the oral manifestations of Cowden's disease consists of surgical removal of lesions (Chapters 138 and 175).

2. E; **3.** E; **4.** D; **5.** D; **6.** E Recurrent aphthous ulcers are the most common of the idiopathic intraoral ulcerations. Initial manifestation can occur in childhood or young adulthood, and lesions may regress somewhat as the patient matures. Early lesions appear as erythematous macules or papules that subsequently undergo central necrosis. The mature lesion is a painful ulcer, 0.5 to 3 cm in diameter, having an erythematous halo.

Aphthae usually occur singly and on unattached mucosa in distinction to the ulcers of herpetic stomatitis. Patients may have more than one ulcer at any given time and may have them continuously in different locations. Based on size and the rare occasional clustering, the ulcers are classified as minor, major, and herpetiform. Although the atypical large ulcers of major aphthae, or Sutton's disease, may take weeks to heal and scar, most aphthae are of the minor variety and will heal uneventfully in 10 to 14 days. Lesions persisting longer than 1 month should be viewed with suspicion.

The etiology of recurrent aphthous stomatitis is unknown, although current investigation suggests an alteration in cell-mediated immunity, namely, activation of cytotoxic T cells, leading to mucosal breakdown. This explanation has naturally led to treatment with topical and in some cases systemic immunosuppressive drugs.

Most patients with recurrent aphthae are managed supportively and symptomatically with topical steroids and/or obtundants. Tetracycline rinse appears to offer some relief and may prevent secondary infection. More severe cases may be treated with steroid-burst therapy, quickly tapering the dose. Refractory cases have been treated with immunosuppressive drugs such as cyclosporine and azathioprine. Retinoids and colchicine have also been used. Thalidomide is the latest addition to the list of therapeutic agents that have been used successfully in patients with HIV-associated aphthae.

Histologically, the ulcer of aphthous stomatitis is characterized by nonspecific inflammation and ulceration with a fibropurulent membrane. Healing proceeds by normal resolution and re-epithelialization with occasional scarring in severe cases.

Since solitary and nonspecific ulcers may occur as part of certain multisystem diseases such as Behçet's and Reiter's syndromes, patients with such lesions should be questioned and examined for lesions of the skin, eye, and genital areas (Chapter 138).

7. E Geographic tongue, or migratory glossitis, is an inflammatory condition affecting approximately 1% to 2% of the population. Clinically, it appears as areas of papillary denudation surrounded by white or yellow margins, involving the dorsum and lateral borders of the tongue. In a cycle of recurrence and healing, the lesions change their configuration constantly, thus the term *migratory*. Should this same condition extend to the buccal or palatal mucosa, the term *ectopic geographic tongue* or *stomatitis areata migrans* is used.

Both migratory glossitis and stomatitis appear more prevalent in patients with psoriasis. Migratory glossitis has also been associated with Reiter's disease, atopy, and psychological stress. Most patients with this entity have no symptoms, but on occasion pain or burning is reported. Histologically, geographic tongue shows loss of filiform papillae, mucosal atrophy, microabscess formation, and an inflammatory infiltrate. Treatment of symptomatic patients has involved the use of topical steroids (Chapter 138).

8. A Mucocele, or mucus retention phenomenon, is a lesion of the minor salivary glands. Predominantly found on the lower lip, the mucocele originates from injury to the duct of a minor salivary gland, causing mucus to extravasate into the submucosa. This results in a dome-shaped, usually superficial, and blue lesion that intermittently ruptures, heals, and then recurs. Mucoceles that lie deeper within the tissue may have a normal-appearing overlying mucosa.

Histologically, the mucocele is a fluid-filled cavity lined by connective tissue with an inflammatory cell infiltrate. It does not have a true epithelial lining; thus the designation *retention cyst* is a misnomer.

Treatment of the mucocele involves surgical excision of the damaged gland and the minor glands surrounding it. Since mucoceles may mimic mucoepidermoid carcinoma, especially when seen on the hard palate, histologic examination is necessary (Chapter 138).

9. C Epulis fissurata is a common intraoral lesion representing an exuberant tissue response to chronic irritation. It is seen most frequently adjacent to or under a poorly fitting denture prosthesis. It is seen most frequently in the maxillary anterior region, although it may manifest anywhere on the residual alveolar ridges and oral vestibule. Lesions are frequently multiple.

Clinically, the epulis occurs as an elongated, exophytic mass. The surface epithelium is covered with normal mucosa if the lesion is long-standing. Chronic trauma from a denture may result in ulceration. The denture flange is frequently seen lying within a cleft in the epulis.

Histologically, the epulis shows fibrous connective tissue covered by normal or thickened epithelium. Pseudoepitheliomatous hyperplasia may be evident. Treatment of this condition involves surgical excision of the epulis and fabrication of new dentures (Chapter 138).

10. D Wegener's granulomatosis involves granulomatous inflammation of small- to medium-sized blood vessels and may involve the skin, oral mucosa, lungs, and kidneys. Superficial involvement of only the skin and oral mucosa appears to have the best prognosis. The cause of this disease is uncertain, but an immunopathologic origin is probable.

The pathognomonic oral manifestation of Wegener's disease is erythematous gingival enlargement with petechial hemorrhage beginning between the teeth. The epithelium has a granular texture. The gingival lesions may begin in a localized area, but eventually spread to other areas of the oral cavity. This results in severe, destructive periodontal disease. Also found in Wegener's granulomatosis are destructive oral ulcerations.

Histologically, the lesions show acute and chronic inflammation, pseudoepitheliomatous hyperplasia and necrotizing vasculitis. Since the oral presentations of any of the forms of Wegener's disease may be the first to appear, characteristic gingival or oral changes should alert the clinician to the necessity of further evaluation (Chapter 59).

11. C; **12.** A *Leukoplakia* is simply a term that denotes a white patch or plaque that cannot be rubbed off. Much confusion has arisen as to the subclassification and malignant potential of leukoplakia. Present opinion favors the designation of all types of leukoplakia as potentially precancerous, thus mandating biopsy and histologic examination of those areas that do not resolve in a reasonable amount of time. Leukoplakia may be either localized or diffuse. It may be homogeneous, nodular, verrucous, or plaque-like. Leukoplakia may have an erythematous or an erosive component; the latter is then designated erythroplakia. It may be present anywhere in the oral cavity with some areas, such as the floor of the mouth, and some varieties, especially erythroplakia, showing a higher incidence of dysplasia than others.

The causes of leukoplakia are multiple. Chronic trauma, tobacco, candidal infection, and electrogalvanism from dental restorations have all been implicated. Those cases without any obvious inciting factors appear to have a higher rate of malignant transformation. Treatment for leukoplakia involves surgical excision and careful follow-up (Chapter 138).

13. E Necrotizing sialometaplasia is a benign lesion of the minor salivary glands. It is most frequently seen on the palate, where it manifests as a deep ulcer 1 to 3 cm in diameter extending down to bone. The ulcer is round and sharply demarcated from the surrounding tissue. Before ulceration, it may initially manifest as an erythematous nodule.

The importance of necrotizing sialometaplasia lies in its frequent confusion with squamous cell carcinoma or mucoepidermoid carcinoma, both of which it closely resembles. Histologically, the tissues show an ulcer base with fibroblastic and angioblastic proliferation, pseudoepitheliomatous hyperplasia of the surface epithelium, squamous metaplasia of salivary gland ducts, and infarctive necrosis of salivary gland acini.

The etiology of necrotizing sialometaplasia is unknown, although some theorize loss of blood supply to the lobules of the salivary glands. The condition heals spontaneously over a course of 6 to 12 weeks (Chapter 138).

14. A Granular cell myoblastoma is a benign tumor usually found in the head and neck region. The oral cavity is commonly involved, the tumor being encountered on the tongue in 30% to 50% of cases. The lesion is symptomless and slow-growing. It is well circumscribed, firm, and covered by normal or whitened mucosa. It is found in all age groups and may have a slight predilection for females. Current theory favors an origin from Schwann's cells, despite the original designation of myoblastoma.

Histologically, the tumor demonstrates large polygonal cells with granules and eosinophilic cytoplasm. The covering epithelium may show pseudoepitheliomatous hyperplasia. Because of the locally infiltrative nature of this lesion, treatment involves excision with a margin of normal tissue and periodic follow-up (Chapters 138 and 149).

15. E Leukoedema is not a disease but a variation in the normal appearance of the oral mucosa. It is frequently seen in blacks—in up to 90% of the population. Clinically, leukoedema manifests as filmy white-to-gray opalescent-appearing buccal or labial mucosa. There may also be wrinkling or folding. Histologically, there is ballooning in the prickle cell layer and a generalized thickening of the epithelium. Leukoedema is frequently mistaken for pathology. No treatment is indicated for this benign condition (Chapter 138).

16. B Oral hairy leukoplakia is an oral lesion associated with the Epstein-Barr virus (EBV) that is commonly seen in HIV-infected patients. It has also been described in non-HIV immunocompromised patients. It appears as a white, corrugated lesion and most often appears on the lateral borders of the tongue, although other oral mucosal surfaces may be involved. The patients usually have no symptoms. Histologically, oral hairy leukoplakia shows hyperkeratosis, acanthotic ballooning degeneration of the superficial prickle cells, and a mild subepithelial inflammatory infiltrate. Superficial keratinocytes show nuclear changes and inclusions reflective of EBV infection. Oral hairy leukoplakia requires no treatment unless the patient has symptoms or is concerned about the appearance. Acyclovir has been shown to be of benefit in these cases. Of particular importance regarding this lesion is the fact that it is not only a marker for HIV seropositivity but also evidence of immune deterioration in an HIV-positive patient (Chapter 125).

17. E Cutaneous fistulae stemming from odontogenic infections, although not common, occur frequently enough to warrant a dental source in the differential diagnosis. The muscles of facial expression and mastication generally confine dental sepsis to the oral cavity, the path of least resistance being through the alveolus and into the oral vestibule. On occasion, the length of the tooth root allows an abscess to fistulate extraorally. The patient usually gives a history of a painful tooth and swelling. Once an egress is given to the infection via the fistula, pain subsides or ceases altogether. Attempts at resolution of the fistula fail until the offending tooth is identified as the source and treated (Chapter 138).

18. E Ectodermal dysplasia, in addition to the well-known manifestations in the skin and its adnexal structures, also demonstrates impressive dental findings. Since the tooth develops from both ectodermal and mesodermal primordia, defective amelogenesis leads to either a partial (oligodontia) or complete (anodontia) absence of teeth. Those teeth that do form are frequently abnormal in contour. Since the alveolar processes of the mandible and maxilla are dependent on normal odontogenesis, they are also hypoplastic. Accessory salivary glands may be affected, leading to xerostomia (Chapter 164).

19. C The overall malignant transformation rate for oral leukoplakia is 3% to 6%. These are subtypes of leukoplakia that however have a higher rate of transformation, such as erythroleukoplakia. There is also a difference in transformation rate related to site, the floor of the mouth displaying the highest rate. Although tobacco and alcohol abuse are known risk factors for development of oral carcinoma, the rate of malignant transformation of leukoplakia seems to be higher in those patients who have no such risk factors (Chapter 138).

20. A Lichen planus is a chronic oral mucosal or mucocutaneous disorder that occurs in about 2% of the population. The condition tends to affect females more often than males, occurs in late middle age, and most commonly involves the buccal mucosa. Oral lichen planus is classified into four major subtypes: reticular, atrophic, erosive, and bullous. Although studies differ as to prevalence of type, a large study conducted at the University of San Francisco demonstrated the erosive type to be the most common entity in patients seeking treatment for lichen planus. The reticular type may be the most common in the general population (Chapter 20).

21. B Nicotinic stomatitis is a palatal lesion induced by chronic exposure to tobacco smoke. It is most frequently seen in pipe smokers. Its distinctive features include gray to white multiple nodules of the palate, each nodule having a red dot at its summit that represents the opening into a minor salivary gland. These minor salivary gland ducts are frequently dilated and/or obstructed. There may be fissures between the nodules. Histologically, nicotinic stomatitis shows hyperkeratosis. The lesions resolve with cessation of pipe smoking (Chapter 138).

22. B; 23. B; 24. E Benign mucous membrane pemphigoid, the most common of the oral vesiculobullous diseases, is also known as cicatricial pemphigoid or mucous membrane pemphigoid. It is an autoimmune disorder, the epithelial basement membrane providing the target antigen. Oral lesions may be the exclusive manifestation of this disorder, or other mucosal surfaces, such as those of the eye, respiratory tract, and genital area, may be involved. Skin lesions are present in about 8% of cases.

The mucosal lesions in mucous membrane pemphigoid are reflective of the separation of the surface epithelium from the underlying connective tissues at the basement membrane level. Gingival lesions frequently manifest as a desquamative gingivitis. The attached gingiva may appear intensely red and is easily wiped off, leaving a denuded surface. Lesions of the oral mucosa are vesiculobullous with bullae rupturing early. Lesions of the conjunctiva may result in scarring, although oral lesions rarely do. Although many patients with mucous membrane pemphigoid are symptom-free, pain is frequently reported. Mucous membrane pemphigoid occurs more frequently in women in the 50- to 80-year-old age group. In some patients, it has been induced by drug therapy and has also been associated with glaucoma. Periods of exacerbation and remission are common. Histologically, direct immunofluorescence shows an even, band-like deposition of immunoglobulin or complement at the basement membrane. C3 and IgG are most commonly found, although IgA and IgM are also reported in a significant number of cases. Patients with cicatricial pemphigoid rarely demonstrate circulating autoantibodies. This is in distinction to bullous pemphigoid, in which up to 80% of patients have circulating antibasement membane antibodies (Chapter 76).

The cause of mucous membrane pemphigoid is unknown, and there is no cure. Corticosteroids have been used both topically and systemically for oral lesions. Use of potent topical steroids such as clobetasol propionate, fluocinonide, and dexamethasone elixir are occasionally effective in controlling exacerbations. Immunosuppressive agents such as azathioprine or cyclophosphamide are frequently required. Other conditions to consider in a patient with similar vesiculobullous oral lesions are bullous pemphigoid, angina bullosa hemorrhagica, epidermolysis bullosa acquisita, linear IgA disease, and dermatitis herpetiformis (Chapters 76 and 138).

25. E The mucous membrane covering the surface of the tongue is special in several respects. It is extremely thin and intimately bound to the underlying muscle. Interspersed among the muscle fibers there are glands whose ducts pass through the submucosa to empty on the tongue's dorsal surface. The tongue mucosa itself is composed of four types of papillae, causing its characteristic roughened appearance. The filiform papillae are tiny projections of cornified epithelium. The fungiform papillae are rounded mushroom-like structures with a thin epithelial covering. They can be seen as small red dots scattered over the dorsal and lateral surfaces of the tongue. The circumvallate papillae are large structures found posteriorly on the tongue, lined up in a V-shaped configuration. There are usually about 10 circumvallate papillae, which house taste buds. They are frequently mistaken for pathology by patients and physicians. The foliate papillae are parallel folds of tissue found along the posterolateral border of the tongue (Chapter 138).

26. E Histologically, lichen planus demonstrates hyperkeratosis, thickening of the granular cell layer; saw-toothed appearance of rete pegs; liquefactive degeneration, necrosis of the basal cell layer, or both; and a subepithelial band of lymphocytes. Civatte and colloid bodies are seen in the basal cell area and dermis, respectively. Subepithelial deposits of fibrinogen and related substances are seen on direct immunofluorescent staining. Occasional staining of immunoglobulins is seen. Differential diagnosis of lichenoid-appearing lesions includes lupus erythematosus, mucous membrane pemphigoid, pemphigus, squamous cell carcinoma, *Candida* infection, erythema multiforme, and graft-versus-host disease. Treatment of oral lichen planus has involved topical or systemic steroids, retinoids, cyclosporine, and cytotoxic drugs. Some patients will experience remissions (Chapter 20).

27. A Eosinophilic ulcer is an uncommon oral lesion of unknown etiology. It most frequently occurs on the lateral border of the tongue in older adults. The median size of the ulcer is 2 cm, the duration, 2 weeks to 6 months. Medical history is most often noncontributory, and allergy does not appear to be an inciting factor. Lesions are isolated, but on rare occasions they may be multiple.

Histologically, the eosinophilic ulcer shows an inflammatory process that extends into the submucosa. Large numbers of eosinophils and histiocytoid cells permeate the lesion. Histiocytic atypicality may suggest malignancy, but these lesions are benign.

Treatment of the eosinophilic ulcer is by excision. Topical steroids have also been used with some success (Chapter 138).

28. A Several oral mucosal conditions share the clinical presentation of desquamative gingivitis. These include lichen planus, mucous membrane pemphigoid, bullous pemphigoid, pemphigus vulgaris, dermatitis herpetiformis, linear immunoglobulin IgA disease, and certain drug reactions.

29. (T); 30. (F); 31. (F); 32. (T) See answer to Question 22.

33. (T); 34. (T); 35. (T); 36. (F) Verruciform xanthoma is a papillary lesion of squamous epithelium usually found in the oral cavity. Extraoral sites have also been described on the penis, vagina, and scrotum. Clinically, the lesion manifests as a raised lesion with a granular surface. It is yellow, red, or gray and may measure up to 2 cm. The most frequent sites of occurrence are the alveolar ridge and gingiva, but other oral sites are involved as well.

Histologically, the verruciform xanthoma displays papillary squamous hyperplasia with hyperparakeratosis and xanthoma cells packing the connective tissue between elongated rete pegs. Verruciform xanthoma is thought to be a reactive lesion and not a neoplasm. Excision is generally curative. Verruciform carcinoma and squamous cell carcinoma should be included in the differential diagnosis (Chapter 138).

37. D The oral lesions encountered in Reiter's syndrome are different from those encountered in Behçet's disease. The lesions are initially vesicular but soon form essentially painless ulcers. Most often, these lesions are found on the buccal and palatal mucosa and the gingiva, tongue, and tonsillar pillars. Their duration is brief. Many ulcers in conjunction give a psoriasiform appearance that may mimic migratory glossitis or stomatitis. Treatment of oral lesions is symptomatic (Chapter 28).

38. A See answer to Question 13.

39. B Granulomatous cheilitis (Miescher's cheilitis) is an uncommon granulomatous disease of the lips of unknown etiology. The lower lip is affected more often than the upper. Clinically, the patient has diffuse soft swelling of the lip that is non-tender. The swelling develops slowly. Miescher's granulomatous cheilitis has been associated with Melkersson-Rosenthal syndrome, Crohn's disease, gingival granulomatosis, and Anderson-Fabry disease.

Histologically, there are noncaseating epithelioid granulomas, Langhans giant cells, edema, and a chronic inflammatory cell infiltrate. Treatment consists of steroid injection or possibly cheiloplasty (Chapter 138).

40. B The most common sign of graft-versus-host disease (GVHD) is increased redness of the oral mucosa with atrophic and lichenoid changes. Some patients may demonstrate erosive lichenoid lesions. The buccal and labial mucosa are usually involved. The histologic changes seen in GVHD range from grade I changes, consisting of an inflammatory cell infiltrate and fibrosis, to grade II changes, demonstrating necrosis of epithelial cells or ducts of the minor salivary gland with goblet cell metaplasia.

Normal mucosa indicates that the patient does not have GVHD. Histologic criteria should be corroborated with clinical findings in making the diagnosis of graft versus host disease.

41. A Morphea, a localized form of scleroderma, has characteristic oral findings. The most common sign is widening of the periodontal ligament space, which can be seen on x-ray film. This does not however lead to loosening of the teeth. Other findings include pale and rigid oral mucosa and fibrotic stricture in the mucogingival areas. Atrophy and induration of the lips, tongue, and soft palate have also been reported. The involved mucosa may be tender. If it occurs at an early age, morphea can lead to many dental problems, including bone resorption, malocclusion, and loss of teeth (Chapters 100 and 138).

42. B Lupus erythematosus (LE) may involve the oral mucosa in both the localized and the systemic forms of the disease. The lesion of lupus consists of a depressed area of erythema with white spots surrounded by a white keratotic border with radiating striae. There may be ulceration and even bleeding, especially with the lesions encountered in systemic lupus. Lesions may be seen on the buccal mucosa, palate, lips, tongue, or gingiva. Lip lesions may start as areas of erythema that then evolve into scaly keratotic patches. These may ulcerate or become atrophic. Lesions may be extremely uncomfortable or painless. Healing occasionally leads to scarring.

Histologically, LE is similar to lichen planus. Differences peculiar to LE include vacuolization of keratinocytes, PAS-positive deposits subepithelially, edema in the upper lamina propria, PAS-positive thickening of blood vessel walls, and severe deep or perivascular infiltrates. Direct immunofluorescence is positive for immunoglobulin as well as fibrinogen and C3 in lesional tissue in discoid lupus and in both lesional and normal tissue in systemic lupus.

Treatment of the oral lesions involves topical or systemic steroid therapy or hydroxychloroquine (Chapter 24).

43. D White sponge nevus is genetically transmitted as an autosomal dominant trait. The oral mucosa is most commonly involved and lesions appear early, sometimes even at birth. The white, thick-appearing mucosa is especially evident at the lateral tongue borders and buccal mucosa. Mucosal changes may intensify until puberty, then stabilize (Chapter 138).

44. E Positive association with xerostomia can be attributed to antihistamines, antidepressants, antihypertensives, antiparkinsonian drugs, diuretics, beta-blockers, and the antipsychotics. Since the intake of these drugs increases with age, with many patients on multidrug regimens there is a positive correlation of xerostomia with age attributable to drug intake (Chapter 138).

45. E The oral lesions of dyskeratosis congenita include vesicles, ulcers, and mucosal atrophy. Mature lesions may appear as white patches. Early lesions may present in childhood. Of special importance is the finding of dysplasia or frank carcinoma, which may develop in long-standing lesions of adults. Periodic follow-up is therefore essential (Chapters 138 and 175).

46. A The autosomal dominant inherited nevoid basal cell carcinoma syndrome includes skin lesions, skeletal abnormalities, intracranial calcifications, and multiple recurrent cysts of the jaws.

The jaw cysts have a keratinized epithelial lining and contain desquamated epithelium. These so-called keratocysts are locally destructive and have a high tendency to recur if incompletely removed. Resection is sometimes necessary with large or recurrent lesions. Cysts may occur in the mandible or maxilla and are frequently picked up incidentally on skull or dental films. Osteomas of the jaws and skull occur in Gardner's syndrome; enamel hypoplasia, in ectodermal dysplasia; and tuberous sclerosis and neurofibromas of the tongue, in von Recklinghausen's syndrome and multiple mucosal neuroma syndrome (Chapter 167).

Bibliography, Part I

Allen CM, Camisa C, Salewski C, et al. Wegener's granulomatosis: Report of three cases with oral lesions. J Oral Maxillofac Surg 1991; 49:294–298.

Barker BF. Lesions of the lips. In: Wood NK, Goaz PW. Differential Diagnosis of Oral Lesions 4th edition. St. Louis: Mosby Year Book 1991:682–683.

Brannon RB, Fowler CB, Hartman KS. Necrotizing sialometaplasia. Oral Surg Oral Med Oral Pathol 1991; 72:317–325.

Doyle JL, Geary W, Baden E. Eosinophilic ulcer. J Oral Maxillofac Surg 1989; 47:349–352.

Gilbert HD, Plezia RA, Pietruk T. Cowden's disease (multiple hamartoma syndrome). J Oral Maxillofac Surg 1985; 43:457–460.

Greenspan D, Greenspan JS, Hearst NG, et al. Relation of oral hairy leukoplakia to infection with the human immunodeficiency virus and the risk of developing AIDS. J Infect Dis 1987; 155:457–481.

Heimdahl A, Johnson G, Danielsson KH, et al. Oral condition of patients with leukemia and severe aplastic anemia. Follow-up 1 year after bone marrow transplantation. Oral Surg Oral Med Oral Pathol 1985; 60:498–504.

Hernandez G, Hernandez F, Lucas M. Miescher's granulomatous cheilitis. J Oral Maxillofac Surg 1986; 44:474–478.

Lynch MA, Brightman VJ, Greenberg MS, eds. Burket's Oral Medicine Diagnosis and Treatment. 8th edition. Philadelphia: JB Lippincott, 1984:308.

Karjalainen TK, Tomich CE. A histopathologic study of oral mucosal lupus erythematosus. Oral Surg Oral Med Oral Pathol 1989; 67:547–554.

Kirschbaum BA, Arm RN. Connective tissue disorders. In: Rose LF, Kaye D. Internal Medicine for Dentistry. 2nd edition. St. Louis: CV Mosby, 1990:806–808.

Klinghoffer JF. Systemic lupus erythematosus. In: Rose LF, Kaye D, eds. Internal Medicine for Dentistry. 2nd edition. St. Louis: CV Mosby, 1990:47–50.

Kramer IRH, Lucas RB, Pindborg JJ, et al. Definition of leukoplakia and related lesions: An aid to studies on oral precancer. WHO Collaborating Centre for Oral Precancerous Lesions, Oral Surg 1978; 46:518–539.

Lamey PJ, Rees TD, Binnie WH, Rankin KV. Mucous membrane pemphigoid. Oral Surg Oral Med Oral Pathol 1992; 74:50–53.

Makoto T, Hikari K. Verruciform xanthoma involving the lip. J Oral Maxillofac Surg 1993; 51:432–434.

Martin JL, Crump EP. Leukoedema of the buccal mucosa in Negro children and youth. Oral Surg 1972; 34:49–58.

Migliorati CA, Jones AC, Baughman PA. Use of exfoliative cytology in the diagnosis of oral hairy leukoplakia. Oral Surg Oral Med Oral Pathol 1993; 76:704–710.

Nisengard RJ, Neiders M. Desquamative lesions of the gingiva. J Periodontol 1981; 52:500–510.

Nowparast B, Howell FV, Rick GM. Verruciform xanthoma. Oral Surg Oral Med Oral Pathol 1981; 51:619–625.

Pogrel MA, Cram D. Intraoral findings in patients with psoriasis with a special reference to ectopic geographic tongue (erythema circinata). Oral Surg Oral Med Oral Pathol 1988; 66:184–189.

Rogers RS, Sheridan PJ, Jordan RE. Desquamative gingivitis. Clinical histopathologic and immunopathologic investigations. Oral Surg Oral Med Oral Pathol 1976; 42:316–320.

Silverman S, Gorsky M, Lozada-Nur F. A prospective follow-up study of 570 patients with oral lichen planus: Persistence in remission and malignant association. Oral Surg Oral Med Oral Pathol 1985; 60:30–34.

Silverman S, Gorsky M, Lozada-Nur F. A prospective study of findings and management in 214 patients with oral lichen planus. Oral Surg Oral Med Oral Pathol 1991; 72:665–670.

Silverman S, Gorsky M, Lozada F. Oral leukoplakia and malignant transformation. Cancer 1984; 53:563–568.

Sreebny LM, Valdin A, Yu A. Xerostomia. Part II. Relationship to nonoral symptoms, drugs, and diseases. Oral Surg Oral Med Oral Pathol 1989; 68:419–427.

Vincent VD, Lilly GE, Baker KA. Clinical historic and therapeutic features of cicatricial pemphigoid. Oral Surg Oral Med Oral Pathol 1993; 76:453–459.

Vincent SD, Lilly, GE. Clinical historic and therapeutic features of aphthous stomatitis: Literature review and open clinical trial employing steroids. Oral Surg Oral Med Oral Pathol 1992; 74:79–86.

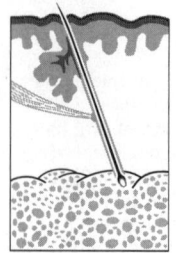

chapter 18, part II

Genital Diseases

MARIA L. TURNER

For each numbered item, choose the most likely associated lettered item. Each numbered item has ONLY ONE answer. Each lettered item may be the answer to one, more than one, or none of the numbered items.

1. Penis
2. Genital fold
3. Scrotum.

A. Labia majora
B. Labia minora
C. Clitoris
D. Vulvar vestibule.

Decide whether EACH of the following statements is TRUE or FALSE. Any combination of answers from all true to all false may occur.

In the middle of August, a heavy-set construction worker complains of itching in the groin area of a month's duration. On examination, there is uniform, tan-to-brown discoloration of both inguinal areas with some maceration within the folds. The borders of the patches are well-defined. The affected areas fluoresced coral-red under Wood's light.

4. The etiologic agent is *Trichosporon beigelii*.
5. Routine fungal cultures will establish the diagnosis.
6. The condition responds to oral erythromycin and the topical azoles.

Regarding vulvovaginal candidiasis,

7. The vaginal carriage rate for *Candida* in asymptomatic women is close to 50%.

8. The most common cause of chronic, recurrent vulvovaginal candidiasis is subclinical diabetes mellitus.
9. The vagina should always be treated in the presence of *Candida* vulvitis.

For each numbered item, choose the most likely associated lettered item. Each numbered item has ONLY ONE answer. Each lettered item may be the answer to one, more than one, or none of the numbered items.

10. *Chlamydia trachomatis* (types D to K)
11. Trichomoniasis
12. Bacterial vaginosis
13. *Neisseria gonorrhoeae*.

A. "Clue" cells seen on wet prep
B. Frothy discharge
C. Occurs with gonorrhea 45% of the time
D. Best treated with ceftriaxone, 250 mg intramuscularly (IM).

Decide whether EACH of the following statements is TRUE or FALSE. Any combination of answers, from all true to all false, may occur.

A 20-year-old man comes for evaluation and treatment of asymptomatic "warts." Examination reveals uniform, finely papillated growths that completely encircle the coronal sulcus.

14. Cryotherapy is indicated, since these are contagious.

---

* All the material in this chapter is in the public domain.

15. Histologically, these are angiofibromas.
16. The etiologic agent is human papillomavirus, type 1.

In the following questions, the set of lettered headings is followed by a list of numbered words or phrases. For each numbered word or phrase, choose

A. If the item is associated with A only
B. If the item is associated with B only
C. If the item is associated with both A and B
D. If the item is associated with neither A nor B.

For each of the following findings, choose whether it describes lichen planus, lichen sclerosus, both, or neither.

17. Orogenital involvement is common
18. Squamous cell carcinoma may occur in 4% to 5% of cases
19. Also known as balanitis xerotica obliterans
20. The papillary dermis appears "homogenized."

A. Lichen sclerosus
B. Lichen planus
C. Both
D. Neither.

For each of the following characteristics, choose whether it describes HSV 1, HSV 2, both, or neither.

21. May cause recurrent painful ulcers in the genital area
22. Currently the most common cause of genital ulcerations
23. Commercially available serologic tests can specifically recognize previous infection.

A. HSV 1
B. HSV 2
C. Both
D. Neither.

Choose the ONE BEST answer to the following question.

24. A 26-year-old woman comes in complaining of increasingly severe introital dyspareunia (pain on penile entry) such as to prevent intercourse most of the time. The pain is confined to the vulvar vestibule, and the only physical findings are erythematous areas in the vestibule that are exquisitely tender on Q-tip palpation. Wet smear, KOH preparation, and cultures for infectious agents are negative. The likeliest diagnosis is

A. Pudendal neuralgia
B. Vulvar Vestibulitis Syndrome
C. Psychosomatic vulvovaginitis.

Decide whether each of the following statements regarding genital HPV infection is TRUE or FALSE.

25. The most common type seen in the general population is type 6/11.
26. Vertical transmission from mother to child has been shown to occur.
27. HPV types 16, 18, 31, and 33 are highly associated with carcinoma of the cervix.
28. Symmetrical, soft, micropapillations on the labia minora are best destroyed to prevent the spread of genital HPV infection.

Decide whether each statement is TRUE or FALSE.

A 50-year-old woman complains of intractable pruritus in the vulvar area of 2 years duration. It has not been responsive to high-potency topical steroids, antihistamines, and good local care. Examination reveals multifocal, thin papules and plaques, portions of which are white and other portions hyperpigmented, involving not only the vulva but the perineum and perianal areas as well. Multiple biopsies reveal varying degrees of nuclear atypia, altered epithelial maturation, cellular crowding, and loss of polarity but no invasion of the basement membrane. Decide whether each statement is TRUE or FALSE.

29. The likely diagnosis is vulvar intraepithelial neoplasia (VIN).
30. The likely diagnosis is extramammary Paget's disease.
31. Synonyms for this condition include carcinoma in situ and Bowen's disease of the vulva.
32. HPV type 16 is frequently associated with this lesion.

ANSWERS

1. C; **2.** B; **3.** A The embryonal cloaca is divided by the urorectal septum into a posterior anorectal canal and an anterior urogenital sinus. The superficial end of the urogenital sinus is known as the phallic portion and consists of an anterior genital tubercle that continues posteriorly toward the perineal body as paired genital folds that are separated from each other by the urogenital slit. Lateral to the genital folds are the genital swellings. The genital tubercle gives rise to the clitoris (penis), the genital folds to the labia minora and the genital swellings to the labia majora (scrotum) (Chapter 139).

4. (F); **5.** (F); **6.** (T) Erythrasma is a superficial infection of the skin caused by *Corynebacterium minutissimum*, which are gram-positive rods. It is likely that more than one species is involved. A warm, humid condition as occurs in the genitocrural area is a predisposing factor. Coral-red fluorescence with Wood's light is attributed to coproporphyrin III, which is water-soluble. If the index of suspicion for erythrasma is high, and the lesion does not fluoresce under Wood's light, have the patient return after not having washed the area for the previous 24 hours. Differential diagnosis includes tinea versicolor, seborrheic dermatitis, and tinea cruris. The infection is responsive to topical azoles, oral erythromycin, and tetracycline. It tends to recur, unless the area is routinely washed with a disinfectant soap and kept as dry as possible (Chapters 105 and 139).

7. (F); **8.** (F); **9.** (T) Currently, vulvovaginal candidiasis is the second most common cause of vaginal infections. About 75% of women will experience this condition at least once during their childbearing years. Of these, 40% to 50% experience a second attack. However, 5% have recurrent, intractable, symptomatic attacks of this infection. *Candida* may be isolated from the genital tract of asymptomatic women about 20% of the time. Increased rates of asymptomatic colonization are seen during pregnancy, with the use of high-estrogen oral contraceptives, with uncontrolled diabetes, and in patients attending sexually transmitted disease (STD) clinics. However, most diabetic patients do not have recurrent infections, and the yield of glucose tolerance tests in all women with recurrent vulvovaginal candidiasis is extremely low. The transition from asymptomatic carriage of *Candida* to symptomatic candidal infection is most likely influenced by loss of local defense mechanisms such as alteration of the normal vaginal flora. *Candida* infection of the female genital tract is almost always a vulvovaginitis (Chapter 139).

10. C; **11.** B; **12.** A; **13.** D Bacterial vaginosis is currently the most common cause of vaginal discharge in the childbearing years. It was previously known as nonspecific vaginitis and was thought to be an infection caused by *Gardnerella vaginalis*. The current consensus is that this entity is not so much an infection as an imbalance of the vaginal flora such that the predominant normal flora, *Lactobacillus acidophilus*, is replaced by anaerobic organisms. The resulting discharge has a "fishy" or "amine" odor, intensified by the addition of KOH, and examination of a wet smear reveals numerous "clue cells" (desquamated epithelial cells covered with bacteria).

Trichomoniasis is an STD caused by *Trichomonas vaginalis*. There is a high prevalence of gonorrhea in both men and women with this condition. *Trichomonas* infection in women can lead to severe acute inflammatory disease characterized by extreme pruritus and a copious, malodorous and frothy discharge. A saline wet smear will show teardrop-shaped motile organisms with numerous white blood cells. Oral metronidazole, 250 mg three times per day for 7 days or a single oral dose of 2 g, achieves comparable clearing.

Chlamydia trachomatis (types D to K) causes most cases of nongonococcal urethritis and mucopurulent cervicitis. It is frequently asymptomatic in women but can give rise to infertility. As much as 45% of patients with gonorrhea have a coexisting chlamydial infection. It is for this reason that simultaneous treatment for *Chlamydia* is administered to patients with gonorrhea, especially if it is not possible to test for *Chlamydia*. The most reliable diagnostic test is a culture. Doxycycline (100 mg orally) twice a day for 7 days or tetracycline (500 mg orally) four times a day is the recommended therapy.

Neisseria gonorrhoeae is a gram-negative diplococcus that can infect the entire genital tract in both men and women. It is a highly contagious STD and is fast developing antibiotic resistance, so that there are now penicillinase-producing and tetracycline-resistant strains. Ceftriaxone (250 mg) in a single intramuscular injection is the current recommendation for gonococcal infection of the genital tract (Chapter 139).

14. (F); **15.** (T); **16.** (F) Pearly penile papules are smooth, dome-shaped, pink papules that may partly or completely encircle the corona of the penis. Although patients may seek treatment because they think that these are warts, on histology, these lesions are found to be benign angiofibromas, and no therapy is necessary (Chapter 139).

17. B; **18.** A; **19.** A; **20.** A Lichen sclerosus may affect both sexes and all ages, although it occurs predominantly on the genitalia of postmenopausal women. It may also be seen on other parts of the body, although reports of oral lesions are rare. Involvement of male genitalia is sometimes known as balanitis xerotica obliterans. At the onset, patchy hypopigmentation to depigmentation accompanied by pruritus is seen. As the disease progresses, sclerosus and narrowing of the orifices in the areas involved begins to occur. Atrophy of the epidermis predisposes the involved areas to erosion and hemorrhages. Histologically, hyalinization or homogenization of collagen in the papillary dermis is characteristic. Prepubertal girls may be affected, and although it was initially thought that these lesions involuted with menarche, this does not appear to be entirely the case. The etiology of lichen sclerosus is still not clear. There is a reported 4% to 6% risk of developing squamous cell carcinoma within genital lesions of lichen sclerosus (Chapter 139).

21. C; **22.** B; **23.** D Genital herpes simplex virus (HSV) infection may be caused by HSV 1 or HSV 2, although most are caused by HSV 2. Primary infections have an incubation period of 3 to 7 days, and recurrences are more common during the first 2 years after the primary infection, with the frequency decreasing with time.

Painful vesicles and small ulcers are the hallmarks of the infection. However, asymptomatic shedding is a well-documented phenomenon, even during acyclovir prophylaxis. Genital HSV infection has to be differentiated from other sexually transmitted diseases, such as syphilis and chancroid, which may in fact accompany a primary infection. A well-done Tzanck smear is a convenient, inexpensive, and fairly accurate test, and a positive culture finding is the "gold standard" for diagnosis. Serologic tests are now available for determining prior exposure to HSV. Current commercial enzyme immunoassays can distinguish seropositive HSV from sero-negative HSV cases. These assays cannot discriminate between HSV 1 and HSV 2 infections. Serologic testing by Western blot or glycoprotein G immunodot enzyme assay can distinguish HSV 1 from HSV 2 exposure, but these are research tools at the moment (Chapters 121 and 139).

24. B Vulvodynia is a problem that dermatologists have only recently managed. It is defined as chronic burning pain or a sensation of rawness in the vulvar area. A simple method of managing this problem is to group patients into three main subsets. In the first subset are women with chronic burning pain caused by dermatologic conditions that give rise to ulcers or erosions. These cases are generally not etiologic or diagnostic problems. The second group of women complain of introital or entry dyspareunia. Physical findings are limited to erythematous patches on the vulvar vestibule (around the openings of Bartholin's and Skene's ducts) that are exquisitely tender to light, Q-Tip palpation. This combination of signs and symptoms constitutes what is known as the vulvar vestibulitis syndrome, the etiology and definitive therapy of which are still under investigation. The third and most problematic group are those patients who have pudendal neuralgia. They complain of dyspareunia and constant burning pain, not only on the vulvar vestibule, but also in the perineal and perianal areas. Additional symptoms include urinary frequency and "sciatica." Involvement of areas outside the vulvar vestibule distinguishes pudendal neuralgia from vulvar vestibulitis syndrome. Small doses of a tricyclic antidepressant, amitryptyline, have been helpful for pudendal neuralgia (Chapter 139).

25. (T); **26.** (T); **27.** (T); **28.** (F) Human papillomavirus (HPV) infection of the genital tract has been increasing rapidly since the 1960s, especially in young, sexually active patients. In a relatively recent study, using the polymerase chain reaction on vulvar samples obtained from women seeking routine gynecologic care at a college campus, 40% to 45% of the samples contained HPV DNA. The most common clinical form of HPV infection is condylomata acuminata, and this is most often associated with HPV types 6 and 11. Recognition of genital HPV infection has become more important because a high percentage of cases of cervical neoplasias (including cervical carcinomas) has been found to harbor DNA from HPV types 16, 18, 31, and 33. Genital HPV infection is mainly transmitted by sexual intercourse, although vertical transmission is known to occur. Genital HPV infection manifesting as cauliflower-like growths (condylomata acuminata) is readily recognized clinically. However, subclinical forms of HPV infection pose problems in diagnosis and therapy. Examples are the soft, micropapillary lesions that may sometimes cover the mucosal surfaces of the inner labia minora and the vulvar vestibule. Some believe that these are manifestations of HPV infection and, as such, should be treated. However, when sensitive techniques, such as polymerase chain reaction, are utilized to isolate HPV DNA, the yield is no higher than that in an asymptomatic, sexually active population. Wholesale treatment of these patients is not warranted (Chapters 123 and 139).

29. (T); **30.** (F); **31.** (T); **32.** (T) Just as in the cervix, vulvar intraepithelial neoplasia is very frequently linked to genital infection with HPV types 16, 18, 31, and 33. These lesions appear as multifocal, pruritic, skin-colored-to-hyperpigmented flat papules or plaques. (They are frequently asymmetric.) There is a tendency to involve contiguous structures such as the perineum, perianal area, and anal canal. When extensive, a biopsy may be necessary to differentiate vulvar intraepithelial neoplasia from lichen simplex chronicus and extramammary Paget's disease. Histology reveals varying degrees of nuclear atypia, altered epithelial maturation, and loss of polarity. The basement membrane is not invaded. Treatment generally consists of laser and/or 5-fluorouracil applications (Chapters 123 and 139).

Bibliography

Ackerman AB, Kornberg R. Pearly penile papules: Acral angiofibromas. Arch Dermatol 1973; 108:673.

Buckley CH, Fox H. Epithelial tumors of the vulva. In: Ridley CM, ed. The Vulva. Edinburgh: Churchill Livingstone, 1988:263.

Drake TE, Maibach HI. Candida and candidiasis: Cultural conditions, epidemiology, and pathogenesis. Postgrad Med 1973; 53:83.

Friedric EG, Jr. Vaginitis. In: Vulvar Disease, 2nd edition. Philadelphia: WB Saunders Co., 1983:22.

Gardner HL, Dukes CD. *Hemophilus vaginalis* vaginitis: A newly defined specific infection previously classified "nonspecific vaginitis." Am J Obstet Gynecol 1955; 69:962.

Highet AS, Hay RJ, Roberts SOB. Bacterial infections. In: Champion RH, Burton JL, Ebling FJG, eds. Textbook of Dermatology. 5th edition. London: Blackwell Scientific Publications, 1992:996.

Judson FN. Gonorrhea. Med Clin North Am 1990; 74:1353.

Judson FN. The importance of coexisting syphilitic, chlamydial, mycoplasmal, and trichomonal infections in the treatment of gonorrhea. Sex Transm Dis 1979; 6:112.

McLean JM. Embryology and congenital anomalies of the vulval areas. In: Ridley CM, ed. The Vulva. 2nd edition. London: Churchill Livingstone, 1988:1.

Ridley CM. Lichen sclerosus. Derm Clin 1992; 10:309.

Sobel JD. Candidal vulvovaginitis. Clin Obstet Gynecol 1993; 36:153.

Sobel JD. Vulvovaginitis. Derm Clin 1992; 10:339.

Villarino ME, Schulte JM. Diagnosis and therapy for common sexually transmitted diseases. Derm Clin 1992; 10:459.

chapter 19

Disorders of Hair, Nails, and Sweat

MARC AVRAM, ARTHUR P. BERTOLINO, and RICHARD K. SCHER

DISEASES OF THE HAIR

Choose the ONE BEST answer to each of the following questions.

1. What is the anagen to telogen ratio of scalp hair?
   A. 90:10
   B. 75:25
   C. 70:30
   D. 60:40
   E. 20:80.

2. What is the rate of growth of hair on the scalp?
   A. 0.1 mm/day
   B. 0.4 mm/day
   C. 0.7 mm/day
   D. 1.0 mm/day.

3. What region of the body normally develops gray hair first in men?
   A. Beard
   B. Scalp
   C. Chest
   D. Pubic region.

4. What age is considered premature for graying in whites and blacks?
   A. Before 4th decade whites and blacks
   B. Before 3rd decade whites and blacks
   C. Before 3rd decade whites and 4th blacks
   D. Before 4th decade whites and 3rd blacks.

5. Menkes' kinky hair syndrome results from a deficiency in
   A. Zinc
   B. Cobalt
   C. Copper
   D. Citrulline.

6. What is the mode of inheritance of Netherton's syndrome?
   A. Autosomal dominant
   B. Autosomal recessive
   C. X-linked recessive
   D. X-linked dominant.

7. Which hair shaft disorder results in elliptical nodes separated at regular intervals?
   A. Pili torti
   B. Monilethrix
   C. Pili annulati
   D. Trichorrhexis nodosa.

8. Trichothiodystrophy is associated with what defect in the hair?
   A. High sulfur content
   B. Low sulfur content

C. High copper content

D. Low copper content.

9. Which of the following hereditary disorders may be associated with permanent alopecia?

    A. Darier's disease

    B. Aplasia cutis congenita

    C. Porokeratosis of Mibelli

    D. All of the above.

10. The majority of cases of nonextensive patch-type alopecia areata display regrowth in

    A. 3 to 6 months

    B. 6 to 12 months

    C. 12 to 18 months

    D. 2 to 3 years.

11. Poor prognostic features for alopecia areata include

    A. Onset prior to puberty

    B. Involvement of the vertex of the scalp

    C. Family history

    D. All of the above.

12. Acquired hypertrichosis lanuginosa is associated with

    A. Diabetes

    B. Syphilis

    C. Underlying malignancy

    D. Polycystic ovarian disease.

13. All the following systems may produce hirsutism EXCEPT

    A. Ovarian

    B. Pituitary

    C. Adrenal

    D. Liver.

For each numbered item choose the most likely associated letter from those provided. Each numbered item has one answer. Within the group, each lettered item may be the answer to one, more than one, or none of the numbered items.

14. Serum luteinizing hormone : follicle-stimulating hormone (LH : FSH) ratio or serum LH

15. Prolactin

16. Serum 17-hydroxyprogesterone

17. Dihydroepiandrosterone sulfate (DHEAS)

18. Dihydrotestosterone.

    A. Potent androgen

    B. 21-β-Hydroxylase deficiency

    C. Polycystic ovarian disease

    D. Adrenal tumor

    E. Pituitary adenoma.

Decide whether EACH of the following questions is TRUE or FALSE. Any combination of answers from all true to all false may occur.

Regarding androgenetic alopecia,

19. Androgenetic alopecia before the fourth decade in either sex is rare.

20. A trichogram may be helpful in making a diagnosis.

21. A punch biopsy may be helpful in distinguishing androgenetic alopecia from other nonscarring alopecias.

22. Residual hair density in women equals that in men over time.

23. Concerning distribution of hair,

    A. The greatest density of hair follicles is in the pubic region

    B. Hair follicles are present throughout the entire integument

    C. The density of hair on the scalp diminishes after birth

    D. Redheads have the greatest density of hair follicles on the scalp.

Concerning folliculitis decalvans,

24. Bacteria are responsible for the condition.

25. It occurs in men and women.

26. Any hair-bearing regions of the body may be affected.

27. On physical examination, expanding groups of pustules and crusts with a central atrophic patch are characteristic.

Choose the ONE BEST answer to EACH of the following questions.

28. All of the following drugs have been associated with telogen effluvium EXCEPT

    A. Allopurinol

    B. Oral contraceptives

    C. Beta-blockers

    D. Lisinopril.

29. Which of the following drugs have been associated with an anagen effluvium?
    A. Methotrexate
    B. Colchicine
    C. Azathioprine
    D. Cyclophosphamide
    E. All of the above.

For the following questions, ONE or MORE of the completions correctly finishes the incomplete statement; choose

    A. If only 1, 2, and 3 are correct
    B. If only 1 and 3 are correct
    C. If only 2 and 4 are correct
    D. If only 4 is correct
    E. If all are correct.

30. Cicatricial alopecia may be caused by
    1. Discoid lupus erythematosus
    2. Lichen planopilaris
    3. Herpes zoster
    4. Oral contraceptives.

31. A scarring alopecia may be associated with
    1. Food deprivation, starvation
    2. Secondary syphilis
    3. Hypothyroidism
    4. Necrobiosis lipoidica diabeticorum.

32. Regarding hair replacement surgery which is TRUE and which, FALSE?
    A. Hair replacement may be performed equally well in all races
    B. Areas of scarring are as suitable as normal skin
    C. Arteriovenous malformations may occur at donor sites
    D. Patches of alopecia areata of less than 3 cm are suitable
    E. Uncontrolled hypertension is a contraindication.

Choose the ONE BEST answer to each of the following questions.

33. Undermining the scalp to close large primary scalp defects should be done in which plane?
    A. Subcutaneous fat
    B. Periosteum
    C. Subgaleal
    D. Subepidermal.

34. Cylindroma has been associated with
    A. Trichilemmoma
    B. Trichoepithelioma
    C. Trichodiscoma
    D. Desmoid tumor.

Decide whether EACH of the following questions is TRUE or FALSE. Any combination of answers from all true to all false may occur.

Regarding hidradenitis suppurativa,

35. The earliest sign of hidradenitis is often a tender, erythematous cystic nodule.
36. Restricted mobility of limbs, rectal fistulas, and squamous cell carcinomas may arise.
37. It occurs predominantly in males.

Choose the ONE BEST answer to each of the following questions.

38. Palmar or plantar hyperhidrosis may be treated by
    A. Topical corticosteroids
    B. Oral corticosteroids
    C. Iontophoresis
    D. Carbon dioxide laser surgery.

39. Fox-Fordyce disease is
    A. An eruption consisting of vascular papules on the scrotum
    B. A pruritic papular eruption in the axillae
    C. Associated with pregnancy in diabetic females
    D. An inherited genodermatosis.

40. All of the following hormones may influence hair growth EXCEPT
    A. Thyroid hormones
    B. Corticosteroids
    C. Sex hormones
    D. Parathyroid hormones.

41. Melanocytes that produce hair color are located in the
    A. Cortex
    B. Medulla

C. Matrix
D. Basement membrane.

In each of the following questions, a set of lettered headings accompanies a list of numbered words or phrases. For each numbered phrase, choose

A. If the item is associated with A only
B. If the item is associated with B only
C. If the item is associated with both A and B
D. If the item is associated with neither A nor B.

42. For each of the statements below, choose whether it is associated with apocrine bromhidrosis, eccrine bromhidrosis, both, or neither.

    1. Occurs only after puberty
    2. Occurs in the axillae
    3. Obesity predisposes to development
    4. Bacteria play a role in the pathogenesis.

    A. Apocrine bromhidrosis
    B. Eccrine bromhidrosis
    C. Both
    D. Neither.

DISEASES OF NAILS

In the following questions, for each numbered item, choose the most likely associated lettered item. Each numbered item has only ONE answer. Within each group, each lettered item may be the answer to one, more than one, or none of the numbered items.

43. Darier's disease
44. Bacterial endocarditis
45. Antimalarials
46. Bronchiectasis
47. Congestive heart failure
48. *Pseudomonas* infection.

    A. Yellow-nail syndrome
    B. Green nails
    C. Red lunula
    D. Linear red and white streaking
    E. Blue nail bed
    F. Splinter hemorrhage.

49. Iron deficiency anemia
50. Marker of recent severe illness
51. Cirrhosis
52. Renal failure
53. Hypoalbuminemia.

    A. Terry's nail
    B. Muehrcke's nails
    C. Half-and-half nails (Lindsay's)
    D. Spoon-shaped nails (koilonychia)
    E. Beau's lines.

Decide whether EACH of the following are TRUE or FALSE. Any combination of answers from all true to all false may occur.

Associated with dyskeratosis congenita,

54. Autosomal dominant inheritance
55. Pancytopenia
56. Keratotic papules
57. Testicular hypoplasia
58. Absence of radial pulse.
59. Associated with the nail-patella syndrome,

    A. Autosomal recessive inheritance
    B. Renal disease may be associated
    C. Onycholysis
    D. Bony abnormalities
    E. Triangular lunulae.

Choose the ONE BEST answer to each of the following questions.

60. Features of pachydermoperiostosis include all of the following EXCEPT

    A. Acromegalic features
    B. Clubbing of digits
    C. Cutis verticis gyrata
    D. Hyperhidrosis
    E. Marfanoid habitus.

61. Dolichonychia (long nails) has been described with each of the following EXCEPT

    A. Hypopituitarism
    B. Marfan's syndrome
    C. Hypohidrotic ectodermal dysplasia
    D. Linear morphea.

62. All of the following may be associated with onycholysis EXCEPT

    A. Reiter's disease
    B. Psoriasis
    C. Pityriasis rotunda
    D. Retinoids.

63. The inheritance of pachyonychia congenita is

    A. Autosomal dominant
    B. Autosomal recessive
    C. X-linked recessive
    D. X-linked dominant.

64. What is the most commonly associated nail change of psoriasis in patients with psoriatic arthritis?
    A. Hyperkeratosis
    B. Oil spot
    C. Onycholysis
    D. Pitting.

65. Fingernails grow at about the rate of
    A. 0.1 cm/month
    B. 0.3 cm/month
    C. 0.5 cm/month
    D. 1.0 cm/month.

66. Carbon monoxide poisoning is associated with which color change of the nail bed?
    A. Brown
    B. Yellow
    C. Blue
    D. Red
    E. Black.

67. The most common epidermal neoplasm of the nail is
    A. Basal cell carcinoma
    B. Squamous cell carcinoma
    C. Malignant melanoma
    D. Cutaneous T-cell lymphoma.

68. Which organism produces blistering distal dactylitis?
    A. *Staphylococcus aureus* type 1
    B. *Candida albicans*
    C. *Pseudomonas aeruginosa*
    D. β-hemolytic streptococcus.

69. Phototoxic reactions of the nail produce what characteristic nail change?
    A. Blue discoloration
    B. Red discoloration
    C. Onycholysis
    D. Longitudinal ridging
    E. Hyperkeratosis.

In each of the following questions a set of lettered headings accompanies a list of numbered words or phrases. For each numbered word or phrase, choose

   A. If the item is associated with A only
   B. If the item is associated with B only
   C. If the item is associated with both A and B
   D. If the item is associated with neither A nor B.

For each of the statements below, choose whether it is associated with hidrotic ectodermal dysplasia, anhidrotic ectodermal dysplasia, both, or neither.

70. Autosomal dominant
71. Significant nail dystrophy
72. X-linked dominant
73. North Americans of French ancestry.

   A. Hidrotic ectodermal dysplasia
   B. Anhidrotic ectodermal dysplasia
   C. Both
   D. Neither.

For each of the statements below, choose whether it is associated with nails in psoriasis, nails in lichen planus, both, or neither.

74. "Oil drop" sign
75. Pterygium formation
76. Onycholysis
77. Subungual hyperkeratosis.

   A. Nails in psoriasis
   B. Nails in lichen planus
   C. Both
   D. Neither.

For the following questions, one or more of the completions correctly finishes the incomplete statement; choose

   A. If only 1, 2, and 3 are correct
   B. If only 1 and 3 are correct
   C. If only 2 and 4 are correct
   D. If only 4 is correct
   E. If all are correct.

78. Which of the following conditions is associated with pitting nails?
    1. Psoriasis
    2. Alopecia areata
    3. Eczema
    4. Keratoderma.

79. Acquired clubbing may be associated with
    1. Intrathoracic neoplasms
    2. Ulcerative colitis
    3. Hyperthyroidism
    4. Cirrhosis.

80. Brachyonychia (short nails) may be associated with
    1. Nail biting
    2. Cirrhosis
    3. Psoriatic arthropathy
    4. Paget's disease.

ANSWERS

1. A There are about 100,000 hairs on the human scalp. The average length of time a follicle remains in anagen (growth stage) is one thousand days and in telogen (resting stage) one hundred days. The anagen:telogen ratio is 90:10. The average number of hairs lost daily is approximately one hundred. The signals involved in transforming a follicle between stages are not well understood (Chapter 133).

2. B The rate of growth varies over different parts of the body. On the scalp, growth averages 0.3 to 0.4 mm/day. Scalp hair in women grows slightly faster than men (Chapter 133).

3. A The onset of graying, canities, is genetically determined and occurs at different ages on different areas of the body. Graying of hair occurs with decreased melanization of melanocytes and subsequent loss of melanocytes. The beard region most often develops graying first, followed by temples and the remainder of the scalp. Chest hair develops graying at a later age. Gray hair in the pubic region is rare (Chapter 133).

4. C Premature graying occurs before the third decade in whites and fourth decade in blacks. Autoimmune diseases such as pernicious anemia and Hashimoto's thyroiditis need to be considered in this setting (Chapter 133).

5. C A partial block in the intestinal absorption of copper results in this X-linked recessive syndrome, which occurs in about one in 35,000 live births. The skin, hair, and central nervous system are principally affected, resulting in short, light-colored, brittle hair; striking pallor of the skin; progressive psychomotor retardation; convulsions; and impaired temperature regulation. Survival beyond 2 years of age is unusual (Chapters 133 and 163).

6. B Patients with Netherton's syndrome are often born with generalized erythema, which improves several weeks after birth. Short, brittle, lusterless hair and characteristic scaly, dry polycyclic plaques on the trunk and extremities are features of this syndrome. Seventy-five per cent of patients have an associated history of atopy. Light microscopy of hair reveals "bamboo-like" nodes in the shaft (Chapter 163).

7. B Monilethrix has been reported to have both autosomal dominant and recessive modes of inheritance. The age of onset and severity varies greatly. Follicular keratosis with short, brittle hair on the scalp is highly characteristic. Eyebrows, eyelashes, and general body hair may be affected. Light microscopy reveals beading (nodes) alternating with constriction of the hair shaft every 0.7 to 1.0 mm. In pili torti, the hairs are flattened and rotated 180 degrees along their long axis. Affected hairs are brittle and break easily with trauma. Nonscalp hairs are rarely affected. In pili annulati, there usually is no hair fragility. Light microscopy reveals alternating light and dark bands. Trichorrhexis nodosa usually results from mechanical or chemical trauma to the hair and creates sporadic fragile nodes and broken shafts (Chapter 163).

8. B Trichothiodystrophy describes brittle hair with low sulfur content. Several clinical syndromes have been associated with trichothiodystrophy, including brittle hair, intellectual impairment, decreased fertility, short stature (BIDS); ichthyosis plus BIDS (IBIDS) and photosensitivity plus IBIDS (PIBIDS) (Chapter 163).

9. D Aplasia cutis congenita is an embryologic defect often localized to the vertex of the scalp. Darier's disease affecting the scalp is not rare; but scarring from the process is unusual, although it does occur. Porokeratosis of Mibelli is a defect in keratinization that may occur anywhere on the body, producing an atrophic plaque with a raised keratotic border (Chapters 135 and 163).

10. B The majority of cases of nonextensive patch-type alopecia areata demonstrate regrowth within 6 to 12 months. Unpigmented fine hair growing from the periphery to the central part of the patch initially occurs, and with time, pigmented, normal diameter hair grows (Chapter 134).

11. A Poor prognostic features in alopecia areata include onset before puberty, multiple episodes, involvement along the scalp margin (ophiasis), atrophy, and progression to total involvement. The presence of a family history of alopecia areata is not related to prognosis (Chapter 134).

12. C Acquired hypertrichosis is a rare syndrome characterized by rapid growth of fine, easily recognized hair all over the body. It is sometimes associated with an underlying malignancy; breast, lung, colon, and pancreatic tumors have been reported. Successful treatment of the tumor has been associated with remission of the hypertrichosis (Chapter 181).

13. D Hirsutism is excessive hair growth in a male-type distribution in women. Ovarian, adrenal, pituitary, and hypothalamic disorders may all be involved in producing hirsutism. A thorough history is the initial step in evaluating hirsute women. Regular menses suggests a nonendocrine etiology. Initial screening tests include dehydroepiandrosterone sulfate (DHEAS), free testosterone, luteinizing hormone:follicle-stimulating hormone ratio (LH:FSH), and prolactin. Endocrinologic and gynecologic consultation helps determine further workup. Idiopathic hirsutism does occur (Chapter 181).

14. C; **15.** E; **16.** B; **17.** D; **18.** A The LH:FSH ratio or serum LH level is elevated with polycystic ovarian disease, which may also result in acne and hirsutism. An elevated prolactin level may result from a pituitary adenoma. Other causes of an elevated prolactin level include hypothyroidism, hepatorenal failure, and phenothiazine use. An elevated serum 17-hydroxyprogesterone is found with 21-hydroxylase deficiency. An elevated DHEAS level indicates an adrenal process that may need further investigation. The potency of androgen hormones can be ordered as follows: dihydrotestosterone > androstenediol > testosterone > androstenedione > dehydroepiandrosterone. Variations in potency may, however, occur in certain tissues (Chapter 181).

19. (F) **20.** (T); **21.** (T); **22.** (F) The process of male or female pattern alopecia may begin any time after puberty. A trichogram may be helpful in making the diagnosis. The normal ratio of anagen to telogen hair is reduced in androgenetic alopecia. A punch biopsy reveals an abundance of telogen-stage follicles that with time may atrophy. The thickness of the epidermis and dermis is often reduced. The decrease in hair density in women is substantially less than men and rarely results in complete balding of the scalp. The reason for this difference is not understood (Chapter 133).

23. A (F); B (F); C (T); D (F) The greatest density of follicles is on the scalp. Hair follicles are found over the entire integument except the palms, soles, and portions of the genitalia. The density of hair follicles diminishes after birth. Individuals with brown or black hair have about 100,000 hair follicles on the scalp. Blondes have about 10% more and redheads about 10% less on average (Chapter 133).

24. (F); **25.** (T); **26.** (T); **27.** (T) The etiology of folliculitis decalvans is unclear. *Staphylococcus aureus* has been grown from pustules, but most often nonpathogenic organisms are grown. Women aged 30 to 60 years are affected, and men from adolescence onward may be affected; there is an overall equal incidence between the sexes. All hairy regions on the body may be affected, and expanding groups of pustules and crust with a central atrophic patch is the typical physical finding (Chapter 135).

28. D When evaluating patients for a possible telogen effluvium, a complete drug history is essential. Common offenders are beta-blockers, anticoagulants, and antithyroid drugs (Chapter 133).

29. E Patients using methotrexate, colchicine, azathioprine, and cyclophosphamide must be told of the possibility of developing a reversible hair loss (Chapter 133).

30. A Early lesions of lichen planopilaris demonstrate keratotic erythematous follicular papules. Follicles are eventually lost, resulting in scarred, hypopigmented, or hyperpigmented smooth areas. In the early active phase, discoid lupus lesions typically manifest as erythematous plaques with follicular plugging. Later, they develop into hypopigmented and hyperpigmented cicatricial patches, making inactive forms of lichen planopilaris and discoid lupus indistinguishable. Herpes zoster may cause scarring on any location that it affects. Oral contraceptives have been associated with a nonscarring alopecia (telogen effluvium) (Chapter 135).

31. D Crash dieting and starvation are associated with a nonscarring alopecia. Other causes of nonscarring alopecia include alopecia areata, endocrine disorders (particularly thyroid), trichotillomania, drugs, hereditary syndromes, and secondary syphilis. Necrobiosis lipoidica diabeticorum rarely occurs on the scalp but may produce a scarring alopecia when it occurs (Chapters 133 to 135).

32. A (T); B (F); C (T); D (F); E (T) Hair replacement surgery has been performed equally well in all races. Hair graft survival is less in areas of scars, presumably as a result of poor vascular supply. Rarely, arteriovenous malformations and pyogenic granulomas may develop at donor sites. Patches of alopecia areata have not proved suitable for hair replacement surgery. The reason is unclear. Uncontrolled hypertension is a contraindication for hair replacement surgery (Chapter 133).

33. C The galea aponeurotica is a strong fibrous attachment between frontal and occipital scalp muscles. Undermining the subcutaneous fat is often bloody and may result in destruction of hair follicles. The subgalea is a bloodless plane that, with undermining, creates enough mobility in the overlying skin to close large primary defects (Chapter 133).

34. B Trichoepithelioma of the face, which has been associated with cylindroma of the scalp, is inherited in an autosomal dominant mode. Tricholemmoma is associated with Cowden's syndrome, which is an autosomal dominant genodermatosis. Other cutaneous features include keratotic lesions resembling warts on the dorsal hands and cobblestoning on the oral mucosa. Patients are at an increased risk of developing breast and thyroid carcinoma. Desmoid tumors may occur with Gardner's syndrome. Other features include osteomas, multiple epidermal inclusion cysts, and intestinal polyposis with a nearly 100% risk of malignant transformation. Trichodiscomas are skin-colored papules that occur on the head and neck (Chapters 142 to 145).

35. (T); **36.** (T); **37.** (F) Cystic erythematous nodules are the earliest lesions found in hidradenitis suppurativa. Their recognition is vital because early aggressive treatment represents the best hope for long-term control. In chronic cases, draining sinus tracts, fibrosis, and tender erythema develop in the involved regions. This may lead to altered limb mobility and fistula formation with perianal hidradenitis, which most often occurs in men. As with other chronic scarred sites, squamous cell carcinomas may arise. The disease occurs in both sexes. It has not been reported before puberty or after menopause, suggesting a role for hormonal changes in the pathogenesis of the disease (Chapter 50).

38. C Iontophoresis has provided a useful alternative to topical aluminum chloride solution treatments (Chapter 137).

39. B Fox-Fordyce disease results from the obstruction and rupture of the intraepidermal component of the apocrine gland. Women are affected more than men, in a ratio of 10:1. Pruritic erythematous papules in the axillae and/or pubes are characteristic (Chapter 137).

40. D Genetic and hormonal influences are the most well-described influences on the regulation of hair growth. Thyroid hormones, sex hormones, and corticosteroids all influence hair growth (Chapters 133 and 181).

41. C Melanocytes located in the matrix of the follicle produce pigment. Eumelanin is the pigment of brown and black hairs, and pheomelanin is the pigment of red and blonde hairs. The intensity of color is related to the amount of pigment in the shaft. Gray hair is produced when there is a markedly decreased transfer of pigment from the melanocytes to the keratinocytes of the hair shaft (Chapter 133).

42. 1 A; 2 C; 3 B; 4 C Apocrine bromhidrosis does not occur before puberty. Both apocrine and eccrine bromhidrosis may occur in the axillae. Individuals with superimposed eccrine bromhidrosis have decreased odor owing to the increased quantity of eccrine sweat. Obesity predisposes an individual to eccrine bromhidrosis due to greater occlusion of the skin in bodyfolds such as the groin and inframammary and intergluteal regions. Bacterial decomposition of both eccrine and apocrine sweat produces a distinctive odor (Chapter 137).

43. D; **44.** (F); **45.** E; **46.** A; **47.** C; **48.** B Darier's disease has distinct nail changes, which include red and white longitudinal streaking and notching of the distal nail plate. Splinter hemorrhages are found in the nail bed and are associated with endocarditis, although they may also be seen with trauma, hypertension, vasculitis, Raynaud's syndrome, and a variety of other processes. Antimalarials are well-known agents that may produce blue discoloration of the nail beds following prolonged use. Argyria, minocycline, and bleomycin have also been associated with blue discoloration of the nail bed. Congestive heart failure may produce red discoloration of the lunula. The yellow-nail syndrome is a combination of (1) thickened, dull, yellow-nails with diminished growth and increased horizontal and vertical curvature; (2) congenitally hypoplastic lymphatics, resulting in lymphedema; (3) respiratory findings, including sinusitis, bronchiectasis, and pleural effusions. *Pseudomonas* nail infection can readily be recognized by a characteristic green discoloration of the nails (Chapter 136).

49. D; **50.** E; **51.** A; **52.** C; **53.** B Koilonychia is a common manifestation of the Plummer-Vinson syndrome and is associated with anemia, glossitis, and dysphagia. In neonates, it has been associated with iron deficiency anemia. It is also associated with thyroid disease, renal dialysis, psoriasis, lichen planus, porphyria, and several congenital syndromes. Beau's lines may be noted after any severe illness or febrile episode. The width of the horizontal depression correlates with the length of disease. The white opacity of the nails associated with cirrhosis is known as Terry's nails. White discoloration of the nail, extending to 1 to 2 mm from the free edge is characteristic of all fingernails and toenails. The half-and-half nail of Lindsay is associated with renal failure. It manifests with a dull-white proximal nail that is sharply demarcated transversely from a pink distal half. Muehrcke's bands are parallel to the lunula and separated by pink nail beds. These bands are a sign of hypoalbuminemia. The presence or absence of the horizontal bands correlates with serum albumin levels (Chapter 136).

54. (F); **55.** (T); **56.** (F); **57.** (T); **58.** (F) Dyskeratosis congenita has been reported to be autosomal recessive and X-linked recessive. Poikilodermatous patches, thin, dystrophic nails, premalignant leukoplakia of the oral mucosa, blepharitis, testicular hypoplasia, and pancytopenia are associated with the genodermatosis. There is an increase in sister chromatid exchanges (Chapters 136 and 175).

59. A (F); B (T); C (F); D (T); E (T) Nail-patella syndrome is an autosomal dominant disorder with abnormalities of the nail, kidney, and bone. Nail changes are present at birth and include a triangular lunula; the patellas are absent or hypoplastic, and nephropathy is found in 30% to 40% of cases. Nail plate abnormalities are the most consistent finding (Chapter 136).

60. E Pachydermoperiostosis is a rare autosomal dominant entity that presents with clubbing of the digits, hyperhidrosis of the palms and soles, acromegalic features, cutis verticis gyrata, subperiosteal calcification of the long bones, and in some cases an underlying bronchogenic carcinoma (Chapters 136 and 175).

61. D Dolichonychia is a condition in which the length of the nail is much greater than the width. It has been associated with Ehlers-Danlos and Marfan's syndromes, hypopituitarism, and hypohidrotic ectodermal dysplasia (Chapter 136).

62. C Retinoid use may result in onycholysis of the nail plates, which resolves with discontinuation of the drug and growth of a new nail plate in 6 months. Pityriasis rotunda is a variant of acquired ichthyosis most often reported in Africans. Circular, scaly, brown patches on the trunk and extremities are characteristic. Hepatocellular carcinoma has been associated (Chapter 136).

63. A Pachyonychia congenita is an autosomal dominant genodermatosis. Clinical features include thickened, yellow nails, paronychial inflammation, recurrent nail shedding, hyperhidrotic palms and soles, keratoderma, oral leukokeratosis, scrotal tongue, and alopecia (Chapters 136 and 175).

64. D All of the findings listed are nail changes seen with psoriasis. Pitting is the most common nail change seen with psoriatic arthritis. Nail changes associated with psoriatic arthritis may or may not improve with control of psoriatic arthritis. There is no easy, clear management of psoriatic nails. Psoralen plus ultraviolet A (PUVA), oral retinoids, topical corticosteroids, and methotrexate have all been used with varying success (Chapters 27 and 136).

65. B Unlike hair, which undergoes resting and growing cycles, the nail matrix continually produces new nails. Nails grow quicker during pregnancy, adolescence, and generally quicker in males than females. Nails grow on average 0.3 cm/month. Fingernails grow faster than toenails. Fingernails grow out in 6 to 8 months and toenails in 12 to 18 months (Chapter 136).

66. D Cherry red discoloration of the lips and nail beds are unusual yet classic features of carbon monoxide poisoning. The increased level of carboxyhemoglobin in the bloodstream is thought to cause the red discoloration (Chapter 136).

67. B Squamous cell carcinoma is the most common epidermal neoplasm of the nail. It commonly manifests as a subungual or a periungual verrucous plaque resembling a common verruca. Any persistent subungual or periungual lesion should be considered for biopsy (Chapter 136).

68. D Blistering distal dactylitis manifests as a tender, blistering plaque on the anterior fat pad of the digit. The eruption may spread and involve the nail, producing a paronychia. It occurs between the ages of 2 and 16 and responds to oral antibiotic therapy (Chapter 136).

69. C Tetracycline, doxycycline, minocycline, and PUVA are commonly used dermatologic treatments that may produce onycholysis when the nails are exposed to ultraviolet light, particularly UVA (Chapter 136).

70. A; **71.** A; **72.** D; **73.** A Hidrotic ectodermal dysplasia is an autosomal dominant disorder manifesting with nail dystrophy; frequent paronychia; hypotrichosis on scalp, eyebrows, and eyelashes; and keratoderma. The majority of cases have involved individuals of French-Canadian ancestry. Hypohidrotic ectodermal dysplasia is X-linked recessive dysplasia. Nail changes rarely occur. Clinical features include an absence of sweating, recurrent sinopulmonary infections, hypotrichosis, defective dentition, and hoarseness (Chapters 136 and 164).

74. A; **75.** B; **76.** C; **77.** C Dorsal pterygium is the loss of the proximal nail fold and subsequent growth of the cuticle onto the nail plate. Ventral pterygium is an extension of hyponychial tissue, thereby eliminating the free distal nail groove. The commonest cause of pterygium is lichen planus. Onycholysis is the detachment of the nail plate from its bed. It is usually asymptomatic. Both psoriasis and lichen planus have been associated with onycholysis. Trauma, fungal infections, Reiter's disease, and drug-induced photo-onycholysis are other common causes of onycholysis. Subungual hyperkeratoses may result from psoriasis, lichen planus, chronic eczema, Reiter's onychomycosis, Darier's disease, fungal infection, and pityriasis rubra pilaris. The "oil drop" sign is pathognomonic for psoriasis (Chapter 136).

78. A Nail pitting is caused by parakeratosis in the nail plate, which is a result of an abnormal matrix. It is most commonly associated with alopecia areata, psoriasis, and eczema (Chapter 136).

79. E Clubbing of the digits may be inherited or acquired. Hereditary clubbing is an autosomal dominant disorder that begins during puberty. It is not associated with systemic disease. Acquired clubbing is a manifestation of a variety of systemic diseases. Bronchopulmonary and cardiovascular diseases are most often associated with clubbing. Cirrhosis, ulcerative colitis, and endocrine disorders may also produce clubbing. Patients with acquired clubbing warrant a thorough history and physical examination (Chapter 136).

80. B Brachyonychia (short nails) may be congenital or acquired. Nail biting is by far the most common cause of acquired brachyonychia. Hyperparathyroidism and psoriatic arthritis have all produced brachyonychia (Chapter 136).

Bibliography

HAIR

Baden HP. Disease of the Hair and Nails. Chicago: Yearbook Medical Publishers, 1987.
Bertolino AP, Freedberg IM. Hair. In: Fitzpatrick TB, Eisen AZ, Wolff K, et al., eds. Dermatology in General Medicine. 4th edition. New York: McGraw-Hill, 1993:671.
Kvedar JC, et al. Hirsutism: Evaluation and treatment. J Am Acad Dermatol 1985; 12:215.
Orentreich N. Autografts in alopecias and other selected dermatologic conditions. Ann N Y Acad Sci 1959; 83:463.
Rook A, Dawber RPR. Diseases of the Hair and Scalp. Oxford: Blackwell Scientific Publications, 1991.

NAILS

Baden, loc. cit.
Lucas GL, Upitz M. The nail-patella syndrome. J Pediatr 1966; 68:273–288.
Scher RK. Punch biopsies of nails: A simple, valuable procedure. J Dermatol Surg Oncol 1978; 4:529.
Scher RK, Daniel CR. Nails: Therapy, Diagnosis, Surgery. Philadelphia: WB Saunders Co., 1990.
Zaias N: Anatomy and Physiology: The Nail in Health and Disease. New York: Spectrum, 1980:6.

section seven

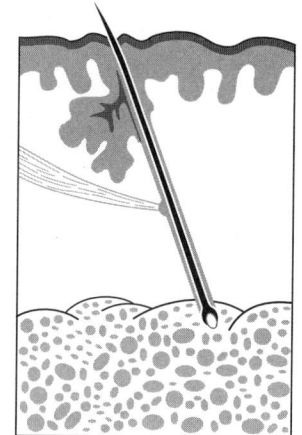

What Benign and Malignant Proliferations of Cells Affect the Skin and How Are They Treated?

chapter 20

Keratinocyte-Derived Tumors

JASON K. RIVERS, LORNE ALBRECHT, and VICTOR TRON

Choose the ONE best answer to each of the following questions.

1. All of the following statements are true of tumor suppressor gene products EXCEPT
   A. They may be bound by viral oncoproteins
   B. They promote cell differentiation
   C. They arrest cells in G1 phase
   D. They promote immune system surveillance
   E. They interact with retinoids.

2. Cutaneous defense mechanisms against ultraviolet radiation (UVR) may include all of the following EXCEPT
   A. Increased stratum corneum thickness
   B. Previtamin D_3
   C. Beta-carotene
   D. Cellular DNA repair mechanisms
   E. Melanin.

3. A 75-year-old woman in poor health has a basal cell carcinoma with a poorly defined inner border on the medial aspect of the lower eyelid. The best approach to treating this lesion is
   A. Surgical excision
   B. Mohs micrographic surgery
   C. Radiation therapy
   D. Intralesional interferon
   E. Cryotherapy.

4. A 43-year-old man presents with a rapidly enlarging 1-cm nodule with a central keratin plug on the shin. Appropriate evaluation includes
   A. Punch biopsy
   B. Shave biopsy
   C. Excisional biopsy
   D. Observation only
   E. None of the above.

5. Recurrence of basal cell carcinoma after Mohs micrographic surgery is most likely to occur in what location?
   A. Periauricular skin
   B. Medial canthus
   C. Nose
   D. Chin
   E. Scalp.

6. A 45-year-old man has a 1.0-cm to 1.5-cm defect on the tip of his nose post Mohs micrographic surgery. The most appropriate repair option would be
   A. Retroauricular skin graft
   B. Split thickness skin graft
   C. Healing by secondary intention

D. A local flap

   E. Side-to-side closure.

7. An 8-year-old girl has a slightly elevated yellowish plaque with alopecia in her scalp. The most appropriate treatment is

   A. Follow-up observation of the lesion annually

   B. Surgical excision

   C. Cryotherapy

   D. Dermabrasion

   E. Electrodesiccation.

8. A 20-year-old woman has an 8-cm-wide, verrucous linear epidermal nevus that extends from the upper thigh to the knee. The best approach to treatment of this lesion is

   A. Electrodesiccation

   B. Cryotherapy

   C. Dermabrasion

   D. Surgical excision

   E. None of the above.

9. A 3-month-old girl presents with a subcutaneous mobile cyst at the midline of the forehead. Appropriate evaluation and treatment includes

   A. Aspiration of cyst contents

   B. Intralesional corticosteroid injection

   C. Punch biopsy of lesion

   D. Incision and drainage

   E. None of the above.

10. The best treatment for an inflamed fluctuant epidermal cyst is

    A. Intralesional triamcinolone 5 mg/mL

    B. Intralesional triamcinolone 10 mg/mL

    C. Excision of the lesion

    D. Incision and drainage

    E. Oral antibiotics.

11. Which of the following is TRUE about a clear-cell acanthoma?

    A. PAS-positive and diastase-resistant

    B. Usually multiple

    C. Has an atrophic epidermis with dyskeratotic cells

    D. Shows neutrophils within the epidermis

    E. Has been linked to diabetes mellitus.

12. An irritated seborrheic keratosis

    A. Mimics a basal cell carcinoma on histology

    B. Shows absence of squamous eddies

    C. Is heavily inflamed

    D. Behaves in a benign fashion

    E. Is also referred to as a follicular hamartoma.

13. The characteristic histologic finding of epidermolytic hyperkeratosis is

    A. Vacuolar changes of cells within the superficial epidermis

    B. Presence of corps ronds and corps grains

    C. Decreased numbers of enlarged keratohyalin granules

    D. The presence of irregular eosinophilic intranuclear inclusions

    E. Superficial epidermal necrosis.

14. A nevus comedonicus

    A. Is a melanocytic nevus with numerous comedones

    B. Is a precursor lesion for malignant melanoma

    C. Histologically shows dermal melanocytes encircling follicles

    D. Is typically a linear lesion

    E. Is more common in women.

15. A pilar cyst

    A. Can be distinguished clinically from an epidermal inclusion cyst

    B. Is otherwise known as a pilar tumor

    C. Shows keratinization analogous to the outer root sheath of hair

    D. Can be transmitted as an autosomal recessive trait

    E. Shows keratinization analogous to the inner root sheath of hair.

16. A surgeon removes a cystic lesion from the forehead of a 4-year-old child. Under the light microscope, the cyst is lined by squamous epithelium with various adnexal structures. The correct diagnosis is

    A. Steatocystoma multiplex

    B. Apocrine hydrocystoma

    C. Benign appendageal cyst

    D. Dermoid cyst

    E. Epidermoid cyst.

17. During examination of a paraffin-embedded histologic section, a cystic invagination of epithelium with numerous dyskeratotic cells and suprabasal splitting is noted. The diagnosis is
    A. Warty dyskeratoma
    B. Warty Darier's disease
    C. Epidermal inclusion cyst
    D. Pilar cyst
    E. Inverted wart.

18. Which of the following cysts typically occurs in the midanterior aspect of the neck?
    A. Steatocytoma multiplex
    B. Eruptive vellous hair cyst
    C. Thyroglossal duct cyst
    D. Dermoid cyst
    E. Apocrine hydrocystoma.

19. A well-circumscribed nodular 1.0-cm primary basal cell carcinoma (BCC) on the forehead is to be excised. The most appropriate surgical margin in mm is
    A. 1.0
    B. 2.0
    C. 4.0
    D. 8.0
    E. 10.0.

For the following questions ONE or MORE of the following completions correctly finishes the incomplete statement; choose
    A. If only 1, 2, and 3 are correct
    B. If only 1 and 3 are correct
    C. If only 2 and 4 are correct
    D. If only 4 is correct
    E. If all are correct.

20. The ozone layer
    1. Absorbs ultraviolet C (UVC) wavelengths
    2. Absorbs ultraviolet A (UVA) wavelengths
    3. Absorbs ultraviolet B (UVB) wavelengths
    4. Is gradually returning to pre-1980 levels.

21. Biologic effects of ultraviolet radiation (UVR) include the following
    1. Shorter wavelengths penetrate the skin least
    2. Erythema due to UVA peaks at 12 to 24 hours post exposure
    3. Shorter wavelengths are more erythemogenic
    4. Erythema due to UVB peaks at 24 to 36 hours post exposure.

22. Mechanisms of ultraviolet radiation (UVR)–induced carcinogenesis may include
    1. Formation of DNA cyclobutane pyrimidine dimers
    2. Increased T-helper cell activity
    3. Oncogene activation
    4. Increased Langerhans cell activity.

23. Which of the following dermatoses have been associated with the development of squamous cell carcinoma (SCC)?
    1. Dystrophic epidermolysis bullosa
    2. Porokeratosis of Mibelli
    3. Erythema ab igne
    4. Lichen sclerosus et atrophicus.

24. Which of the following characteristics apply to aggressive growth of basal cell carcinomas (BCC)?
    1. Associated with morpheaform histology
    2. More likely to be found in patients over age of 35 years
    3. Associated with infiltrating histology
    4. Associated with primary tumors.

25. Which of the following statements regarding photodynamic therapy using porfimer sodium (Photofrin) for treatment of basal cell carcinoma are true?
    1. Photodestruction of the photosensitizer occurs during treatment
    2. Yellow laser light is employed
    3. Photosensitizer is selectively retained in tumor versus normal skin
    4. Generalized cutaneous photosensitivity resolves by 2 weeks post therapy.

26. Which of the following statements regarding intralesional interferon alfa-2B in the treatment of basal cell carcinoma (BCC) are true?
    1. Usual dosage is 1.5 million units 3 times weekly for 3 weeks
    2. Systemic side effects include headache, fever, and myalgia
    3. Complete response rate of 80% can be obtained
    4. Main immune response involves humoral antibody protection.

27. Treatment of superficial basal cell carcinoma (BCC) with liquid nitrogen (LN$_2$) spray cryosurgery should employ
    1. A freeze time of 15 seconds
    2. A halo measuring 2 mm
    3. A depth of freeze of 2 mm
    4. A lateral spread of freeze of 5 mm.

28. Microcystic adnexal carcinoma is characterized by which of the following?
    1. Can resemble syringoma histologically
    2. Capable of widespread metastases
    3. Best treated with Mohs micrographic surgery
    4. Occurs most commonly on the leg.

29. Accepted treatment options for actinic cheilitis include
    1. Vermilionectomy
    2. Carbon dioxide laser ablation
    3. Cryosurgery
    4. Electrosurgery.

30. A small nodular basal cell carcinoma (BCC) is excised. The pathology report indicates that there is tumor involving the lateral margins of the specimen. Appropriate management includes
    1. Re-excision of the treated site
    2. Close observation only
    3. Initial follow-up in 3 months
    4. Intralesional interferon at the treated site.

31. Mohs micrographic surgery would be considered the best treatment for which of the following tumors?
    1. A 2.0-cm primary nodular basal cell carcinoma (BCC) of the medial canthus
    2. A 2.0-cm primary nodular BCC of the forehead
    3. A 1.0-cm recurrent BCC of the ear following repeat electrosurgery
    4. A 2.0-cm, primary, well-defined squamous cell carcinoma (SCC) of the forehead.

32. Etiologic factors associated with the development of keratoacanthoma include
    1. Human papillomavirus
    2. Trauma
    3. Immunosuppression
    4. Polycyclic aromatic hydrocarbons.

33. Bowen's disease is discovered on a non–sun exposed site. The patient should be evaluated for the presence of
    1. Keratoses of the palms and soles
    2. Peripheral neuropathy
    3. Pigmentation of the axillae and groin
    4. Jaw cysts.

34. A very thick, hyperkeratotic nodule with an overlying horn is discovered on the ear of an elderly patient. Your initial management should be
    1. Shave biopsy
    2. Cryosurgery alone
    3. Curettage and electrodesiccation
    4. Topical 5-fluorouracil.

35. Sebaceous gland carcinoma is
    1. Often metastatic when it occurs on the scalp
    2. Found most often on the eyelid
    3. Associated with chronic actinic damage
    4. Associated with the Muir-Torre syndrome.

36. Electrosurgery (electrodesiccation and curettage) has been chosen to treat a skin tumor. Which of the following lesions would be appropriate for this modality?
    1. A 1.0-cm nodular basal cell carcinoma (BCC) on the cheek of a 45-year-old woman
    2. A 1.0-cm nodular BCC on the ala nasi of a 70-year-old man
    3. A 1.0-cm squamous cell carcinoma on the ear of a renal transplant patient
    4. A 1.0-cm nodular BCC on the forehead of a 70-year-old man.

37. Merkel cell carcinoma is
    1. Most frequently found on the legs
    2. Associated with a high rate of nodal metastasis
    3. Usually S-100–positive on histochemical staining
    4. Associated with squamous cell carcinoma.

Decide whether EACH of the following questions is TRUE or FALSE. Any combination of answers from all true to all false may occur.

38. Oncogenes control normal cellular growth.
39. Oncogene products can serve as growth factors or growth factor receptors.

40. Viral oncogenes and cellular oncogenes are identical.
41. Viral oncogenes derive from cellular counterparts termed proto-oncogenes.

Regarding precursor lesions to invasive squamous cell carcinoma (SCC),

42. Bowenoid papulosis is associated with human papillomavirus infection.
43. The diagnosis of Bowen's disease should prompt an investigation for internal malignancy.
44. The risk of malignant transformation of an actinic keratosis to invasive squamous cell carcinoma is 1:1000 per year.
45. Oral leukoplakia undergoes malignant transformation in the majority of individuals.
46. Erythroplasia of Queyrat is associated with human papillomavirus infection.
47. Regarding basal cell carcinoma,
    A. Actinic keratoses are a major predictor of risk
    B. Nodular basal cell carcinoma is the most common variant
    C. This malignancy occurs most often on the nose
    D. It rarely affects the eyelids
    E. Metastases occur in 1% to 2% of cases.
48. Basal cell and squamous cell carcinoma may be seen in association with the following genodermatoses:
    A. Gorlin's syndrome
    B. Oculocutaneous albinism
    C. Cockayne's syndrome
    D. Bloom's syndrome
    E. Xeroderma pigmentosum.
49. The following agents are useful in the management of advanced basal cell and/or squamous cell carcinoma.
    A. 13 *cis*-retinoic acid
    B. α-Interferon
    C. *Cis*-platin
    D. 5-Fluorouracil
    E. Carmustine (BCNU).
50. High recurrence rates of treated primary basal cell carcinoma (BCC) are associated with
    A. Increasing lesion diameter
    B. Tumors of the nose
    C. Patient's age
    D. Patient's sex
    E. Tumors of the upper extremities.
51. Radiation therapy for basal cell carcinoma (BCC) is contraindicated in the following situations.
    A. Tumor invading cartilage
    B. Tumor invading muscle
    C. Tumor invading bone
    D. Recurrent BCC
    E. Patients less than 40 years of age.
52. The following factors may place patients with cutaneous squamous cell carcinoma (SCC) in a high-risk group
    A. Tumor size greater than 2 cm in diameter
    B. Origin in a scar, chronic ulcer, or sinus tract
    C. Immunosuppression
    D. Rapid growth
    E. Anatomic site (ear).
53. The epidermal nevus syndrome is associated with
    A. Hemangiomata
    B. Cutaneous malignancies
    C. Seizures
    D. Spina bifida
    E. Pulmonary fibrosis.

In each of the following questions, a set of lettered headings accompanies a list of numbered words or phrases. For each numbered word or phrase, choose

A. If the item is associated with A only
B. If the item is associated with B only
C. If the item is associated with both A and B
D. If the item is associated with neither A or B.

For each of the following characteristics, choose whether it describes squamous cell carcinoma, basal cell carcinoma, both, or neither.

54. Increased incidence in renal transplant patients   A. Squamous cell carcinoma
55. Can occur in chronic ulcers   B. Basal cell carcinoma
56. Increased incidence in acquired immunodeficiency syndrome (AIDS)   C. Both
                                                               D. Neither
57. Associated with human papillomavirus (HPV) infection.

For each of the following characteristics, choose whether it describes clear-cell acanthoma, warty dyskeratoma, both, or neither.

58. Occurs on the head and neck most frequently
59. Prone to spontaneous regression
60. May undergo malignant degeneration
61. Liquid nitrogen cryotherapy is effective treatment.

A. Clear-cell acanthoma
B. Warty dyskeratoma
C. Both
D. Neither.

For each of the following characteristics, choose whether it describes epidermal cyst, trichilemmal cyst, both, or neither.

62. Often shows an autosomal recessive inheritance
63. Associated with Gardner's syndrome
64. The trunk is most commonly affected.

A. Epidermal cyst
B. Trichilemmal cyst
C. Both
D. Neither.

For each of the following characteristics, choose whether it describes eccrine poroma, eccrine spiradenoma, both, or neither.

65. Malignant degeneration is known to occur
66. Characteristically are painful
67. Characteristically are found on the palm and sole
68. Histochemical stains are positive for amylophosphorylase.

A. Eccrine poroma
B. Eccrine spiradenoma
C. Both
D. Neither.

For each numbered item, choose the most likely associated lettered item. Each numbered item has only ONE answer. Within each group, each lettered item may be the answer to one, more than one, or none of the numbered items.

For each of the following listed tumors, choose the therapeutic modality with which it is best treated.

69. Nodular basal cell carcinoma of the trunk
70. Recurrent basal cell carcinoma of the scalp
71. A 1.0- to 1.5-cm, well-differentiated primary squamous cell carcinoma of the arm
72. A 1.5-cm superficial basal cell carcinoma of the back.

A. Cryotherapy
B. Surgical excision
C. Curettage and electrodesiccation
D. None of the above
E. All of the above.

For each of the numbered cutaneous tumors, choose the one lettered histologic feature with which it is most closely associated. Each lettered item may be used once, more than once, or not at all.

73. Desmoplastic trichoepithelioma
74. Pilomatricoma
75. Trichilemmoma
76. Trichofolliculoma.

A. Primary follicle with surrounding secondary follicles
B. Ghost cells
C. Abundant glycogen
D. Narrow strands of tumor
E. Squamous eddies.

77. Syringocystadenoma papilliferum
78. Cylindroma
79. Syringoma
80. Chondroid syringoma.

A. Small tadpole-like ducts
B. "Jigsaw puzzle" pattern
C. Numerous plasma cells
D. Numerous foamy histiocytes
E. Mixed tumor.

ANSWERS

1. D Tumor suppressor genes, also known as antioncogenes, act on normal cell cycling to promote growth arrest and cellular differentiation. Their protein products (e.g., p53 and p105Rb proteins) in their unphosphorylated forms bind to DNA transcription factors, thus maintaining cells in G0 and G1 growth phases. Human papillomavirus (HPV) 16 E7 oncoprotein may bind to both p105Rb and p53 proteins and this mechanism likely plays a role in HPV-associated cancers. Differentiating agents such as retinoic acid inhibit the phosphorylation of p105Rb, thus maintaining growth arrest and cellular differentiation (Chapter 140).

2. B Ultraviolet radiation (UVR)-induced cutaneous damage results in an increase in epidermal and stratum corneum thickness and an increase in epidermal melanization. Other epidermal constituents that may protect against UVR include urocanic acid, beta-carotene, and skin surface lipids. The repair of damaged cellular DNA is another important defense mechanism. Melanin acts to scatter and absorb UVR and serves as a free radical "trap." Tanning is divided into immediate and delayed phases. Immediate pigment darkening appears after ultraviolet A (UVA) and visible light exposure and occurs through melanin oxidation and a redistribution of melanosomes. Delayed tanning occurs mainly after UVB exposure and results from melanin synthesis (Chapters 83, 129, and 140).

3. C Radiation therapy still has a major role to play in the treatment of malignant neoplasia of the skin, especially when the patient is incapable of undergoing surgery. Although Mohs surgery is a consideration in this case, the tumor's location would necessitate the reconstruction of the lacrimal apparatus, which would make this a technically difficult problem. Lesions that have extended into the medial canthus to an extent that the inner border cannot be clearly identified should not be treated with cryosurgery. Furthermore, this process requires experience and a thermocouple needle to be done properly. Interferon is still considered investigational (Chapter 141).

4. C The most likely diagnosis is keratoacanthoma (KA). However, the architecture of the entire lesion is required for the pathologist to make this diagnosis. Both punch and shave biopsy techniques may not provide the pathologist with adequate tissue for evaluation. Because squamous cell carcinoma can be mistaken for a lesion that has the classic appearance of KA both on clinical and histologic examination, all KAs should be removed in toto, not left to regress spontaneously (Chapter 141).

5. A The periauricular skin is an area from which it is difficult to eradicate neoplasms because of anatomic structures and numerous contours. Tumor cells tend to creep below the mastoid process and traverse along tissue planes (Chapter 141).

6. D On the nasal tip, a local flap is preferred, since this area has an abundance of pilosebaceous units, and one would like to preserve the cosmetic appearance as much as possible. A retroauricular skin graft would not provide a good color/texture match for this anatomic area, and a split thickness graft would end in a similar result. The lesion is probably too large for side-to-side closure, and healing by secondary intention would result in a poor cosmetic outcome (Chapter 141).

7. B The lesion described is typical for nevus sebaceous. Treatment modalities that remove the superficial portion of the tumor such as cryotherapy, dermabrasion, or electrodesiccation will not completely eradicate the lesion. Surgical excision is recommended because of the high potential for developing basal cell carcinoma (5%). The procedure should be done in childhood because nevus sebaceous enlarges after puberty and the risk for malignancy increases substantially after this time (Chapters 142 and 174).

8. E Although surgical excision is the best way of permanently eliminating these lesions, the extent of the nevus precludes this approach. Excision must extend to the deep dermis, otherwise the lesion may recur. Other forms of treatments have been tried, but because they only remove the superficial portion of the nevus, recurrence is common. Linear epidermal nevi are associated with a small risk of malignancy. Therefore, suspicious areas should be biopsied and excised when necessary (Chapter 142).

9. E Any midline lesion that appears at birth or in early childhood should be evaluated by noninvasive techniques before any treatment is attempted. In this situation, the most likely diagnosis, given the lesion's early age of onset and location, is dermoid cyst. Dermoid cysts can become inflamed and infected. Infection may be produced iatrogenically through aspirations, biopsies, or injections. Since there may be intracranial extension of these lesions, appropriate preoperative evaluation is mandatory. Imaging studies include MRI or CT scans as well as polytomography of the base of the skull. Treatment of a dermoid cyst is by excision with removal of any underlying sinus tract to prevent recurrence (Chapter 142).

10. D An inflamed, noninfected cyst can be treated by intralesional triamcinolone 5 mg/mL. A fluctuant, probably infected, cyst, should be incised, drained, and cultured. If there is no improvement, then antibiotic treatment can be initiated. Removal of the cyst is usually deferred until the inflammation and infection have cleared. A cyst that has never been inflamed can often be enucleated easily through a simple incision, whereas a cyst with a history of previous inflammation and scarring may need to be carefully dissected out. In order to prevent recurrence, the entire cyst lining must be removed or destroyed (Chapter 143).

11. D The clear cell acanthoma is a relatively uncommon but distinctive neoplasm. It characteristically manifests as a solitary lesion and is typically 1 to 2 cm in greatest diameter. It is said to have a seborrheic keratosis–like appearance and may exude some fluid. On histology, the epidermis is markedly hyperplastic. Although individual cells are slightly enlarged, they fail to show cytologic atypia. The cells contain a clear substance, which is glycogen that stains positively with PAS and is eliminated when diastase is used. Numerous neutrophils are noted within the epidermis, a rather characteristic finding (Chapter 142).

12. D An irritated seborrheic keratosis mimics a squamous cell carcinoma on clinical and histologic examination. The lesion can either be exophytic or endophytic. The endophytic variant has been called an inverted follicular keratosis. The characteristic histologic finding is the presence of squamous "eddies." These are eosinophilic, flattened, squamous cells, arranged in layers in an onion peel fashion. Typically, an irritated seborrheic keratosis shows little in the way of inflammation. These are benign tumors, with no malignant potential (Chapters 141 and 142).

13. A Epidermolytic hyperkeratosis is a histologic pattern that is seen in cases of bullous congenital ichthyosiform erythroderma and is also typically seen in benign epidermal tumors. This pattern may be seen in solitary epidermal nevi, as an incidental finding, or in a disseminated epidermolytic acanthoma. Its salient histologic findings are the presence of perinuclear vacuolization of epidermal cells in the superficial layer and increased numbers of irregularly shaped keratohyalin granules. Corps ronds and corps grains are typical findings of

Darier's disease and are dyskeratotic cells. Eosinophilic nuclear inclusions are not present in epidermolytic keratosis and generally signify a viral inclusion such as herpes (Chapter 142).

14. D A nevus comedonicus is not a melanocytic nevus but rather a set of closely clustered papules with hyperkeratotic plugs resembling comedones arranged in a linear fashion. These lesions are most often solitary. On histology, the comedones are epidermal invaginations filled with keratin—an appearance identical to the open comedones of acne vulgaris (Chapter 142).

15. C A pilar cyst, otherwise known as a tricholemmal cyst, is indistinguishable from an epidermal inclusion cyst on clinical examination. They can be inherited in an autosomal dominant pattern. On excision, they are easily enucleated and have a smooth capsule. A pilar tumor is an uncommon lesion occurring on the head and neck in elderly individuals that can mimic a squamous cell carcinoma. Pilar cysts arise from the outer root sheath and show tricholemmal keratinization. Calcification is a rather common feature in pilar cysts (Chapter 143).

16. D Dermoid cysts typically occur on the head and neck in children. They can measure up to 5 cm in diameter. Histologically, they are composed of a simple squamous epithelium with appendageal structures, including hair follicles and sebaceous, eccrine, and apocrine glands. Steatocystoma multiplex appears as numerous small cystic nodules, typically on the trunk. On histology, only sebaceous glands are seen within the cyst wall. An apocrine hydrocystoma develops on the head and is composed of a single layer of cuboid cells of apocrine type. Benign appendageal cyst and epidermoid cyst are fictitious entities (Chapters 143 and 145).

17. A The correct diagnosis is a warty dyskeratoma. This is a solitary keratotic papule with an umbilicated center most often found on the head and neck. The histology is reminiscent of Darier's disease with the presence of a suprabasal split and numerous dyskeratotic cells. However, Darier's disease does not show epithelial invagination. Neither epidermal inclusion cysts nor pilar cysts show suprabasal splitting with dyskeratotic cells (Chapter 142).

18. C The thyroglossal duct cyst is the most common developmental cyst occurring in the neck. It arises secondary to an abnormal descent of thyroid tissue into the neck. Most thyroglossal duct cysts are asymptomatic and retract on swallowing or extension of the tongue. On histology, these cysts are lined by stratified squamous epithelium. Occasionally, thyroid tissue may be seen arising within the connective tissue wall. Steatocystoma multiplex and eruptive villous hair cyst typically occur on the trunk, whereas dermoid cysts and apocrine hydrocystomas are confined to the head (Chapter 142).

19. C Excisional surgery, cryosurgery, and radiotherapy rely on a visual estimate of the tumor margin prior to treatment. For well-circumscribed, previously untreated basal cell carcinoma (BCC) with a diameter of less than 2.0 cm, a surgical excision margin of 4.0-mm eradicates the tumor in more than 95% of cases. For poorly circumscribed BCC (i.e., morpheaform) and for high risk anatomic sites (eyelids, canthi, pinnae, nasolabial folds, and ala nasi), a 4.0-mm treatment margin may not be adequate since subclinical lateral spread may exist (Chapter 141).

20. B Ozone (O_3) is formed naturally when high energy solar ultraviolet radiation (UVR) acts on molecular oxygen (O_2) to form singlet oxygen (O). Singlet oxygen then reacts with O_2 to form more ozone. Ozone levels vary with season and with latitude. Ozone effectively absorbs UV wavelengths below 300 nm. Therefore, it screens all UVC radiation (200 to 290 nm) and the majority of UVB radiation (290 to 320 nm). It does not significantly alter UVA transmission. It is estimated that a 1% decrease in ozone thickness increases the biologically effective UVB by 1.3 to 1.5% (Chapters 83 and 140).

21. E All parts of the ultraviolet spectrum (UVC, UVB, and UVA) are capable of inducing a biologic response. One aspect of this is the minimal erythema dose (MED). MED is the minimum amount of energy required to produce clearly marginated erythema in the irradiated area at 24 hours. The most erythemogenic wavelengths fall within the UVC and UVB ranges with a peak absorption within the UVB spectrum at 297 nm.

Ultraviolet C penetrates only the upper epidermis and creates an erythema with little or no effect on melanogenesis. UVC-induced erythema begins 4 to 6 hours after exposure and peaks at 8 hours. UVB (290 to 320 nm) penetrates into the epidermis and upper dermis and creates both erythema and pigmentation. UVB erythema begins at 2 to 6 hours and peaks at 24 to 36 hours post exposure. UVA (320 to 400 nm) creates both erythema and pigmentation with pigmentation more easily induced than erythema in dark-skinned individuals. UVA-induced erythema begins immediately or within a few hours and peaks at 12 to 24 hours post exposure (Chapters 83 and 140).

22. B Ultraviolet radiation (UVR) acts as a complete carcinogen capable of both tumor initiation and promotion. Initiation may occur through mutations arising from direct DNA damage (e.g., cyclobutane pyrimidine dimers) with resultant sister chromatid exchange and cell transformation. Promotion is most likely influenced by UVR-induced alterations in immune surveillance. Exposure to UVB leads to decreased CD1+ Langerhans cell density with the appearance of CD1− epidermal macrophage antigen–presenting cells. These cells preferentially activate pathways in which suppression dominates, leading to the presence of tumor antigen specific suppressor T cells. This in turn may lead to immunologic tolerance and tumor promotion. Alterations in oncogene function also seem to occur. Amplification of the c-*ras* oncogene and consequent overexpression of c-*ras* RNA transcripts in murine UVB-induced epidermal neoplasms have been demonstrated. Thus, abnormal oncogene function may play a role in UV-induced tumor initiation and promotion (Chapters 83 and 140).

23. E Pre-existing chronic dermatoses are associated with development of squamous cell carcinoma (SCC). Processes that result in chronic inflammation and scarring most often give rise to SCC. Some examples include porokeratosis of Mibelli, disseminated superficial actinic porokeratosis, discoid lesions of lupus erythematosus, lichen planus, lichen sclerosus et atrophicus, dystrophic epidermolysis bullosa, erythema ab igne, dissecting perifolliculitis of the scalp, hidradenitis suppurativa and acne conglobata, nevus sebaceus, and linear epidermal nevus (Chapter 141).

24. B Aggressive-growth basal cell carcinoma (BCC) is a subgroup of BCCs that are clinically and histologically aggressive in their capacity for local spread and tissue destruction. They include morpheaform, infiltrating, and recurrent BCCs. They are often easily overlooked on clinical examination. BCCs are seen most often in patients less than 35 years old (Chapter 141).

25. B Photodynamic therapy (PDT) involves the interaction of light with a photosensitizing agent. Photofrin is a mixture of porphyrins administered systemically that on exposure to red light at 630 nm ultimately produces singlet oxygen and a biologic effect. Photofrin is administered systemically and is selectively retained in tumor tissue, although the mechanism for this is unknown. Photodestruction of the Photofrin occurs during treatment. Photobleaching (photoinactivation) of the remaining drug in normal skin occurs after treatment owing to exposure to ambient light. The major limitation of PDT using Photofrin is a persistent generalized cutaneous photosensitivity to visible light that can last up to 8 weeks. Photosensitivity reactions to new porphyrin derivatives such as benzoporphyrin-derivative monoacid ring A are significantly less (1 week) and may allow PDT to become a practical therapeutic modality in future. Although PDT is currently limited to investigational status for the treatment of basal cell carcinoma (BCC) and squamous cell carcinoma, its use might be considered in the following situations: (1) in patients with nevoid BCC syndrome, (2) in patients unfit to undergo surgery, (3) in patients in whom surgery would be disfiguring, (4) in patients previously treated with radiotherapy who would not be surgical candidates (Chapter 141).

26. A A large multicenter trial, using intralesional α-interferon in a dosage of 1.5 million units 3 times weekly for 3 weeks, achieved a cure rate of over 80% for superficial and noduloulcerative basal cell carcinomas (BCCs) measuring less than 2.0 and 1.5 cm, respectively. Short-term systemic side effects of interferon therapy include influenza-like symptoms and, less commonly, dizziness and confusion. Leukopenia, increased liver enzymes, and fluid and electrolyte disturbances have been reported. The exact mechanism of action of interferon on BCC is unknown but involves a cellular immune response, including increased natural killer cell activity. Also, antiproliferative and prodifferentiation effects have been demonstrated (Chapter 141).

27. D Superficial basal cell carcinoma (BCC) can be treated successfully with cryosurgery using liquid nitrogen (LN_2) therapy ($-196°$ C). For spray techniques, the lateral spread of freeze corresponds directly (1:1) with the depth of freeze. The lateral spread of freeze is measured from the outer margin of the treated area to the outer margin of visible freezing and is also termed the halo. This halo should extend 5 mm beyond the tumor margin to result in a 5-mm depth of freeze to ensure the destruction of a superficial BCC. The rate of freezing should be as rapid as possible to ensure that appropriate temperatures are achieved at the base of the lesion. The BCC should remain frozen for a total of 60 to 90 seconds (in single or multiple freeze-thaw cycles). For this reason, cryosurgery using a cotton swab is not suitable in the management of BCC. Using the proper technique, a 5-year cure rate of 95% to 97% can be anticipated for selected cases of BCC (Chapter 141).

28. B Microcystic adnexal carcinoma is a slow-growing adnexal tumor with histologic findings suggestive of syringoma, trichoadenoma, or desmoplastic trichoepithelioma. Although this neoplasm has not been reported to metastasize, it is capable of extensive local tissue destruction with invasion into surrounding soft tissue and nerves. On clinical examination, microcystic adnexal carcinoma appears as a plaque or nodule on the head and neck, especially on the upper lip. Mohs micrographic surgery is the treatment of choice (Chapter 141).

29. E Actinic cheilitis is the mucosal equivalent of cutaneous actinic heliodermatosis and manifests as wrinkling, dyspigmentation, and irregular hyperkeratosis with occasional erosions, usually of the lower lip. Actinic cheilitis is thought to be a precursor lesion to squamous cell carcinoma (SCC), and adequate treatment therefore is important. Of note, 90% of SCCs of the lip develop on the lower lip, and these tumors are associated with a significant rate of metastasis. Accepted treatment modalities include cryosurgery with liquid nitrogen, electrosurgery, and scalpel excision. Best results may however be obtained with vermilionectomy, topical fluorouracil, and carbon dioxide laser ablation (Chapter 141).

30. A Recurrence rates for incompletely excised basal cell carcinoma (BCC) range from 12% to 41% in various series. A recent study employing Mohs surgery to determine residual tumor for incompletely excised BCCs showed residual tumor in 55% of the cases. Because of this, some clinicians recommend only close serial observation of the tumor site, whereas others suggest a re-excision. Close follow-up of all patients is important to detect recurrent disease and new primary tumors. An initial follow-up interval at 3 to 6 months has been suggested (Chapter 141).

31. B A well-defined primary basal cell (BCC) or squamous cell (SCC) on the forehead measuring 2.0 cm or less can be treated equally well with excision or radiation therapy. Mohs surgery for the treatment of basal cell (BCC) and squamous cell carcinomas (SCC) should be considered in the following situations: lesions occurring

in anatomic areas known for a high rate of recurrence (i.e., nasal ala, periocular area, scalp, nasolabial fold, ear, preauricular area, and retroauricular sulcus), recurrent or poorly defined tumors, tumors arising in areas in which maximal tissue conservation is essential (e.g., periocular area, penis, digit), morphea-type or infiltrating BCCs or BCCs with an aggressive-appearing histology, thick or poorly differentiated SCC, primary BCC/SCC greater than 2 cm in diameter (the latter indication is not absolute and depends on the location and type of tumor) (Chapter 141).

32. E Keratoacanthoma is a benign neoplasm that may mimic SCC both on clinical and histologic examination. Suspected etiologic factors include ultraviolet radiation (UVR), chemical carcinogens (pitch and coal tar), mechanical trauma, human papillomavirus, immunosuppression, pre-existing dermatoses (e.g., radiation dermatitis, lichen planus, eczema, psoriasis), and the Muir-Torre syndrome (Chapter 141).

33. A The possibility of arsenic exposure should be suspected when Bowen's disease is discovered on a non–sun-exposed site. Other cutaneous stigmata of chronic arsenicism include arsenical keratoses, pigmentary changes, Mees' lines, and alopecia. Arsenical keratoses are multiple punctate keratoses usually developing on sites of friction such as palms and soles. Hyperpigmented patches with small depigmented areas ("rain drops") may occur on nipples, axillae, groin, and other pressure points. Mees' lines are seen in both acute and chronic arsenicism. Noncutaneous stigmata include peripheral neuropathy, anemia, leukopenia, and thrombocytopenia. Chronic arsenicism may lead to development of cancers of the nasorespiratory, gastrointestinal, and genitourinary tracts (Chapter 141).

34. B A large number of processes may produce a cutaneous horn, including actinic keratoses, seborrheic keratoses, filiform warts, basal and squamous cell carcinomas and, rarely, metastatic renal carcinoma, granular cell tumor, sebaceous carcinoma, and Kaposi's sarcoma. In the elderly, most cutaneous horns that develop on sun-exposed sites are actinic keratoses. In this case, however, histologic examination is necessary for exclusion, and shave biopsy with curettage is appropriate management (Chapter 141).

35. C Sebaceous gland carcinoma usually manifests as a solitary ulcerated nodule. These often occur on the eyelids, and it is from this site that widespread metastases most frequently develop. Indeed, metastatic disease is rare from tumors arising from other sites. There is no predilection of this tumor to develop on sun-damaged skin.

Muir-Torre syndrome is the association of internal malignancies with sebaceous tumors of the skin with or without keratoacanthomas. Multiple sebaceous adenomas are usually found, although sebaceous hyperplasia and sebaceous epitheliomas and carcinomas have also been recorded. Visceral neoplasms are often multiple and include tumors of the colon, gastrointestinal tract, larynx, and endometrium (Chapters 141 and 144).

36. D Electrodesiccation and curettage is appropriate treatment for well-defined primary exophytic basal cell carcinomas (BCC) or squamous cell carcinomas (SCC) measuring ≤1.0 cm in diameter. Superficial BCC and SCC in situ measuring greater than 1.0 cm are also appropriately treated with electrosurgery. Electrosurgery is best used on areas such as the forehead and cheek. It may not be an appropriate treatment for younger patients in whom excision would result in better cosmesis. Tumors that should not be treated with electrosurgery include morpheaform BCC; BCC or SCC greater than 1.0 cm (excluding superficial BCC and SCC in situ); recurrent, ill-defined, or poorly differentiated tumors; tumor present in immunosuppressed patients; and tumor present in anatomic areas known for a high rate of recurrence, such as the nasal ala, nasolabial fold, periocular region, and ear (Chapter 141).

37. C Merkel cell carcinoma affects older patients and usually manifests as a rapidly growing nodule most commonly found on the head and neck, although extremities, buttocks, and trunk are also affected. Associations with squamous cell and basal cell carcinomas, Bowen's disease, actinic keratoses, and adnexal neoplasms have been demonstrated. Two main histologic patterns are found: (1) nodular or diffuse pattern resembling lymphoma and (2) sheets of cells forming cords, nests, and trabeculae. Electron microscopy shows the presence of peripherally arranged neurosecretory granules. Tumor cells usually stain positive with neuron-specific enolase and chromogranin A, and negative with S-100 protein and vimentin.

Merkel cell carcinoma is a high-grade malignant tumor. Regional lymph node metastases develop in approximately 50% of patients, and the 3-year survival rate is only 55%. Wide local excision (1- to 2-cm margins) of the primary lesion should be performed along with a regional lymph node dissection (Chapter 141).

38. (T); 39. (T); 40. (F); 41. (T) Oncogenes are genes whose abnormal expression converts a cell toward the malignant phenotype. Oncogenes were originally discovered through the actions of transforming retroviruses. These RNA retroviruses contain oncogenes that transform a cell to a malignant phenotype when inserted into the cellular genome. Viral oncogenes (v-onc) share a large degree of homology with corresponding normal genes in the cellular genome termed cellular oncogenes (c-onc) or proto-oncogenes. C-onc differ from v-onc by not being capable of transforming a cell toward malignancy unless altered by point mutations within the gene, leading to an altered protein product; multiplication of the gene within the chromosome, leading to increased product activity (amplification); or by chromosomal rearrangements such that normal control of oncogene expression is lost. Oncogenes code for proteins that are essential in normal cellular growth and differentiation. Oncogene products include the following: extracellular growth factors, transmembrane receptors with protein kinase activity, membrane-associated guanosine triphosphate (GTP)-binding proteins, and intranuclear proteins that affect DNA transcription (Chapter 140).

42. (T); **43.** (F); **44.** (T); **45.** (F); **46.** (F) Bowenoid papulosis is an eruption of pigmented genital papules, resembling seborrheic keratoses, which show histologic changes consistent with squamous cell carcinoma (SCC) in situ. Bowenoid papulosis has been associated with a number of human papillomavirus (HPV) oncogenic types, including HPV-16 and -18. Individual lesions may regress spontaneously or persist for years. There is an increased tendency to develop invasive SCC in immunocompromised and older patients. The presence of these lesions places women at increased risk for cervical and vulvar neoplasia.

A recent population-based study showed no overall association between Bowen's disease and internal malignancy. The subgroup of Bowen's disease occurring on non–sun-exposed skin also showed no increased incidence of internal malignancy. Therefore, extensive workup is not indicated, especially in the young.

Spontaneous regression may occur in approximately 30% of actinic keratoses (AKs). However, studies have suggested that over a 10-year period, the risk of malignant transformation of AK to SCC may be as high as 10%, although the risk of transformation for an individual lesion is only 1:1000 per year.

Leukoplakia may be a precursor lesion to oral SCC. However, oral SCC is more likely to be associated with erythroplasia or erythroleukoplakia than with leukoplakia alone. Nonetheless, leukoplakia should be biopsied when it occurs at high-risk sites for oral SCC such as the floor of the mouth, side of the tongue, or the soft palate.

Erythroplasia of Queyrat presents as a sharply demarcated velvety plaque on the glans penis of uncircumcised males. Histologic changes may be identical to those of cutaneous SCC in situ. There has been no definite association of erythroplasia of Queyrat with human papillomavirus. Etiologic factors may include irritation, smegma, poor local hygiene, genital herpes simplex, heat, friction, and trauma (Chapters 123 and 141).

47. A (T); B (T); C (T); D (F); E (F) Fair-skinned individuals who burn easily and do not tan are at high risk for both basal cell carcinoma (BCC) and squamous cell carcinoma (SCC). Although actinic keratoses may be precursor lesions to SCC, they are also strongly associated with subsequent risk for developing BCC. Of the clinical variants, BCC most often manifests as a well-defined nodule with surface telangiectasias. The nose is the site of predilection for BCC, and BCC is also the most common malignancy on the eyelid. This diagnosis should especially be considered when there is an enlarging or nonhealing papule of the lower eyelid. The incidence of metastases for BCC has been estimated to be slightly less than 0.1%. Median age at first sign of metastases is 59 years, and median survival is only 8 months after systemic metastases have been detected (Chapter 141).

48. A (T); B (T); C (F); D (F); E (T) Xeroderma pigmentosum (XP), Cockayne's syndrome, and Bloom's syndrome are all autosomal recessive disorders in which patients display significant sun sensitivity. XP patients under 20 years of age have more than a 1000-fold increased risk to develop cutaneous basal cell carcinoma (BCC) or squamous cell carcinoma (SCC). Patients with Cockayne's syndrome show cellular abnormalities similar to those of XP patients; however, the cells from Cockayne's syndrome patients do not have the same DNA repair defects as XP cells, and the usual tests for DNA-excision repair are normal. These patients are not at increased risk of neoplasia. Patients with Bloom's syndrome, on the other hand, are at increased risk of neoplasia of the hematopoietic system (leukemia). People with tyrosinase-negative oculocutaneous albinism are at increased risk for nonmelanoma skin cancer, but, perhaps surprisingly, the risk for melanoma is not substantially increased above that for the general population. Finally, patients with basal cell nevus syndrome (Gorlin's syndrome) show autosomal dominant transmission with variable penetrance. In this condition, BCCs occur early in life and can cause extensive local tissue destruction. These tumors usually have their onset between puberty and 35 years of age and occur predominantly on skin exposed to sunlight (Chapters 141, 167, and 168).

49. A (T); B (T); C (T); D (T); E (F) There has been some success in the management of advanced or metastatic basal cell and squamous cell carcinomas with different antineoplastic drugs. However, cures are uncommon, underscoring the importance of early detection and treatment of these malignancies (Chapter 141).

50. A (T); B (T); C (F); D (T); E (F) If basal cell carcinoma (BCC) recurs, it usually does so beginning in the first year post treatment with the majority of lesions having recurred by 5 years. In general, lesions greater than 1 cm in diameter tend to have a higher recurrence rate compared with smaller tumors. BCC of the nose and other areas in which there are embryonal closure planes are also at high risk for recurrence. The patient's age has no bearing on recurrence rate, but conclusions from the results of one large study were that being male is associated with BCC recurrence, at least when tumors are treated by excisional surgery. Primary tumors of the upper extremities have a low risk of recurrence, and any treatment modality can therefore be used in this setting (Chapter 141).

51. A (F); B (F); C (F); D (F); E (F) The surgical literature in the 1950s and 1960s suggested that radiation therapy was contraindicated for basal cell carcinoma (BCC) invading cartilage, skeletal muscle, or bone because it resulted in a high incidence of necrosis. The literature addressing modern fractionated radiation therapy does not support this view. Several investigators have found an acceptable cure rate with x-ray therapy on recurrent BCCs. However, Mohs surgery has emerged as the most common treatment modality for recurrent disease. Patient age is a relative contraindication to radiotherapy as cosmetic results deteriorate with time. However, there are situations in which patients are not surgical candidates, and x-ray therapy can be used as an effective alternative (Chapter 141).

52. A (T); B (T); C (T); D (T); E (T) For squamous cell carcinoma (SCC) greater than 2 cm in diameter, local recurrence and metastatic rates are significantly higher than those for lesions less than 2 cm. One study on growth rate found that lesions with rapid growth on the ear or eyelid had a 33% metastatic rate compared with a rate of 5% to 10% for lesions with a slower growth. Tumors that develop in the setting of inflammation appear after a long latency and can be aggressive in biologic activity. Excluding the lip, SCC on the ear is the only site consistently reported to have a higher risk of metastasis. Finally, the immunocompromised patient is at increased risk of developing SCC, and in this situation tumors may metastasize in a substantial number of cases (Chapter 141).

53. A (T); B (T); C (T); D (T); E (F) The epidermal nevus syndrome is a disease complex consisting of an association of epidermal nevus with various developmental anomalies of the skin and the nervous, skeletal, cardiovascular, and urogenital systems. Depending on the abnormalities detected by a physical examination, further investigations would include computed tomography and magnetic resonance imaging scans, intravenous pyelogram, and radiographic evaluation of bones. These patients should be seen on a regular basis for follow-up purposes (Chapter 142).

54. C; **55.** C; **56.** D; **57.** A Chronic immunosuppression increases the risk for both squamous cell (SCC) and basal cell carcinomas (BCC). In this environment, these cancers appear earlier in life than in nonimmunosuppressed individuals, and the tumors occur predominantly on sun-exposed skin. Any chronic inflammatory state can result in the development of BCC or SCC. Therefore, the margin of any long-standing, nonhealing ulcer should be biopsied to exclude malignancy. The development of BCC and SCC has been reported in AIDS patients, and in this setting, these tumors may act aggressively. However, the incidence is not significantly increased compared with that of the general population. Although human papillomavirus (HPV) sequences have been seen in the occasional BCC, they are recognized to play a significant role in the pathogenesis of the Buschke-Lowenstein tumor and other verrucous squamous carcinomas. Epidermodysplasia verruciformis is a good model for viral carcinogenesis in which SCC develops in association with a number of HPV types (Chapters 123, 140, and 141).

58. B; **59.** D; **60.** D; **61.** A Clear-cell acanthoma is an uncommon tumor that usually affects the lower extremity. This tumor can be removed by simple excision, curettage, or by liquid nitrogen cryotherapy. By contrast, warty dyskeratoma is a lesion most commonly located on the head or neck. This epithelial neoplasm is characterized by a nodule with a central keratotic plug and measures between 1 and 2 cm. It is best treated by saucerization or elliptical excision, which allows histologic examination of the entire lesion. Neither clear-cell acanthoma nor warty dyskeratoma has any tendency to involute spontaneously, and these lesions are not associated with malignant transformation (Chapter 142).

62. D; **63.** A; **64.** D Epidermal cysts are common and usually occur sporadically. However, they can be seen in large numbers in association with Gardner's syndrome or Gorlin's syndrome (nevoid basal cell carcinoma syndrome). Trichilemmal cysts are often inherited in an autosomal dominant pattern. The distribution of these cysts helps to differentiate them clinically. Trichilemmal cysts occur most commonly on the scalp, whereas epidermal cysts develop on the face and neck (Chapters 143 and 144).

65. C; **66.** B; **67.** A; **68.** C Eccrine poroma occurs as a solitary lesion, usually on the sole or palm of a person over the age of 40. It may be skin-colored to erythematous with a smooth, often lobulated surface. Ulceration may occur at points of pressure. Solid masses or anastomosing tracts of tumor cells embedded in a vascular stroma extend from the epidermis into the deep dermis. The cells are uniform, basophilic, and contain large amounts of glycogen. They are differentiating in the direction of intraepidermal eccrine duct cells. Malignant degeneration has been described.

Eccrine spiradenoma occurs in young patients as a solitary nodule, usually slightly to severely tender to palpation. Tumor cells consisting of small basophilic cells and relatively large pale cells are arranged in lobules and strands and are surrounded by a capsule of compressed connective tissue. The cells appear to be differentiating in the direction of both ductal and secretory segments of the eccrine sweat gland. Malignant degeneration has been reported. Cells of eccrine differentiation characteristically stain with a number of histochemical stains, including amylophosphorylase, succinic dehydrogenase, leucine aminopeptidase, and periodic acid–Schiff (PAS) (Chapter 145).

69. E; **70.** D; **71.** B; **72.** C Depending on the size and location, primary basal cell carcinoma (BCC) can be treated by a number of different modalities, all of which show similar cure rates. However, large lesions or recurrent tumors, especially of the scalp, should be treated exclusively by Mohs surgery when available. Superficial BCC can be effectively treated by any of the methods outlined above. However, for a relatively small, superficial BCC on the back, curettage would be the preferred treatment of most dermatologists because the curette can easily ferret out tumor cells, and the final cosmetic result is generally very good (Chapter 141).

73. D; **74.** B; **75.** C; **76.** A Types of tumors of the pilosebaceous unit are numerous. The desmoplastic trichoepithelioma is generally solitary, occurring in younger patients. It is a benign lesion; however, it can closely mimic a sclerosing basal cell carcinoma (BCC). The presence of small strands of basaloid cells in a desmoplastic stroma is highly reminiscent of a morpheaform BCC. However, there are numerous horn cysts within the lesion, and it fails to show the retraction artifact that is present in BCCs. A pilomatricoma is a distinctive tumor that histologically shows ghost cells. The ghost cells, also known as shadow cells, have a washed-out appearance. In addition to ghost cells, basaloid cells and foreign body giant cells are seen. Abundant glycogen is characteristic of a trichilemmoma. This lesion is important because of its association with Cowden's disease, an autosomal dominant genodermatosis associated with a high incidence of breast cancer in women. Trichofolliculoma has a central primary hair follicle with surrounding smaller secondary hair follicles. Small groups of sebaceous glands may be embedded in the walls of the secondary follicles. In general, the importance of recognizing tumors of pilosebaceous origin lies in differentiating them from malignant neoplasms (Chapter 144).

77. C; **78.** B; **79.** A; **80.** E Syringomata often occur as multiple lesions located near the eyes. Numerous small "tadpole-like" ducts are a characteristic histologic finding. The ducts are embedded in a fibrous stroma and have comma-like tails that resemble tadpoles. Occasionally, the cells may contain abundant glycogen. The jigsaw pattern aptly describes the cylindroma. This neoplasm occurs on the scalp and has been called the "turban" tumor. Histologically, it is composed of islands of epithelial cells that seem to fit together like pieces of a jigsaw puzzle. Numerous plasma cells are characteristic of syringocystadenoma papilliferum. It often develops within a nevus sebaceus. The plasma cells are located within the stroma, adjacent to the columnar cells. The epithelium shows apocrine differentiation. Because a chondroid syringoma shows mesenchymal and epithelial differentiation, it is often referred to as a mixed tumor. The epithelium consists of small aggregates of ducts, the lumina of which often contain PAS-positive material. The stroma has a chondroid appearance. Chondroid syringomas appear as solitary intradermal nodules and most commonly occur on the head and neck (Chapters 142 and 145).

Bibliography

Albright SD. Treatment of skin cancer using multiple modalities. J Am Acad Dermatol 1982; 7:143–171.

Bieley HC, Kirsner RS, Reyes BA. The use of Mohs micrographic surgery for determination of residual tumor in incompletely excised basal cell carcinoma. J Am Acad Dermatol 1992; 26:754–756.

Bishop J. Molecular themes in oncogenesis. Cell 1991; 64:235–248.

Brownstein MH. The genodermatology of adnexal tumors. J Cutan Pathol 1985; 11:457–465.

Brownstein MH, Fernando S, Shapiro L. Clear cell acanthoma. Am J Clin Pathol 1973; 59:306–311.

Coldiron BM. Thinning of the ozone layer: facts and consequences. J Am Acad Dermatol 1992; 27:653–662.

Cornell RC, Greenway HT, Tucker SB, et al. Intralesional interferon therapy for basal cell carcinoma. J Am Acad Dermatol 1990; 23:694–700.

Dodson JM, DeSpain J, Hewett JE, et al. Malignant potential of actinic keratoses and the controversy over treatment. Arch Dermatol 1991; 127:1029–1031.

Feldman SR, Yaar M. Oncogenes, the growth control genes. Arch Dermatol 1991; 127:707–711.

Frankel DH, Hanusa BH, Zitelli JA. New primary nonmelanoma skin cancer in patients with a history of squamous cell carcinoma of the skin. J Am Acad Dermatol 1992; 26:720–726.

Hashimoto K, Lever WF. Tumors of skin appendages. In: Fitzpatrick TB, Eisen AZ, Wolff K, et al., eds. Dermatology in General Medicine, vol. 4. New York: McGraw-Hill, 1993:873.

Headington JT. Tumors of the hair follicle. Am J Pathol 1976; 85:480–515.

Ho VCY, McLean DI. Benign epithelial tumors. In: Fitzpatrick TB, Eisen AZ, Wolff K, et al., eds. Dermatology in General Medicine, vol. 4. New York: McGraw-Hill, 1993:855.

Johnson TH, Rowe DE, Nelson BR, et al. Squamous cell carcinoma of the skin (excluding lip and oral mucosa). J Am Acad Dermatol 1992; 26:467–484.

Kwa R, Campan K, Moy RL. Biology of cutaneous squamous cell carcinoma. J Am Acad Dermatol 1992; 26:1–26.

Lee N. Tumor suppressor genes. Head Neck Surg 1992; 14:407–414.

Lefell DJ, Headington JT, Wong DS, et al. Aggressive-growth basal cell carcinoma in young adults. Arch Dermatol 1991; 127:1663–1667.

Lui H, Anderson RR. Photodynamic therapy in dermatology. Arch Dermatol 1992; 128:1631–1636.

Miller SJ. Biology of basal ce‡K carcinoma. Part 1. J Am Acad Dermatol 1991; 24:1–13.

Miller SJ. Biology of basal cell carcinoma. Part 2. J Am Acad Dermatol 1991; 24:161–175.

Picascia DD, Robinson JK. Actinic cheilitis: A review of the etiology, differential diagnosis, and treatment. J Am Acad Dermatol 1987; 17:255–264.

Pinkus H. "Sebaceous cysts" are trichilemmal cysts. Arch Dermatol 1969; 99:544–555.

Preston DS, Stern RS. Nonmelanoma cancers of the skin. N Engl J Med 1992; 327:1649–1662.

Roenigk RK, Roenigk HH. Current surgical management of skin cancer in dermatology. J Dermatol Surg Oncol 1990; 16:136–151.

Rowe DE, Carroll RJ, Day CL. Prognostic factors for local recurrence, metastasis, and survival rates in squamous cell carcinoma of the skin, ear, and lip. J Am Acad Dermatol 1992; 26:976–990.

Rowe DE, Carroll RJ, Day CL. Long-term recurrence rates in previously untreated (primary) basal cell carcinoma: Implications for patients' follow-up. J Dermatol Surg Oncol 1989; 15:315–328.

Silverman, MK, Kopf AW, Bart RS, et al. Recurrence rates of treated basal cell carcinomas. Part 3: Surgical excision. J Dermatol Surg Oncol 1992; 18:471–476.

Silverman MK, Kopf AW, Gladstein AH, et al. Recurrence rates of treated basal cell carcinomas. Part 4: X-ray therapy. J Dermatol Surg Oncol 1992; 18:549–554.

Spiller WF, Spiller RF. Treatment of basal cell epithelioma by curettage and electrodesiccation. J Am Acad Dermatol 1984; 11:808–814.

Torre D. Cryosurgery of basal cell carcinoma. J Am Acad Dermatol 1986; 15:917–927.

Weinberg R. Tumor suppressor genes. Science 1991; 254:1138–1146.

Wolf DJ, Zitelli JA. Surgical margins for basal cell carcinoma. Arch Dermatol 1987; 123:340–344.

chapter 21

Mesenchymal Tumors

RINO CERIO

Choose the ONE BEST answer to the following question:

1. All the following characteristics are typical features of cutaneous blood supply EXCEPT:
   A. Skin receives its blood supply from vessels within subcutaneous fat
   B. Two vascular plexuses arise from subcutaneous vessels linked by intercommunicating veins
   C. Capillaries enter the epidermis from the superficial vascular plexus to supply the epidermis
   D. The dermis is supplied by arteriovenous anastomoses called glomus bodies. The arterial fragment is called the Sucquet-Hoyer canal
   E. Cutaneous blood flow control is medicated by the autonomic nervous system.

For the following questions, ONE or MORE of the completions correctly finishes the incomplete statement; choose

   A. If only 1, 2, and 3 are correct
   B. If only 1 and 3 are correct
   C. If only 2 and 4 are correct
   D. If only 4 is correct
   E. If all are correct.

2. The following represent(s) proliferation of cellular elements relating to vessels:
   1. Pyogenic granuloma
   2. Kaposi's sarcoma
   3. Hemangiopericytoma
   4. Glomangioma.

3. Which of the following is (are) characteristic of angioma serpiginosum?
   1. Typically occurs in childhood
   2. Characterized by multiple, tiny, punctate, red or purple lesions about the size of a pinhead, arranged in a gyrate or serpiginous pattern
   3. May be familial
   4. Regresses spontaneously with age.

4. Which of the following is (are) type(s) of lymphangioma?
   1. Cavernous lymphangioma
   2. Glomangioma
   3. Cystic hygroma
   4. Pyogenic granuloma.

5. Which of the following represent(s) benign tumors?
   1. Lipoma
   2. Angiolipoma
   3. Hibernoma
   4. Lipoblastoma.

6. Which of the following describe(s) the clinicopathologic features of nevus lipomatosis superficialis?
   1. This connective tissue nevus is typically solitary, occurring on the lower back and upper thigh
   2. It can be readily distinguished from a large acrochordon

3. Its histology is undistinguishable from the cutaneous nodule of focal dermal hypoplasia
4. It can progress to malignancy.

7. Which of the following represent(s) typical characteristics of lipoblasts?
   1. Variable in size
   2. Irregular hyperchromatic, sometimes multiple, nuclei
   3. Contains fat droplets
   4. Contains cross striations.

8. Which of the following describe(s) the features of an extraskeletal osteosarcoma?
   1. It occurs in both sexes in the fifth and sixth decades
   2. It is a primary bone tumor
   3. The legs are particularly affected
   4. Eighty per cent are associated with previous radiotherapy
   5. The 5-year survival rate is 75%.

9. The histogenesis of which of the following tumors is from synovial tissue?
   1. Clear-cell sarcoma
   2. Alveolar soft-part sarcoma
   3. Epithelioid sarcoma of Enzinger
   4. Synovial sarcoma.

10. Which of the following describe(s) the histologic features of nodular fasciitis?
    1. Cells are plump, spindle-shaped, and set in a loose myxoid and collagenous stroma
    2. Numerous thin-walled blood vessels are found
    3. There may be an accompanying chronic inflammatory infiltrate
    4. One mitosis per high-power field is often observed.

11. Which of the following statements regarding keloids is (are) correct?
    1. They commonly occur in young adults, especially in blacks and Asians
    2. Spontaneous resolution is common
    3. They typically extend beyond the site of original injury
    4. Re-excision is often curative.

12. Which of the following features is (are) characteristic of infantile digital fibroma?
    1. The tumor affects infants up to 3 years of age, but adult cases have been reported
    2. It manifests as a dermal or subcutaneous, rapidly growing nodule on the dorsal or lateral aspect of the digit
    3. Multiple lesions on more than one digit are not uncommon
    4. It is associated with underlying arthropathy.

13. Which of the following describe(s) the clinical features of infantile myofibromatosis?
    1. It is a rare hamartomatous condition previously termed congenital generalized fibromatosis
    2. Firm nodules usually occur subcutaneously
    3. It is a condition more frequently found in males
    4. The condition does not have systemic effects as a result of visceral involvement.

14. Which of the following conditions is (are) variant(s) of the same condition?
    1. Fibrous histiocytoma
    2. Dermatofibroma
    3. Sclerosing hemangioma
    4. Reticulohistiocytoma.

15. Which of the following suggest(s) malignant transformation of cutaneous leiomyoma?
    1. Pleomorphism
    2. Mitotic figures
    3. Inflammation
    4. Large size (greater than 5 cm).

In the following questions, decide whether EACH choice is TRUE or FALSE. Any combination of answers from all true to all false may occur.

16. Regarding the following vascular tumors,
    A. Lymphangiomas, unlike hemangiomas, do not contain erythrocytes
    B. Telangiectasia macularis eruptiva perstans is a form of mastocytosis
    C. Angiokeratoma is an acquired disorder with no systemic sequelae
    D. Satellitosis may occur following surgical removal of a granuloma pyogenicum

E. Bacillary epithelioid angiomatosis is an acquired infection.

17. Regarding angiolymphoid hyperplasia,
    A. Angiolymphoid hyperplasia with eosinophilia has been called epithelioid hemangioma
    B. A subtype occurs in male Asian children and is called Kimura's disease
    C. It is a type of lymphoma
    D. It can be associated with an underlying arteriovenous malformation
    E. The adult form tends to affect females in the head and neck region.

18. Regarding these vascular tumors,
    A. Lymphangioma circumscriptum most often manifests in infancy
    B. Recurrence of lymphangioma circumscriptum following excision is not uncommon
    C. Angiosarcoma has also been called hemangiosarcoma, malignant hemangioendothelioma, hemangioblastoma, and lymphangiosarcoma
    D. Prognosis for angiosarcoma affecting the skin is good
    E. Angiosarcoma of the limb often manifests with lymphedema.

19. Regarding angiolipomas,
    A. Angiolipomas are often tender or painful
    B. They occur in young adults on the distal limbs
    C. The tumors are encapsulated
    D. They are rarely multiple
    E. They progress to liposarcoma if left untreated.

20. Regarding soft tissue chondromas,
    A. Soft tissue chondromas typically affect the distal limbs
    B. These tumors most commonly affect children
    C. Lesions are small and easily excised
    D. Malignant change is a recognized complication
    E. Lesions may be both intradermal and subcutaneous.

21. Regarding synovial sarcomas,
    A. They often arise in the legs of teenage males
    B. The tumors can involve the dermis
    C. Local excision is usually sufficient treatment
    D. Histology is characterized by a biphasic pattern of spindle cells and pseudoglandular spaces
    E. Calcification of the tumor can occur.

22. Regarding nodular fasciitis,
    A. Nodular fasciitis often manifests on the forearms of young adults
    B. Lesions can reach 4 to 5 cm in diameter within 2 to 3 months
    C. The condition has malignant potential and can metastasize
    D. This is a florid reactive process and not a true tumor
    E. A metaplastic formation that rarely occurs in neurofibromatosis is known as fasciitis ossificans.

23. Regarding calcifying aponeurotic fibromas,
    A. Calcifying aponeurotic fibroma may be confused with palmar fibromatosis
    B. This subcutaneous lesion may arise at any site
    C. Preoperative radiologic examination may reveal soft tissue calcification
    D. Local recurrence, particularly in younger patients, is common
    E. Invasion of underlying muscle is not infrequent.

24. Regarding fibrous hamartomas of infancy,
    A. Myofibroblast can be demonstrated by phosphotungstic acid–hematoxylin (PTAH) staining
    B. Fibrous hamartoma of infancy manifests with multiple subcutaneous nodules
    C. It is inherited as a sex-linked trait
    D. Lesions can grow to as much as 10 cm in diameter
    E. Surgical excision is usually curative.

25. Regarding the following fibromatoses,
    A. Metaplastic ossification is a rare complication of penile fibromatosis
    B. Plantar fibromatosis is essentially the equivalent of palmar fibromatosis in the foot
    C. In plantar fibromatosis, a single nodule or multiple nodules occur on the medial aspect of the sole

D. Intralesional steroids and/or radiotherapy is (are) recognized form(s) of treatment for the fibromatoses.

26. Regarding the following histiocytic disorders,
    A. Juvenile xanthogranuloma can involve the iris
    B. Juvenile xanthogranuloma can occur in both infants and adults
    C. Reticulohistiocytoma can be associated with destructive arthritis
    D. Generalized eruptive histiocytoma may involve mucous membrane, unlike histiocytoma cutis
    E. Atypical fibroxanthoma occurs only in elderly patients.

27. Regarding granular cell tumors,
    A. Granular cell tumors most frequently occur in the tongue
    B. Granular cell tumors are a proliferation of myofibroblasts
    C. The histologic picture is characteristic
    D. The eosinophilia granular cytoplasm in granular cell tumor brightly stains with periodic acid–Schiff.

28. Regarding the following skin tumors,
    A. Cells in neural tumors are "wavy" in shape
    B. Cells in smooth muscle tumors are cigar-shaped
    C. Cells in histiocytoma/dermatofibroma are characteristically histiocytic in nature
    D. Cutaneous leiomyomas may be inherited as an autosomal dominant trait.

29. Regarding liposarcomas,
    A. Histologically, pleomorphic liposarcoma can be difficult to distinguish
    B. Liposarcoma most commonly occurs in the subcutis, particularly on the legs and trunk
    C. Liposarcomas affect males more than females
    D. The tumors affect children more frequently than elderly adults
    E. Patients with liposarcoma have a good prognosis.

30. The following are benign neural tumors:
    1. Ancient schwannoma
    2. Pacinian neurofibroma
    3. Neurothekoma (dermal sheath myxoma)
    4. Granular cell tumor.

In each of the following questions, a set of lettered headings accompanies a list of numbered words or phrases. For each numbered word or phrase, choose

   A. If the item is associated with A only
   B. If the item is associated with B only
   C. If the item is associated with both A and B
   D. If the item is associated with neither A nor B.

31. For each of the following characteristics, choose whether it describes Kaposi's sarcoma, angiosarcoma, both, or neither.

    i. Occur(s) in HIV-positive patients
    ii. Is (are) associated with Stewart-Treves syndrome
    iii. Histology shows numerous spindle and cleft-like vascular spaces
    iv. Can affect other organs as well as skin
    v. May respond to radiotherapy.

    A. Kaposi's sarcoma
    B. Angiosarcoma
    C. Both
    D. Neither.

32. For each of the following characteristics, choose whether it describes angiolymphoid hyperplasia with eosinophilia, Kimura's disease, both, or neither.

    i. Represent(s) a reactive condition classified as pseudolymphoma
    ii. Occurs mainly in children
    iii. Is (are) associated with systemic disease and poor prognosis
    iv. Skin lesions have symptoms of tenderness and pruritus
    v. Lesions are prone to ulceration and secondary bleeding.

    A. Angiolymphoid hyperplasia with eosinophilia
    B. Kimura's disease
    C. Both
    D. Neither.

33. For each of the following characteristics, choose whether it describes factor VIII–related antigens, *Ulex europaeus* agglutinin 1, both, or neither.

   i. Identify(ies) blood vessels by immunohistochemical techniques in skin
   ii. Represent(s) panendothelial cell markers
   iii. Useful diagnostically in all forms of Kaposi's sarcoma
   iv. Can be used on routine paraffin sections
   v. Can differentiate Kaposi's sarcoma from angiosarcoma.

   A. Factor VIII–related antigens
   B. *Ulex europaeus* agglutinin 1
   C. Both
   D. Neither.

34. For each of the following characteristics, choose whether it describes lipoma, angiolipoma, both, or neither.

   i. More often occur(s) in adults
   ii. Painful and tender
   iii. Progress(es) to liposarcoma
   iv. Can be multiple
   v. Associated with internal disease.

   A. Lipoma
   B. Angiolipoma
   C. Both
   D. Neither.

35. For each of the following characteristics, choose whether it describes lipoblastoma, hibernoma, both, or neither.

   i. Occur(s) in infants rather than adults
   ii. Occur(s) in the interscapular region, axillae, or chest wall
   iii. Malignant adipose tumor
   iv. Made up of brown fat
   v. Adipocytes are large, containing granular cytoplasm.

   A. Lipoblastoma
   B. Hibernoma
   C. Both
   D. Neither.

36. For each of the following characteristics, choose whether it describes lipoblastoma, liposarcoma, both, or neither.

   i. Is (are) malignant
   ii. Can involve muscle
   iii. Often present(s) in the skin
   iv. Occur(s) in children
   v. Histology shows mitotic figures.

   A. Lipoblastoma
   B. Liposarcoma
   C. Both
   D. Neither.

37. For each of the following characteristics, choose whether it describes soft tissue chondroma, chondroid sarcoma, both, or neither.

   i. Occur(s) in childhood
   ii. Affect(s) distal limbs
   iii. Present(s) with a slow-growing soft tissue
   iv. Arise(s) from cartilage-formatting tissue
   v. Ten to fifteen per cent metastasize.

   A. Soft tissue chondroma
   B. Chondroid sarcoma (extraskeletal myxoid chondrosarcoma)
   C. Both
   D. Neither.

38. For each of the following characteristics, choose whether it describes synovial sarcoma, epithelioid sarcoma of Enzinger, both, or neither.

   i. Occur(s) in distal limbs of young adults
   ii. Good prognosis
   iii. Histology shows a spindle cell and epithelioid pattern
   iv. Tissue expresses both vimentin and keratin
   v. Can be confused with metastatic necrotic adenocarcinoma.

   A. Synovial sarcoma
   B. Epithelioid sarcoma of Enzinger
   C. Both
   D. Neither.

39. For each of the following characteristics, choose whether it describes nodular fasciitis, proliferative myositis, both, or neither.

    i. The condition occurs in young adults
    ii. It is entirely benign
    iii. It occurs as a deep, intramuscular lesion
    iv. The common occurrence of mitoses can lead to misdiagnosis of malignancy
    v. Local recurrence is common following excision.

    A. Nodular fasciitis
    B. Proliferative myositis
    C. Both
    D. Neither.

40. For each of the following characteristics, choose whether it describes keloids, hypertrophic scars, both, or neither.

    i. Occur(s) mainly on the head and neck
    ii. Show(s) no race predilection
    iii. Can be distinguished clinically and histologically
    iv. Prone to recurrence
    v. Is (are) due to a proliferation of elastic fibers.

    A. Keloids
    B. Hypertrophic scars
    C. Both
    D. Neither.

41. For each of the following characteristics, choose whether it describes fibroma of the tendon sheath, calcifying aponeurotic fibroma, both, or neither.

    i. Occur(s) in adults rather than children
    ii. Most often affect(s) the distal extremities, especially the hands
    iii. Local calcification is typical
    iv. Local recurrence is not uncommon
    v. Has (have) histologic appearance(s) similar to giant cell tumors of tendon sheath.

    A. Fibroma of the tendon sheath
    B. Calcifying aponeurotic fibroma
    C. Both
    D. Neither.

42. For each of the following characteristics, choose whether it describes fibrous hamartoma of infancy, juvenile hyaline fibromatosis, both, or neither.

    i. Manifest(s) with multiple dermal masses
    ii. The trunk can be involved
    iii. Surgical intervention is the treatment of choice
    iv. Malignant transformation is a well-recognized, rare complication
    v. Either sex can be affected.

    A. Fibrous hamartoma of infancy
    B. Juvenile hyaline fibromatosis
    C. Both
    D. Neither.

43. For each of the following characteristics, choose whether it describes atypical fibroxanthoma, dermatofibrosarcoma protuberans, both, or neither.

    i. Occur(s) in sun-exposed skin
    ii. Manifest(s) as a spindle cell dermal tumor
    iii. May contain melanin
    iv. Cells are bizarre and pleomorphic with numerous atypical figures
    v. Local recurrence is not uncommon.

    A. Atypical fibroxanthoma
    B. Dermatofibrosarcoma protuberans
    C. Both
    D. Neither.

44. For each of the following characteristics, choose whether it describes cutaneous leiomyoma, angioleiomyoma, both, or neither.

    i. Often occur(s) as painful tender nodules
    ii. Can be multiple
    iii. Malignant transformation is recognized
    iv. Can involve the genitals of both sexes
    v. Tumor stains with Masson's trichrome and phosphotungstic acid–hematoxylin stains.

    A. Cutaneous leiomyoma
    B. Angioleiomyoma
    C. Both
    D. Neither.

Choose the ONE BEST answer to each of the following questions.

45. Angiolymphoid hyperplasia with eosinophilia has the following pathologic features:
    A. The vessels are lined by large endothelial cells with marked histiocytoid appearances
    B. There is an intense neutrophilic infiltrate in the dermis
    C. Atypical lymphocytes are present
    D. All of these
    E. None of these.

46. Intravascular papillary endothelial hyperplasia (Masson's tumor) has the following features EXCEPT:
    A. Affects patients in their fourth and fifth decades (a slight predilection for females)
    B. Manifests as slow-growing, elevated cysts and nodules measuring less than 2 cm in diameter
    C. A malignant vascular tumor
    D. Its histology cannot be distinguished from features seen in an organizing thrombus
    E. The clinicopathologic differential diagnosis must include angiosarcoma.

47. All of the following are features of lipoma EXCEPT:
    A. The single most common connective tissue tumor
    B. Often affects obese females on the trunk in mid adult life
    C. Should be excised because it can progress to liposarcoma
    D. Usually encapsulated and lobulated and composed of univacuolated, mature adipocytes
    E. It may occur multiply.

48. Lipomas and angiolipomas are best treated as follows:
    A. Surgery
    B. Intralesional steroids
    C. Radiotherapy
    D. All of these
    E. None of these.

49. The following describe the features of benign symmetrical lipomatosis EXCEPT:
    A. HLA-B8, DR3–related.
    B. Characterized by disfiguring unencapsulated overgrowth of adipose tissue and manifests in several forms
    C. Can be inherited in an autosomal dominant fashion
    D. Localized form affects the cervical region and is called Madelung's disease
    E. Only radical surgery can prevent recurrence.

50. The following stain(s) demonstrate adipose tissue in routine paraffin sections:
    A. Periodic acid–Schiff
    B. Oil Red O
    C. Sudan black B
    D. All of these
    E. None of these.

51. All of the following are characteristic and are typical of liposarcoma EXCEPT:
    A. Liposarcoma can be divided into two histologic well-differentiated subtypes (adipocytic and sclerosing)
    B. The single most important feature in diagnosing liposarcoma is the presence of lipoblasts
    C. Peripheral tumors have a better prognosis than retroperitoneal lipomas
    D. Metastases rarely occur
    E. Overall 5-year survival rate ranges from 30% to 50%.

52. Radiotherapy causes which of the following tumors?
    A. Angiosarcoma
    B. Osteosarcoma
    C. Fibroepithelial tumor of Pinkus
    D. All of these
    E. None of these.

53. About 10% of which of the following tumors is associated with previous radiotherapy?
    A. Extraskeletal osteosarcoma
    B. Extraskeletal myxoid chondrosarcoma
    C. Extraskeletal mesenchymal chondrosarcoma
    D. All of these
    E. None of these.

54. All of the following are characteristic of giant cell tumors of tendon sheaths EXCEPT:
    A. Affect adults in their fourth and fifth decade
    B. Manifest as slow-growing, painless nodules
    C. Wide excision is the treatment of choice because of malignant potential
    D. Underlying bone can be focally involved.

55. All of the following are true regarding nodular fasciitis EXCEPT:
    A. It can easily be misdiagnosed clinically and histologically
    B. Proliferative myositis is a variant
    C. It is most often seen in young and middle-aged adults
    D. It typically is painless
    E. The lesions tend to occur distally, except on the forearm.

56. This pseudotumor is thought to represent degenerative and reactive changes in elastic fibrous tissue.
    A. Elastofibroma
    B. Keloid
    C. Hypertrophic scar
    D. Shagreen patch
    E. Elastosis perforans serpiginosa.

57. The following are true regarding elastofibroma EXCEPT:
    A. Develops in females more often than in males
    B. This pseudotumor occurs on the distal limbs
    C. Cause may be explained as chronic frictional trauma
    D. Elastic fibers become coarse, thick, globular, and irregular in distribution
    E. Biochemical and ultrastructural studies reveal features of both elastotic collagenous degeneration and elastic proliferation.

58. Keloids are best treated in which of the following ways?
    A. Surgery
    B. Cryotherapy
    C. Radiotherapy
    D. All of the above
    E. None of the above.

59. All of the following are true of fibromas of tendon sheath EXCEPT:
    A. They are painful subcutaneous nodules
    B. Benign tumors confined to distal extremities
    C. Rarely exceed 2 cm in diameter
    D. Local recurrence may be seen in up to 25% of patients
    E. Histology shows fibrous proliferation and numerous slit-like vascular spaces.

60. Fibroma of tendon sheath should be treated with which of the following modalities?
    A. Surgery
    B. Chemotherapy
    C. Radiotherapy
    D. All of the above
    E. None of the above.

61. All of the following are true regarding palmar fibromatosis EXCEPT:
    A. Comparatively uncommon in dark-skinned races
    B. More common in alcoholics and epileptics
    C. Bilateral involvement occurs frequently
    D. The ring finger is usually affected
    E. An association with trauma and occupation is well known.

62. Regarding neural tumors, all of the following characteristics are typical EXCEPT:
    A. Traumatic neuroma is a hyperplastic response of axons and Schwann cells to peripheral nerve injury

B. Morton's neuroma (metatarsalgia) often manifests as pain over the dorsal aspect of the foot

C. Both neurilemoma (schwannoma) and neurofibroma are associated with von Recklinghausen's neurofibromatosis

D. The biphasic histologic pattern is characteristic of neurofibroma

E. S-100 protein immunolabeling is positive in both neurilemoma and neurofibroma.

63. All of the following characteristics of muscle tumors are typical EXCEPT:

A. Leiomyosarcoma in the skin arises from either arrector muscles of hair or muscles in blood vessels

B. Rhabdomyomas are invariably confined to the skin

C. Rhabdomyosarcoma and rhabdomyoma may occur on the genitals

D. Rhabdomyosarcomas are divided into four subtypes: embryonal, botryoid, alveolar, and pleomorphic

E. Cross-striations are not always demonstrated in rhabdomyosarcoma.

64. Which of the following lesions is tender to palpation?

A. Glomus tumor
B. Angiolipoma
C. Leiomyoma
D. All of the above
E. None of the above.

65. Which ONE of the following conditions is treatable with antibiotics?

A. Kaposi's sarcoma
B. Sclerosing hemangioma
C. Bacillary epithelioid angiomatosis
D. All of the above
E. None of the above.

66. Kaposi's sarcoma of the classic and epidemic (HIV) types responds to the following treatment:

A. Surgery
B. Chemotherapy
C. Radiotherapy
D. All of the above
E. None of the above.

67. Strawberry hemangiomas have the following features EXCEPT:

A. Associated with consumption coagulopathy resulting from deposition of platelets within the lesion (Kasabach-Merritt syndrome)

B. Associated with multiple enchondromas (Maffucci's syndrome)

C. Shows a tendency to regress spontaneously

D. Associated with Sturge-Weber syndrome

E. Composed of numerous dilated vessels with flattened endothelium and large, almost sinusoid lumina.

ANSWERS

1. C The skin receives a rich supply from vessels within the subcutaneous fat. Most of the blood flow is directed to the epidermis and appendages; the dermal papillae are richly vascularized. No capillaries actually enter the epidermis, which absorbs nutrition by diffusion (Chapter 146).

2. E Pyogenic granuloma and granuloma telangiectaticum are the same lesion, which is not infective but reactive. It resembles granuloma tissue. Kaposi's sarcoma is divided into four clinical subtypes: classical, immunosuppression related, African (endemic), and AIDS related (epidemic). Glomangioma, a glomus tumor—hemangiopericytoma, arises from pericytes (Chapter 146).

3. A Angioma serpiginosum, which may be familial, typically occurs in childhood, appearing most commonly in the extremities. It is characterized by multiple tiny, punctate, red or purple lesions about the size of a pinhead. They may be arranged in a gyrate or serpiginous pattern. More lesions form, and they tend to expand with age (Chapter 146).

4. B Pyogenic granulomas are not lymphangiomas but proliferative vascular lesions. Glomus tumors arise from within the muscle coat of the Suquet-Hoyer, a canal in which there is a prominent vascular component (Chapter 146).

5. E Hibernoma is a benign but rare tumor arising from vestigial foci of brown fat. It typically occurs in adults of either sex, often in the intrascapular region in the axillae or on the chest wall. Lipoblastoma is the subcutaneous counterpart of lipoma seen in children and is hamartomatous in nature (Chapter 147).

6. B Nevus lipomatosis superficialis, thought by many to be a fatty skin tag, represents a connective tissue nevus. It can grow up to 2 cm in diameter, often starting in childhood or adolescence. Histologically, it is indistinguishable from focal dermal hypoplasia (Chapter 147).

7. A The single most important feature required to make the diagnosis of liposarcoma is the presence of lipoblasts. Typically, the cells are highly comparable in size; contain more than one well-defined fat droplet; and have irregular, hypochromatic, and sometimes multiple nuclei. Cross-striations are found in muscle cells (Chapter 147).

8. B Extraskeletal osteosarcoma often results in rapid local recurrence and widespread systemic dissemination. More than 25% of patients are dead within 3 years. Up to 10% of cases are associated with previous irradiation of the affected site (Chapter 178).

9. D Clear-cell sarcoma, epithelioid sarcoma of Enzinger, and alveolar soft part sarcoma are tumors of unknown histogenesis.

10. E; **11.** B Keloids are common reactive lesions that may arise at any age but are most common in adolescence. They are most common in blacks and Asians, occurring most frequently on the ear, upper chest, and arms. They become progressively more indurated as time passes and can be pruritic or even tender. Not all are associated with previous trauma. Local recurrence after surgical excision is characteristic (Chapter 101).

12. A Infantile digital fibroma occurs on fingers and toes of youngsters before the age of 3 years, although adult cases involving other sites apart from the digits have been reported. Typically, lesions are small, rapidly growing, and either dermal or subcutaneous. It is not associated with any underlying condition, and the condition is completely benign. Histologically, the presence of eosinophilic inclusion bodies makes the microscopic appearances diagnostic (Chapter 149).

13. A Infantile myofibromatosis is a rare hamartomatous condition manifesting most often in the first year of life, usually as a solitary dermal subcutaneous or intramuscular nodule. It affects males most often, especially over the head and neck. The lesions are firm or rubbery. If multiple, they are associated with bony or visceral tumors of a similar nature. Recent evidence suggests an autosomal dominant inheritance (Chapter 149).

14. A Fibrous histiocytoma, otherwise known as dermatofibroma and histiocytoma cutis, is one of the most common benign soft tissue tumors with no malignant potential. Because the histology embraces a variety of appearances, various terms have been used to describe this spectrum of lesions, and all are likely to have the same unknown etiology. The least common variant, sclerosing hemangioma, which has a prominent vascular pattern with hemosiderin deposition, is probably more closely related to juvenile xanthogranuloma (Chapter 149).

15. E Mitotic activity and a degree of pleomorphism is acceptable in the histology of the uterine leiomyoma but not in cutaneous leiomyoma. Leiomyosarcoma accounts for about 3% of all superficial soft tissue sarcomas, although it is more common in deep locations and is especially common on the legs, arising from subcutaneous blood vessel walls (Chapters 147 and 149).

16. A (F); B (T); C (F); D (T); E (T) Due to the connection between blood vessels, lymphangiomas, particularly lymphangioma circumscriptum, often contain blood. Telangiectasia macularis eruptiva perstans is a telangiectatic form of cutaneous mastocytosis. Angiokeratomas are associated with an inherited deficiency of α-galactosidase and deposition of ceramide trihexocidase in Anderson-Fabry disease. A frightening but harmless occurrence is the formation of multiple satellites after surgical removal of granuloma pyogenicum. Bacillary epithelioid angiomatosis closely resembles granuloma pyogenicum both clinically and histologically. It has been recognized to occur almost exclusively in patients with AIDS and is due to a *Bartonella*-like organism that is susceptible to antibiotic treatment (Chapter 146).

17. A (T); B (T); C (F); D (T); E (T) Angiolymphoid hyperplasia of eosinophilia typically affects females in the third and fourth decades. It manifests with painless, dull-red nodules on the head and neck region, particularly around the ear. There are superficial and deep types. Only a small proportion of patients have concomitant lymphadenopathy and circulating eosinophilia. In Asians, however, the condition affects children and teenagers, especially males, and is associated with widespread lymphadenopathy and circulating eosinophilia (Chapter 146).

18. A (T); B (T); C (T); D (F); E (T) Lymphangioma circumscriptum, which usually manifests in infancy, has a deep component, which explains frequent recurrences after excision or carbon dioxide laser surgery. The prognosis of angiosarcoma is very poor, since the tumor often manifests late and excision is difficult. Repeated local recurrences, rapid dissemination, and death occur in up to 80% of cases, often within a fairly short time. Patients, especially females, with small, early lesions, occurring midface may respond to radical radiotherapy (Chapter 146).

19. A (T); B (T); C (T); D (F); E (F) Angiolipomas are typically tender or painful in contrast to simple lipomas. These encapsulated tumors, which are often multiple, may occasionally be locally infiltrative. Histologically, the proportion of angiomatous component may vary greatly. Luminal microthrombi are a frequent finding. Progression to liposarcoma never occurs (Chapter 147).

20. A (T); B (F); C (F); D (T); E (T) Soft tissue chondromas are uncommon, most often affecting middle-aged to elderly patients, particularly males. They occur almost exclusively on the hands and feet. The tumor manifests as a slow-growing mass, usually less than 2 cm in diameter, that may calcify. Ten per cent recur after excision, but malignant change does not occur (Chapter 178).

21. A (T); B (T); C (F); D (T); E (T) Synovial sarcoma is an uncommon tumor typically occurring on the legs of young adults, especially in males. Lesions on the hands and feet are more likely to manifest in the dermis. The prognosis is poor with metastatic spread and death occurring in at least 50% of patients. Tumors that calcify tend to do slightly better (Chapter 178).

22. A (T); B (T); C (F); D (T); E (T) Nodular fasciitis is an unusual, but not uncommon, lesion of unknown etiology which occurs in young adults, particularly on the forearms, as a rapidly growing, typically painful or tender, subcutaneous nodule. Local recurrence is unusual after excision and should raise the possibility of misdiagnosis (Chapter 149).

23. A (T); B (T); C (T); D (T); E (T) Calcifying aponeurotic fibroma is a rare condition particularly affecting males. It manifests as a small nodule or infiltrative mass, occurring most often in the hands or feet, especially palms and soles. Soft tissue calcification can be seen on radiography. Local recurrence is common and tends to be focal, surrounded by chondrocytes and occasional osteo-like giant cells (Chapter 149).

24. A (T); B (F); C (F); D (T); E (T) Phosphotungstic acid–hematoxylin is a useful stain for myofibrils. These can be seen in infantile myofibromatosis. Electron-microscopic studies confirm that the tumor cells are myofibroblasts. This hamartoma is a rare, benign tumor manifesting in childhood in the first years of life as a solitary subcutaneous mass. Males are particularly affected around the shoulder region or trunk. The tumor can grow up to 10 cm in diameter. There is no family history (Chapter 147).

25. A (T); B (T); C (T); D (T)

26. A (T); B (T); C (T); D (T); E (F) Juvenile xanthogranuloma occurs in crops but most lesions involute spontaneously. They may occasionally involve the iris. Multicentric reticular histiocytoma is associated with a seronegative destructive arthropathy. Lesions are multiple, occurring on the dorsum of the hands. Generalized eruptive histiocytoma is an extremely rare tumor of adults that may occur at any age. Innumerable pale reddish-blue papules occur on the trunk, proximal limbs, and mucous membranes and continue to form for many years. Some early lesions may involute. Atypical fibroxanthoma can be divided into two main groups. The first is much more common, arising on the head and neck of geriatric patients. The second occurs on the limbs of middle-aged patients. Both are associated with sun exposure. Other malignant spindle cell tumors, either primary or secondary, particularly amelanotic spindle cell melanoma and spindle cell carcinoma, should be excluded. Histocytochemistry can be essential in these circumstances to differentiate these tumors (Chapter 147).

27. A (T); B (F); C (T); D (T) Granular cell tumors, previously termed myoblastoma, derive not from myofibroblasts but from the neuroectoderm. They are fairly common tumors occurring in middle age, particularly in females, on the tongue, trunk, and limbs. About 10% of patients have multiple tumors. Recurrence and malignant change is rare. The tumors have a characteristic granular pattern in the cytoplasm. Tumor cells are periodic acid–Schiff-positive, and diastase-resistant S-100 protein is also positive (Chapter 148).

28. A (T); B (T); C (F); D (T) The nuclear morphology of spindle cells can help to differentiate them. Histiocytoma-dermatofibroma is composed largely of undulating fascicles of slender spindle cells, sometimes in focal storiform arrangement, with occasional foamy histiocytes or multinuclear cells. The majority of the peripheral cells are dermal dendritic in origin (Chapters 147, 148, and 149).

29. A (T); B (T); C (T); D (F); E (F) Liposarcoma is one of the most common soft tissue sarcomas. It is primarily a subcutaneous lesion occurring on the thighs and trunk, most often in elderly males. The overall 5-year survival rate ranges from 30% to 50%, reflecting the comparatively rare nature of true, well-differentiated liposarcoma (Chapter 147).

30. A (T); B (T); C (T); D (T) Neurofibromas are composed of an admixture of Schwann cells and perineural fibroblasts. Patients frequently present with single lesions. Multiple lesions are the cardinal feature of von Recklinghausen's neurofibromatosis. There are many variants, including ancient plexiform, diffuse myxoid epithelioid, and Pacinian types. Neurothekoma has no association with neurofibromatosis and manifests as a solitary, raised dermal lesion in young adults, occurring particularly on the face and arms. It tends to recur but has no malignant potential. It is composed of a well-defined, lobulated mass in the dermis that is often S-100 protein–negative (Chapter 148).

31. i A; ii B; iii C; iv C; v C The term *angiosarcoma* is synonymous with hemangiosarcoma and lymphangiosarcoma. It occurs in two distinct forms—with and without lymphedema. Lesions in males, usually found on the head and neck, are without lymphedema. Lesions in females are usually a complication following mastectomy with axillary lymph node dissection or radiotherapy and subsequent lymphedema (Stewart-Treves syndrome). The prognosis in both sexes is extremely poor. Early, aggressive radiotherapy, particularly electron beam therapy, is occasionally successful (Chapter 146).

32. i C; ii B; iii D; iv C; v C See the answer to Question 17.

33. i C; ii D; iii D; iv C; v D *Ulex europaeus* agglutinin 1 is a panendothelial lectin marker. Factor VIII–related antigen labels blood vessels rather than lymphatics. Kaposi's sarcoma and angiosarcoma are probably of lymphatic origin. The Factor VIII–related antigen may be negative in these tumors (Chapter 146).

34. i C; ii B; iii C; iv C; v D See the answer to Question 19.

35. i A; ii B; iii D; iv B; v A See the answer to Question 5.

36. i B; ii C; iii D; iv A; v C See the answer to Question 29.

37. i A; ii C; iii B; iv C; v D Extraskeletal myxoid chondrosarcoma (chondroid sarcoma) is a most uncommon tumor affecting adults, particularly on the legs, and is slightly more common in males. It occurs as a large painless mass. Ten to fifteen per cent of the lesions recur or metastasize after excision (Chapter 178).

38. i C; ii D; iii C; iv C; v C Epithelioid sarcoma of Enzinger is a tumor occurring on the distal limbs, especially the hands, of young male adults. It is slow-growing and nontender, and ulceration is a common feature. Because of histologic appearance, there can be confusion with granulomatous inflammatory lesion. Up to 75% of cases recur locally, but less than half metastasize. Metastases to lymph nodes, an unusual feature in sarcomas, is common. The overall 5-year survival is more than 75%. Also see answer to Question 21.

39. i A; ii C; iii B; iv C; v D Proliferative myositis is closely allied to nodular fasciitis but involves deep muscle and therefore is rarely presented to the dermatologist. It occurs in patients aged 50 to 60 years and is also thought to be reactive and entirely benign (Chapters 147 and 149).

40. i C; ii B; iii C; iv A; v D Hypertrophic scars can be distinguished both clinically and pathologically from keloids; they are less raised and do not extend beyond the boundaries of the initiating injury. In addition, they consist of dermal fibrosis; are often associated with epidermal atrophy; tend to be more cellular than keloids; and hyalinized collagen fibers are far less prominent. Evidence of a foreign body granulomatous reaction may sometimes manifest in hypertrophic scars (Chapter 101).

41. i C; ii C; iii B; iv C; v D See the answers to Question 23.

42. i D; ii C; iii C; iv D; v C Juvenile hyaline fibromatosis is a rare, disfiguring condition of children occurring with multiple dermal masses about the head and neck. Some individuals are mentally retarded. The lesions are thought to be a genetic abnormality of collagen production. The only treatment is surgical excision of each lesion, but new tumors tend to develop into adulthood (Chapter 149).

43. i A; ii C; iii B; iv A; v C Dermatofibrosarcoma typically occurs on the trunk as a multinodular, slow-growing dermal mass and infiltrates the underlying fat. Tumors containing cells pigmented by melanin describe the variant so-called Bednar's tumor. Other variants include myxoid dermatosis fibrosarcoma. Recurrence is common, but metastatic potential is unusual. Compared with atypical fibroxanthoma, the morphology is rather bland, and there is an extremely low mitotic activity (Chapter 149).

44. i C; ii C; iii D; iv A; v C Cutaneous leiomyoma tends to occur in the dermis, whereas angioleiomyoma is a subcutaneous benign tumor originating from blood vessel walls. Both are typically painful, particularly when compressed. The most common variant of leiomyoma arises from arrector hair muscles and often multiplies. The other variant is genital, originating from musculature of the scrotum, vulva, or nipple. Both types of lesion are prone to local recurrence but have no malignant potential whatsoever. Myofibromas can be demonstrated using Masson's trichrome or phosphotungstic acid–hematoxylin stain (Chapter 147).

45. A The histology of angiolymphoid hyperplasia with eosinophilia is characteristically composed of an ill-defined, lobulated mass centered around numerous vascular spaces. These are lined with rounded endothelial cells with copious rather than eosinophilic cytoplasms and oval nuclei. There is no pleomorphism or mitotic activity. There is often an intense eosinophilic infiltrate in the surrounding stroma. Lymphoid follicle formation is a common feature, particularly in the subcutaneous type (Chapter 146).

46. C Intravascular capillary endothelial hyperplasia (Masson's tumor) is a relatively uncommon lesion arising in the fourth and fifth decades, particularly in females. It occurs in the head and neck region or on the hand and is a slow-growing, elevated, rather nodular, cystic lesion measuring up to 2 cm in diameter. The histology of this benign lesion is essentially that of an organizing thrombus (Chapter 146).

47. C Lipomas are entirely benign, and local excision is nearly always curative. Recurrence is infrequent and progression to liposarcoma never occurs. Several variants include angiolipoma, spindle cell lipoma, and pleomorphic lipoma (Chapter 147).

48. A Surgical excision is the treatment of choice in both lipomas and angiolipomas. Both tend to be encapsulated and lobulated on surgical removal (Chapter 147).

49. A Benign symmetrical lipomatosis is an extremely rare condition that may occur in localized and diffuse forms. It is a disfiguring, encapsulated overgrowth of mature adipose tissue. Only surgery can prevent local recurrence. However, extensive surgery can be performed only if there is no functional impairment (Chapter 147).

50. E Fat stains cannot be performed on routine paraffin sections. Fresh frozen material is required, since the fat is lost in routine paraffin processing, especially at the xylene cleaning stage (Chapter 147).

51. D See the answer to Question 29.

52. D The link between radiotherapy and angiosarcoma is well known, particularly when angiosarcoma may develop on the perineum after radiation treatment of a gynecologic malignancy. Up to 10% of cases of extraskeletal osteosarcoma are associated with previous irradiation to the affected site (Chapter 146).

53. A Only extraskeletal osteosarcoma is associated with previous radiotherapy.

54. D Giant cell tumors have no malignant potential, but they may recur locally in up to 15% of cases. Normal mitotic figures are commonly seen on histologic examination (Chapter 147).

55. D See the answer to Question 22.

56. A; **57.** B Elastofibroma is an uncommon, deep-seated tumor thought to be a degenerative condition of elastic fibrous tissue. It almost always arises in the infrascapular region, particularly in females. It can be bilateral and may be related to heavy manual labor (Chapter 149).

58. E Keloids are best treated with intralesional steroids. Surgery alone invariably makes the condition worse. A combination of surgery immediately followed by radiotherapy or intralesional corticosteroid injections has been beneficial in some patients. Silastic foam applied directly to the keloid appears to be at least somewhat effective treatment (Chapter 101).

59. A Fibroma of tendon sheath is a not uncommon, solitary, usually painless, subcutaneous nodule occurring in middle-aged individuals, particularly males. It is attached to an underlying tendon on the flexor aspect of the wrist or hand. It rarely exceeds 2 cm in diameter. Twenty-five per cent of cases recur locally (Chapter 149).

60. A Fibroma of tendon sheath should be treated surgically, but local recurrence may be seen in 25% of cases (Chapter 149).

61. E Palmar fibromatosis, like Dupuytren's contracture and Peyronie's disease, tends to occur in adults, especially male. It increases in incidence with age. There is no evidence of any relationship to either occupation or trauma.

62. B Morton's neuroma (metatarsalgia) is not a true neoplasm but probably represents a degenerative response to chronic, low-grade tissue damage. It often occurs in adults, who complain of pain in the distal sole of the foot when walking. Females are affected more commonly than males. Histology shows a localized, rather fusiform expansion on one of the plantar digital nerves. Compared with neurofibroma, neurilemoma (schwannoma) is far less common. This dermal tumor is encapsulated and is characterized by a biphasic pattern of Antoni's A and B areas. The former are more cellular being composed of spindle cells with rather wavy nuclei and nuclear palisading (Verocay's bodies). Antoni's B areas show scattered spindle cells in abundant myxoid stroma, giving a "honeycomb" appearance. The histogenesis is from Schwann cells (Chapter 148).

63. B Rhabdomyomas are rare, deep, cutaneous lesions that are not usually limited to the skin. Cardiac rhabdomyomas are seen in tuberous sclerosis. There are adult and fetal cellular types that arise on the head and neck and occur behind the ears. Strap-like cells with cross-striations are diagnostic on microscopy. Lack of mitotic activity and nuclear pleomorphism distinguishes rhabdomyoma from rhabdomyosarcoma. Electron microscopy can be helpful in identifying components of the sarcomere system in both benign and malignant tumors of striated muscle (Chapter 147).

64. D Other painful cutaneous nodules include blue rubber bleb nevus, eccrine spiradenoma, neurofibroma, glomus tumor, angiolipoma, and leiomyoma (BENGAL) (Chapters 146 to 149).

65. C Bacillary epithelioid angiomatosis has been shown to be caused by a *Bartonella*-like organism that can be isolated in lesions and identified with silver stain (Chapter 115).

66. D All forms of Kaposi's sarcoma are sensitive to both chemotherapy and radiotherapy. Although early lesions can be surgically excised, it is not the treatment of choice (Chapter 125).

67. D Cavernous hemangiomas may be associated with sequestration of platelets and DIC. There is no association with multiple cutaneous or visceral hemangiomas (Maffucci's syndrome) or hemangiomas of the elementary tract (blue rubber bleb nevus syndrome). Sturge-Weber syndrome and nevus flammeus (port-wine stain) are associated with ipsilateral or meningovascular lesions. Unlike cavernous hemangioma, nevus flammeus does not tend to regress (Chapter 146).

Bibliography

Enzinger FM, Weiss SW. Soft Tissue Tumor. 2nd edition. St. Louis: CV Mosby, 1988.
McKee PH. Pathology of the Skin. London: Gower, 1989.
Mehregan AH, Hashimoto K. Pinkus' Guide to Dermatohistopathology. London: Prentice-Hall International (UK), 1991.
Rook, A. Textbook of Dermatology, 4th ed. St. Louis: Mosby Year Book, 1986.
Rosai J. Ackerman's Surgical Pathology. 7th edition. vols. I and II. St. Louis: CV Mosby, 1989.

chapter 22

Melanocytic Disorders

DAVID M. ZLOTY, AND VINCENT C. HO

Choose the ONE BEST answer to each of the following questions.

1. All of the following statements are true of malignant blue nevi EXCEPT
   A. Can arise de novo or from cellular blue nevi
   B. Exhibit a characteristic clinical appearance
   C. Absence of junctional activity, presence of dendritic atypical melanocytes, and areas of necrosis are the primary histologic features
   D. Histologic differentiation from metastatic malignant melanoma may be difficult
   E. Treatment is the same as for melanoma.

2. Malignant degeneration in a giant congenital melanocytic nevus most commonly manifests as
   A. Increase in diameter
   B. Border irregularity
   C. Nodular thickening
   D. Marked variegation in pigmentation.

3. All of the following statements concerning melanoacanthoma are true EXCEPT
   A. It represents a rare variant of seborrheic keratosis
   B. It is characterized by the presence of large melanocytes scattered throughout an acanthotic epidermis
   C. It is histologically indistinguishable from a pigmented acanthotic seborrheic keratosis
   D. It may clinically resemble a melanoma.

4. All of the following statements relating to age at onset of Spitz nevus (spindle and epithelioid cell nevus) are true EXCEPT
   A. Onset after the age of 60 has not been documented
   B. The majority of lesions occur before age 20
   C. The nevus may be present at birth
   D. The incidence of Spitz nevus decreases with increasing age.

5. Which one of the following statements concerning malignant melanoma is true?
   A. The current incidence of melanoma in the United States is approximately 1:100 population
   B. The incidence of melanoma in the United States has reached a plateau
   C. The mortality rate for melanoma in the United States has decreased
   D. Five-year survival rates for melanoma in the United States have increased
   E. Median age at diagnosis for melanoma is 70 to 75 years.

6. Which of the clinical warning signs for melanoma listed is the LEAST reliable?
   A. Variegated color, or colors of blue, red, and white
   B. Borders that are notched or irregular
   C. Lesion asymmetry
   D. Diameter exceeding 6 mm.

7. Choose the ONE correct statement concerning melanoma and pregnancy.
   A. Pregnancy is a negative prognostic factor
   B. Melanoma during pregnancy should be treated promptly and adequately
   C. A pregnant patient with melanoma should be advised to terminate the pregnancy
   D. Subsequent pregnancy increases the chance of recurrence
   E. The use of oral contraceptive agents in patients with melanoma is absolutely contraindicated.

For the following questions, ONE or MORE of the completions correctly finishes the incomplete statement; choose
   A. If only 1, 2, and 3 are correct
   B. If only 1 and 3 are correct
   C. If only 2 and 4 are correct
   D. If only 4 is correct
   E. If all are correct.

8. Which of the following statements can be used to describe balloon cell nevi?
   1. They can be clinically differentiated from common acquired melanocytic nevi
   2. They are common
   3. They should be treated with wide excision
   4. They are characterized histologically by large cells with small nucleus and abundant finely granular cytoplasm.

9. The epidemiology of common acquired melanocytic nevi is correctly described as
   1. They are more common in whites compared with other races
   2. In nonwhites, nevi density corresponds to areas of maximal ultraviolet (UV) exposure
   3. In white males and females, the number of nevi correlates with melanoma risk
   4. New nevi appear maximally during mid to late adulthood in all ethnic groups.

10. Which of the following statements concerning the relationship of congenital melanocytic nevi to melanoma is (are) correct?
    1. The risk of melanoma in small congenital nevi is greatest after puberty
    2. The lifetime risk of melanoma in giant congenital nevi is less than 2%
    3. Giant congenital nevi may be associated with melanoma of the nervous system
    4. Melanoma arising from giant congenital nevi has a favorable prognosis.

11. Which of the following statements regarding halo nevi is (are) correct?
    1. Most commonly occur on the trunk
    2. Multiple lesions may develop
    3. May be associated with leukotrichia
    4. May be associated with vitiligo or melanoma.

12. Clinical features of speckled and lentiginous nevus (nevus spilus) include
    1. Commonly located on face and neck
    2. May have a dermatomal (zosteriform) configuration
    3. Predilection for older males
    4. Early lesions can resemble café-au-lait macules.

13. The histology of atypical (dysplastic) nevi is characterized by
    1. Lentiginous melanocytic proliferation
    2. Pagetoid spread of atypical melanocytes
    3. Variable and discontinuous cellular atypia of melanocytes
    4. Epidermal ulceration.

14. Which of the following statements is (are) correct concerning familial melanoma syndromes?
    1. Familial retinoblastoma is associated with an increased risk of melanoma
    2. The gene for the familial atypical mole syndrome resides on the short arm of chromosome 1
    3. The Lynch type II syndrome and the Li-Fraumeni syndrome are associated with an increased familial melanoma risk
    4. The mode of inheritance of the familial melanoma syndromes is autosomal recessive.

15. Which of the following features is (are) characteristic of desmoplastic melanoma?
    1. Commonly found on the face
    2. Often occurs in or around cutaneous nerves
    3. High risk of local recurrence following excision
    4. Often amelanotic.

16. Which of the following statements is (are) true regarding a patient with nodal or distant metastases of melanoma?
    1. Male patients have a better prognosis
    2. Survival in patients with nodal metastases correlates well with the number of involved lymph nodes
    3. Anatomic location of the primary melanoma is an important prognostic variable in patients with distant metastases
    4. Survival in patients with distant metastases correlates inversely with the number of metastatic sites.

17. From these statements concerning distant metastases of melanoma, choose those that are correct:
    1. Brain metastases are common
    2. Kidney metastases are common
    3. Surgical excision of liver metastases is seldom of value
    4. Surgical resection of isolated metastases has not been shown to improve survival.

Decide whether EACH of the following questions is TRUE or FALSE.

Regarding Becker's nevus,

18. It is found only in males.
19. It commonly appears within first year of life.
20. Hypertrichosis is the most prominent clinical feature.
21. There is an association with smooth muscle hamartoma and connective tissue nevi.

Regarding congenital nevi,

22. Giant congenital nevi occur in 1% of newborns.
23. Giant congenital nevi most commonly occur over the proximal limbs.
24. Congenital nevi on the scalp, palms, and soles are rare.
25. Giant congenital nevi on the scalp may be associated with hydrocephalus and seizures.
26. Small congenital nevi on the limbs can be associated with clubfoot or hypertrophy of the deep structures of the limb.

Regarding the clinical features of a Spitz nevus (spindle and epithelioid cell nevus),

27. It occurs most frequently on the trunk.
28. Ulceration is uncommon.
29. Differential diagnoses may include melanoma or pyogenic granuloma.
30. May spontaneously resolve.
31. It occurs as a solitary lesion only.

Regarding atypical (dysplastic) melanocytic nevi,

32. They are uncommon in the general population.
33. They may be associated with familial melanoma.
34. They are markers of increased melanoma risk.
35. Atypical nevi are potential precursors of melanoma.
36. They occur only in sun-sensitive individuals.

Regarding the treatment of patients with the atypical (dysplastic) nevus syndrome,

37. Prophylactic removal of all atypical nevi is recommended.
38. Excision of atypical nevi on the hairy scalp is recommended.
39. Periodic follow-up is not necessary.
40. Surgical excision with 1-cm margins is recommended.
41. Assessment of first-degree family members is recommended.

Regarding the biology of malignant melanoma,

42. Basic fibroblast growth factor is an important mitogen for melanocytes.
43. Nerve growth factor receptors are found on melanocytes but not on melanoma cells.
44. The *ras* oncogene has been shown to be pivotal in melanoma formation.
45. Karyotypic abnormalities involving chromosomes 1, 6, 7, and 11 have been described.
46. Mutant p53 suppressor genes are commonly found in metastatic melanoma cell lines.

Regarding prognosis in clinical stage I melanoma,

47. Lentigo maligna melanoma is associated with a poorer prognosis than superficial spreading melanoma.
48. Increased mitotic activity is associated with decreased survival.
49. The presence of microscopic satellites correlates with increased risk of local recurrence but not with decreased survival.
50. The presence of an intense host inflammatory response is associated with improved survival.

51. Increased expression of HLA-A, -B, and -C antigens correlates with decreased survival.

Regarding the treatment of stage I melanoma,

52. The fascia underlying the primary melanoma should be excised even if it is not grossly involved.

53. A melanoma with a 3.75-mm Breslow thickness should be excised with 5.0-cm margins.

54. Elective regional lymph node dissection is recommended for melanomas with Breslow thickess of less than 0.75 mm.

55. A melanoma with a 0.95-mm Breslow thickness should be excised with 1-cm margins.

56. The surgical resection margin may be influenced by anatomic site.

For the following questions decide whether EACH choice is TRUE or FALSE. Any combination of answers from all true to all false may occur.

57. Regarding halo nevi,
    A. The halo phenomenon may occur in benign or malignant lesions
    B. The density of the peripheral inflammatory infiltrate correlates with the extent of leucoderma
    C. Late-stage halo nevi may histologically resemble vitiligo.

58. Regarding speckled and lentiginous nevus (nevus spilus),
    A. The tan macules or patches are characterized histologically by increased basilar melanization
    B. Darker macules within the tan patch histologically show elongation of rete ridges, increased melanization, and increased melanocyte number
    C. Melanophages are commonly found in the dermis.

59. Regarding melanoma risk factors,
    A. Age of less than 15 is a significant risk factor
    B. Melanoma risk correlates with the number of melanocyte nevi
    C. Exposure to ultraviolet radiation increases melanoma risk
    D. The presence of multiple atypical nevi increases melanoma risk
    E. Inability to tan is a melanoma risk factor.

60. Regarding epiluminescence microscopy (ELM),
    A. The use of oil immersion reduces light reflectance from the stratum corneum, rendering it relatively translucent
    B. ELM has been shown to increase the sensitivity and specificity for the clinical diagnosis of thin melanomas
    C. ELM can reliably detect early melanoma in situ
    D. ELM morphologic variables have not been found to have reproducible histologic correlates
    E. ELM permits in vivo visualization of pigment patterns only within the epidermis.

61. Regarding radiation therapy for melanoma,
    A. Melanoma is not responsive to radiotherapy
    B. Adjuvant radiotherapy is indicated for localized (stage I) melanoma
    C. Radiotherapy may be used to treat melanoma brain metastases
    D. High dose per fraction protocols are commonly used
    E. Hyperthermia may enhance the effect of radiation.

62. Regarding dacarbazine (DTIC) chemotherapy for melanoma,
    A. The treatment response rate is more than 80%
    B. It is the most effective single agent
    C. Prominent side effects include flu-like symptoms, nausea, and vomiting
    D. The treatment response is usually partial
    E. Effective in treating central nervous system metastases.

For each of the following questions, the set of lettered headings accompanies a list of numbered words or phrases. For each numbered word or phrase, choose

A. If the item is associated with A only
B. If the item is associated with B only
C. If the item is associated with both A and B
D. If the item is associated with neither A nor B.

63. For each of the following characteristics, choose whether it describes common blue nevus, cellular blue nevus, both, or neither.

    1. Arise(s) through embryologic arrest
    A. Common blue nevus

of melanocytes bound for the dermoepidermal junction
2. Most common site of occurrence is the buttocks and sacrococcygeal region
3. The nevus most commonly presents as a small slate-grey or blue-black papule.
4. Histologically shows elongated heavily melanized melanocytes and large spindle-shaped melanocytes with abundant pale cytoplasm.
5. Malignant melanoma may arise from the lesion.

B. Cellular blue nevus
C. Both
D. Neither.

64. For each of the following characteristics, choose whether it describes halo nevus, melanoma, both, or neither.
   1. May develop scaling, crusting, pruritus, or variegated pigmentation
   2. May show a dense dermal lymphocytic infiltrate histologically
   3. Circulating antimelanocyte antibodies may develop
   4. Spontaneous involution may occur
   5. Mean age of appearance is 50 years.

   A. Halo nevus
   B. Melanoma
   C. Both
   D. Neither.

65. For each of the following characteristics, choose whether it describes Spitz nevus, melanoma, both, or neither.
   1. Sharp circumscription of the tumor
   2. Symmetrical configuration
   3. Maturation of melanocytes with increasing depth of dermal penetration
   4. Mitotic figures are common
   5. Presence of atypical melanocytes in the dermis.

   A. Spitz nevus
   B. Melanoma
   C. Both
   D. Neither.

66. For each of the following characteristics, choose whether it describes common acquired melanocytic nevi, atypical nevi, both, or neither.
   1. Lesion asymmetry
   2. Irregular shape
   3. Irregularity of borders
   4. Disordered and haphazard pigmentation pattern
   5. Relative sparing of sun-protected sites.

   A. Common acquired melanocytic nevi
   B. Atypical nevi
   C. Both
   D. Neither.

67. For each of the following characteristics, choose whether it describes superficial spreading melanoma, atypical mole, both, or neither.
   1. Radial streaming
   2. Homogeneous blue global pigment pattern
   3. Pseudopods
   4. Irregular pigment network with blue-grey veil
   5. Irregularly distributed, variably sized, brown globules.

   A. Superficial spreading melanoma
   B. Atypical mole
   C. Both
   D. Neither.

68. For each of the following characteristics, choose whether it describes superficial spreading melanoma, lentigo maligna melanoma, both, or neither.
   1. Most common clinical variant in patients over 60 years of age
   2. Variegated pigmentation is common

   A. Superficial spreading melanoma
   B. Lentigo maligna melanoma
   C. Both
   D. Neither.

3. Predilection for sun-damaged skin
4. Prominent horizontal (radial) growth phase
5. Does not undergo a vertical growth phase.

69. For each of the following characteristics, choose whether it describes acral-lentiginous melanoma, nodular melanoma, both, or neither.

    1. Minimal or no horizontal (radial) growth phase
    2. Common variant in blacks, Asians, and Hispanics
    3. Rarely metastasizes
    4. Vertical growth is a hallmark
    5. Sunlight exposure is not a significant etiologic factor.

    A. Acral-lentiginous melanoma
    B. Nodular melanoma
    C. Both
    D. Neither.

70. For each of the following characteristics, choose whether it describes Clark's level of invasion, Breslow's tumor thickness, both, or neither.

    1. Single most important predictor of survival in localized melanoma
    2. Good interobserver correlation
    3. Interpretation may be difficult because of regional variation in cutaneous microanatomy
    4. Is measured from the basal cell layer
    5. Interpretation may be difficult because of exophytic growth patterns.

    A. Clark's level of invasion
    B. Breslow's tumor thickness
    C. Both
    D. Neither

71. For each of the following characteristics, choose whether it is described by junctional, compound, intradermal, all, or none.

    1. Nevus cells present in both epidermis and dermis
    2. Nevus cells present in epidermis only
    3. Histologically may resemble a neurofibroma
    4. Pagetoid spread of nevus cells in epidermis
    5. Increasing size of nevus cells with maturation of the nevus.

    A. Junctional
    B. Compound
    C. Intradermal
    D. All of the above
    E. None of the above.

72. For each of the following characteristics, choose whether it describes acquired intradermal melanocytic nevus, cellular blue nevus, giant congenital melanocytic nevus, all, or none.

    1. Presence of a narrow Grenz zone
    2. Prominent nuclear atypicality of nevus cells
    3. Melanophages are present in abundance
    4. Nevus cells infiltrate skin appendages, nerves, and blood vessels
    5. Presence of dendritic melanocytes in the dermis.

    A. Acquired intradermal melanocytic nevus
    B. Cellular blue nevus
    C. Giant congenital melanocytic nevus
    D. All of the above
    E. None of the above.

73. For each of the following characteristics, choose whether it describes pigmented spindle cell nevus, Spitz nevus, nodular melanoma, all, or none.

    1. Commonly occurs as a dark brown papule on the legs of women
    2. Mean age of onset is 25 years
    3. Presence of, uniform, sharply marginated, junctional nests of heavily pigmented spindle-shaped melanocytes is characteristic

    A. Pigmented spindle cell nevus
    B. Spitz nevus
    C. Nodular melanoma
    D. All of the above
    E. None of the above.

4. Mitotic figures may be present
5. Should be treated by wide local excision.

74. For each of the following characteristics, choose whether it describes superficial spreading melanoma, nodular melanoma, lentigo maligna melanoma, all, or none.

    1. Incisional biopsy is contraindicated
    2. There is little tendency for horizontal (radial) growth
    3. There is frequent extension of atypical melanocytes along basal cell layer of hair follicles
    4. Atypical melanocytes are scattered in a pagetoid pattern throughout the epidermis
    5. There is epidermal atrophy.

    A. Superficial spreading melanoma
    B. Nodular melanoma
    C. Lentigo maligna melanoma
    D. All of the above
    E. None of the above.

75. For each of the following characteristics, choose whether it describes flow cytometry, AgNOR, HMB-45, S-100, or none.

    1. Is used to analyze the DNA content of cells
    2. Detects loops of DNA that transcribe ribosomal RNA
    3. Differentiates between Spitz nevus (spindle and epithelioid cell nevus) and melanoma
    4. Specific for the detection of cells of melanocytic origin
    5. Useful in determining the histogenesis of skin tumors.

    A. Flow cytometry
    B. Silver-staining organizing regions (AgNOR)
    C. Homatropine methyl bromide (HMB)-45
    D. S-100 antibody
    E. None of the above.

76. Match each of the following epiluminescence microscopy (ELM) features with the correct histologic correlate.

    1. Pigmented and elongated rete ridges with an increased number of melanocytes in the basal layer
    2. Large collections of melanocytes and/or melanin in the cornified layer
    3. Compact orthokeratosis and hypergranulosis
    4. Confluent pigmented junctional nests of melanocytes
    5. Nests of melanocytes.

    A. Pigment network pattern
    B. Pseudopods and radial streaming
    C. Whitish veil (Milky Way)
    D. Brown globules
    E. Black dots.

77. For each of the histologic stains listed, choose the disease with which it is most closely associated.

    1. Fontana-Masson stain
    2. Dopa stain
    3. S-100 antibody staining
    4. Homatropine methyl bromide (HMB)-45 antibody staining
    5. Cytokeratin antibody staining

    A. Malignant melanoma
    B. Squamous cell carcinoma
    C. Large cell lymphoma
    D. Soft tissue sarcoma
    E. Merkel cell carcinoma.

78. For each of the following characteristics choose whether it describes negative prognostic variable, positive prognostic variable, or variable of no prognostic significance in clinical stage I melanoma.

    1. Asian ancestry
    2. Age more than 60 years
    3. Polypoid configuration
    4. Female sex
    5. Location on the upper back.

    A. Negative prognostic variable
    B. Positive prognostic variable
    C. Of no prognostic significance.

79. Concerning the treatment of melanoma, select the ONE lettered item that is most closely related to EACH numbered item.

1. May be used to target chemotherapy for melanoma
2. May be used intralesionally for the treatment of intradermal metastases
3. Most common agent combined with immuno-stimulants in chemoimmuno-therapy
4. May produce a severe vascular hyperpermeability syndrome
5. Has been used as a melanoma tumor vaccine.

A. Bacille Calmette-Guerin (BCG)
B. Interleukin-2 (IL-2)
C. Neuraminidase-treated melanoma cells
D. Melanoma antigens GD2, GD3, GM2
E. Dacarbazine (DTIC).

ANSWERS

1. B Malignant blue nevi may arise de novo or from cellular blue nevi. There is no diagnostic morphologic appearance, but ulceration or sudden enlargement of a blue-grey dermal nodule should suggest the possibility of a malignant blue nevus. The definitive diagnosis is based on histologic examination. There are atypical dendritic melanocytes in the dermis, and necrosis of the tumor may be present. These tumors arise from dermal melanocytes and abnormal cells at the dermoepidermal junction are not found. Differentiation from metastatic malignant melanoma may be difficult. The presence of dendritic cells favors the diagnosis of malignant blue nevus. Treatment follows general guidelines for malignant melanoma of an equivalent clinical stage and Breslow thickness (Chapters 150 and 151).

2. C Malignant degeneration of a giant congenital melanocytic nevus (CMN) to a melanoma may be associated with itching, pain, bleeding, ulceration, deepening of pigmentation, or the new appearance of a dermal or subcutaneous nodule. The classic signs of melanoma, namely, asymmetry, border irregularity, pigment variegation, may not be evident. A melanoma developing in a CMN may first manifest as a dermal or subcutaneous nodule (Chapters 150 and 151).

3. C A melanoacanthoma is characterized by the presence of large dendritic melanocytes throughout an acanthotic epidermis, whereas in a pigmented acanthotic seborrheic keratosis, the melanocytes remain confined to the basal layer. However, some authors believe that a melanoacanthoma represents an irritated or inflamed pigmented acanthotic seborrheic keratosis. Although it may clinically be difficult to differentiate a melanoacanthoma from a melanoma, the absence of dysplastic melanocytes makes histologic differentiation simple (Chapter 150).

4. A Spitz nevi may develop at any age. The incidence decreases with increasing age. Fifty per cent of Spitz nevi occur before age 15, 80% before age 20, and 90% before age 45. The diagnosis of Spitz nevus after age 45 should be accepted only after a careful review of the pathology to exclude melanoma (Chapter 150).

5. D The incidence rate of melanoma is currently 10 to 15 per one hundred thousand population in the United States. It is estimated that the current lifetime risk of melanoma is approximately 1 in 100, with an expected increase to about 1 in 75 by the year 2000. Accompanying this rise in incidence rates is an increase in mortality rates. However, there is a general trend to earlier diagnosis and the 5-year survival rates have increased to 80% versus 50% in the early 1950s. The median age at time of diagnosis is 50 years (Chapter 151).

6. D The ABCD acronym is helpful in assessing pigmented lesions suspected of being malignant. *A* refers to the presence of lesion asymmetry, *B* refers to border irregularity, *C* is for color variegation, and *D* stands for diameter greater than 6 mm. Lesion asymmetry is the most helpful clinical sign for the diagnosis of melanoma. The least helpful distinguishing feature is size greater than 6 mm, since melanomas of less than 6 mm have been documented (Chapter 151).

7. B Large retrospective studies have failed to document that pregnancy is a negative prognostic factor. In addition, subsequent pregnancies do not influence survival or recurrence after successful treatment of a melanoma. Melanoma diagnosed during pregnancy should be treated per standard protocol. Pregnancy should be terminated only if the patient's melanoma or its treatment threatens the health of the fetus. The effect of estrogen supplements, including oral contraceptive agents, on melanoma is controversial, and their use is not absolutely contraindicated, but patients should be informed of the theoretical risks (Chapter 151).

8. D This uncommon nevus occurs equally in both sexes. It manifests as a small, soft, skin-colored papule that cannot clinically be distinguished from a common melanocytic nevus. Balloon cell nevus gets its name from its histologic appearance in which the majority of melanocytes are large, ballooned cells with a centrally placed small nucleus and empty or finely granular cytoplasm. Balloon cell nevus has no systemic associations and no malignant potential (Chapter 150).

9. B Common acquired melanocytic nevi begin to appear in early childhood, new lesions appearing most rapidly during puberty and early adulthood. The maximum number of nevi is reached by midadulthood; following that there is a gradual decrease in number, so that by age 80, most individuals have few remaining nevi. Whites have more nevi compared with nonwhites. In whites, the density of nevi is in areas of highest ultraviolet (UV) exposure, that is, the back in men and both the back and legs in women. These are also the sites of predilection for melanoma. Indeed, increased number of nevi is the most important risk factor for melanoma. In nonwhites, there does not appear to be a direct correlation between number of nevi and UV exposure (Chapter 150).

10. B Melanoma may develop in a small congenital melanocytic nevus. This usually occurs after puberty. The risk of melanoma arising from a small congenital nevus remains unknown. For giant congenital melanocytic nevi, the risk of melanoma is estimated to be about 6% to 9%. Melanoma arising from giant congenital nevi originate in the deep dermis, are difficult to detect, and have a poor prognosis. Giant congenital nevi on the scalp or posterior midline may be associated with leptomeningeal melanosis, which can transform into melanomas. In addition to melanomas, malignant schwannomas, liposarcomas, or rhabdomyosarcomas may develop in giant congenital nevi (Chapters 150 and 151).

11. E Halo nevi occur most commonly on the trunk. Location in a hairy area may be associated with leukotrichia. Multiple lesions may develop. Antimelanocyte antibodies may be found in these patients, and association with vitiligo is not uncommon. The most important differential diagnosis of halo nevi is a regressed primary melanoma (Chapter 150).

12. C Speckled and lentiginous nevi (nevus spilus) affect the sexes equally. They usually appear at birth or in early childhood. The trunk and lower extremities are the favored sites; the face and neck are rarely involved. Lesions may begin as café-au-lait–like macules that over time acquire central, darker, lentigo-like macules and/or nevi. Lesions may be multiple and vary in size from 1 cm to large zosteriform lesions (Chapter 150).

13. B Most dermatologists and dermatopathologists agree that atypical melanocytic nevus (AMN) is a distinct clinicohistologic entity. AMN may occur at any site, including sun-protected areas. Morphologic features of AMN include lesion asymmetry, border irregularity, color variegation, and a diameter greater than 5 mm. The most important differential diagnosis is melanoma. Any lesion suspected of being malignant should be excised for histologic examination. Histologic features of AMN include variable and discontinuous cellular atypia of melanocytes and lentiginous melanocytic proliferation. In contrast, melanoma shows *continuous* basilar proliferation of atypical melanocytes and/or pagetoid spread of melanocytes (Chapter 150).

14. B The familial melanoma syndromes include the familial atypical mole—malignant melanoma (FAMMM syndrome), Lynch type II syndrome, Li-Fraumeni syndrome, and the familial retinoblastoma melanoma syndrome. All are believed to be inherited in an autosomal dominant fashion. The gene for the FAMMM syndrome has been linked to the short arm of chromosome 9. Members of families with these familial melanoma syndromes have an increased risk of melanoma, but the degree of risk has not been fully determined. The lifetime risk of melanoma in family members of patients with the FAMMM syndrome is believed to approach 100% (Chapter 151).

15. E Desmoplastic melanoma is an uncommon variant of melanoma. It commonly occurs on the face. Histologically, it is characterized by spindle-shaped malignant melanocytes in a fibrous stroma that may be difficult to differentiate from fibrosarcoma. Desmoplastic melanoma is an aggressive tumor. It infiltrates widely and tends to track along neurovascular bundles. The risk of local recurrence and metastasis is high (Chapter 151).

16. C The most important prognostic factor for patients with melanoma metastatic to the lymph nodes is the number of involved lymph nodes. One study documented a 10-year survival rate of 40% in patients with 1 nodal metastasis, 25% with 2 to 4 nodes involved, and 15% when 5 or more nodes are involved. For patients with distant metastases, the number of metastatic sites and the location of the metastases are important; nonvisceral, that is, soft tissue metastases, are associated with a better prognosis than visceral metastases (Chapter 151).

17. B Malignant melanoma can metastasize to any site, with skin, soft tissue, brain, lung, and liver being most common. Surgery is the best palliative treatment for solitary lesions in accessible locations such as lung or brain and may be associated with prolonged survival. For multiple brain metastases or symptomatic bone metastases, radiotherapy is the treatment of choice. Liver metastases are frequently multiple and are generally associated with short survival and thus surgery is seldom of value. Isolated gastrointestinal (GI) metastases may manifest as GI bleeding, obstructions, or intussusception. Surgery may be indicated for these complications (Chapter 151).

18. (F); **19.** (F); **20.** (F); **21.** (T) Becker's nevus occurs primarily in males with a male-to-female ratio of 5 to 10:1. The lesion usually appears at puberty as a unilateral hyperpigmented patch involving the shoulder, anterior chest, and proximal upper limb. Hypertrichosis is commonly present, and the involved skin may become slightly thickened. Histologic changes that may be seen include epidermal thickening, basal layer hyperpigmentation, and increased numbers of smooth muscle fibers. Associations with smooth muscle hamartoma and connective tissue nevi have been documented (Chapter 150).

22. (F); **23.** (F); **24.** (T); **25.** (T); **26.** (F) Congenital melanocytic nevi occur in approximately 1% of newborns, the great majority being small lesions of less than 1.5 cm. Giant congenital nevi greater than 20 cm are rare, occurring in less than 1 in fifty thousand live births. They often occur on the trunk. The scalp, palms, and soles are uncommon sites for congenital nevi. Giant congenital nevi on the scalp may be associated with leptomeningeal melanosis, leading to hydrocephalus, seizures, or melanoma; those over the lower posterior midline may be associated with spina bifida; and those over the limbs may be associated with clubfoot, soft tissue hypertrophy, or soft tissue hamartomas. Small congenital nevi have no associated systemic abnormalities (Chapter 150).

27. (F); **28.** (T); **29.** (T); **30.** (T); **31.** (F) Although Spitz nevi may occur at any site, truncal lesions are uncommon. They usually manifest as solitary, dome-shaped, 0.5- to 1.0-cm nodules that may be pink, brown, or black. A variant called agminated Spitz nevus occurs as multiple lesions arranged in a group. Ulceration is not a usual feature of Spitz nevus, and its presence should arouse suspicion of a melanoma. Other lesions that may be confused clinically with a Spitz nevus are common melanocytic nevi, pyogenic granuloma, dermatofibroma, and keloids. Spitz nevi usually spontaneously resolve, but this may take months to years (Chapter 150).

32. (F); **33.** (T); **34.** (T); **35.** (T); **36.** (F) Atypical (dysplastic) nevi are common, occurring in 2% to 5% of the adult white population. The number of atypical nevi correlates well with melanoma risk. Histologic continuity of atypical nevi with melanoma has been shown, and it is believed that atypical nevi may be precursors of melanoma. Familial aggregation of atypical nevi and melanoma has been well documented. Atypical nevi occur in individuals of any skin phototype (Chapter 150).

37. (F); **38.** (T); **39.** (F); **40.** (F); **41.** (T) The management of patients with the atypical nevus syndrome remains controversial. Most agree that prophylactic removal of all nevi is not indicated. Some authors recommend excision of atypical nevi on the scalp or perianal area that are difficult to monitor. Any nevus suspected of malignant transformation must be excised for histologic examination. The recommended method of removal is surgical excision with narrow margins (1 to 3 mm). Follow-up of all patients with the atypical nevus syndrome is advised; the interval depends on the number of nevi, rate of change of nevi, and other melanoma risk factors and may vary from 4 to 12 months. It is advisable to examine first-degree family members who may also be at risk for developing melanoma. Patients should be educated on the features of melanoma, sun protection, and skin self-examination techniques (Chapter 150).

42. (T); **43.** (F); **44.** (F); **45.** (T); **46.** (F) The biology of malignant transformation of melanoma has not been fully elucidated. Growth factors such as basic fibroblast growth factor (BFGF) and nerve growth factor (NGF) may participate in malignant transformation. BFGF is a melanocyte mitogen and has been implicated in unregulated melanocyte proliferation. NGF may favor growth of melanoma because the NGF receptor, but not melanocytes, has been found on melanoma cells. The *ras* oncogene and karyotypic abnormalities of chromosomes 1, 6, 7, and 11 have been described in melanoma cells but their role in malignant transformation has not been elucidated. Mutation of the p53 tumor suppressor gene is uncommon in melanoma cells (Chapter 151).

47. (F); **48.** (T); **49.** (F); **50.** (T); **51.** (F) A number of histologic variables have been found to have prognostic significance in clinical stage I melanoma. Tumor thickness (the Breslow measurement) is the most important prognostic indicator. Tumor volume is a more accurate predictor of prognosis but is too tedious for clinical utility. The prognostic importance of histologic growth patterns is somewhat controversial; in multivariate analysis, it has not been shown to be an important independent prognostic indicator. Increased tumor mitotic activity, absence of host inflammatory response, increased expression of HLA-DR antigens and reduced expression of HLA-A, -B, or -C antigens, and the presence of microscopic satellites have all been shown to be negative prognostic variables (Chapter 151).

52. (F); **53.** (F); **54.** (F); **55.** (T); **56.** (T) Surgery is the mainstay of therapy for localized melanoma. The trend is toward narrower surgical margins. The current recommendation is to use a 1-cm margin for melanomas with a Breslow thickness less than 1 mm, a 2- to 3-cm margin for melanomas between 1 and 4 mm thick, and a 3-cm margin for melanomas greater than 4 mm thick. It has been found that there is no difference in survival or local recurrence rate when comparing surgical margins of 3 cm versus 5 cm, even for melanomas thicker than 4 mm.

Excision of the fascia is not necessary, unless it is infiltrated with tumor. Elective regional lymph node dissection (ERLND) is not recommended for melanomas less than 1.5 mm in the Breslow thickness. The role of ERLND for melanomas larger than 1.5 mm in thickness remains controversial (Chapter 151).

57. A(T); B(F); C(T) The primary histologic change in halo nevi is nevus cells within the dermis or at the dermoepidermal junction, embedded in a dense lymphocytic inflammatory infiltrate. Uncommonly, however, halo nevi may have no infiltrate (noninflammatory halo nevus). As a halo nevus continues to evolve, the nevus may completely regress, leaving a depigmented patch that may be clinically and histologically indistinguishable from vitiligo (Chapter 150).

58. A(T); B(T); C(T) The tan background of nevus spilus is characterized histologically by increased basilar melanization. The darker macules within the tan patch show increased basal layer melanization, increased melanocyte number, and elongation of the rete ridges. Papules present in nevus spilus may show histologic features of a benign nevus, an atypical nevus, a blue nevus, or a Spitz nevus. Melanophages are commonly found in a nevus spilus (Chapter 150).

59. A(F); B(T); C(T); D(T); E(T) The risk of melanoma increases with age. Melanoma is rare before age 15. The most important melanoma risk factor is increased numbers of common, acquired melanocytic nevi. Additional risk factors for melanoma include history of intense ultraviolet radiation exposure (particularly in childhood), inability to tan, the presence of multiple atypical melanocytic nevi, and a family history of melanoma (Chapter 151).

60. A(T); B(T); C(F); D(F); E(F) Epiluminescence microscopy (ELM) involves the application of oil to the skin, illumination, and examination under magnification. The oil reduces light reflectance from the stratum corneum and renders it translucent. This allows in vivo visualization of pigment patterns in the epidermis, dermoepidermal junction, and papillary dermis. These patterns have been shown to correlate with histologic changes that are associated with benign and malignant pigmented lesions. ELM can aid in the diagnosis of melanoma, atypical nevi, Spitz nevi, thrombosed hemangioma, blue nevus, seborrheic keratoses, and pigmented basal cell carcinoma. At this time, ELM cannot reliably detect early melanoma in situ (Chapter 151).

61. A (F); B (F); C (T); D (T); E (T) Melanoma has traditionally been considered a radioresistant tumor, but recent use of high dose per fraction protocols has demonstrated that some melanomas do respond to radiotherapy. The primary use of radiotherapy has been for the treatment of lentigo maligna melanomas not suitable for surgery and for the palliative treatment of bone and brain metastases. Radiotherapy also has palliative value in locally recurrent disease, nonresectable soft tissue metastases, and metastases causing spinal cord compression. In an attempt to improve the efficacy of radiation, combination protocols using tissue hyperthermia and radiosensitizers have been employed (Chapter 151).

62. A (F); B (T); C (T); D (T); E (F) The overall response rate of metastatic melanoma to dacarbazine (DTIC) chemotherapy is about 15% to 25%. The response is usually partial and of short duration. Skin, soft tissue, nodal, or lung metastases respond better than metastases elsewhere. DTIC is the most effective single agent for the treatment of advanced metastases. The most common adverse effects of DTIC are low-grade fevers, chills, and gastrointestinal upset. Occasionally, mild bone marrow toxicity may develop. DTIC does not penetrate the blood-brain barrier well and has no significant effect on central nervous system metastases (Chapter 151).

63. 1 C; 2 B; 3 A; 4 B; 5 B Blue nevi can be divided into three types: common, cellular, and combined. All arise through embryologic arrest of melanocytes bound for the dermoepidermal junction. Over 50% of common blue nevi are located on the face or distal extremities. Cellular blue nevi have a predilection for the buttocks and sacrococcygeal region. The most common clinical presentation of common blue nevi is a small blue papule, which is usually less than 8 mm in diameter. Cellular blue nevi classically manifest as firm dermal nodules larger than 1 cm.

Histologically, both forms are characterized by the presence of dendritic, heavily melanized melanocytes in the dermis. Cellular blue nevi have, in addition, islands of large spindle-shaped cells with abundant pale cytoplasm. Both the common and cellular blue nevi usually remain stable throughout life. However, the cellular blue nevus can rarely transform into a malignant melanoma (Chapter 150).

64. 1 C; 2 C; 3 C; 4 A; 5 B Halo nevi and melanoma may have similar clinical and histologic features. Both may be accompanied by pruritus. Surrounding leukoderma (i.e., "halo phenomenon") is a characteristic feature of halo nevi and may also be seen in melanoma. This may be associated with circulating antimelanocyte antibodies. Scaling, crusting, and erythema may be present in both. Halo nevi appear at a mean age of 15 years, in contrast to melanoma, for which the mean age is 50 years (Chapters 150 and 151).

65. 1 A; 2 A; 3 A; 4 C; 5 C Spitz nevi and melanoma share many common histologic features, and their distinction may be difficult. Nests of atypical melanocytes and mitoses are present in both conditions. Features that are helpful in distinguishing the two include the following: (1) Spitz nevi are usually less than 6 mm in diameter, whereas melanoma are usually bigger; (2) Spitz nevi do not show intraepidermal pagetoid spread of atypical melanocytes; (3) Spitz nevi have symmetrical configuration, whereas melanoma is usually asymmetrical; (4) maturation of nevus cells with depth suggests a benign lesion; (5) mitoses are present in both, but atypical mitoses or mitoses located deep in the tumor suggest melanoma; (6) artifactual clefts above melanocytic nests at the dermoepidermal junction are more prevalent in Spitz nevi; (7) eosinophilic globules known as Kamino bodies are found at the dermoepidermal junction in 60% to 80% of Spitz nevi and in only 2% of melanoma (Chapter 150).

66. 1 B; 2 B; 3 B; 4 B; 5 A Most dermatologists and dermatopathologists agree that atypical melanocytic nevi (AMN) are a distinct clinicohistologic entity. AMN may occur at any site without sparing sun-protected areas. Morphologic features of AMN include lesion asymmetry, border irregularity, color variegation, and a diameter greater than 5 mm. The most important differential diagnosis is melanoma. Any suspicion of malignancy requires excision and histologic examination. Histologic features of AMN include variable and discontinuous cellular atypia of melanocytes, and lentiginous or epithelial cell patterns of intraepidermal melanocytic proliferation. Melanoma shows *continuous* basilar proliferation of atypical melanocytes and/or pagetoid spread of melanocytes (Chapter 151).

67. 1 A; 2 D; 3 A; 4 A; 5 C Radial streaming, pseudopods, and a whitish veil are epiluminescence microscopy (ELM) features suggestive of the diagnosis of melanoma. Radial streaming and pseudopods are seen as irregular finger-like projections of dark pigment at the periphery of the lesion. Histologically, they correspond to confluent pigmented junctional nests of atypical melanocytes. A whitish veil (milky way) is a ground-glass–appearing haze over a region of the lesion. The histologic correlate is an area of compact orthokeratosis and hypergranulosis. A white veil occurring in association with a pigment network may be seen in melanoma.

Pigment network patterns, brown globules, and black dots are ELM features that may be seen in most melanocytic lesions. Pigment networks are seen as reticulated pigmented lines with hypopigmented holes. Histologically, a pigment network shows pigmented and elongated rete ridges with an increased number of melanocytes in the basal layer. Brown globules are uniform pigmented spots. Brown globules represent nests of melanocytes in the epidermis or dermis. Irregularly distributed, variably sized, brown globules may be seen in atypical nevi and melanoma. Black dots are punctate, extremely dark pigment concentrations. Histologically, large collections of melanocytes and/or melanin can be seen in the cornified layer (Chapter 151).

68. 1 A; 2 C; 3 B; 4 C; 5 D The four major clinicohistologic subtypes of melanoma are superficial spreading melanoma (SSM), lentigo maligna melanoma (LMM), acral-lentiginous melanoma (ALM), and nodular melanoma (NM). SSM accounts for 70% of melanoma and in whites is the most common variant in all age groups. Variegated pigmentation is common in SSM, and colors of gray or white may indicate areas of tumor regression. The SSM growth pattern is characterized by radial extension before dermal invasion occurs. LMM occurs primarily in elderly patients in areas of marked actinic damage, most commonly the head and neck. The radial growth phase of this variant is generally slow. NM may occur at any anatomic site, most commonly the trunk in men and the legs in women. Vertical growth is a hallmark of NM. NM commonly presents as a pigmented nodule that may be misdiagnosed as a pyogenic granuloma, or thrombosed hemangioma. NM demonstrates minimal, if any, horizontal (radial) growth. ALM is an uncommon variant in whites but is the most common form of melanoma in dark-skinned individuals. Sunlight exposure is not believed to be an important etiologic factor for ALM (Chapter 151).

69. 1 B; 2 A; 3 D; 4 B; 5 A The four major clinicohistologic subtypes of melanoma are superficial spreading melanoma (SSM), lentigo-maligna melanoma (LMM), acral-lentiginous melanoma (ALM), and nodular melanoma (NM). SSM accounts for 70% of melanoma and in whites is the most common variant in all age groups. Variegated pigmentation is common in SSM and colors of grey or white may indicate areas of tumor regression. The SSM growth pattern is characterized by radial extension before dermal invasion occurs. LMM occurs primarily in elderly patients in areas of marked actinic damage, most commonly the head and neck. The radial growth phase of this variant is generally slow. NM may occur at any anatomic site, most commonly the trunk in men and the legs in women. Vertical growth is a hallmark of NM. NM commonly presents as a pigmented nodule which may be misdiagnosed as a pyogenic granuloma, or thrombosed hemangioma. NM demonstrates minimal, if any, horizontal (radial) growth. ALM is an uncommon variant in whites but is the most common form of melanoma is dark-skinned individuals. Sunlight exposure is not believed to be an important etiologic factor for ALM (Chapter 151).

70. 1 B; 2 B; 3 A; 4 D; 5 A The Breslow thickness and the Clark level are both used to predict survival in localized melanoma. Currently, the Breslow thickness is the most important predictor of survival in localized melanoma. Breslow's method measures depth of invasion (in millimeters) from the top of the granular cell layer to the deepest invasive tumor cell. Clark's method subdivides the level of invasion as follows: level I, intraepidermal; level II, into the papillary dermis; level III, fills the papillary dermis; level IV, invasion into reticular dermis; and level V, extension into subcutaneous fat. The Breslow thickness is now the preferred prognostic indicator because there is good interobserver correlation, and interpretation is not limited by variation in cutaneous anatomy or exophytic growth patterns. Five-year survival figures for melanomas using Breslow's method are less than 0.76 mm, 95%; 0.76 to 1.49 mm, 85%; 1.50 to 2.49 mm, 75%; 2.50 to 3.99 mm, 65%; and greater than 4 mm, 45% (Chapter 151).

71. 1 B; 2 A; 3 C; 4 E; 5 D Common acquired melanocytic nevi are characterized by the presence of clusters of melanocytes (nevus cells). They are subdivided histologically by the location of the nevus cells. In a junctional nevus, the nevus cells are present in the lower epidermis or dermoepidermal junction. A compound nevus has nevus cells in both the epidermis and the dermis. An intradermal nevus has nevus cells in the dermis only. The nevus cells are generally bigger, or "epithelioid," in the upper dermis and become smaller and more spindle shaped as they move deeper into the dermis. This process is called maturation and implies benignity. Intradermal nevi may exhibit nests and cords of multinucleated giant cells. They may resemble a neurofibroma. Pagetoid spread and nuclear atypicality suggest melanoma and are not features of common melanocytic nevi (Chapter 150).

72. 1 C; 2 E; 3 E; 4 C; 5 B Intradermal melanocytic nevi are characterized by the presence of epithelioid or spindle-shaped melanocytes in the dermis. Cellular blue nevi show both dendritic melanocytes and islands of spindle-shaped cells. Giant congenital nevi differ from common acquired nevi by having deeper extension of the nevus cells into the reticular dermis and subcutaneous fat. These nevus cells typically infiltrate skin appendages, nerves, blood vessels, and collagen bundles. Prominent nuclear atypicality or abundant melanophages are not characteristic of any of these nevi (Chapter 150).

73. 1 A; 2 A; 3 A; 4 D; 5 C Pigmented spindle cell nevus (PSCN) is thought by most to represent an entity distinct from Spitz nevus (spindle and epithelioid cell nevus). It commonly occurs as a small brown or black, dome-shaped papule on the legs of women. The mean age of onset for PSCN is 25 years. Histologically, PSCN is characterized by the presence of prominent, uniform, sharply marginated, junctional nests of heavily pigmented spindle-shaped melanocytes. These features distinguish PSCN from Spitz nevus, which typically has a more infiltrative growth pattern, more vascular stroma, and less heavily pigmented melanocytes. PSCN can be distinguished from nodular melanoma, since the latter displays lesion asymmetry, atypical melanocytes, and lack of maturation. Mitotic figures may be present in PSCN, Spitz nevus, and melanoma and therefore cannot be used to differentiate these lesions. PSCN is a benign lesion, and treatment is excision with narrow margins. Treatment of Spitz nevus is also by narrow excision. A nodular melanoma is treated by wide excision (Chapter 150).

74. 1 E; 2 B; 3 C; 4 A; 5 C A biopsy of any lesion suspected to be melanoma should be done for histologic examination. Excisional biopsy is the preferred method, if possible, but if the lesion is too big, an incisional biopsy is acceptable and has not been shown to worsen the prognosis. Superficial spreading melanoma histologically shows pagetoid distribution of large atypical melanocytes throughout the epidermis. The histology of lentigo maligna (LM) is characterized by an increased number of atypical melanocytes along the basal layer. Epidermal atrophy and extension of atypical melanocytes along the basal layer of hair follicles are also prominent histologic features of LM. These melanocytes may be elongated or spindle shaped. When an LM assumes a vertical growth phase and invades the dermis, it is called a lentigo maligna melanoma. Nodular melanoma (NM) exhibits minimal, if any, intraepidermal growth. Dermal invasion of epithelioid or spindle-shaped melanocytes occurs early. Any intraepidermal involvement in NM occurs through upward extension of tumor cells from the dermis. The histopathology of acral-lentiginous melanoma exhibits basilar proliferation of large, atypical dendritic melanocytes (Chapter 151).

75. 1 A; 2 B; 3 E; 4 C; 5 D The molecular and immunohistochemical techniques listed have all been unsuccessfully used to differentiate between Spitz nevus and melanoma. Flow cytometry analyzes the DNA content of cells. Malignant cells may be aneuploid, but unfortunately this feature is not specific enough to reliably distinguish melanoma from Spitz nevus.

Silver-staining nucleolar organizing regions (AgNOR) detects loops of DNA that transcribe ribosomal RNA. The number of loops correlates with cellular activity, and an increase in AgNORs may imply malignancy.

The S-100 antibody stains melanocytes, Langerhans cells, Schwann cells, and cells of eccrine and apocrine glands. Consequently, it is useful in determining the histogenesis of skin tumors but cannot separate Spitz nevus from melanoma. Homatropine methyl bromide (HMB)-45 is a monoclonal antibody specific for the detection of cells of melanocytic origin, and since both Spitz nevus and melanoma arise from melanocytes, but this stain is not useful in differentiating between Spitz nevus and melanoma (Chapter 151).

76. 1 A; 2 E; 3 C; 4 B; 5 D Radial streaming, pseudopods, and a whitish veil are epiluminescence microscopy (ELM) features suggestive of the diagnosis of melanoma. Radial streaming and pseudopods are seen as irregular finger-like projections of dark pigment at the periphery of the lesion. Histologically, they correspond to confluent pigmented junctional nests of atypical melanocytes. A whitish veil (milky way) is a ground-glass–appearing haze over a region of the lesion. The histologic correlate is an area of compact orthokeratosis and hypergranulosis. A white veil occurring in association with a pigment network may be seen in melanoma.

Pigment network patterns, brown globules, and black dots are ELM features that may be seen in most melanocytic lesions. Pigment networks are reticulated pigmented lines with hypopigmented holes. Histologically, a pigment network shows pigmented and elongated rete ridges with an increased number of melanocytes in the basal layer with ELM. Brown globules manifest as uniform pigmented spots. Brown globules represent nests of melanocytes in the epidermis or dermis. Black dots are punctate, extremely dark pigment concentrations. Histologically, one sees large collections of melanocytes and/or melanin in the cornified layer (Chapter 151).

77. 1 A; 2 A; 3 A; 4 A; 5 B Highly undifferentiated melanomas can histologically resemble a number of other anaplastic tumors, including squamous cell carcinoma, large cell lymphomas, or soft tissue sarcomas. Special stains are helpful in differentiating these tumors. The Fontana-Masson stain identifies melanin, reticulum fibers, and nerves. The dopa stain takes advantage of the fact that tyrosinase present in melanocytes oxidizes colorless dopa to dopa-melanin, which is black. S-100 is a polyclonal antibody that stains melanocytes, Langerhans cells, Schwann cells, and nerves. Homatropine methyl bromide (HMB)-45 is a monoclonal antibody that is specific for melanocytes. The cytokeratin antibody stain is specific for squamous epithelium and can be used to separate squamous cell carcinoma from melanoma (Chapter 151).

78. 1 C; 2 A; 3 C; 4 B; 5 A For stage I melanoma, the only clinical factors shown to have negative prognostic significance independent of tumor thickness are advancing age, male sex, tumor ulceration, and lesions in the BANS (upper back, posterior arm, postlateral neck, and occipital scalp) locations (Chapter 151).

79. 1 D; 2 A; 3 E; 4 B; 5 C Bacille Calmette-Guerin (BCG) injected directly into intradermal melanoma metastases results in tumor regression in up to 50% of nodules. A combination of dacarbazine and BCG (chemoimmunotherapy) improves remission rates over either agent alone but does not impact on survival. The cytokine interleukin-2 (IL-2) has been used alone and in combination with patients' own lymphocytes to treat metastatic melanoma. Severe side effects, including a severe vascular hyperpermeability syndrome, limits the clinical use of IL-2. The melanoma antigens GD2, GD3, and GM2 may be used to target chemotherapy toward melanoma. Neuraminidase-treated melanoma cells have been used to create melanoma tumor vaccines (Chapter 151).

Bibliography

Barnhill RL, Mihm MC Jr, Fitzpatrick TB, Sober AJ. Neoplasms: Malignant melanoma. In: Fitzpatrick TB, Eisen AZ, Wolff K, et al., eds. Dermatology in General Medicine. New York: McGraw-Hill, 1993:1078–1116.

Casso EM, Grin-Jorgensen CA, Grant-Kels JM. Spitz nevi. J Am Acad Dermatol 1992; 27:901–913.

Goldsmith LA, Askin FB, Chang AE, et al. NIH Consensus Conference. Diagnosis and treatment of early melanoma. JAMA 1992; 268:1314–1319.

Friedman RJ, Heilman ER, Gottlieb GJ, et al. Malignant melanoma: Clinicopathologic correlations. In: Friedman RJ, Rigel DS, Kopf AW, et al., eds. Cancer of the Skin. Philadelphia: WB Saunders Co., 1991:148–176.

Harris MN, Roses DF. Malignant melanoma treatment. In: Friedman RJ, Rigel DS, Kopf AW, et al., eds. Cancer of the Skin. Philadelphia: WB Saunders Co., 1991:177–197.

Ho VC, Sober AJ. Therapy for cutaneous melanoma: An update. J Am Acad Dermatol 1990; 22:159–176.

Hoffman SJ, Yohn JJ, Norris DA, et al. Cutaneous malignant melanoma. Curr Probl Dermatol 1993; 5:1–44.

Koh HK. Cutaneous melanoma. New Engl J Med 1991; 325;171–182.

Kopf AW, Rivers JK, Friedman RJ, et al. Dysplastic nevi. In: Friedman RJ, Rigel DS, Kopf AW, et al., eds. Cancer of the Skin. Philadelphia: WB Saunders Co., 1991:125–141.

Rhodes AR. Neoplasms: Benign neoplasia, hyperplasias, and dysplasia of melanocytes. In: Fitzpatrick TB, Eisen AZ, Wolff K, et al., eds. Dermatology in General Medicine. New York: McGraw-Hill, 1993:996–1077.

Rivers JK, Ho VC. Malignant melanoma. Who shall live and who shall die? Arch Dermatol 1992; 128:537–542.

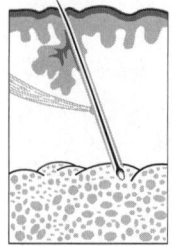

chapter 23

Mast Cell and Langerhans Cell Proliferative Disorders, Lymphocytic Proliferative Disorders, and Metastatic Disease

DONALD ROSENTHAL

Choose the ONE BEST answer to the following question.

1. Patients with Jessner's lymphocytic infiltration of the skin are most likely to present with
   A. Chronic cyclic episodes of papules and plaques on face, chest, and back
   B. Palpable purpura associated with sun exposure on face, chest, and back
   C. Atrophic, scaling, tender plaques on extremities
   D. Pruritic progressive nodules on chest, back, and face
   E. None of the above.

In the following questions, ONE or MORE of the following completions correctly finishes the incomplete statement; choose

A. If only 1, 2, and 3 are correct
B. If only 1 and 3 are correct
C. If only 2 and 4 are correct
D. If only 4 is correct
E. If all are correct.

2. The pathologic and immunopathologic features characteristic of Jessner's lymphocytic infiltration of the skin include
   1. Perivascular infiltrates of normal-appearing lymphocytes
   2. Civatte bodies in epidermis
   3. Negative immunofluorescence
   4. Parakeratosis.

3. Preferred management of Jessner's lymphocytic infiltration of the skin includes
   1. Careful monitoring of the patient to rule out transition into lupus erythematosus or malignant lymphoma
   2. Reassurance of the patient that this is almost always a benign condition
   3. Intermittent use of topical steroids
   4. Long-term, low-dose oral dapsone therapy.

Choose the ONE BEST answer for the following questions.

4. All of the following statements are true of telangiectasia macularis eruptiva perstans EXCEPT

    A. Darier's sign is often not well demonstrated

    B. Mainly occurs in adults

    C. Commonly progresses to or is associated with hepatosplenomegaly

    D. Dermal mast cell proliferation is often subtle or minimal

    E. Significant pruritus is uncommon.

5. The most common clinical characteristics of cutaneous lesions in patients with mastocytosis are

    A. Bullae or vesicles

    B. Telangiectasia and petechiae

    C. Macules and papules

    D. Pruritus or tenderness

    E. Solitary tumors.

Decide whether EACH choice in the following questions is TRUE or FALSE. Any combination of answers from all true to all false may occur.

6. Concerning urticaria pigmentosa,

    A. Cutaneous lesions tend to occur early in life

    B. An autosomal dominant pattern of inheritance is a common feature

    C. Cutaneous lesions are seen in 10% to 20% of patients with systemic mastocytosis

    D. Giemsa and Hale stains are preferred to demonstrate the characteristic metachromasia of mast cells

    E. Nonlesional skin also shows increased numbers of mast cells.

7. Concerning mastocytosis, mast cell mediator release may result in

    A. Hypotension

    B. Pruritus

    C. Urticaria

    D. Flushing

    E. Wheezing.

8. Concerning lymphocytoma cutis,

    A. It is one of the disorders that is commonly described as paraneoplastic

    B. It is a true malignant neoplasm of lymphocytes, occurring initially in the skin

    C. The most common clinical presentation is that of disseminated, discrete papules

    D. Oral lesions are common

    E. Persistence of the skin lesions for many years is often seen.

For the following question, one or more of the following completions correctly finishes the incomplete statement; choose

  A. If only 1, 2, and 3 are correct
  B. If only 1 and 3 are correct
  C. If only 2 and 4 are correct
  D. If only 4 is correct
  E. If all are correct.

9. Cutaneous pseudolymphomas

    1. Clinically can mimic B-cell or T-cell lymphoma

    2. Are rarely associated with fever and lymphadenopathy

    3. May be caused by contact allergy

    4. Most cases resolve spontaneously

    5. Drug-induced cases are most commonly caused by anticonvulsant medication.

Decide whether EACH of the following questions is TRUE or FALSE. Any combination of answers for all true to all false may occur.

10. Concerning cutaneous lymphoma,

    A. Pseudolymphomas are characterized by polyclonal proliferations of T or B cells

    B. Mycosis fungoides is one subtype of cutaneous T-cell lymphoma

    C. Cutaneous T-cell lymphomas other than mycosis fungoides are characterized by expression of the CD30 antigen by the neoplastic cells

    D. "Blastic transformation" in tumor-stage mycosis fungoides is always associated with a poor prognosis

    E. CD8+, CD4− phenotype cutaneous T-cell lymphoma is almost always associated with a poor prognosis.

11. Concerning cutaneous B-cell lymphoma,

    A. Primary cutaneous B-cell lymphoma is a biologically aggressive neoplasm with a poor prognosis

B. Primary cutaneous B-cell lymphoma commonly manifests clinically either as discrete nodules or erythroderma
C. Conventional radiotherapy is palliative treatment in primary cutaneous B-cell lymphoma
D. Chemotherapy is the treatment of choice in therapy of primary cutaneous B-cell lymphoma
E. Primary cutaneous B-cell lymphoma neoplastic cells do not demonstrate any consistent immunophenotypic pattern.

12. Concerning the Ki1 antigen,
    A. The Ki1 antigen was initially described in Reed-Sternberg cells
    B. The Ki1 antigen has been demonstrated on activated T and B cells
    C. The Ki1 antigen has been demonstrated in some cases of non-Hodgkin's lymphoma
    D. Ki1 anaplastic large-cell lymphoma has a poor prognosis
    E. Ki1 anaplastic large-cell lymphoma was formerly known as regressing atypical histiocytosis.

13. Concerning leukemia and lymphoma cutis,
    A. Specific cutaneous involvement (neoplastic cellular proliferation in the skin) is less common in leukemia and lymphoma than in carcinomas
    B. Twenty-five to fifty per cent of patients with leukemia and lymphoma have cutaneous changes related to their disease sometime in the course of their disease
    C. Erythroderma often (more than 25%) occurs in patients with chronic lymphocytic leukemia
    D. The histology of leukemic cells in the skin commonly mimics that seen in bone marrow and/or blood
    E. Leukemia cutis is statistically not a poor prognostic factor.

14. Concerning the skin and Hodgkin's disease,
    A. Reed-Sternberg cells are thought to derive from T cells
    B. Nonspecific cutaneous signs are much more common than specific cellular infiltrates
    C. Specific cutaneous involvement in Hodgkin's disease is seen in patients with highly aggressive disease

D. Patients with Hodgkin's lymphoma tend to be older than patients with non-Hodgkin's lymphoma
E. The histologic classification of specific cutaneous infiltrates is generally the same as that of involved lymph nodes.

Choose the ONE BEST answer to each of the following questions.

15. All of the following statements are TRUE concerning T-cell receptor gene rearrangement analysis EXCEPT:
    A. Detects clonality in skin and blood
    B. The detection of clonal rearrangement is not synonymous with malignant neoplasia
    C. Clonal rearrangements are often seen in skin biopsies of dilantin-induced drug reactions
    D. Patients with early stage mycosis fungoides or cutaneous T-cell lymphoma often have no detectable clonal rearrangement
    E. T-cell receptor gene rearrangement–analysis of lymphoid tissue is a useful technique in establishing lineage of lymphoid infiltrates.

16. All of the following characteristics are typical of the histologic features of *plaque-stage* mycosis fungoides EXCEPT:
    A. Band-like mononuclear infiltrate
    B. Fibrosis of papillary dermis
    C. Epidermal spongiosis
    D. Medium-sized and large atypical cells
    E. Epidermotropism.

17. Regarding mycosis fungoides,
    A. Mycosis fungoides is only one of several cutaneous T-cell lymphomas
    B. Mycosis fungoides may develop from or coexist with lymphomatoid papulosis
    C. If untreated, mycosis fungoides almost always clinically involves lymph nodes, spleen, and liver
    D. Tumor formation is a poor prognostic sign in mycosis fungoides
    E. Woringer-Kolopp disease is a rare variant of mycosis fungoides.

18. Regarding mycosis fungoides,
    A. Mycosis fungoides is significantly more common in women than in men

B. In the United States, blacks are more likely to be affected than whites

C. Environmental contaminants have been shown to be a common cause of mycosis fungoides

D. Sézary's syndrome is the leukemic phase of mycosis fungoides

E. Mycosis fungoides is a T-helper cell malignancy de novo.

For the following question, ONE or MORE of the completions correctly finishes the incomplete statement; choose

A. If only 1, 2, and 3 are correct
B. If only 1 and 3 are correct
C. If only 2 and 4 are correct
D. If only 4 is correct
E. If all are correct.

19. Appropriate therapy for early stage mycosis fungoides includes
    1. Conventional ultraviolet B therapy
    2. Psoralen ultraviolet A (PUVA) therapy
    3. Total-skin electron radiation
    4. High-dose infusions of gamma globulin
    5. Pulse therapy with methyl prednisolone.

Decide whether EACH choice in the following questions is TRUE or FALSE. Any combination of answers from all true to all false may occur.

20. Regarding the histopathology of mycosis fungoides,
    A. A Grenz zone is almost always found in biopsies of plaque-stage mycosis fungoides
    B. Atypical cerebriform lymphocytes, histiocytes, plasma cells, and eosinophils are commonly found in biopsies of plaque-stage mycosis fungoides
    C. Spongiosis is a common epidermal finding in biopsies of plaque-stage mycosis fungoides
    D. Superficial (papillary) dermal fibrosis is a common finding in biopsies of plaque-stage mycosis fungoides
    E. The "mycosis cell" is pathognomonic of mycosis fungoides.

21. Concerning parapsoriasis en plaque,
    A. Large-plaque parapsoriasis is thought to be a pre–mycosis fungoides stage
    B. Ulceration is commonly seen in the transition from pre–mycosis fungoides to frank plaque-stage mycosis fungoides
    C. Guttate parapsoriasis is thought not to be a pre–mycosis fungoides stage
    D. Poikiloderma atrophicans vasculare is a clinical syndrome that often is mycosis fungoides
    E. Poikiloderma of Civatte is a localized variant of poikiloderma atrophicans vasculare occurring most commonly on the neck.

Choose the ONE BEST answer to each of the following questions.

22. All of the following are unusual clinical features of cutaneous T-cell lymphoma EXCEPT
    A. Pustules
    B. Solitary tumor
    C. Urticaria
    D. Erythroderma
    E. Sharply circumscribed plaques.

23. Tumors in mycosis fungoides
    A. Always arise in plaques of mycosis fungoides
    B. May arise in previously uninvolved skin
    C. Are seen only in the terminal stage of mycosis fungoides
    D. Rarely ulcerate
    E. Rarely occur in erythrodermatous skin.

24. Regarding the immunologic status of patients with mycosis fungoides,
    A. In early-stage mycosis fungoides, there is commonly an elevated level of circulating B cells
    B. Immunoglobulin G (IgG) is significantly elevated in late-stage mycosis fungoides
    C. Skin tests to detect delayed hypersensitivity to common antigens such as nickel, tuberculin, and so on are similar to normal populations in early-stage disease
    D. Induction of contact sensitivity to common antigens (e.g., DNCB) is commonly depressed in early-stage disease
    E. Significant impairment of macrophage function is commonly seen in plaque-stage mycosis fungoides.

Decide whether EACH choice in the following questions is TRUE or FALSE. Any combination of answers from all true to all false may occur.

25. In the prognosis for patients with clinical and pathologic evidence of mycosis fungoides,

    A. There is a subset of patients who undergo spontaneous remission

    B. Patients do not die from mycosis fungoides unless they develop lymphadenopathy or tumors or ulcerations

    C. Spontaneous remissions in patients with mycosis fungoides is predicted by absence of eosinophils in skin biopsy

    D. Early treatment of patients with early-stage mycosis fungoides by any of the approved forms of treatment significantly prolongs survival

    E. Patients who develop mycosis fungoides before the age of 25 tend to have a benign clinical course.

26. Concerning lymphomatoid papulosis,

    A. The disease is caused by a retrovirus infection

    B. Fifty per cent of cases evolve into a frank lymphoma within 5 years of diagnosis

    C. Lymphomatoid papulosis has been shown to exhibit clonal rearrangements of the T-cell receptor gene

    D. Lymphomatoid papulosis may be an adult variant of pityriasis lichenoides et varioliformis acuta (PLEVA)

    E. Leukocytoclastic vasculitis is a common finding in skin biopsies of lymphomatoid papulosis.

27. **For each numbered item, choose the most likely associated lettered item. Within the group each lettered item may be the answer to one, more than one, or none of the numbered items.**

    1. Malignant potential increases over the age of 40 years
    2. High tendency toward spontaneous regression
    3. Cellular infiltrate is predominantly epidermal
    4. Reticulated morphology is characteristic.

    A. Lymphomatoid papulosis
    B. Woringer-Kolopp disease
    C. Alopecia mucinosa
    D. Parapsoriasis variegata.

For the following question, ONE or MORE of the following completions correctly finishes the incomplete statement; choose

A. If only 1, 2, and 3 are correct
B. If only 1 and 3 are correct
C. If only 2 and 4 are correct
D. If only 4 is correct
E. If all are correct.

28. Which of the following clinical features are characteristic of the Sézary syndrome?

    1. Generalized pruritus and erythroderma
    2. Alopecia and dystrophic nails
    3. Keratodermia of the palms and soles
    4. Ectropion and cataracts
    5. Recalcitrant bacterial pyoderma.

29. **Decide whether EACH of the following questions is TRUE or FALSE. Any combination of answers from all true to all false may occur.**

    The Sézary cell is

    A. Also known as the Lutzner cell

    B. Rarely seen in the leukocytosis of Sézary syndrome patients

    C. Small- and large-cell variants exist

    D. Seen commonly in bone marrow aspirates

    E. Not found in skin biopsies of patients with Sézary syndrome.

30. **Choose the ONE BEST answer to the following question.**

    Concerning the treatment of cutaneous T-cell lymphoma (CTCL),

    A. Extracorporeal photochemotherapy (extracorporeal photophoresis) is an established form of therapy for tumor-stage CTCL

    B. A common adverse effect associated with extracorporeal photochemotherapy (photophoresis) is bone marrow suppression

    C. Extracorporeal photophoresis (photochemotherapy) is an established form of therapy for erythrodermic CTCL

    D. Clinical improvement in patients treated with extracorporeal photophoresis correlates well with significant changes in T-cell subsets

    E. Extracorporeal photophoresis (photochemotherapy) is currently the treatment of choice in pemphigus vegetans.

For the following questions, one or more of the following completions correctly finishes the incomplete statement; choose

A. If only 1, 2, and 3 are correct
B. If only 1 and 3 are correct
C. If only 2 and 4 are correct
D. If only 4 is correct
E. If all are correct.

31. Langerhans cell histiocytosis
    1. Is the proliferative cell in regressing atypical histiocytosis
    2. Contains a characteristic trilaminar cytoplasmic organelle
    3. Is likely derived from dermal dendrocytes
    4. Plays an important role in generation of T-cell–dependent immune responses
    5. Originates from neural crest precursor cells.

32. Langerhans cell histiocytosis
    1. Is a synonym for histiocytosis X
    2. Characteristically begins in adolescence
    3. Vinblastine, prednisone, and methotrexate combination therapy is recommended in patients with multiple organ involvement
    4. Petechiae are a poor prognostic sign
    5. Occurs in 90% of patients with otitis externa.

Choose the ONE BEST answer to EACH of the following questions:

33. The prognosis for disseminated Langerhans cell histiocytosis is dependent on
    A. Age at diagnosis
    B. Histologic findings
    C. Extent of the lesions
    D. Severity of anemia at time of diagnosis
    E. Presence and severity of diabetes insipidus.

34. In children with cutaneous or multisystem Langerhans cell histiocytosis, which of the following clinical signs or symptoms is LEAST likely to be found?
    A. Erythematous papules
    B. Mucous membrane ulcerations
    C. Xanthomas
    D. Crusting of the scalp
    E. Otitis externa.

35. In children with multiorgan Langerhans cell histiocytosis, which of the following organs is LEAST likely to be involved?
    A. Kidneys
    B. Liver
    C. Lymph nodes
    D. Lungs
    E. Bone.

36. A 56-year-old man presents with a 3-week history of a generalized nodular eruption associated with fever and malaise. A nodule biopsy reveals a dense superficial and deep dermal infiltrate of large mononuclear cells with eosinophilic periodic acid–Schiff (PAS)–positive cytoplasm and eccentric pale staining of notched nuclei. Immunohistochemical studies reveal that the majority of cells express Ia and S-100 antigens. The most likely diagnosis is
    A. Syphilis
    B. B-cell lymphoma
    C. Mastocytosis
    D. Langerhans cell histiocytosis
    E. Pseudolymphoma.

37. All of the following statements are correct with regard to malignant histiocytosis EXCEPT
    A. Also known as histiocytic medullary reticulosis
    B. The atypical histiocytes contain S-100 protein
    C. The atypical histiocytes contain Birbeck granules
    D. Skin lesions are an integral part of this disease in children
    E. Malignant histiocytosis has an extremely poor prognosis with a median survival of less than 1 year.

Decide whether EACH choice in the following questions is TRUE or FALSE. Any combination of answers from all true to all false may occur.

38. Regarding the histopathology of Langerhans cell histiocytosis,
    A. The atypical cell has eosinophilic cytoplasm
    B. The atypical cell has a cerebriform nucleus
    C. Most of the infiltrating cells have typical Langerhans granules

D. The majority of cells are negative for CD1 antigen

E. Most of the infiltrating cells are S-100–positive.

39. Concerning metastases of internal malignancy to the skin,

   A. In comparison with the liver, the skin is more commonly involved

   B. Roughly 20% of patients with internal malignancy are affected with cutaneous metastases

   C. Lung cancer in males and breast cancer in females are the commonest internal malignancies to cause cutaneous metastases

   D. Cutaneous metastases often occur as ulcerated multiple papulovesicles

   E. Carcinoma en cuirasse is a scirrhous form of cutaneous metastases, usually seen with hypernephroma.

40. **For each numbered item, choose the most likely associated lettered item. Within the group, each lettered item may be the answer to one, more than one, or none of the numbered items.**

   1. Umbilical nodule
   2. Renal cell carcinoma
   3. Cutaneous lymphatic spread from breast carcinoma
   4. Carcinoma of the lung
   5. Sclerotic clinical appearance.

   A. Alopecia neoplastica
   B. Sister Mary Joseph's nodule
   C. Carcinoma erysipelatoides
   D. Chest wall cutaneous metastases
   E. Vascular cutaneous metastases.

ANSWERS

1. A; **2.** B; **3.** A Although some argue that Jessner's lymphocytic infiltrate rarely progresses to systemic lupus erythematosus (SLE), or lymphoma, most clinicians monitor such patients routinely, at the same time reassuring them that this is a benign but chronic cutaneous disorder. The pathology is classic but there are many instances when the dermatopathologist hedges between SLE, Jessner's lymphocytic infiltrate, and lupus erythematosus profundus. Although antimalarials may be beneficial, there is not enough data to routinely recommend their long-term use in this entity.

Most clinicians would agree that this is a benign reactive process but what is the skin reacting to? Equally frustrating to the clinician is the lack of consistent clinical response to therapeutic measures such as topical corticosteroids, or long-term use of antimalarial therapy.

Recent attempts to characterize the nature of the dermal infiltrate in Jessner's lymphocytic infiltrate of the skin, polymorphous light eruption, and cutaneous lupus erythematosus have not been very helpful. In all of these conditions, there is a similar phenotypic T-cell population. There is, however, an absence of HLA-DR–positive T cells in lymphocytic infiltrate of the skin and polymorphous light eruption compared with those in cutaneous lupus erythematosus (Chapter 156).

4. C; **5.** C; **6.** A (T); B (F); C (F); D (F); E (T) **7.** A (T); B (T); C (T); D (T); E (F) How extensive an investigation is warranted in patients with cutaneous mastocytosis is debatable. Finding of sclerotic bone lesions doesn't really change therapy. Symptomatic therapy is mandatory because cure is not obtainable and in children the vast majority of skin lesions will improve with or without therapy.

In telangiectasia macularis eruptive perstans (TMEP), biopsy and special stains with Giemsa and toluidine blue often show only a subtle increase in the number of dermal mast cells. Often, the dermatopathologist has great difficulty in giving a clearcut diagnosis in this condition. The number of dermal mast cells varies often from field to field, and there is really no "gold standard" upon which to rely for a diagnosis of TMEP. It is prudent for the clinician to biopsy three or four characteristic clinical lesions to give the dermatopathologist more material from which to work in an attempt to make a clearcut diagnosis. Because of the subtle increase in mast cells, the erythema and wheal formation and so forth may also be minimal. In most cases, there is no good evidence of systemic involvement.

Mast cell growth factor has recently been implicated as a possible cause both for the accumulation of dermal mast cells and the somewhat characteristic pigmentation seen in patients with cutaneous mastocytosis. This theory argues that some forms of mastocytosis may represent reactive hyperplasia rather than mast cell neoplasia. How this helps the patient or the clinician is uncertain (Chapter 152).

8. A (F); B (F); C (F); D (F); E (T) **9.** E; **10.** A (T); B (T); C (T); D (T); E (F) **11.** A (F); B (F); C (F); D (F); E (F) **12.** A (T); B (T); C (T); D (F); E (T) **13.** A (T); B (T); C (F); D (F); E (F)

14. A (F); B (T); C (T); D (F); E (T) **15.** C Cutaneous lymphomatous infiltrates clinically suspected because of persistent nodules, often on head and neck, and confirmed as "atypical lymphocytic infiltrates" by dermatopathology present a real dilemma to the clinician. Differentiation of "true" lymphoma from benign (reactive) pseudolymphoma, despite such modern achievements as immunoperoxidase techniques and gene rearrangement studies, is often difficult. To confound the clinician still further, it is now recognized that clonality is not necessarily the sine qua non of aggressive biologic behavior; that "true lymphoma" can stay localized to the skin for very long intervals, if not forever, and that relatively simple therapy such as excision or local orthovoltage radiation may be preferable to aggressive chemotherapy. For example, it is recognized that most patients

PROLIFERATIVE DISORDERS AND METASTATIC DISEASE **281**

with primary cutaneous B-cell lymphoma, that is, those without evidence of systemic involvement, often have a long benign course with some studies reporting a 10- to 30-year interval before systemic infiltration occurs. With such a relatively good prognosis and prolonged clinical course, the dermatologist's dilemma is Who should be treated, and how aggressive should treatment be?

It is apparent that the unpredictability of the behavior of such infiltrates mandates careful explanation to the patient and even more careful clinical and investigative monitoring (Chapters 156, 159, and 160).

16. C; **17.** A (T); B (T); C (F); D (T); E (T) **18.** A (T); B (T); C (F); D (T); E (T)

19. A; **20.** A (F); B (T); C (F); D (T); E (F) **21.** A (T); B (F); C (T); D (T); E (F)

22. E; **23.** B; **24.** C; **25.** A (T); B (T); C (F); D (F); E (F)

26. A (F); B (F); C (T); D (T); E (F) **27.** 1 C; 2 A; 3 B; 4 D

28. A; **29.** A (T); B (F); C (T); D (F); E (F) **30.** C Different subsets of cutaneous T-cell lymphomas continue to be identified. Mycosis fungoides, the commonest cutaneous T-cell lymphoma, has its own clinical subsets, which are difficult to distinguish in the early stages. Among these subsets are a small group of patients who go into clinical remission with minimum or no therapy and a larger group whose skin lesions remain static for many years and who do not appear to progress to multisystem disease.

The optimal management of mycosis fungoides remains controversial. The merits of topical nitrogen mustard, carmustine, total-skin electron radiation and psoralen ultraviolet A (PUVA) therapy continue to be debated by their proponents in the literature. Mycosis fungoides is not a rare disease. It is therefore difficult to understand why a multicenter prospective randomized trial of therapy has not been done in North America. The literature is still full of such comments as "we prefer" and "the management of mycosis fungoides continues to be controversial." It is clear that the experts are still baffled. Preferred forms of therapy are yet not supported by good evidence–based decision making. The literature clearly tells us that all of the previously mentioned forms of therapy are helpful in significant numbers of patients so treated. Definitely, a well-designed randomized trial comparing different modalities of therapy is needed.

Extracorporeal photophoresis appears to be the treatment of choice for Sézary syndrome, but it is expensive and at present is available only in certain tertiary care centers. Interferon therapy appears to hold promise as monotherapy even in early-stage disease but studies confirming this promise are not yet completed. To confuse the interferon issue further, different groups are using different interferons. A recent *Journal of the National Cancer Institute* reported trials with human interferon gamma, whereas earlier trials described encouraging results with recombinant human interferon-α-2A.

In the excitement of using newer more sophisticated forms of therapy, the clinician must remember that there have been reasonable studies suggesting that, in at least the early stage of mycosis fungoides, in minimal scattered patch disease, routine ultraviolet B therapy may be extremely helpful in the majority of patients so treated (Chapters 18 and 158).

31. C; **32.** B; **33.** C; **34.** C; **35.** A; **36.** D; **37.** C

38. A (T); B (F); C (T); D (F); E (T) It is not unusual for dermatologists to make the diagnosis of Langerhans cell histiocytosis in a child with seborrheic-like scalp dermatitis, a widespread petechial dermatitis, or persistent "external otitis." Careful examination of mucous membranes is important, since mouth lesions in particular are not uncommon. Although Langerhans cell histiocytosis affects similar areas of the body as do seborrheic and atopic dermatitis, the clinician should suspect Langerhans cell histiocytosis if purpura or scarring is noted in the persistent plaques. Furthermore, if compliant therapy with topical corticosteroids results in only marginal improvement, the clinician should be increasingly concerned, and appropriate biopsies should be done. In most centers, therapy is directed by the pediatric oncologist after the diagnosis is made.

Clearly, since the skin is involved in roughly 85% of patients, adequate and multiple skin biopsies are the diagnostic procedures of choice. The characteristic pathology varies from granulomatous through xanthomatous to proliferative in nature. Marker studies and electron microscopy are vital to identify the proliferating Langerhans cell, an epidermal bone marrow–derived histiocyte that has a vital role in epidermal immunity.

Although it is less common than in children, Langerhans cell histiocytosis can occur in adults both as single system disease of bone, skin, or lungs or as multisystem involvement. It appears that adults fare better than children, as least in one study. Systemic steroids are suggested as the best form of therapy for multisystem histiocytosis X in adults (Chapter 153).

39. A (F); B (F); C (T); D (F); E (F) **40.** 1 (B); 2 (E); 3 (C); 4 (D); 5 (A) It is not often that a dermatologist is the initial physician to diagnose systemic malignancy from the biopsy of a suspect nodule, the commonest morphology of skin metastases. However, distinctive clinical patterns of cutaneous metastases should be recognized, and umbilical nodules, morphea form plaques, cellulitic or lymphangitic patterns, and alopecia should arouse the dermatologist's suspicions. Cutaneous metastases, by and large, suggest a dismal prognosis.

Histology, although not always absolutely diagnostic of the primary site, almost always points the way to the most likely possibilities (Chapter 161).

Bibliography

Banerjee SS, et al. Twelve cases of Ki1-positive anaplastic large cell lymphoma of skin. J Clin Pathol 1991; 44:119–125.
Esterly N, et al. Histiocytosis X: A seven-year experience at a children's hospital. J Am Acad Dermatol 1985; 13:3:481–496.

Longley B, et al. Altered metabolism of mast cell growth factor in cutaneous mastocytosis. N Engl J Med 1993; 328:1302–1307.

Pimpinelli N, et al. Cutaneous lymphoma: A clinically relevant classification (review). Int J Dermatol 1993; 32:10:695–700.

Rijlaarsdam JU, et al. Characterization of the dermal infiltrates in Jessner's lymphocytic infiltrate of the skin, polymorphous light eruption and cutaneous lupus erythematosus: Differential diagnostic and pathogenetic aspects. J Cutan Pathol 1990; 17:2–8.

Smolle J, et al. Immunohistochemical classification of cutaneous pseudolymphomas: Delineation of distinct patterns. J Cutan Pathol 1990; 17:149–159.

Soter N. The skin in mastocytosis. J Invest Dermatol 1991; 96:32S–39S.

Stingl G, et al. Adv Dermatol 1989; 2:269.

Toonstra J, et al. Jessner's lymphocytic infiltration of the skin. Arch Dermatol 1989; 125:1525–1530.

Watsky J, et al. Primary cutaneous B-cell lymphoma: Diagnosis, treatment and prognosis. J Dermatol Surg Oncol 1992; 18:951–954.

section eight

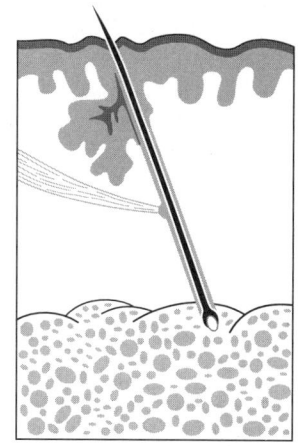

What Diseases of the Skin Are Malformations or Are Predominantly Inherited?

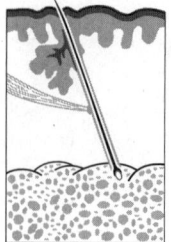

chapter 24

Inherited Diseases and Malformations of the Skin

LARISA KELLEY, and KAREN WISS

Choose the ONE BEST answer to each of the following questions.

1. The ichthyosiform syndrome that is characterized by a sharp midline demarcation of a unilateral ichthyosiform erythroderma and limb, nail, and hair deformities is
   A. CHILD syndrome
   B. Sjögren-Larsson syndrome
   C. Chanarin-Dorfman syndrome
   D. Refsum disease
   E. KID syndrome.

2. Menkes' kinky hair syndrome
   A. Is X-linked dominant
   B. Is not commonly associated with CNS impairment
   C. Has been related to a defect in intestinal iron transport
   D. Exhibits decreased free sulfhydryl content of hair
   E. Is associated with cutaneous and deep blood vessels that contain spiral twists.

3. The fragile hair condition that is evidenced by bamboo-shaped hairs is
   A. Netherton's syndrome
   B. Trichorrhexis nodosa
   C. Marinesco-Sjögren syndrome
   D. Monilethrix
   E. Pili torti.

4. All of the following criteria support the diagnosis of neurofibromatosis 1 EXCEPT
   A. Presence of two of more café-au-lait macules with diameter greater than 5 mm in a child less than 6 years of age
   B. Two or more neurofibromas
   C. Freckling of the axillary region
   D. An optic nerve glioma
   E. Two or more Lisch's nodules (iris hamartomas).

5. The neurocutaneous condition that is associated with recurrent epistaxis, pulmonary arteriovenous anastomoses, and spinal angiomas is
   A. Hereditary hemorrhagic telangiectasia
   B. Leopard syndrome
   C. Sturge-Weber syndrome
   D. Lindau-von Hippel syndrome
   E. Russell-Silver syndrome.

6. The autosomal dominant palmoplantar keratoderma (PPK) that is characterized by diffuse peripheral keratotic papules and hyperhidrosis is
   A. Unna-Thost syndrome
   B. Epidermolytic keratoderma

C. Keratoderma climactericum

D. Keratoderma blennorrhagicum

E. Acrokeratoelastoidosis.

7. All of the following statements are true of oculocutaneous albinism (OCA) EXCEPT

   A. Chédiak-Higashi syndrome, a variant of OCA, is clinically manifested by recurrent bacterial infections in a patient with lightly pigmented skin, hair, and eyes

   B. Tyrosinase-negative OCA is more common

   C. Visual acuity and nystagmus are more severe in tyrosinase-negative OCA

   D. Patients with tyrosinase-positive OCA develop mild pigmentation with increasing age

   E. Inheritance is autosomal recessive.

8. All of the following statements about hypohidrotic ectodermal dysplasia are true EXCEPT

   A. A normal number of eccrine glands is seen histologically, although physiologically they are nonfunctional

   B. Infants usually have episodes of unexplained fever

   C. Hypoplasia of mucous and mammary glands is seen

   D. Most infants have frequent respiratory infections

   E. Females frequently have aplastic breast tissue.

9. A firm plaque on the forehead, shown in Figure 24–1, may be the manifesting cutaneous feature of this disorder.

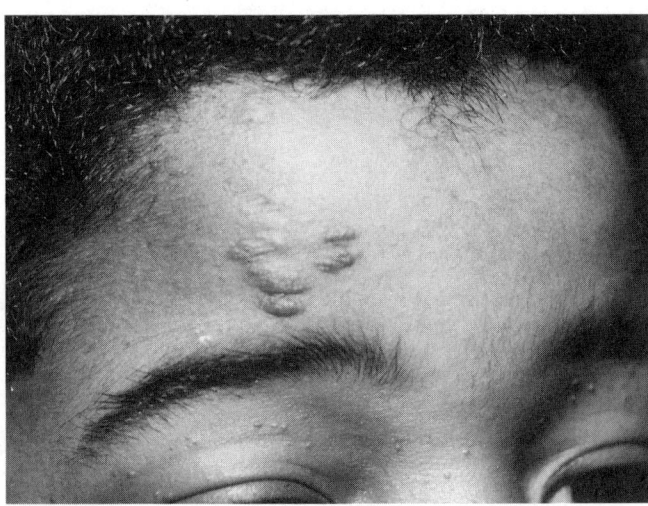

FIGURE 24–1.

   A. Neurofibromatosis

   B. Rapp-Hodgkin syndrome

   C. Tuberous sclerosis

   D. Cockayne's syndrome

   E. Rothmund-Thomson syndrome.

10. Four weeks after weaning from breast milk, a 6-month-old infant developed patchy alopecia, diarrhea, and an erythematous vesiculobullous dermatitis, mainly around his mouth and diaper area. The best treatment for the infant would be to

    A. Start supplemental iron

    B. Give oral zinc sulfate daily

    C. Tell the mother that as she introduces more foods the symptoms will disappear

    D. Continue breast feeding

    E. Substitute with a higher-calorie formula.

11. All of the following are commonly seen with nevoid basal cell carcinoma syndrome EXCEPT

    A. Hypertelorism

    B. Jaw cysts

    C. Neuroblastoma

    D. Calcification of the falx cerebri

    E. Bifid ribs.

12. Appropriate treatment for a 20-year-old with nevoid basal cell carcinoma syndrome who has approximately 50 tumors covering his arms, face, and back would include all of the following EXCEPT

    A. Excision

    B. Mohs' surgery for suspected aggressive tumors

    C. Radiotherapy to cover large areas of tumor involvement

    D. Cryotherapy

    E. Electrodesiccation and curettage.

13. All of the following are features of dyskeratosis congenita EXCEPT

    A. Oral leukoplakia

    B. Nail dystrophy

    C. Brittle, sparse hair

    D. Reticulated hyperpigmentation

    E. Fanconi-type pancytopenia.

14. The condition in which dermal papules and plaques composed of increased elastic and/or collagen fibers appear on the trunk is called
    A. Cutix laxa
    B. Pseudoainhum
    C. Buschke-Ollendorff syndrome
    D. Steatocystoma multiplex
    E. Ehlers-Danlos syndrome.

15. The most important reason to excise a nevus sebaceus is the
    A. Potential to enlarge to the point of becoming cosmetically disfiguring
    B. Foul odor
    C. Potential for malignant degeneration
    D. Potential intracranial extension
    E. Growth at puberty.

16. All of the following are features of the condition shown in Figure 24–2 EXCEPT
    A. Eighty per cent of cases involve the scalp
    B. Thirty per cent of scalp lesions have involvement of underlying bone
    C. Subcutaneous fat herniates into the hypoplastic dermis
    D. Surgically excising the area, if possible, is the treatment of choice
    E. The larger scalp lesions are associated with greater risk of extension into the meninges or dura.

17. A 6-month-old infant is brought for evaluation. Clinical examination reveals linear atrophic bands following Blaschko's lines, with scattered telangiectases, several soft reddish-yellow nodules, and a "lobster claw"-type deformity of her left hand. You assume that she has
    A. Cornelia de Lange's syndrome
    B. Rubinstein-Taybi syndrome
    C. Omenn's syndrome
    D. Goltz syndrome
    E. None of the above.

18. Primary cutaneous bone formation is commonly seen in
    A. Subcutaneous fat necrosis of the newborn
    B. Albright's hereditary osteodystrophy
    C. Pseudoxanthoma elasticum
    D. Systemic lupus erythematosus
    E. Ehlers-Danlos syndrome.

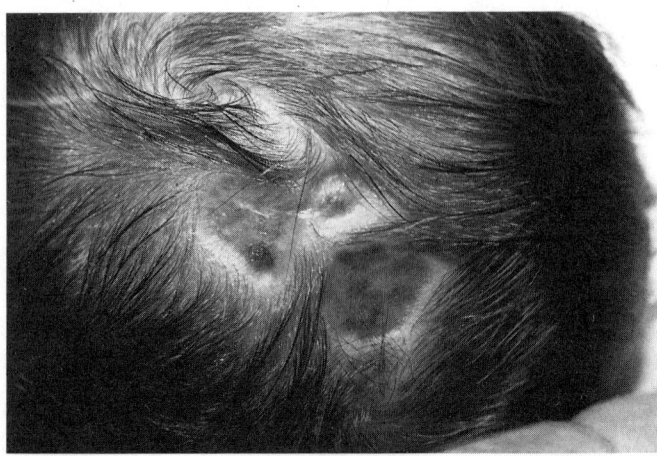

FIGURE 24–2.

For the following questions, ONE or MORE of the following completions may correctly finish the incomplete statement; choose

  A. If only 1, 2, and 3 are correct
  B. If only 1 and 3 are correct
  C. If only 2 and 4 are correct
  D. If only 4 is correct
  E. If all are correct.

19. An absent granular cell layer is seen in which of the following primary ichthyosiform disorders?
    1. Lamellar ichthyosis
    2. X-linked ichthyosis
    3. Epidermolytic hyperkeratosis
    4. Ichthyosis vulgaris.

20. Ichthyoses are often classified based on their rates of epidermal turnover. Of the listed ichthyosiform disorders, which show retention hyperkeratosis (as opposed to increased epidermal proliferation)?
    1. Ichthyosis vulgaris
    2. Lamellar ichthyosis
    3. X-linked ichthyosis
    4. Congenital ichthyosiform erythroderma.

21. Poliosis is seen in which of the following disorders?
    1. Piebaldism
    2. Tuberous sclerosis
    3. Vogt-Koyanagi-Harada syndrome
    4. Alezzandrini syndrome.

22. Trichothiodystrophy occurs with brittle hair in addition to
    1. Decreased fertility
    2. Short stature
    3. Mental retardation
    4. Renal malformations.

23. In tuberous sclerosis
    1. Inheritance is autosomal dominant with less than one third of all cases being new mutations
    2. About one third of the familial cases are linked to a locus on 9q34 near the locus for ABO blood group
    3. Angiofibromas are usually the presenting cutaneous feature
    4. There is a normal number of melanocytes in the hypopigmented ash-leaf macules.

24. Which of the following is associated with Hunter's syndrome?
    1. Generalized hypertrichosis
    2. White papules and nodules on the inferior angle of the scapula
    3. X-linked inheritance
    4. Deficient iduronate sulfatase.

25. Which of the following are (is) associated with pseudoxanthoma elasticum?
    1. Severe lung disease
    2. Retinal angioid streaks
    3. D-penicillamine is a common treatment
    4. Calcification and fragmentation of elastic fibers in the mid and lower dermis.

26. Which of the following are (is) characteristics of lipoid proteinosis?
    1. Hoarseness
    2. Enlarged tongue
    3. Yellow papules beaded along the eyelid margins
    4. Increased extracellular hyaline in the dermis EXCEPT around eccrine coils.

27. Calcinosis cutis is commonly seen in which of the following disorders?
    1. Systemic amyloidosis
    2. CREST syndrome
    3. Henoch-Schönlein purpura
    4. Dermatomyositis.

28. Patients with chylomicronemia (types 1 and 5 hyperlipoproteinemia) often have
    1. Eruptive xanthomas
    2. Lipemia retinalis
    3. Pancreatitis
    4. Xanthoma disseminatum.

29. Metabolic diseases that can cause secondary dyslipoproteinemia include
    1. Diabetes mellitus
    2. Hypothyroidism
    3. Primary biliary cirrhosis
    4. Multiple myeloma.

30. Familial hypercholesterolemia is associated with
    1. Tendon xanthomas
    2. Early coronary artery disease
    3. Xanthelasma palpebrum
    4. Defect in HDL receptor.

Decide whether EACH of the following questions is TRUE or FALSE.

Regarding ichthyosis,

31. Ichthyosis vulgaris is associated with relative flexural sparing and hyperlinear palms and soles.

32. Lamellar ichthyosis is associated with a steroid sulfatase deficiency.

33. X-linked ichthyosis manifests cryptorchidism as well as adult-onset corneal opacities.

34. Verrucous keratotic plaques in flexural areas, which frequently become macerated and secondarily colonized with bacteria, are typical of epidermolytic hyperkeratosis.

35. The most characteristic hair abnormality seen in patients with ichthyosis linearis circumflexa is trichorrhexis nodosa.

Regarding congenital disorders of connective tissue,

36. Skin changes associated with Marfan's syndrome include striae distensae and elastosis perforans serpiginosa.

37. The genetic defect in Marfan's syndrome is postulated to be a mutation within the fibrilin gene.

38. Ehlers-Danlos syndrome (EDS) type IV is associated with an abnormality in type 3 collagen.

39. Joint hyperextensibility in EDS produces a protective effect on future development of osteoarthritis.

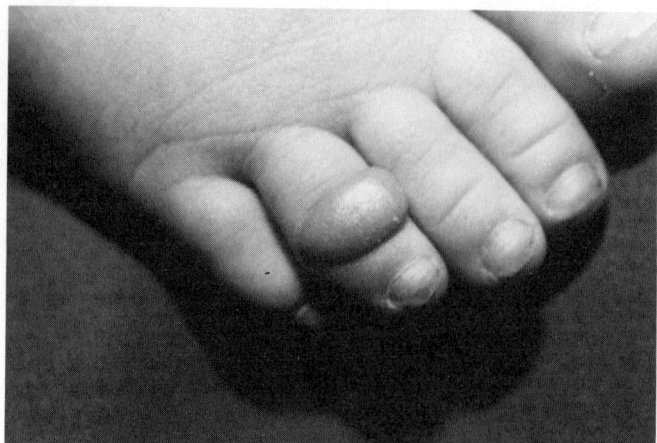

FIGURE 24–3.

40. Thrombotic events are the most common cause of death in patients with homocystinuria.
41. In addition to loose skin, patients with cutis laxa manifest poor wound healing and excessive skin fragility.
42. Blue sclerae and multiple pathologic fractures are hallmarks of EDS.

Regarding lesions of supporting tissue,

43. Infantile digital fibroma (Reye's tumor), as depicted in Figure 24–3, has a tendency to recur despite excision.
44. Infantile myofibromatosis is a condition in which multiple fibrous nodules are found in the skin, subcutis, muscle, and bone with sparing of visceral structures.
45. The hallmark of Peyronie's disease is a contracting fibrosis of the palmar fascia over the fourth metacarpal head.
46. Pruritus in hypertrophic scars and keloids is most likely due to an increased number of mast cells.
47. Joint deformities, gingival hyperplasia, and perianal papillomas are seen in juvenile hyaline fibromatosis.

For the following questions, the set of lettered headings is followed by a list of numbered words or phrases. For each numbered word or phrase, choose

    A. If the item is associated with A only
    B. If the item is associated with B only
    C. If the item is associated with both A and B
    D. If the item is associated with neither A nor B

For each of the following characteristics, choose whether it describes hidrotic ectodermal dysplasia, hypohidrotic ectodermal dysplasia, both, or neither.

48. Autosomal dominant inheritance
49. Thick, everted lips
50. Nail dystrophy
51. Alopecia
52. Hyperthermia.

    A. Hidrotic ectodermal dysplasia
    B. Hypohidrotic ectodermal dysplasia
    C. Both
    D. Neither.

For each of the following characteristics, choose whether it describes neurofibromatosis I, McCune-Albright's syndrome, both, or neither.

53. Multiple café-au-lait macules
54. Elevated serum alkaline phosphatase
55. Increased incidence of Wilms' tumor, rhabdomyosarcoma, leukemia
56. Skeletal abnormalities
57. Precocious puberty.

    A. Neurofibromatosis I
    B. McCune-Albright's syndrome
    C. Both
    D. Neither.

For each of the following characteristics, choose whether it describes incontinentia pigmenti, hypomelanosis of Ito, both, or neither.

58. X-linked dominant inheritance
59. Early linear vesiculation and verrucous changes
60. Hypopigmented swirls
61. Seizures.

    A. Incontinentia pigmenti
    B. Hypomelanosis of Ito
    C. Both
    D. Neither.

For each numbered item in the following questions choose the most likely associated lettered item. Each numbered item has ONLY ONE answer. Within each group, each lettered item may be the answer to one, more than one, or none of the numbered items.

For each of the following disorders, choose the most appropriate histologic description.

62. Porokeratosis
63. Hailey-Hailey disease

    A. Suprabasal location of vesicles and bullae with large numbers of cells in

64. Darier's syndrome
65. Pemphigus vulgaris.

the bullae cavity. The detached epidermis, devoid of most intercellular bridges, is loosely held together and resembles a dilapidated brick wall

B. Keratin-filled invagination of the epidermis with a tightly packed column of parakeratotic cells arising from the center of this invagination

C. Suprabasal bullae, acantholysis, and positive immunofluorescence for epidermal intercellular antibodies

D. Acantholysis leading to suprabasal clefts and lacunae with a peculiar form of dyskeratosis that results in the formation of corps ronds and grains.

For each of the following characteristics of metabolic disease, choose the most appropriate disorder.

66. Deficiency of hypoxanthine phosphoribosyltransferase
67. Enzyme defect in the metabolism and function of catecholamines
68. Associated with a deficiency in niacin
69. Multiple angiokeratomas
70. Untreated patients have depigmentation of hair and/or skin.

A. Riley-Day syndrome
B. Fabry's disease
C. Lesch-Nyhan syndrome
D. Phenylketonuria
E. Pellagra.

For each of the following inherited immunodeficiency syndromes, choose the associated clinical or laboratory manifestation.

71. DiGeorge's syndrome
72. Wiskott-Aldrich syndrome
73. Selective IgA deficiency
74. Hyperimmunoglobulin E syndrome
75. Ataxia-telangiectasia
76. Chronic granulomatous disease.

A. Thrombocytopenia
B. Cold abscesses
C. Defective nitroblue tetrazolium reduction
D. Tetany
E. Defective DNA repair
F. Lupus-like syndrome

For each of the following malignancies, choose the most commonly seen paraneoplastic syndrome.

77. Pancreatic tumor
78. Adenocarcinoma of the colon
79. Multiple myeloma
80. Oropharyngeal squamous cell carcinoma
81. Breast and lung cancer.

A. Bazex's syndrome
B. Amyloidosis
C. Dermatomyositis
D. Muir-Torre syndrome
E. Necrolytic migratory erythema.

ANSWERS

1. A CHILD is an acronym for a syndrome that includes congenital hemidysplasia with ichthyosiform erythroderma and limb defects. The hallmark of this syndrome is a sharp midline demarcation of an ichthyosiform erythroderma. There usually are other ipsilateral deformities, including unilateral alopecia, severe nail dystrophy, hypoplastic limbs, and organ defects. All of the other ichthyosiform disorders listed have generalized ichthyosis.

Sjögren-Larsson syndrome includes a triad of congenital ichthyosis, mental retardation, and motor spasticity. The ichthyosis phenotypically resembles lamellar ichthyosis or congenital ichthyosiform erythroderma.

Chanarin-Dorfman syndrome results from a rare autosomal recessive error of lipid metabolism. Generalized ichthyosis, along with myopathy and vacuolated leukocytes, are seen in persons of Middle Eastern or Mediterranean descent.

Refsum disease is characterized by motor and sensory polyneuropathy, neural deafness, retinitis pigmentosa and ichthyosis vulgaris–like skin changes. The full spectrum is usually not manifested until 10 to 20 years of age. It is due to an autosomal recessive deficiency in the α-hydroxylation of phytanic acid and therefore an inability to break down dietary phytanic acid, which accumulates in tissues.

KID syndrome is an acronym for a disorder with keratitis, ichthyosis, and deafness (Chapter 162).

2. E Menkes' kinky hair syndrome is an X-linked recessive, neurodegenerative syndrome with twists along the hair shafts (pili torti) reflecting twists in the hair follicle. Spiral twists in blood vessels are also seen, presumably due to abnormalities in elastic tissue. Severe cognitive and motor cerebral deficits are common as well as an increased susceptibility to infections. A defect in intestinal copper transport with resultant low serum and tissue copper levels is seen as well as increased free sulfhydryl content of hair. Copper treatment has been tried with disappointing results (Chapter 163).

3. A Netherton's syndrome is an autosomal recessive disorder with three main features: brittle hair, ichthyosis linearis circumflexa, and atopy. The fragile hair results from trichorrhexis invaginata, or bamboo hair, which is a nodular defect caused by abnormal intussusception along the shaft. The hair appears dry and lusterless, and easily fractures.

Trichorrhexis nodosa is the most common hair shaft abnormality. Hairs are broken and have grayish-white nodules along the shaft. The nodules are weakened points, usually the result of acquired damage to hair shaft cuticular cells. Trichorrhexis nodosa has also been associated with argininosuccinic aciduria and congenital ectodermal dysplasias.

Marinesco-Sjögren syndrome is a fragile hair syndrome due to transverse shaft fractures (tracheoschisis). Cerebellar ataxia, dysarthria, congenital cataracts, mental and physical retardation, abnormal teeth, fragile nails, and autosomal recessive inheritance are features.

Monilethrix is a fragile hair disorder in which the hair shaft has a beaded appearance. The beading corresponds to variation in follicular diameter, not intussusception of the hair shaft. The abnormal hairs arise from horny follicular papules and are most commonly found in the occipital area.

Pili torti is a description for flat, twisted hair shafts caused by curvature of the hair follicle (Chapter 163).

4. A Neurofibromatosis 1 (NF1) is an autosomal dominant neurocutaneous disorder with its gene locus mapped to chromosome 17. New mutations and variable phenotypic expression are common. Café-au-lait macules (CALM) are often the first sign. However, approximately 10% of the normal population has one or two CALM. More than six CALM in a young child is suggestive of NF1. Other findings strongly suggestive of NF1 include the presence of two or more neurofibromas, freckling of the axillary and inguinal regions (Crowe's sign), optic nerve gliomas, two or more Lisch's nodules, and a family history of similar findings (Chapter 166).

5. A Hereditary hemorrhagic telangiectasia (HHT, familial telangiectasia, Osler-Rendu-Weber disease) is an autosomal dominant condition of blood vessels in the skin, mucous membranes, and visceral organs. Recurrent epistaxis is the most common presenting sign, but any area of telangiectasia has an increased tendency to bleed. The lesions can occur diffusely but are usually found on the face, lips, ears, conjunctivae, trunk, and forearms. The lesions start as vascular papules and evolve into spider-like telangiectases by adult life. This disease is the most common cause of pulmonary arteriovenous anastomosis. Brain and/or spinal angiomas are seen, but infrequently.

LEOPARD syndrome is a condition characterized by multiple lentigines, electrocardiographic abnormalities, ocular hypertelorism, pulmonary stenosis, abnormalities of the genitalia, retardation of growth, and deafness.

Sturge-Weber syndrome is the association of a facial port wine stain involving the ophthalmic branch of the trigeminal nerve and ipsilateral leptomeningeal angiomatosis.

Lindau-von Hippel syndrome demonstrates a benign cerebellar tumor composed of a cystic mass of capillaries. Retinal angiomas are seen in about 20% of patients.

Russell-Silver is a syndrome of dwarfed stature and multiple CALM. Limb asymmetry is also seen (Chapter 175).

6. E Acrokeratoelastoidosis is clinically characterized by keratotic papules at the periphery of the hands and feet, diffuse palmoplantar hyperkeratosis, and hyperhidrosis. Fragmented elastic fibers are seen in the dermis.

Unna-Thost syndrome is a diffuse, symmetrical palmoplantar keratoderma with sharp margins, inherited in an autosomal dominant fashion. Histologically, orthokeratosis is seen.

Epidermolytic keratoderma is an autosomal dominant diffuse palmoplantar keratoderma that is clinically similar to Unna-Thost. Histologically, as in epidermolytic hyperkeratosis, epidermal vacuolization is seen.

Keratoderma climactericum is an acquired keratoderma, usually seen in women over 40 years of age. Oval plaques of hyperkeratosis enlarge and become confluent. The plantar surfaces are usually affected first.

Keratoderma blennorrhagicum is an acquired palmoplantar keratoderma associated with Reiter's disease. Clinically, it can appear identical to pustular psoriasis or a more diffuse keratoderma. Histologically, it is identical to pustular psoriasis (Chapter 162).

7. B Oculocutaneous albinism (OCA) is an autosomal recessive condition of lightened to absent ocular and cutaneous pigmentation. There are approximately nine subtypes, which are classified by the presence or absence of the enzyme tyrosinase. Tyrosinase-positive types are characterized by the ability of hair bulbs to darken after incubation with tyrosine. Tyrosinase-negative types do not. Tyrosinase-positive OCA is more common than tyrosinase-negative. Visual acuity and nystagmus are features in most forms of OCA but are worse in tyrosinase-negative. Tyrosinase-positive patients frequently develop mild pigmentation by adulthood, with mild freckling and yellow hair.

Chédiak-Higashi syndrome is a variant of OCA in which giant granules accumulate in various cells. These granules are marked in leukocytes. Neutrophil function is impeded, and bacterial killing decreases. Giant melanosomes, seen in melanocytes, cannot be transported effectively out of the cells, leading to hypopigmentation. The mechanism of the giant granule formation is not known (Chapter 131).

8. A Hypohidrotic ectodermal dysplasia histologically reveals absent or decreased numbers of eccrine glands. The glands that are present are presumed to be functioning properly. Thermoregulation is markedly disturbed because of decreased sweating. This often leads to unexplained fever. Mucous glands are commonly hypoplastic, causing decreased sputum production and therefore impaired clearing of respiratory organisms. Females show aplasia or hyperplasia of breast tissue (Chapter 164).

9. C Tuberous sclerosis has many cutaneous manifestations. These include angiofibromas, periungual fibromas (Koebner's tumors), shagreen patches, hypopigmented macules, and fibromatous plaques. Most of the cutaneous signs of this disease are not fully manifested until puberty. Hypopigmented macules and fibromatous forehead plaques are two of the earliest cutaneous findings and frequently are diagnostic in a child with seizures and developmental delay.

Neurofibromatosis has as its most prominent cutaneous findings neurofibromas, CALM, and intertriginous freckling.

Rapp-Hodgkin syndrome is an autosomal dominant ectodermal dysplasia in which hypohidrosis and alopecia are the main features. Pili torti, narrow dystrophic nails, cleft lip and palate, hypospadias, conical teeth, and aplastic lacrimal puncta are associated findings.

Cockayne's syndrome consists of short stature, mental retardation, photosensitivity, large hands and feet, ocular abnormalities, and extensive demyelination.

Rothmund-Thomson syndrome is a rare condition in which poikilodermatous plaques appear during infancy. The face and hands have pronounced telangiectases. Photosensitivity is common. Cataracts, alopecia, and short stature are evident. By adolescence, large warty keratomas develop on acral surfaces (Chapters 164, 166).

10. B The baby has signs and symptoms consistent with acrodermatitis enteropathica, which results from the inability to absorb sufficient zinc from the diet. It can be easily reversed by adding supraphysiologic doses of zinc to the diet. Zinc in human milk is much more available to infants than that in cow's milk. Continuing to breast feed would help temporarily but is not a good long-term solution. Symptoms would only worsen if no treatment was initiated and could lead to CNS damage. Advancing the diet to more solid foods would not give the adequate excess of zinc needed to correct the deficiency. Iron deficiency usually has an insidious presentation. Anemia, alopecia, pruritus, and koilonychia are seen with long-term iron deficiency.

Besides zinc deficiency, an acrodermatitis enteropathica–like syndrome can also be seen with cystic fibrosis, essential fatty acid deficiency, multiple carboxylase deficiency, methylmalonic acidemia, kwashiorkor, and maple syrup urine disease (Chapter 170).

11. C Nevoid basal cell carcinoma (NBCC) is transmitted in an autosomal dominant fashion with variable expressivity. The most common phenotypic findings are multiple basal cell carcinomas, palmoplantar pits, jaw and dental cysts, rib and vertebral abnormalities, and a characteristic facies (broad nasal root, hypertelorism, frontal bossing). The palmoplantar pits are due to premature shedding of abnormal keratin caused by a delay in maturation of basal cells. The basal cell carcinomas are histologically typical; however, clinically they often resemble nevi, neurofibromas, or skin tags (smooth, flesh-colored to pigmented papules). Other findings include short fourth metacarpals, lamellar calcification of the falx cerebri, and agenesis of the corpus callosum. Medulloblastomas, seen in 2% to 3% of patients, and ovarian fibromas are commonly associated tumors. Neuroblastomas are not reported with increased frequency (Chapter 167).

12. C Radiotherapy (XRT) is not an appropriate treatment, since it has been shown to induce multiple basal cell carcinomas when used as therapy for central nervous system tumors or as treatment of multiple basal cell carcinomas (BCCs) in these patients. Patients with nevoid BCC (NBCC) have been shown to have defective repair of normal cells after XRT and therefore produce new tumors after radiotherapy at an exponential rate compared with normal individuals. Mohs' micrographic surgery is recommended for clinically or histologically aggressive BCCs. Cryotherapy or electrodesiccation and curettage are desirable options for treating numerous superficial tumors (Chapter 167).

13. C Dyskeratosis congenita is a rare X-linked recessive disorder characterized by leukoplakia, nail dystrophy (thin, ridged, fissured nails or pterygium), and hyper- and hypopigmented reticulated macules. The pigmentary changes may also be associated with atrophy and telangiectasia resembling poikiloderma. Approximately 50% of affected individuals have bone marrow failure by 20 years of age, leading to anemia or a Fanconi-type pancytopenia. There is an increased risk of neoplasms, most notably squamous cell carcinomas, which arise in the areas of leukoplakia. The incidence of Hodgkin's disease and adenocarcinoma of the pancreas is also increased. There is no associated hair abnormality (Chapter 175).

14. C Patients with Buschke-Ollendorff syndrome (BOS) have an asymmetrical distribution of yellowish dermal papules and plaques on the trunk and limbs. Histologically, the lesions reveal increased numbers of elastic and/or collagen fibers. Diagnosis of BOS can be confirmed by the radiographic findings of focal round or oval densities (osteopoikilosis) on long bones.

Cutis laxa has a diffuse paucity of elastic fibers, giving the skin a loose appearance.

Pseudoainhum is a condition in which connective tissue bands cause annular constriction of the digits. Various disorders can cause pseudoainhum (e.g., pityriasis rubra pilaris, pachyonychia congenita, leprosy, Raynaud's phenomenon).

Steatocystoma multiplex consists of multiple cysts lined with epithelium that is studded with flattened sebaceous lobules.

In Ehlers-Danlos syndrome, there is decreased collagen synthesis, leading to fragile skin, poor wound healing, easy bruisability (Chapters 104, 172).

15. C Lesions of nevus sebaceus have an approximately 10% chance of developing basal cell carcinoma and/or appendageal tumors. Squamous cell carcinoma has also been reported to arise within a nevus sebaceus. Excision prior to puberty is recommended because of pubertal hormone influence on the size of the sebaceous

glands with subsequent nevus enlargement. Enlargement to the point of cosmetic disfigurement is unusual. Foul odor and intracranial extension are not seen (Chapters 144, 174).

16. C Aplasia cutis is a congenital disorder of localized absence of skin. Eighty per cent of cases have involvement of the scalp in the parietal area. The defect ranges from only epidermal loss to defects in the underlying soft tissue and bone. Up to 30% of scalp lesions extend into the skull. Larger lesions have a greater tendency to extend deeper into the dura and meninges. Spontaneous re-epithelialization occurs; however, the result is an absence of appendageal structures and scars. In contrast to focal dermal hypoplasia (Goltz syndrome), subcutaneous fat herniation into the dermis does not occur. However, subcutaneous fat can be exposed. Surgical excision is a good therapeutic option when anatomically possible (Chapter 173).

17. B Goltz syndrome, or focal dermal hypoplasia, is an X-linked dominant that is lethal in homozygous males. The dermis is markedly reduced in thickness, resulting in superficial placement of subcutaneous fat. The classic skin findings in the patient are described. Atrophic linear bands or streaks with telangiectases, red-yellow soft nodules due to herniation of subcutaneous fat, and ulcers are commonly seen. The most typical skeletal defect is the "lobster claw" deformity that results from syndactyly plus absent digits. Osteopathia striata, or vertical striations on radiographs of long bones are diagnostic. In addition to skin and skeletal lesions, hypoplastic hair, nails, and teeth are seen.

Cornelia de Lange's syndrome is best noted by the classic facies—bushy, confluent eyebrows, low hair line, small nose with anteverted nostrils, thin lips, and receding chin. Cutaneous findings include hirsutism and cutis marmorata. Mental retardation and short stature are common.

Rubinstein-Taybi syndrome is characterized by broad thumbs and great toes, microcephaly, capillary malformation of the forehead or nape of neck, hypertrichosis, and mental retardation.

Omenn's syndrome is a type of severe combined immunodeficiency that manifests with exfoliative erythroderma and profound adenopathy. Successful bone marrow transplantation is the only hope for survival (Chapter 173).

18. B Patients with Albright's hereditary osteodystrophy have osteoblastic activity within the skin which leads to formation of bone spicules in the dermis and subcutaneous fat, whereas calcinosis cutis is not organized by osteoblasts. Clinically, Albright's patients have short stature, skeletal anomalies (short metacarpals and metatarsals), short, broad nails, soft tissue calcification and bone formation, pseudohypoparathyroidism, and pseudopseudohypoparathyroidism.

Subcutaneous fat necrosis of the newborn, pseudoxanthoma elasticum, systemic lupus erythematosus, and Ehler-Danlos syndrome all may manifest calcinosis cutis, but primary cutaneous ossification would be very unusual (Chapter 178).

19. D Ichthyosis vulgaris is histopathologically characterized by moderate hyperkeratosis with a thin to absent granular cell layer; all the other primary ichthyosiform disorders listed have a normal to increased granular cell layer (Chapter 162).

20. B Ichthyosis vulgaris and X-linked ichthyosis have normal rates of epidermal turnover. The hyperkeratosis is considered a retention hyperkeratosis because of increased adhesiveness of the corneocytes, delayed desquamation, and eventual shedding in large clumps. In congenital ichthyosiform erythroderma and lamellar ichthyosis, there is evidence of increased epidermal proliferation (Chapter 162).

21. E Poliosis is a localized loss of hair pigment that can be associated with a variety of disorders.

Piebaldism, an autosomal dominant syndrome, is manifested by a white forelock and symmetrically located amelanotic macules. Hyperpigmented macules are often also seen within the amelanotic macules and on normal skin.

Tuberous sclerosis manifests poliosis in about 50% of patients. It is usually seen in the scalp and occasionally in the eyelashes.

Vogt-Koyanagi-Harada syndrome is a rare disease that displays uveitis, dysacousia, alopecia, poliosis, and vitiligo. This disease typically appears in three phases: meningoencephalitic, ophthalmic, and convalescent. It is during the convalescent phase that alopecia, vitiligo, and poliosis become prominent.

Alezzandrini's syndrome includes facial vitiligo, eyebrow and eyelash poliosis, deafness, and unilateral tapetoretinal degeneration (Chapters 131, 163, and 166).

22. A Trichothiodystrophy is an autosomal recessive syndrome in which patients have sparse, short, brittle hair with variable alopecia resulting from an abnormally low sulfur content. Individual hairs show clean transverse fractures and alternating birefringence. Associated features include cerebellar ataxia, dysarthria, retarded physical and cognitive development, dystrophic nails, cataracts, and decreased fertility. Renal malformations are not common. The acronyms BIDS (brittle hair, intellectual impairment, decreased fertility, and short stature) and IBIDS (when ichthyosis is a feature) have been used to describe trichothiodystrophy (Chapter 163).

23. C Tuberous sclerosis (TS) is a neurocutaneous disorder with autosomal dominant inheritance and 50% to 75% spontaneous mutations. The disease has marked variability in expression. The most common clinical manifestations are hypopigmented macules, adenoma sebaceum (angiofibromas), seizures, and mental retardation. Hamartomas are seen in the skin, nervous tissue, heart, and kidneys. Multiple genetic loci have been found for expression of TS; however, one third of familial cases have been linked to a locus on 9q34. The facial angiofibromas are usually not seen until over 5 years of age and are often mistaken for acneiform lesions. Ash-leaf macules may be seen at birth and become diagnostic in an infant with developmental delay and seizures. Hypopigmented macules are seen in 87% of affected indi-

viduals. Although a polygonal "thumbprint" pattern is most common, the lance-ovate, or ash-leaf macule, is the most characteristic. The size of the hypopigmented macules ranges from a few millimeters to several centimeters and one or many may be visible. Histologically, there are a normal number of melanocytes with fewer and smaller melanosomes (Chapter 166).

24. E Hunter's syndrome is a mucopolysaccharidosis (MPS) in which the lysosomal enzyme, iduronate sulphatase, is deficient. This results in accumulation of dermatan and heparin sulfate in organs and tissues. There are 13 syndromes associated with deficient breakdown of mucopolysaccharides. All are autosomal recessive except Hunter's, which is X-linked recessive. Universal findings of MPS include hypertrichosis and thickened skin. Hunter's syndrome in particular shows "pebbly" white papules and nodules on the inferior angle of the scapula. Death occurs by the third decade as a result of severe organ infiltration (heart, liver, brain) (Chapter 175).

25. C Pseudoxanthoma elasticum (PXE) is an idiopathic disorder of progressive calcification and fragmentation of elastic fibers in the dermis. Cardinal features include retinal angioid streaks caused by breaks in Bruch's membrane; ischemic cardiac and peripheral vascular disease, hypertension from renal artery involvement, and gastrointestinal hemorrhage. The elastic media of blood vessels calcifies. The typical skin findings are clustered, pebbly, yellow papules in flexural regions, giving a "plucked chicken" appearance. Skin biopsy demonstrates calcified, fragmented elastic fibers in the mid to deep dermis. Lung involvement is fortunately not seen. An acquired PXE-like picture has been described in patients being treated with penicillamine for other reasons (Chapter 172).

26. A Lipoid proteinosis (hyalinosis cutis et mucosae) is a rare autosomal recessive disorder of increased extracellular hyaline that infiltrates into various organs. Classic findings are hoarseness, swollen tongue, and yellow waxy papules and nodules caused by hyaline accumulation in the respective organ. Cutaneous lesions tend to have a hyperkeratotic scale. Yellow waxy papules along eyelid margins and face are extremely typical features and often are diagnostic.

Histologically, there is markedly increased hyaline in the dermis, especially around blood vessels, eccrine ducts, and the arrector pili apparatus. The abnormal hyaline material has a lipid component; hence the name lipoid proteinosis. Like lipoid proteinosis, porphyria shows increased hyaline deposition around superficial dermal blood vessels but lacks the deeper dermal involvement. The hyaline in porphyria is only present in sun-exposed areas (Chapter 169).

27. C CREST syndrome and dermatomyositis both have associated calcinosis cutis. In both cases, it is due to dystrophic mineralization rather than to a systemic abnormality of calcium and phosphate metabolism.

CREST syndrome represents an acronym for calcinosis cutis, Raynaud's phenomenon, esophageal dysfunction, sclerodactyly, and telangiectasias. Anticentromere antibodies are seen in more than 50% of patients. Patients with CREST have a more favorable prognosis; visceral involvement is infrequent.

In dermatomyositis, calcinosis cutis is most commonly seen in the pediatric population with extensive ectopic calcium involving the dermis, subcutaneous tissue, and muscle. Occasionally, areas of cutaneous calcification over extensor surfaces ulcerate. Henoch-Schönlein purpura and systemic amyloidosis are not commonly associated with calcinosis cutis (Chapter 178).

28. A Chylomicronemia, seen in types 1 and 5 hyperlipoproteinemia, is manifested clinically by eruptive xanthomas, lipemia retinalis, and chronic pancreatitis. Triglyceride concentrations are greater than 1500 mg/dL. Some patients with severe elevations of plasma triglycerides also have neuropsychiatric symptoms.

Xanthoma disseminatum is a normolipemic histiocytic disorder that affects the skin and mucous membranes and is associated with diabetes insipidus (Chapters 155, 176).

29. E Secondary lipoproteinemias may result in xanthomas because of metabolic disease. Eruptive xanthomas have been described with diabetes mellitus, diffuse plane xanthomas with multiple myeloma, and various types of xanthomas with primary biliary cirrhosis and hypothyroidism (Chapter 176).

30. A In familial hypercholesterolemia, one of a variety of low-density lipoprotein (LDL)-receptor defects leads to reduced cellular uptake of LDL and therefore increased circulating plasma LDL. Tendon, palpebral, and intertriginous xanthomas may all be seen with this condition. Early development of severe coronary artery disease is characteristic of homozygous and heterozygous disease (Chapter 176).

31. (T) Ichthyosis vulgaris has the most pronounced flexural sparing of the primary ichthyosiform disorders except when it is concomitantly associated with atopic dermatitis. Hyperlinear palms are indicative of mild hyperkeratosis. Fine white scales are present on extensor surfaces (Chapter 162).

32. (F) X-linked ichthyosis is due to a deficiency of the enzyme steroid sulfatase. The diagnosis can be confirmed by measuring steroid sulfatase activity in cultured keratinocytes, fibroblasts, leukocytes, or keratotic scale. One could also measure excessive cholesterol sulfate in the serum by noting excessive mobility of beta-lipoproteins with serum electrophoresis. The defect in lamellar ichthyosis is not clear (Chapter 162).

33. (T) Comma-shaped corneal opacities on the posterior capsule or Descemet's membrane appear in adulthood. There exists a 25% chance of cryptorchidism with X-linked ichthyosis (Chapter 162).

34. (T) The disease manifests with blistering at or shortly after birth. Eventually, the skin becomes verrucous and keratotic, especially in the flexural regions.

Bacterial overgrowth and infection are significant problems in these individuals (Chapter 162).

35. (F) Ichthyosis linearis circumflexa (ILC) is a migratory, polycyclic, erythematous, scaly eruption with a thick hyperkeratotic margin. Many patients also have an associated hair abnormality called trichorrhexis invaginata (bamboo hairs). The association of trichorrhexis invaginata with ILC is termed Netherton's syndrome. Trichorrhexis nodosa can be seen with Netherton's syndrome but is much less common than trichorrhexis invaginata (Chapter 162).

36. (T); **37.** (T) Marfan's syndrome displays autosomal dominant transmission. The characteristic phenotype consists of tall stature with abnormally long extremities, loose joints, large hands, and kyphoscoliosis. The typical skin finding is striae distensae. Occasionally, elastosis perforans serpiginosa is seen. The other organ systems commonly involved are the eye (ectopia lentis and retinal detachment) and the cardiovascular system (diffuse aneurysms). The defect in Marfan's syndrome has been shown to be due to mutations in the fibrillin gene (chromosome 15). Fibrillin is an elastin-associated microfibril that is present in increased concentration in the organs affected in Marfan's syndrome (Chapter 172).

38. (T); **39.** (F) The Ehlers-Danlos syndrome is a group of inherited disorders of collagen synthesis. Ten subtypes are commonly described, the unifying features being joint laxity, skin hyperextensibility, poor wound healing, and easy bruisability. In contrast to cutis laxa, the skin promptly recoils to its normal position after stretching. Clinically, the differences lie in the degree of clinical symptoms. The biochemical defect in collagen synthesis in most cases is still unknown. EDS type IV has been shown to be due to abnormal type III collagen synthesis. This type has mild joint laxity and skin hyperextensibility but an increased incidence of artery and bowel rupture. EDS type VI is postulated to be due to lysyl hydroxylase deficiency. In type VII, there is a defect in the conversion of procollagen to collagen, and type IX is due to abnormal copper utilization with deficient lysyl oxidase. Joint hypermobility in most types leads to premature-onset osteoarthritis (Chapter 172).

40. (T) Homocystinuria is a metabolic disorder with autosomal recessive inheritance in which patients have a body habitus similar to those with Marfan's syndrome. The enzyme β-cystathionine synthase is defective. Homocysteine is converted to homocystine in excess. The exact defect in collagen synthesis and structure is not completely known, but it is postulated that increased homocystine interferes with collagen cross-linking. Features of homocystinuria that distinguish it from Marfan's syndrome include arterial and venous thrombosis, joint limitation, osteopenia, and mental retardation. Arterial and venous thrombosis is the main cause of premature death. The typical skin changes include malar flush, thinned hair, and cutis reticulata. As in Marfan's syndrome, ectopia lentis, dolichostenomelia (long, narrow extremities), pectus excavatum, pectus carinatum, and kyphoscoliosis are features (Chapter 182).

41. (F) Cutis laxa is a disorder of loose, sagging skin resulting from decreased numbers and fragmentation of elastic fibers. Collagen fibers are also noted to be defective. When the skin is stretched, it slowly returns to its normal position. The disorder does not manifest the excessive skin fragility, poor wound healing, and joint hypermobility that Ehlers-Danlos syndrome does. Other features include emphysema and tortuous blood vessels (Chapter 104).

42. (F) Blue sclerae and multiple pathologic fractures are hallmarks of osteogenesis imperfecta. Type I collagen is abnormal, leading to the main feature of this disorder—osseous fragility, or brittle bones. There are four types described; type I shows mild disease and types II, III, and IV more severe disease (Chapter 178).

43. (T) Infantile digital fibromatosis is a condition of solitary or multiple digital dermal nodules, usually located on the extensor or lateral surfaces of the finger or toes. Histologically, there is a dermal infiltrate of spindle-shaped fibroblasts and collagen bundles with eosinophilic cytoplasmic inclusions. Recurrence is common after surgical excision and spontaneous remission usually occurs if left alone (Chapter 184).

44. (F) Infantile myofibromatosis encompasses two fibrous disorders—congenital multiple myofibromatosis and congenital generalized myofibromatosis. In congenital multiple myofibromatosis, fibrous nodules composed of myofibroblasts are present at birth or shortly after in the skin, subcutaneous fat, skeletal muscle, and bone. Prognosis is excellent with spontaneous resolution by 2 years of age. Visceral involvement occurs in those patients with congenital generalized myofibromatosis with a mortality rate of 80% caused by obstruction of the lungs, gastrointestinal tract, or the central nervous system (Chapter 184).

45. (F) Bilateral contracting fibrosis of the palmar fascia over the fourth metacarpal head is the hallmark of Dupuytren's contracture. Peyronie's disease is a similar contracting fibrosis of the fibrous septa on the dorsal penis (Chapter 102).

46. (T) Hypertrophic scars and keloids are both due to an abnormal healing response in which fibrous tissue and fibroblasts consolidate to form a thickened, haphazard arrangement. There are a paucity of elastin fibers and an increase in mast cells and plasma cells. The increase in mast cells likely leads to the common symptom of pruritus (Chapter 101).

47. (T) Juvenile hyaline fibromatosis is a disorder that consists of soft, translucent, dermal papules and nodules concentrated on the face, scalp, and extremities in association with flexion contractures, gingival hyperplasia, osteolytic bone lesions, and growth retardation. Histologically, "chondroid" cells are embedded in eosinophilic hyaline ground substance (Chapter 149).

48. A; **49.** B; **50.** C; **51.** C; **52.** B Hidrotic ectodermal dysplasia is autosomal dominantly inherited and displays marked nail dystrophy. Slow-growing, thick, striated, discolored nail plates are common (onychauxis). Periun-

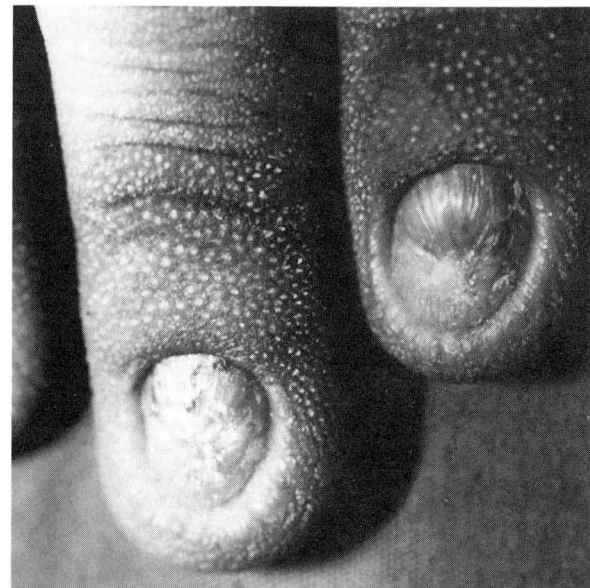

FIGURE 24-4.

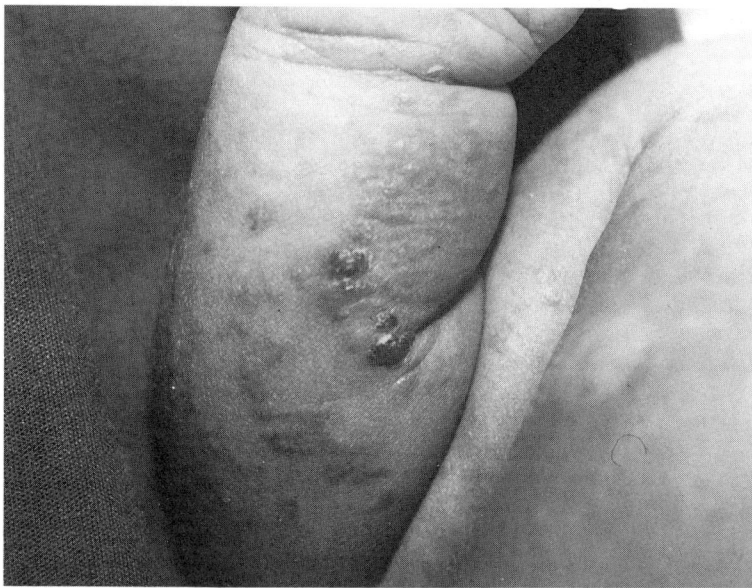

FIGURE 24-5.

gual hypertrophy with a mamillated appearance (as depicted in Fig. 24-4) is typical. Paronychial infections are frequent. Palmoplantar keratoderma is commonly seen. Scalp hair is sparse and brittle. Normal facies, normal dentition, and normal sweating distinguish this condition from hypohidrotic ectodermal dysplasia.

Hypohidrotic ectodermal dysplasia is usually X-linked recessive. It is characterized by partial or complete absence of sweat glands, hypotrichosis, hypodontia, and occasionally brittle, thin, ridged nails. There is also a characteristic facies associated with this syndrome: frontal bossing, prominent chin, saddle nose, sunken cheeks, thick, everted lips, sparse hair, and small, pointed ears. Reduced sweating leads to hyperthermia (Chapter 164).

53. C; **54.** B; **55.** A; **56.** C; **57.** C Both NF1 and McCune-Albright syndrome typically have numerous large café-au-lait macules (CALM). Several clinical features however help to distinguish the two. CALM in NF1 usually have smooth borders and are typically 2 to 5 cm (can be larger); they are scattered across the body and usually show increased numbers of melanocytes with melanin macroglobules. CALM in McCune-Albright's classically are larger than 10 cm, usually unilateral, do not cross the midline, and have irregular, serrated borders (like the "coast of Maine"). Histologically, they typically do not have increased numbers of melanocytes or melanin macroglobulins.

McCune-Albright's syndrome is characterized by a triad of CALM, polyostotic fibrous dysplasia of bone, and precocious puberty. Serum calcium and phosphorus are usually normal; however, serum alkaline phosphatase is usually elevated. The bone lesions arise from replacement of normal bone by fibrous connective tissue. Clinically, pain and pathologic fractures are seen. Precocious puberty is most pronounced in females.

The skeletal abnormalities in NF1 include scoliosis, short stature, pseudoarthrosis, and macrocephaly. Precocious puberty due to hamartomas in the hypothalamus is seen. Malignant transformation occurs in about 5% of NF1 patients. The most common tumor is neurofibrosarcoma; however, Wilm's tumor, rhabdomyosarcoma, and leukemia have been described (Chapter 166).

58. A; **59.** A; **60.** C; **61.** C Incontinentia pigmenti (IP) is X-linked dominant (lethal to males), the most notable characteristic being swirls of brown pigmentation. This disease has four stages: (1) linear vesiculobullous lesions on the trunk and extremities that appear from birth to 1 month of age (Fig. 24-5); (2) a verrucous stage that replaces the vesicles and bullae; (3) whorls of pigment that appear by 3 to 7 months of age that do not directly correspond to the areas of vesiculobullous lesions but frequently follow Blaschko's lines, this stage giving the condition its name; pigment intensifies during childhood and starts fading by adolescence; (4) hypopigmented swirls often remain where the original pigmented swirls had been.

Approximately 30% of affected individuals have mental retardation and seizures. Histologically, the pigmented stage reveals decreased melanin in basal cells with increased melanin in the dermis, free or within dermal melanophages.

Hypomelanosis of Ito (incontinentia pigmenti achromians) is a neurocutaneous disorder that is likely the result of genetic mosaicism of two cell lines with different pigment potential. The characteristic hypopigmented swirls arise from birth to 1 year of age. There is no preceding vesiculobullous or verrucous stage. Clinically, this resembles a negative image of IP. Up to 75% of patients have other anomalies—specifically, mental and motor retardation, skeletal abnormalities, and seizures (Chapters 131, 132, 175).

62. B In porokeratosis, the diagnostic clinical finding is a peripheral keratotic ridge of which the clinicopathologic correlate is the cornoid lamella. The cornoid lamella is composed of a keratin-filled invagination of the epidermis with a central parakeratotic column. There is no granular layer in the area in which the cornoid lamella arises. There are five different forms of porokeratosis, all of which have a cornoid lamella of varying degrees (Chapter 162).

63. A In Hailey-Hailey disease (benign familial pemphigus), the main histologic feature is acantholysis of full-thickness epidermis. There are resulting lacunae, vesicles, and bullae. Many of the acantholytic cells are loosely held together because of a few intact intercellular bridges. This gives Hailey-Hailey a classic appearance that resembles a dilapidated brick wall. Occasionally, corps ronds and grains are seen (Chapters 162 and 174).

64. D The histologic findings in Darier's disease (keratosis follicularis) include dyskeratotic cells termed corps ronds and grains, suprabasal acantholysis with resulting suprabasal clefts or lacunae, and elongated dermal papillae that are lined with a single layer of basal cells protruding into the lacunae. In contrast to Hailey-Hailey disease, acantholysis is usually limited to the lower epidermis, and dyskeratosis is an extremely prominent feature (Chapter 162).

65. C Histologically, pemphigus vulgaris evolves from intercellular edema to suprabasilar bullae. The distinguishing features from Hailey-Hailey disease are the suprabasal acantholysis with a normal-appearing detached epidermis, eosinophils in the bullae, and positive direct immunofluorescence for IgG in the intercellular spaces (Chapter 74).

66. C; 67. A; 68. E; 69. B; 70. D Riley-Day is a syndrome of autonomic dysfunction with autosomal recessive inheritance that is caused by an enzyme defect in the metabolism and function of catecholamines. Patients have defective lacrimation, cutaneous blotchy erythematous patches, hyperhidrosis, and excessive drooling. It is most prevalent in Ashkenazi Jews.

Fabry's disease (angiokeratoderma corporis diffusum) is due to a deficiency of the enzyme α-galactosidase A that results in accumulation of trihexosyl ceramide in endothelium and smooth muscle. The most obvious cutaneous findings are multiple telangiectatic macules and papules with or without hyperkeratosis. Clustering tends to occur on the hips, buttocks, lower trunk, and shaft of the penis. Histologically, the lesions are angiokeratomas. Glycolipid accumulates in the media and intima of blood vessels.

Lesch-Nyhan syndrome is an X-linked recessive disorder manifested by mental retardation, motor spasticity, choreoathetosis, and self-mutilation (especially of the face and lower lip). This syndrome is due to a deficiency of the enzyme hypoxanthine guanine phosphoribosyltransferase, which results in elevated blood uric acid levels.

Phenylketonuria is a metabolic disorder characterized by mental retardation, seizures, and decreased pigmentation of the hair and skin. There is a block in the conversion of phenylalanine to tyrosine, often due to a deficiency of phenylalanine hydroxylase. Treatment depends on early detection and low dietary intake of phenylalanine.

Pellagra is due to a deficiency in nicotinic acid, which is mainly found in green vegetables and red meat. Clinical symptoms are frequently referred to as the three Ds. dermatitis, which is photodistributed, erythematous, and vesicular; diarrhea; and dementia. Replacement therapy reverses the symptoms (Chapter 182).

71. D DiGeorge's syndrome, or congenital thymic aplasia, is the result of a congenital malformation of the third and fourth pharyngeal pouches. Infants have candidiasis and are susceptible to overwhelming viral, fungal, or bacterial infections. They present with tetany in the neonatal period because of an absence of parathyroid glands. These infants have profound defects in cell-mediated immunity (Chapter 125).

72. A Wiskott-Aldrich syndrome is an X-linked recessive disorder with defective T-cell and B-cell function. The most common presenting signs are thrombocytopenia, recurrent pyogenic infections, and atopic dermatitis, all within the first few months of life. Fungal, viral, and opportunistic infections arise as T-cell function diminishes. The lymphocyte and platelet abnormalities are thought to be due to a defective surface glycoprotein. Palliative treatment consists of platelet transfusion and intravenous gammaglobulin. Definitive treatment is bone marrow transplantation. In those who survive to adulthood, leukemia and lymphoma are common (Chapter 125).

73. F Selective IgA deficiency is one of the most common immunodeficiencies. The vast majority of affected individuals are healthy. However, allergies, asthma, lupus erythematosus, dermatomyositis, pernicious anemia, and rheumatoid arthritis have been described. Besides IgA deficiency, a variety of complement deficiencies (C1r, C1s, C1q, C2, C4, C5, C6, C7, C8, C1 inhibitor) have been associated with a lupus-like syndrome (Chapter 125).

74. B Hyperimmunoglobulin E syndrome consists of recurrent sinopulmonary infections, repeated cutaneous furuncles, coarse facial features, and an eczematous dermatitis. Patients have markedly high serum IgE levels and impaired neutrophil chemotaxis. They have high levels of *Staphylococcus aureus*–specific IgE. The cutaneous abscesses lack the warmth, tenderness, and erythema typically seen and have been referred to as "cold abscesses." Job's syndrome, described in fair, red-haired girls, is identical to hyper-IgE syndrome (Chapter 125).

75. E Ataxia-telangiectasia is a combined T and B cell–deficiency syndrome. Recurrent bacterial and viral infections are the rule in particular sinopulmonary infections. Cutaneous findings, which begin in late childhood, include telangiectases of the bulbar conjunctivae, cheeks, and ears. Scleroderma-like atrophy, ulcers, and premature graying are also seen. Ataxia, choreoathetosis, and dysarthric speech usually arise in early childhood, before the cutaneous signs. Lymphoreticular malignancies are seen in 10% to 15% of patients by adolescence. Most patients have decreased serum IgE, IgA, and cell-mediated immunity. There is a defect in DNA repair with frequent chromosomal breaks and translocations (Chapter 125).

76. C Chronic granulomatous disease is a congenital immunodeficiency in which the function of phagocytic leukocytes is impaired, as a result of a defective nicotinamide-adenine dinucleotide phosphate (NADPH) oxidase system. Superoxide and other cytopathic oxygen metabolites that are necessary to kill catalase-positive intracellular organisms (*Staphylococcus aureus, Salmonella, Aspergillus*) are not produced. Within the first several years of life, patients develop multiple staphylococcal abscesses, both cutaneous and internal (in lymph nodes, lungs, liver, gastrointestinal (GI) tract). Because of intracellular survival of these bacteria, granulomas are formed in the GI tract and genitourinary system. Treatment consists of prophylactic antibiotics, incision and drainage of abscesses, bone marrow transplantation, and α-interferon.

One screening test for the disease is the nitroblue tetrazolium (NBT) reduction assay. Neutrophils are unable to reduce NBT dye after phagocytosis because the respiratory burst does not occur (Chapter 125).

77. E Necrolytic migratory erythema consists of scaly papules and plaques most concentrated around the perineum, thighs, and buttocks that coalesce into annular serpiginous plaques. The epidermis becomes necrotic and desquamates. This eruption is associated with glucagon-secreting alpha cell tumors of the pancreas. Alleviation of cutaneous symptoms is seen when the tumor is excised. Protein- and zinc-supplemented diets also help abate symptoms (Chapter 180).

78. D Muir-Torre syndrome is autosomal dominant with the essential cutaneous findings of multiple sebaceous neoplasms (benign and malignant) and, occasionally, keratoacanthomas. Besides the sebaceous tumors, patients may have multiple visceral neoplasms, in particular adenocarcinoma of the colon. Malignancies in Muir-Torre syndrome have a tendency to be low grade (Chapter 180).

79. B Primary amyloidosis is associated with multiple myeloma in about 30% of cases. Localized and secondary forms of amyloidosis are not typically associated with malignancy. Amyloidosis is a disorder in which fibrillar material is deposited in various organs, in particular the heart, tongue, gastrointestinal tract, nerves, and skin. The fibrillar material (amyloid) consists of immunoglobulin light chains. Diagnosis lies in demonstrating amyloid in tissue biopsy. Presenting symptoms include enlarged tongue, periorbital or "pinch purpura," weight loss, hepatomegaly, edema, and paresthesias (Chapter 177).

80. A Cutaneous signs of Bazex's syndrome (paraneoplastic acrokeratosis) are psoriasiform plaques on the feet, dorsal hands, nose, and ears; and nail dystrophy. It is unresponsive to routine therapy. All patients are eventually found to have a malignant neoplasm, usually squamous cell carcinoma of the oral cavity, upper respiratory system, tongue, or esophagus. The cutaneous symptoms persist unless the underlying malignancy is treated (Chapter 180).

81. C Dermatomyositis is clinically manifested by proximal muscle weakness, periorbital heliotrope, Gottron's papules, periungual telangiectasia, and poikiloderma. In contrast to juvenile-onset disease, adult-onset dermatomyositis is associated with malignancy. Adult patients that have eroded, ulcerated, or necrotic lesions have an even higher incidence of malignancy. Various malignancies have been reported; lung and breast carcinomas are the most frequent. Diagnosis is confirmed by elevated creatine phosphokinase, aldolase, serum glutamic oxaloacetic transferase, abnormal muscle biopsy, and abnormal electromyography in a patient with the previously mentioned skin findings. Screening tests in a patient with adult-onset dermatomyositis should include mammogram, stool guaiac, chest x-ray, chemistry profile, and complete blood count (Chapter 180).

Bibliography

Bertolino AP, Freedberg IM. Hair. In: Fitzpatrick TB, Eisen AZ, Wolff K, et al., eds. Dermatology in General Medicine. 4th edition. vol. I. New York: McGraw-Hill, 1993:671.

Black MM, Gawkrodger DJ, Seymour CA, et al. Metabolic and nutritional disorders. In: Champion RH, Burton JL, Ebling FJG, eds. Rook/Wilkinson/Ebling Textbook of Dermatology. 5th edition. vol. IV. Oxford: Blackwell Scientific Publications, 1992:2295.

Dawber RPR, Ebling FJG, Wojnarowska FT. Disorders of hair. In: Champion RH, Burton JC, Ebling FJG, eds. Rook/Wilkinson/Ebling Textbook of Dermatology. 5th edition. vol. IV. Oxford: Blackwell Scientific Publications, 1992:2533.

Giacoia GP, Berry GT: Acrodermatitis enteropathica–like syndrome secondary to isoleucine deficiency during treatment of maple syrup urine disease. Am J Dis Child 1993; 147:954.

Griffiths WAD, Leigh IM, Marks R: Disorders of keratinization. In: Champion RH, Burton JL, Ebling FJG, eds. Rook/Wilkinson/Ebling Textbook of Dermatology. 5th edition. vol. II. Oxford: Blackwell Scientific Publications, 1992:1325.

Harper J. Genetics and genodermatoses. In: Champion RH, Burton JL, Ebling FJG, eds. Rook/Wilkinson/Ebling Textbook of Dermatology. 5th edition. vol I. Oxford: Blackwell Scientific Publications, 1992:305.

Hurwitz S. Cutaneous tumors in childhood. In: Hurwitz S, ed. Clinical Pediatric Dermatology. 2nd edition. vol. I. Philadelphia: WB Saunders Co., 1993:230.

Kraemer KH. Heritable diseases with increased sensitivity to cellular injury. In: Fitzpatrick TB, Eisen AZ, Wolff K, et al., eds. Dermatology in General Medicine, 4th edition. vol. II. New York: McGraw-Hill, 1993:1974.

Lever WF, Schaumburg-Lever G. Congenital disease/genodermatoses. In: Lever WF, Schaumburg-Lever G, eds. Histopathology of the Skin. 7th edition. Philadelphia: JB Lippincott, 1990:65.

Paller AS. Genetic immunodeficiency diseases. In: Fitzpatrick TB, Eisen AZ, Wolff K, et al., eds. Dermatology in General Medicine. 4th edition. vol. II. New York: McGraw-Hill, 1993:1950.

Phillips SB, Baden HP: Ichthyosiform dermatoses. In: Fitzpatrick TB, Eisen AZ, Wolff K, et al., eds. Dermatology in General Medicine. 4th edition. vol. I. New York: McGraw-Hill, 1993:531.

Poole S, Fenske NA. Cutaneous markers of internal malignancy. I. Malignant involvement of the skin and the genodermatoses. J Am Acad Dermatol 1993; 28:1.

Poole S, Fenske NA. Cutaneous markers of internal malignancy. II. Paraneoplastic dermatoses and environmental carcinogens. J Am Acad Dermatol 1993; 28:147.

Short MP, Adams RD: Neurocutaneous diseases. In: Fitzpatrick TB, Eisen AZ, Wolff K, et al., eds. Dermatology in General Medicine. 4th edition. vol. II. New York: McGraw-Hill, 1993:2249.

Weston WL, Lane AT. Neonatal dermatology. In: Fitzpatrick TB, Eisen AZ, Wolff K, et al., eds. Dermatology in General Medicine. 4th edition. vol. II. New York: McGraw-Hill, 1993:2941.

Williams ML. Ichthyosis and disorders of cornification. In: Schachner LA, Hansen RC, eds. Pediatric Dermatology. vol. I. New York: Churchill Livingstone, 1988:389.

section nine

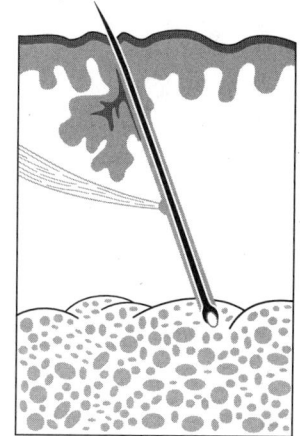

What Are the Pathologic Findings in Skin Disease?

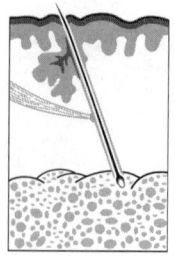

chapter 25

Dermatopathology

JULIE K. DESCH, and BRUCE R. SMOLLER

BENIGN CUTANEOUS NEOPLASMS

For the following questions, ONE or MORE of the following completions correctly finishes the incomplete sentence; choose

- A. If only 1, 2, and 3 are correct
- B. If only 1 and 3 are correct
- C. If only 2 and 4 are correct
- D. If only 4 is correct
- E. If all are correct.

1. The histologic differential diagnosis of oral white sponge nevus includes
   1. Oral lesion of pachyonychia congenita
   2. Leukoedema of the oral mucosa
   3. Oral focal epithelial hyperplasia
   4. Oral lichen planus.

2. The histologic differential diagnosis of Paget's disease includes all but
   1. Bowen's disease
   2. Erythema multiforme
   3. Malignant melanoma
   4. Verrucous carcinoma.

3. The following statements are true concerning the lesion shown in Figure 25–1; it
   1. Occurs most commonly on the face and upper extremities

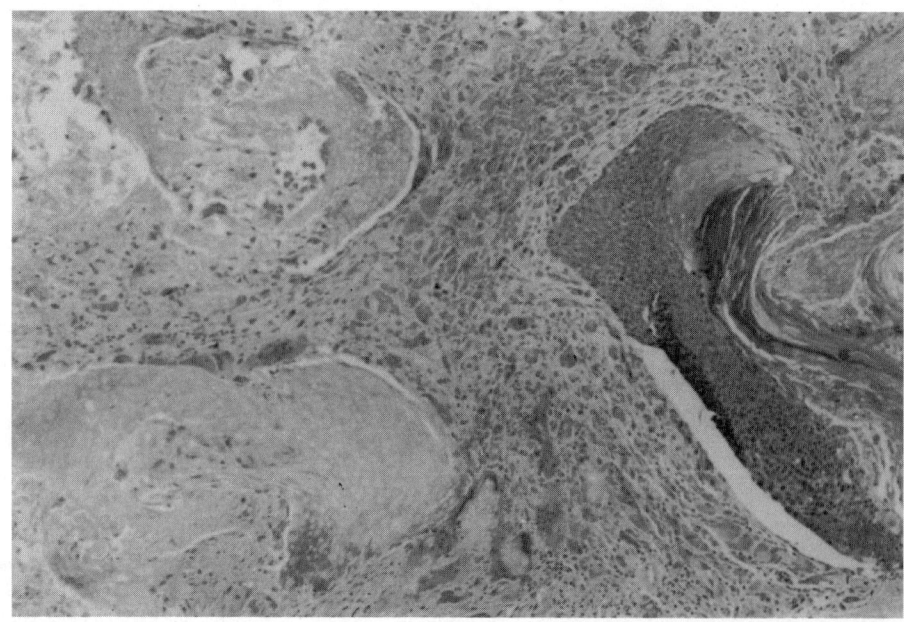

FIGURE 25–1.

2. Is not usually hereditary
3. Usually occurs in children and young adults
4. May rarely be associated with myotonic dystrophy.

4. Multiple trichilemmomas are associated with a genodermatosis having which of the following features?
   1. Autosomal recessive
   2. Autosomal dominant
   3. Colonic polyposis with high risk of adenocarcinoma
   4. High incidence of breast carcinoma in women.

5. Multiple trichoepitheliomas can be distinguished from the basal cell nevus syndrome by which of the following?
   1. Histologic findings of hair follicle differentiation, peripheral palisading of basaloid cells, and circumscription
   2. Location of tumors
   3. Dominant inheritance
   4. Absence of central nervous system disorders.

6. A subcutaneous, slowly growing asymptomatic tumor is located on the posterior neck of an elderly man. It is excised, revealing a grossly encapsulated, soft, glistening, yellowish tumor. Based on this information, the differential diagnosis should include
   1. Dermatofibrosarcoma protuberans
   2. Fibrous hamartoma
   3. Well-differentiated liposarcoma
   4. Spindle cell lipoma.

7. The cell of origin in a tumor composed of Antoni A and Antoni B areas would show which ultrastructural features?
   1. Intact basal lamina completely surrounding the plasma membrane
   2. No basal lamina, indicating endoneurial differentiation
   3. Axons entrapped in cytoplasmic invaginations
   4. Dense-core secretory granules.

8. Lobular neuromyxomas are distinguished from pacinian neurofibromas by
   1. Site of predilection
   2. Cell of origin
   3. Presence of mucin
   4. Size.

9. Histologic findings in recurrent infantile digital fibroma are
   1. Dermal fibroblasts and collagen bundles in interlacing fascicles
   2. Perinuclear eosinophilic inclusion bodies
   3. Extension of the tumor into subcutaneous fat
   4. Multinucleated giant cells.

Decide whether EACH of the following questions is TRUE or FALSE. Any combination of answers from all true to all false may occur.

10. The stellate multinucleated dermal cells characteristic of fibrous papules are
    A. S-100–negative
    B. Cytokeratin-positive
    C. Factor XIIIA–positive
    D. CEA-positive
    E. Leukocyte common antigen–positive.

11. Atypical fibroxanthomas
    A. Arise within the retroperitoneum
    B. Arise within the subcutaneous fat but may grow into the deep dermis
    C. Are characterized by Kamino bodies in the papillary dermis
    D. Are histologically malignant.

Choose the ONE BEST answer to each of the following questions.

12. Histochemical examination reveals a deficiency of what enzyme in the cells composing this lesion from the leg of a 45-year-old woman (Figure 25-2)?
    A. Homogentisic acid oxidase
    B. Uroporphyrinogen decarboxylase
    C. Phosphorylase
    D. Steroid sulfatase
    E. Lysyl oxidase.

13. Granular cell tumors
    A. Are commonly malignant
    B. Are multiple in 50% of cases
    C. Originate from immature striated muscle cells

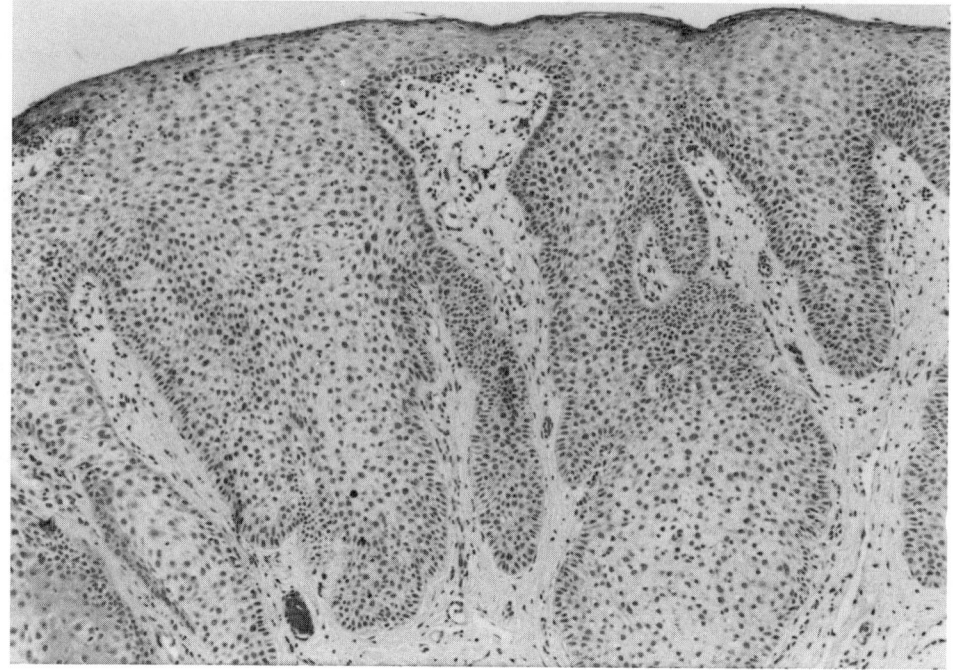

FIGURE 25–2.

    D. Often incite an overlying squamous cell carcinoma

    E. None of the above.

14. Multiple perifollicular fibromas may be associated with

    A. Tuberous sclerosis

    B. HLA-B8

    C. Colonic polyps

    D. Trichodiscomas and acrochordons

    E. Acquired ichthyosis.

15. The multinucleated giant cells in a reparative granuloma (giant cell epulis) stain immunophenotypically as

    A. Osteoblasts

    B. Osteoclasts

    C. Myofibroblasts

    D. Bone marrow–derived histiocytes

    E. Foreign body giant cells.

16. Cell-poor fibrous trabeculae, whorls of immature spindle cells in a mucoid matrix, and mature adipose tissue constitute

    A. Nodular fasciitis

    B. Fibrous hamartoma of infancy

    C. Dermatofibrosarcoma protuberans

    D. Giant cell tumor of tendon sheath

    E. Angiomyolipoma.

17. Occurring in a young adult, having a rapid onset, a size of 1 to 5 cm, common location in an upper extremity, and tenderness describe

    A. Dermatofibrosarcoma protuberans

    B. Fibrous hamartoma of infancy

    C. A tumor characterized by increased numbers of abnormally oriented collagen bundles

    D. A tumor composed of abundant multinucleated giant cells

    E. Nodular fasciitis.

MALIGNANT TUMORS OF THE SKIN

For the following questions, ONE or MORE of the following completions correctly finishes the incomplete sentence; choose

    A. If only 1, 2, and 3 are correct
    B. If only 1 and 3 are correct
    C. If only 2 and 4 are correct
    D. If only 4 is correct
    E. If all are correct.

18. Regarding leiomyosarcoma,

    1. Its location is not related to prognosis

    2. Histologic malignancy correlates with metastatic capacity

3. The malignant cells label for Factor VIII–related antigen

4. A basal lamina surrounds the malignant cells.

19. Reed-Sternberg cells in classic nodular sclerosing Hodgkin's disease stain positively with

    1. Leu 22
    2. Leukocyte common antigen (LCA)
    3. S-100
    4. Ber H2 (Ki-1; CD30).

20. Epidermotropism of malignant lymphocytes in mycosis fungoides is distinguished from exocytosis of lymphocytes in a subacute allergic contact dermatitis by

    1. The presence of eosinophils
    2. The absence of significant spongiosis
    3. Epidermal hyperplasia
    4. Cytologic atypia.

Decide whether EACH choice of the following question is TRUE or FALSE. Any combination of answers from all true to all false may occur.

21. The following is(are) true for a person with intermittent flushing, diarrhea, and abdominal pain:

    A. Metastases to the liver are common
    B. A tumor is often located in the small intestine
    C. Pellagra is occasionally an associated problem
    D. There is excessive excretion of 5-hydroxyindoleacetic acid
    E. An occult Merkel cell carcinoma is usually present.

Choose the ONE BEST answer to each of the following questions.

22. Sister Mary Joseph's nodule refers to

    A. A solitary scalp metastasis, usually from breast carcinoma
    B. Chronic callus formation of bilateral patellae
    C. Periumbilical cutaneous metastasis from intra-abdominal adenocarcinoma
    D. Rosary-associated prurigo nodularis between thumb and first finger
    E. None of the above.

23. The incidence of metastasis of a dermatofibrosarcoma protuberans is estimated to be

    A. Less than 1.0%
    B. Between 1 and 5%
    C. Ten per cent
    D. Fifteen per cent
    E. Twenty-five per cent.

24. Gingival hypertrophy and granulocytic sarcomas are characteristic of which hematologic malignancy?

    A. Chronic lymphocytic leukemia (CLL)
    B. Acute myeloblastic leukemia (AML)
    C. Non-Hodgkin's lymphoma
    D. Acute lymphoblastic leukemia (ALL)
    E. Nodular sclerosing Hodgkin's disease.

PIGMENTATION AND MELANOCYTIC LESIONS

For the following questions, ONE or MORE of the following completions correctly finishes the incomplete sentence; choose

A. If only 1, 2, and 3 are correct
B. If only 1 and 3 are correct
C. If only 2 and 4 are correct
D. If only 4 is correct
E. If all are correct.

25. The following is true concerning the lesion in Figure 25–3). It

    1. Is usually a single lesion, often on the face or lower extremity
    2. Commonly metastasizes to brain, liver, or lymph nodes
    3. Commonly contains Kamino bodies
    4. Usually measures more than 1.0 cm.

26. A Mongolian spot differs from a common blue nevus in the following way(s).

    1. Intensity of pigment alteration seen clinically
    2. Concentration of cells in the lesion
    3. Site of predilection
    4. Presence of dermal dendritic melanocytes as the cause of the pigmentation alteration.

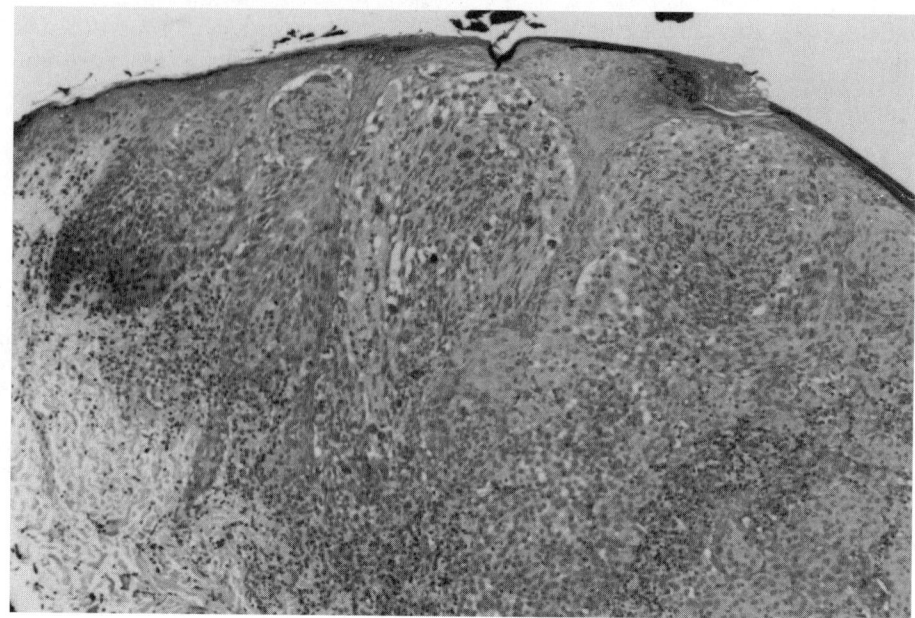

FIGURE 25–3.

Choose the ONE BEST answer to each of the following questions.

27. The histologic characteristics of melasma are found within the
    A. Dermis
    B. Epidermis
    C. Both
    D. Neither.

28. The increase in pigmentation in Addison's disease can be traced to
    A. Increased endogenous ACTH
    B. Decreased pituitary secretion of melanocyte-stimulating hormone (MSH)
    C. Increased pituitary secretion of MSH
    D. Exogenous administration of corticosteroids.
    E. Endogenous extra-adrenal corticosteroid production.

29. Melanosomes of these stage(s) are found within melanocytes in tyrosinase-negative albinism:
    A. Types 1 and 2
    B. Types 3 and 4
    C. No melanosomes are produced
    D. Types 1 to 4
    E. No melanocytes are present in albinism.

NONINFECTIOUS, ERYTHEMATOUS, PAPULOSQUAMOUS DISEASES

For the following question, ONE or MORE of the following completions correctly finishes the incomplete sentence; choose

A. If only 1, 2, and 3 are correct
B. If only 1 and 3 are correct
C. If only 2 and 4 are correct
D. If only 4 is correct
E. If all are correct.

30. The histologic features of pityriasis rosea are distinguished from those of a subacute or chronic dermatitis by the presence of
    1. Parakeratosis
    2. Necrotic keratinocytes
    3. Focal spongiosis
    4. Extravasated erythrocytes.

Choose the ONE BEST answer to each of the following questions.

31. Pustulosis palmaris et plantaris can be distinguished from acrodermatitis continua of Hallopeau by the fact that in the former
    A. Acral portions of fingers and toes are involved
    B. Acral portions of fingers and toes are spared
    C. There is a family history of psoriasis
    D. There is an association with HLA-B28

32. Ulcerative lichen planus may consist of
    A. Atrophic scarring on feet and toes
    B. Loss of toenails
    C. Atrophic alopecia
    D. Cutaneous and oral lesions
    E. All of the above.

33. In early lichen planus, the number of Langerhans cells in the epidermis is
    A. Increased
    B. Decreased
    C. Unchanged.

34. Colloid bodies in lichen planus stain mainly with
    A. IgG
    B. IgM
    C. IgA
    D. Complement 3 (C3)
    E. Fibrin.

35. The immunoperoxidase study(ies) most helpful in distinguishing pityriasis lichenoides varioliformis acuta (PLEVA) from lymphomatoid papulosis are
    A. Leukocyte common antigen (LCA)
    B. L26
    C. Leu 22
    D. Leu 2 (T cytotoxic/suppressor) and Leu 3 (T helper/inducer)
    E. None of the above.

36. A "claw clutching a ball" describes the histologic findings in
    A. Lichen planopilaris
    B. Lichen nitidus
    C. Lichen striatus
    D. Lichen aureus
    E. Lichen planus.

NONINFECTIOUS BULLOUS DISEASES OF THE SKIN

For the following questions, ONE or MORE of the following completions correctly finishes the incomplete sentence; choose

   A. If only 1, 2, and 3 are correct
   B. If only 1 and 3 are correct
   C. If only 2 and 4 are correct
   D. If only 4 is correct
   E. If all are correct.

37. An increased CD4:CD8 ratio is seen in the following:
    1. Atopic dermatitis
    2. Mycosis fungoides
    3. Alopecia areata
    4. PLEVA
    5. Actinic reticuloid.

38. Intraepidermal microabscesses composed of eosinophils are characteristic of
    1. Pemphigus vegetans
    2. Bullous pemphigoid
    3. Pyoderma vegetans
    4. Sweet's syndrome.

Decide whether EACH choice of the following question is TRUE or FALSE. Any combination of answers from all true to all false may occur.

39. Acantholysis in the upper epidermis is characteristic of the following disease(s):
    A. Pemphigus foliaceus
    B. Pemphigus erythematosis
    C. Fogo selvagem
    D. Pemphigus vulgaris
    E. Pemphigus vegetans.

Choose the ONE BEST answer to each of the following questions.

40. Blister formation due to primary acantholysis is seen in all but
    A. Pemphigus vulgaris
    B. Darier's disease
    C. Familial benign pemphigus
    D. Herpes simplex
    E. Transient acantholytic dermatosis (Grover's disease).

41. A spongiotic intraepidermal infiltrate rich in eosinophils can be seen in all but
    A. Erythema toxicum neonatorum
    B. Incontinentia pigmentosa
    C. Psoriasis
    D. Herpes gestationis
    E. Pemphigus vegetans.

42. A vesicular lesion of dermatitis herpetiformis most frequently shows
    A. Granular IgA at the dermoepidermal junction (DEJ)
    B. Linear IgA at the DEJ
    C. Granular IgG at the DEJ
    D. Linear IgG at the DEJ
    E. Negative immunofluorescence.

43. The bullous pemphigoid antigen is located
    A. Within the intraepidermal ground substance
    B. In the lamina lucida, associated with the hemidesmosomes
    C. In the sublamina densa
    D. Within the anchoring fibrils.

DISEASES OF THE CUTANEOUS VESSELS

For the following questions, ONE or MORE of the following completions correctly finishes the incomplete sentence; choose

A. If only 1, 2, and 3 are correct
B. If only 1 and 3 are correct
C. If only 2 and 4 are correct
D. If only 4 is correct
E. If all are correct.

44. A defect in proline hydroxylation is clinically characterized by
    1. Follicular hyperkeratosis
    2. "Corkscrew hairs"
    3. Perifollicular petechiae
    4. Periorificial erythema.

45. The direct immunofluorescence findings in autoerythrocyte sensitization syndrome include
    1. Perivascular IgM
    2. Granular IgM at the dermoepidermal junction
    3. Perivascular C3
    4. C3 at dermoepidermal junction
    5. Negative immunofluorescence.

46. Purpura fulminans is distinguished from coumadin necrosis by
    1. Involvement of extracutaneous sites
    2. Presence of disseminated intravascular coagulation
    3. Response to heparin therapy
    4. Histologic findings on skin biopsy.

47. In a biopsy taken to distinguish purpura pigmentosa chronica (pigmented purpuric eruption) from stasis dermatitis it is best to examine
    1. The presence of siderophages in dermis
    2. The depth of dermal extension of vascular changes
    3. The presence of fibrinoid material within vessel walls
    4. The presence of epidermal changes and dermal fibrosis.

48. Granuloma faciale is distinguished from erythema elevatum diutinum by
    1. Presence of a Grenz zone and eosinophils
    2. Immunofluorescence findings
    3. The site of lesions
    4. Histologic evidence of vasculitis
    5. Foreign body giant cells.

Decide whether EACH choice of the following questions is TRUE or FALSE. Any combination of answers from all true to all false may occur.

49. Which of the following is(are) helpful in distinguishing between lymphomatoid granulomatosis (angiocentric T-cell lymphoma) and midline granuloma of the face?
    A. Cutaneous histologic features
    B. The presence of atypical lymphocytes in the dermis
    C. Immunoperoxidase studies performed on skin biopsy material
    D. The clinical presentation.

50. Solitary glomus tumors are distinguished histologically from multiple glomangiomas by
    A. Circumscription by a fibrous capsule
    B. Larger vascular spaces
    C. More perilesional nerve fibers
    D. Less numerous glomus cells.

51. The cell of origin in Kaposi's sarcoma reacts positively with
    A. *Ulex europaeus*
    B. S-100
    C. Factor VIII–related antigen
    D. Desmin.

DERMATOPATHOLOGY 307

Choose the ONE BEST answer to each of the following questions.

52. The best histologic criterion to use in differentiating between acute febrile neutrophilic dermatosis and erythema elevatum diutinum is
    A. The presence of eosinophils
    B. The presence of vasculitis
    C. Leukocytoclasis
    D. Ulceration
    E. All of the above.

53. A cutaneous biopsy diagnostic of systemic polyarteritis nodosa demonstrates
    A. Leukocytoclastic vasculitis
    B. Occlusion of small vessels by fibrin thrombi
    C. Involvement of subcutaneous vessels
    D. None of the above
    E. All of the above.

54. Hemangiopericytoma is a tumor of cells that originate
    A. From endothelium
    B. Between endothelium and adventitia
    C. From the wall of the arterial Suquet-Hoyer canal
    D. From perivascular fibroblasts
    E. From metaplastic glomus cells.

55. Weibel-Palade bodies in pyogenic granulomas (lobular capillary hemangiomas) are
    A. Increased
    B. Decreased
    C. Unchanged
    D. Malformed.

INFECTIOUS DISEASES OF THE SKIN

For the following questions, ONE or MORE of the following completions correctly finishes the incomplete sentence; choose

A. If only 1, 2, and 3 are correct
B. If only 1 and 3 are correct
C. If only 2 and 4 are correct
D. If only 4 is correct
E. If all are correct.

56. Masses of organisms resembling "sulfur granules" most commonly are seen involving the
    1. Periorificial area
    2. Anogenital area
    3. Scalp
    4. Cervicofacial area.

57. The histologic differential diagnosis of sporotrichosis includes
    1. Tularemia
    2. *Mycobacterium marinum*
    3. Cat-scratch disease
    4. Actinomycosis
    5. Botryomycosis.

58. Cerebral chromomycosis can be distinguished from cutaneous or subcutaneous chromomycosis because
    1. It is caused by a different agent
    2. Both mycelia and spores are found
    3. Cerebral lesions are often seen in the absence of skin lesions
    4. Necrosis is absent in biopsies of cerebral lesions.

59. Endothelial cell swelling and hyperplasia, together with a perivascular inflammatory infiltrate in the superficial dermis of lymphocytes and numerous plasma cells, prompt a differential diagnosis including
    1. Pityriasis lichenoides et varioliformis acuta (PLEVA)
    2. Primary syphilis
    3. Tertiary syphilis
    4. Secondary syphilis.

Decide whether EACH choice of the following questions is TRUE or FALSE. Any combination of answers from all true to all false may occur.

60. Multinucleated giant cells and intranuclear (Cowdry type A) inclusions are characteristic of infection with the following virus(es):
    A. Herpes simplex virus
    B. Herpes varicella virus
    C. Cytomegalovirus
    D. Vaccinia virus
    E. Poxvirus.

61. Inclusion bodies are found in the following group(s) of viruses:
    A. Herpesvirus

B. Poxvirus

C. Papillomavirus

D. Picornavirus.

Choose the ONE BEST answer to each of the following.

62. Michaelis-Gutman bodies are diagnostic of _____ and are best seen with a _____ stain.

    A. Granuloma inguinale; Giemsa

    B. Sarcoidosis; periodic acid–Schiff (PAS)

    C. Malacoplakia; von Kossa

    D. Rhinoscleroma; PAS

    E. Sarcoidosis; hematoxylin and eosin.

63. A systemic infection with *Cryptococcus neoformans* is suspected by clinical history, but only scattered papules and occasional pustules are present. An urgent skin biopsy is performed before initiating antifungal treatment. Which is the best special stain to be requested along with the initial hematoxylin and eosin?

    A. Periodic acid–Schiff (PAS)

    B. Gram

    C. Mucicarmine

    D. Trichrome

    E. Reticulin.

64. Biopsy of a destructive intranasal lesion reveals numerous large histiocytes containing multiple organisms 2 to 4 microns in diameter that do not appear to be encapsulated. The inflammatory infiltrate is otherwise nonspecific. A Giemsa stain shows a central nucleus and a paranuclear kinetoplast within each organism. Which organism is responsible?

    A. *Klebsiella rhinoscleromatis*

    B. *Leishmania tropica*

    C. *Leishmania braziliensis*

    D. *Histoplasma capsulatum*

    E. *Leishmania mexicana*.

65. The kinetoplast of *Leishmania* species is located

    A. Within the nucleus

    B. Within an intracellular lysosome

    C. Just outside the parasite, within an invagination of the plasma membrane

    D. Within large mitochondria

    E. Within the Golgi apparatus.

66. Bone lesions, palmar and plantar hyperkeratosis, and rhinopharyngitis mutilans are suggestive of

    A. Tertiary syphilis

    B. Tertiary yaws

    C. Tertiary pinta

    D. Secondary syphilis

    E. Rhinoscleroma.

67. Acrodermatitis chronica atrophicans is a manifestation of infection with which organism?

    A. *Treponema carateum*

    B. *Borrelia burgdorferi*

    C. *Rickettsia rickettsii*

    D. *Klebsiella rhinoscleromatis*

    E. *Leishmania tropica*.

68. Replication of the varicella-zoster virus takes place almost exclusively in

    A. Keratinocytes of affected epidermis

    B. The dorsal root ganglion

    C. Dermal capillary endothelium

    D. Axons of dermal nerves.

CONNECTIVE TISSUE DISEASES

For the following question, ONE or MORE of the following completions correctly finishes the incomplete sentence; choose

A. If only 1, 2, and 3 are correct
B. If only 1 and 3 are correct
C. If only 2 and 4 are correct
D. If only 4 is correct
E. If all are correct.

69. The direct immunofluorescence findings in the syndrome characterized by Raynaud's phenomenon, polyarthralgia, sclerodactyly, and swelling of hands that results in a "sausage" appearance of fingers, esophageal hypomotility, proximal myopathy, and pulmonary disease include

    1. Linear IgA at the dermoepidermal junction

    2. A positive "lupus band" test in most cases

    3. Negative staining for all immunoglobulins and complement

    4. Speckled pattern of IgG within epidermal keratinocyte nuclei.

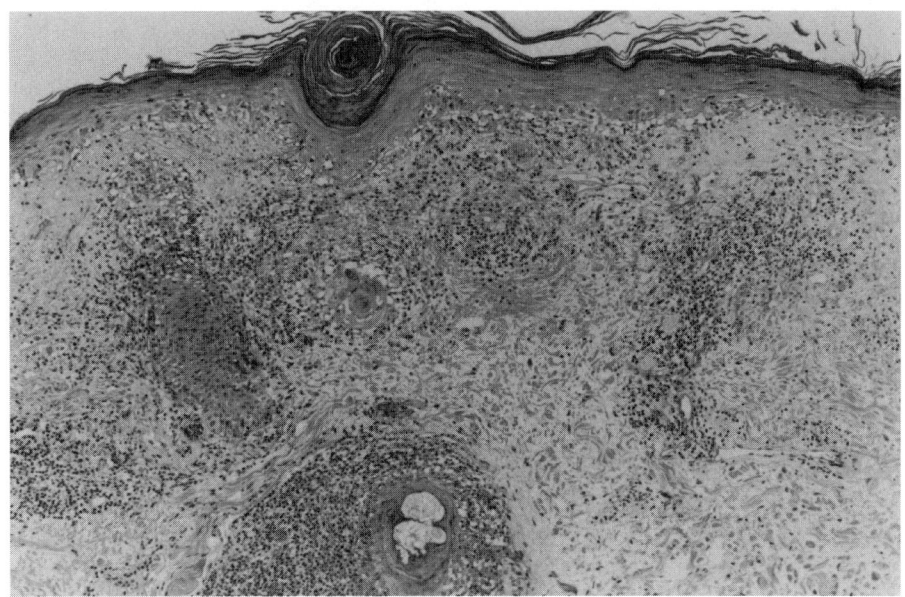

FIGURE 25-4.

Choose the ONE BEST answer to each of the following questions.

70. The histologic features of this biopsy suggest which diagnosis (Figure 25-4)?

    A. Lichen planus
    B. Late sclerotic morphea
    C. Lupus erythematosus
    D. Polymorphous light eruption
    E. Lymphocytic lymphoma.

71. Prominent cutaneous manifestations occur as a feature in what per cent of patients with systemic lupus erythematosus?

    A. Five
    B. Twenty
    C. Forty
    D. Sixty
    E. Eighty.

INFLAMMATORY DISEASES OF FAT, APPENDAGES, AND CARTILAGE

For the following questions, ONE or MORE of the following completions correctly finishes the incomplete sentence; choose

A. If only 1, 2, and 3 are correct
B. If only 1 and 3 are correct
C. If only 2 and 4 are correct
D. If only 4 is correct
E. If all are correct.

72. Alopecia areata is characterized by which of the following?

    1. Increased lesional CD8:CD4 lymphocyte ratio
    2. Early loss of sebaceous glands
    3. An excess of androgenic hormones
    4. Presence of intrabulbar Langerhans cells.

73. Relapsing polychondritis and chondrodermatitis nodularis helicis share

    1. Common involvement of nasal cartilage
    2. Vasculitis
    3. Circulating antibodies to type II cartilage
    4. Degeneration of cartilage

Decide whether EACH choice of the following questions is TRUE or FALSE. Any combination of answers from all true to all false may occur.

74. A cutaneous biopsy reveals a subcutaneous lobular panniculitis, showing areas of caseous necrosis surrounded by palisading lymphocytes, histiocytes, and giant cells. An extensive vasculitis is present, involving small and medium-sized vessels. The differential diagnosis includes

    A. The chronic form of erythema nodosum
    B. Infection
    C. Superficial migratory thrombophlebitis
    D. Erythema induratum.

Choose the ONE BEST answer to each of the following questions.

75. Given a biopsy of a cutaneous lesion, which additional test would be most helpful in distinguishing between erythema nodosum and benign cutaneous periarteritis nodosa?

    A. Renal biopsy

    B. Elastic tissue stain

    C. Immunoperoxidase stain for *Ulex europaeus*

    D. Fluorescent antinuclear antibody (FANA)

    E. Elevated anti-streptolysin-O titer.

76. The histologic feature on which the diagnosis of Weber-Christian disease depends is the presence of

    A. Neutrophils

    B. Foam cells

    C. Vasculitis

    D. Necrobiotic "ghost-like" adipocytes

    E. Caseating granulomas.

HISTIOCYTIC PROCESSES

For the following questions, ONE or MORE of the following completions correctly finishes the incomplete sentence; choose

A. If only 1, 2, and 3 are correct
B. If only 1 and 3 are correct
C. If only 2 and 4 are correct
D. If only 4 is correct
E. If all are correct.

77. The syndrome including erythema nodosum, hilar adenopathy, fever, migratory polyarthritis, and acute iritis

    1. Shows well-formed, "naked" collections of epithelioid histiocytes located in the mid–reticular dermis

    2. Is associated with lung involvement in 50% of cases and with ocular involvement in 25% of cases

    3. Is associated with the electron microscopic findings of complex laminated bodies and "asteroid bodies"

    4. Is a subacute, transient syndrome that subsides within months without cutaneous lesions other than erythema nodosum.

78. Which of the following is helpful in distinguishing sarcoidosis from lupus vulgaris?

    1. Caseous central necrosis

    2. Culture studies

    3. Atrophy without areas of ulceration, acanthosis, and pseudocarcinomatous hyperplasia

    4. Positive lupus band on direct immunofluorescence.

79. Cheilitis granulomatosa may histologically be confused with

    1. Cheilitis glandularis

    2. Tuberculosis

    3. Sarcoidosis

    4. Erythema induratum.

80. Multiple small, soft, yellow papules, occurring on the buttocks and posterior thighs, that come and go with fluctuation of plasma triglyceride concentration are associated with which subtype(s) of hyperlipoproteinemia?

    1. I

    2. IIb

    3. III

    4. IV.

Decide whether EACH choice of the following question is TRUE or FALSE. Any combination of answers from all true to all false may occur.

81. Ultrastructural findings of electron-dense deposits in endothelial cells, pericytes, and fibroblasts with a lamellar structure having a periodicity of 5 nm is diagnostic of a disease that

    A. Is inherited as an X-linked recessive trait

    B. Is due to a deficiency of ceramidase

    C. Shows vascular cutaneous lesions

    D. Is inherited as an autosomal dominant trait.

Choose the ONE BEST answer to the following question.

82. The histologic features of this biopsy from the dorsal hand of a 65-year-old woman (Fig. 25–5) are diagnostic of what disorder? Which stain would be most helpful in confirming the diagnosis?

    A. Rheumatoid nodule; fibrin stain

    B. Necrobiosis lipoidica; trichrome stain

    C. Granuloma annulare; mucin stain

    D. Rheumatoid nodule; no stain helpful

    E. Tuberculosis; acid-fast stain.

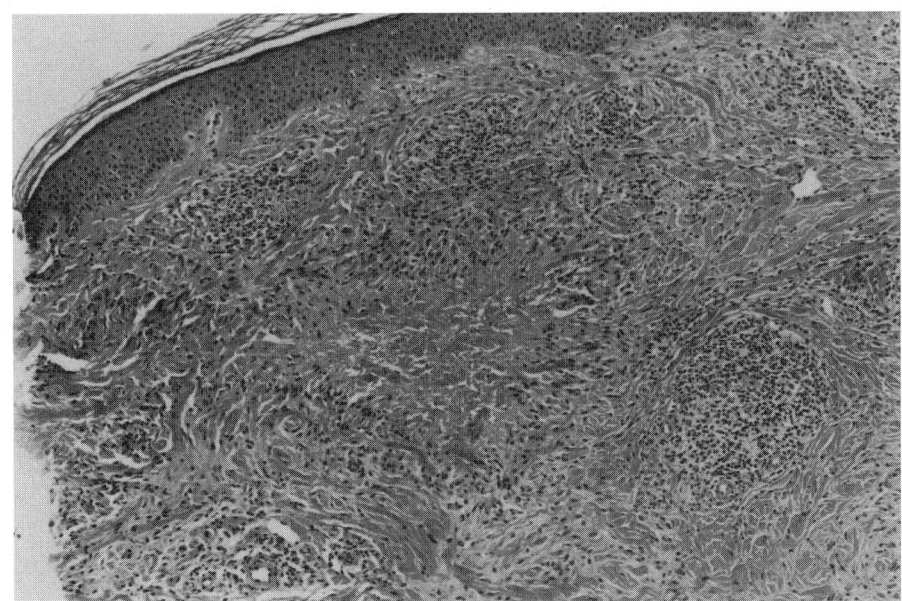

FIGURE 25-5.

DRUG ERUPTIONS AND METABOLIC DISORDERS

For the following questions, ONE or MORE of the following completions correctly finishes the incomplete sentence; choose

- A. If only 1, 2, and 3 are correct
- B. If only 1 and 3 are correct
- C. If only 2 and 4 are correct
- D. If only 4 is correct
- E. If all are correct.

83. Histologic differences between a photoallergic and a phototoxic eruption include

   1. Eosinophils are more common in a phototoxic eruption
   2. Necrotic keratinocytes are more common in a photoallergic eruption
   3. A lymphocytic vasculitis is seen in photoallergic eruptions
   4. Epidermal spongiosis and microvesiculation is seen in photoallergic eruptions.

84. The electron-dense bodies seen in chlorpromazine pigmentation

   1. React histochemically like melanin
   2. Are iron-containing drug-metabolite-protein complexes
   3. Are complexes of melanin and chlorpromazine
   4. Are located only within dermal macrophages.

85. Penicillamine administration may induce which of the following?

   1. Characteristic changes of elastic fibers, including "lateral budding"
   2. Hyperplasia of elastic fibers
   3. Diminution or absence of elastic tissue
   4. Production of subepidermal deposition of IgG on direct immunofluorescence.

Decide whether EACH choice of the following questions is TRUE or FALSE. Any combination of answers from all true to all false may occur.

86. The histologic features seen in Figure 25-6 should elicit a differential diagnosis that includes which of the following?

   A. Pemphigus vegetans
   B. Bromoderma
   C. Deep fungal infection
   D. Invasive squamous cell carcinoma.

87. Distinguishing the juvenile form of colloid milium from adult colloid milium or nodular colloid degeneration can be made by

   A. Ultrastructural studies
   B. Hematoxylin and eosin
   C. Clinical history

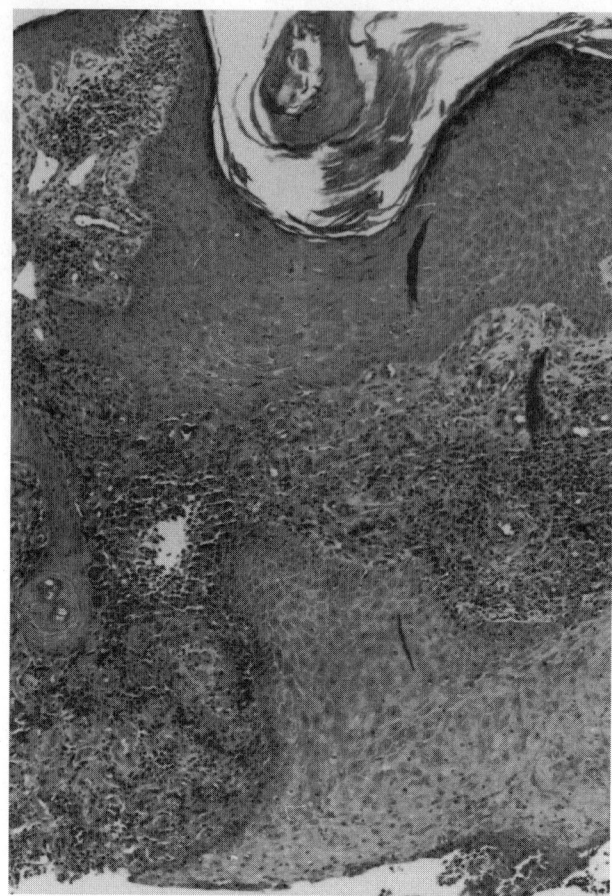

FIGURE 25–6.

D. Periodic acid–Schiff with and without prior digestion with diastase

E. Electrophoresis studies.

88. The electron microscopic findings in lipoid proteinosis include

   A. Basal lamina multiplication
   B. Dermal accumulation of amorphous hyaline material
   C. Decrease in number of collagen fibrils
   D. Decrease in size of collagen fibrils.

DEGENERATIVE DISEASES AND THOSE RELATED TO SUNLIGHT AND HEAT

For the following questions, ONE or MORE of the following completions correctly finishes the incomplete sentence; choose

   A. If only 1, 2, and 3 are correct
   B. If only 1 and 3 are correct
   C. If only 2 and 4 are correct
   D. If only 4 is correct
   E. If all are correct.

89. Polymorphous light eruption can be differentiated from discoid lupus erythematosus by
   1. Direct immunofluorescence
   2. Clinical presentation
   3. Lack of basal vacuolar change
   4. Presence of solar elastosis.

90. The histologic differential diagnosis of a persistent arthropod response includes all of the following EXCEPT
   1. Mycosis fungoides
   2. Hodgkin's disease
   3. Lymphomatoid papulosis
   4. Polymorphous light eruption.

91. Which of the following diseases show(s) a central keratotic plug and a perforation through which degenerated elastic fibers are extruded?
   1. Reactive perforating collagenosis
   2. Elastosis perforans serpiginosa
   3. Kyrle's disease
   4. Perforating folliculitis.

92. In bullosis diabeticorum, electron microscopy reveals the split to occur at what level?
   1. Within the basal keratinocytes
   2. Below the lamina densa
   3. Within the lamina densa
   4. Within the lamina lucida.

Decide whether EACH choice of the following question is TRUE or FALSE. Any combination of answers from all true to all false may occur.

93. Which histologic features are helpful in distinguishing lichen sclerosus et atrophicus from morphea?

   A. Presence of hydropic degeneration of basal keratinocytes
   B. Presence of elastic fibers in the upper dermis
   C. Superficial dermal zone of edema with homogenization of collagen
   D. Thickening and hyperchromasia of collagen bundles in the mid and lower dermis with a minimal inflammatory infiltrate.

Choose the ONE BEST answer to each of the following questions.

94. Actinic reticuloid
    A. Is a CD8-mediated process
    B. Is a CD4-mediated process
    C. Often eventuates in mycosis fungoides
    D. Results from a hypersensitivity to ultraviolet A radiation only
    E. None of the above.

95. Erythema ab igne is characterized by
    A. Homogenization of elastic tissue with loss of fibrous structure
    B. Predominantly affected sun-exposed areas
    C. Decreased elastic tissue
    D. A lack of epidermal changes
    E. None of the above.

GENODERMATOSES

For the following questions, ONE or MORE of the following completions correctly finishes the incomplete sentence; choose

A. If only 1, 2, and 3 are correct
B. If only 1 and 3 are correct
C. If only 2 and 4 are correct
D. If only 4 is correct
E. If all are correct.

96. Trichorrhexis invaginata is seen with which ichthyosis in Netherton's syndrome?
    1. Ichthyosis linearis circumflexa
    2. Epidermolytic hyperkeratosis
    3. Lamellar ichthyosis
    4. Erythrokeratoderma variabilis
    5. X-linked ichthyosis.

97. The histologic differential diagnosis of keratosis palmaris et plantaris could include all EXCEPT
    1. Psoriasis vulgaris
    2. Lichen simplex chronicus
    3. Lichen planus
    4. Epidermolytic hyperkeratosis
    5. Verruca vulgaris.

Decide whether EACH choice of the following question is TRUE or FALSE. Any combination of answers from all true to all false may occur.

98. The histologic differential diagnosis of acrokeratosis verruciformis of Hopf includes
    A. Seborrheic keratosis
    B. Linear epidermal nevus
    C. Acanthosis nigricans
    D. Verruca vulgaris
    E. Clear-cell acanthoma.

Choose the ONE BEST answer to each of the following questions.

99. The following ichthyosis is due to which known enzymatic deficiency?
    A. Ichthyosis vulgaris
    B. X-linked ichthyosis
    C. Bullous congenital ichthyosiform erythroderma
    D. Lamellar ichthyosis
    E. Ichthyosis linearis circumflexa.

100. Immunosuppression has been associated most commonly with which porokeratosis subtype?
    A. Punctate porokeratosis
    B. Disseminated superficial actinic porokeratosis
    C. Mibelli's porokeratosis
    D. Linear porokeratosis
    E. Porokeratosis palmaris et plantaris disseminata.

101. A deficiency of type 3 collagen results in the syndrome(s) of
    A. Ehlers-Danlos type 7
    B. Ehlers-Danlos type 3
    C. Ehlers-Danlos type 9
    D. Ehlers-Danlos type 1
    E. Ehlers-Danlos type 4.

ANSWERS

BENIGN CUTANEOUS NEOPLASMS

1. A The histologic features are epithelial hyperplasia with marked hydropic swelling of the epithelial cells. Swelling is seen in cells extending down rete ridges, but

it spares the basilar layer. Parakeratosis is seen at the surface. These findings are identical to those seen in leukoedema and oral focal epithelial hyperplasia. Lichen planus of the oral mucosa shows parakeratosis, but there is usually thinning of the epithelial surface, damage to the basal layer, and a band-like infiltrate along the mucosal-submucosal junction (Chapter 20).

2. C The epidermis in Paget's disease contains scattered atypical "pagetoid cells"—large, rounded cells without intercellular bridges that contain a large nucleus and abundant cytoplasm. These cells may occur singly or in clusters. Flattened basal cells are often seen between the tumor cells and the dermis. Single atypical cells extending upward throughout the epidermis are also a feature of malignant melanoma, termed "pagetoid extension" of malignant melanocytes. In this case, nests of these atypical cells are also often seen at the dermoepidermal junction. Bowen's disease, or squamous cell carcinoma in situ, may also have atypical cells, both singly and in clusters, extending through the epidermis and surrounded by normal-appearing keratinocytes. In this case, the presence of intercellular bridges is helpful in making the diagnosis. Erythema multiforme demonstrates scattered dyskeratotic keratinocytes, but they represent dying cells, not a clonal proliferation (Chapters 22, 141, and 151).

3. E The lesion shown in Figure 25–1 is a pilomatricoma, a tumor of cells differentiating toward hair cells. The diagnostic features include basophilic and shadow cells with abundant calcium deposits and foreign body giant cells also prominent. These are tumors that usually occur on the face and upper extremities in children and young adults (60% in the first two decades of life). Usually, they are not hereditary, although rare cases of familial occurrence have been reported. Some of these cases have been associated with myotonic dystrophy (Chapter 144).

4. C Multiple trichilemmomas are seen in Cowden's disease, or the multiple hamartoma syndrome. This disease is transmitted in an autosomal dominant fashion and is important to recognize because of the high incidence of breast cancer in women with this syndrome. Other tumors seen in this syndrome are fibrous hamartomas, usually of the breasts, thyroid, and gastrointestinal tract (Chapter 144).

5. C Both the basal cell nevus syndrome and multiple trichoepitheliomas are transmitted as an autosomal dominant trait. The histologic features of trichoepitheliomas and keratotic basal cell carcinomas are similar, and the two syndromes possibly cannot be distinguished on biopsy alone. Multiple trichoepitheliomas tend to occur mainly on the face, particularly in the nasolabial fold; they are small and do not ulcerate. The lesions of the basal cell nevus syndrome are widely distributed over the face and body. They may become extremely large, and they occasionally ulcerate. The disease sometimes enters a "neoplastic" stage late in life, when the lesions, especially those on the face, become destructive and mutilating and may even metastasize. Patients with the basal cell nevus syndrome have other abnormalities, including palmar and plantar pits and skeletal and central nervous system anomalies (Chapters 141 and 144).

6. D The clinical history in this case is the classic one for a spindle cell lipoma, although a usual lipoma would also be in the clinical differential. Dermatofibrosarcoma protuberans, although slow-growing, is grossly encapsulated and looks grossly fibrous, not fatty. The diagnosis of a well-differentiated liposarcoma in a superficial location would be most unusual. These are usually deep tumors, often in the retroperitoneum, and although they may kill by local invasion, they rarely metastasize before dedifferentiating into an obviously cytologically malignant tumor. In the skin, even cytologically malignant fatty tumors do not often behave aggressively, and the diagnosis of liposarcoma should be avoided if at all possible. Certainly, an encapsulated tumor of well-differentiated lipocytes located in the skin is not malignant. Fibrous hamartomas are tumors of infancy (Chapters 147 and 149).

7. B Antoni A and Antoni B areas are the two types of tissue comprising a schwannoma, or neurilemoma. These are tumors of Schwann's cells and as such have a basal lamina peripheral to the plasma membrane. This is present around all of the tumor cells other than in Antoni B areas in which degenerated cells may show detachment of some portions of their basal lamina. Schwann's cells may also contain axons surrounded by a basal lamina within invaginations of their cytoplasm. Dense-core secretory granules are not seen in normal Schwann's cells or in the tumor cells of a schwannoma (Chapter 148).

8. B Both lobular neuromyxomas (neurothekeomas) and pacinian neurofibromas are thought to have the same cell of origin, the perineurial cell. They are also similar in usual size, occurring as solitary nodules that measure less than 1 cm. Lobular neuromyxomas occur most commonly on the face and upper extremities, whereas pacinian neurofibromas occur most commonly on the hands and feet. Histologically, both are well circumscribed and lobulated, and the cells of each are similar, having a spindle-shaped nucleus and long cytoplasmic extension. Characteristically, lobular neuromyxomas contain abundant mucin, whereas pacinian neurofibromas contain lamellar formations and little or no mucin (Chapter 148).

9. A Infantile digital fibromas manifest at birth or appear during the first year of life with single or multiple subcutaneous nodules on the fingers or toes. They involute spontaneously but may recur. Histologically, the tumors show fibroblasts and collagen arranged in interlacing bundles, often extending into the subcutaneous fat. The presence of intracytoplasmic (usually paranuclear) eosinophilic inclusion bodies clinches the diagnosis. By electron microscopy, these are electron-dense filaments with no limiting membrane that form by accretion of myofilaments (Chapter 149).

10. A (T); B (F); C (T); D (F); E (F) Fibrous papules were originally thought to be involuting nevi, but immunoperoxidase staining fails to reveal staining with S-100.

Instead, these cells stain with Factor XIIIA, a marker for dermal dendrocytes. Cytokeratins and carcinoembryonic antigen are markers of epithelial differentiation and do not stain dermal dendrocytes. Leukocyte common antigen is a lymphoid marker and does not stain in dermal dendrocytes (Chapter 149).

11. A (F); B (F); C (F); D (T) Atypical fibroxanthomas arise within the dermis and are centered there. They may extend into the subcutaneous fat. They are neoplasms of histiocytes and cytologically are quite malignant. The same lesion arising within the subcutis or deeper tissues is termed a malignant fibrous histiocytoma. These tumors do have metastatic potential, albeit quite low, mainly because of their small size and superficial location. Kamino bodies are seen in the papillary dermis of spindle and epithelioid cell (Spitz) nevi and are not described in atypical fibroxanthomas (Chapter 149).

12. C The clear cells in clear-cell acanthoma are deficient in phosphorylase. This results in the inability to digest glycogen, and the accumulation of glycogen gives the cells their clear appearance. The histologic features of this lesion include elongation of rete ridges with striking clear-cell change of the keratinocytes, slight spongiosis, and the presence of numerous neutrophils, many of which show fragmentation of their nuclei (Chapter 142).

13. E Granular cell tumors are thought to originate from Schwann's cells and not myoblasts, as was originally proposed. These tumors are only multiple in 10% of cases and only rarely are they malignant. They occur most commonly on the tongue but can also be seen in numerous other sites. They often incite a proliferation of the overlying squamous epithelium, and this "pseudocarcinomatous hyperplasia" has been mistaken for carcinoma. There is no known increased incidence of true squamous cell carcinoma (Chapter 148).

14. C There exists a rare and sometimes familial syndrome with generalized perifollicular, flesh-colored papules and colonic polyps. More commonly, perifollicular papules often with a central comedo are seen limited to the face and neck or possibly extending to the upper trunk. Histologically, normal or dilated follicles are surrounded by concentrically arranged loose collagen. Trichodiscomas and acrochordons are associated with trichofolliculomas (not perifolliculomas) in the Birt-Hogg-Dube syndrome (Chapters 142 and 144).

15. B Reparative granuloma occurs mainly in children and young adults as a solitary tumor of the gingiva near deciduous teeth. Histologically, it is a well-circumscribed, benign-appearing lesion in which bland-appearing fibroblasts are admixed with numerous large, multinucleated giant cells. These giant cells stain with osteoclast-specific monoclonal antibodies (Chapter 178).

16. B This tumor has an organoid appearance and consists of three separate distinct components, namely, fibrous trabeculae that separate whorls of loose mesenchymal tissue containing immature spindle cells and varying amounts of mature adipose tissue. They classically occur in infants, when one or two subcutaneous nodules are present at birth or develop shortly thereafter. The importance of recognizing this tumor is that it is not an aggressive fibromatosis and is usually cured by simple excision (Chapter 149).

17. E This is the classic presentation, and features suggesting its benign nature are the small size and rapid onset. Histologically, nodular fasciitis may appear extremely cellular and is classically quite proliferative, with numerous mitotic figures. The nuclei are bland, however, and atypical mitoses are absent. The growth pattern may be quite infiltrative, and confusion with fibrosarcoma may occur. Dermatofibrosarcoma protuberans is usually slow-growing and occurs most commonly on the trunk. It is extremely cellular with a distinct storiform pattern, and atypical mitoses are common. Giant cell epulis, which contains many multinucleated giant cells, is an oral lesion and a hypertrophic scar that has increased numbers of abnormally oriented collagen bundles and a history of prior trauma. Fibrous hamartoma of infancy is congenital or arises in the first year of life (Chapter 149).

MALIGNANT TUMORS OF THE SKIN

18. D Leiomyosarcomas located in the skin almost never metastasize, whereas those located in the subcutis do so in one third of cases. If present in the deep soft tissues, they are nearly always fatal. Histologic features of malignancy do not seem to correlate with clinical behavior. The tumor cells are not endothelial but are of smooth muscle origin. Therefore, they do not stain with Factor VIII–related antigen. Smooth muscle cells do have a complete basal lamina seen ultrastructurally, and this usually holds true in leiomyosarcoma, although the basal lamina may be incomplete (Chapter 147).

19. D The large atypical Reed-Sternberg cells in nodular sclerosing Hodgkin's disease typically are positive for the Ki-1 antigen and not for leukocyte common antigen. Leu 22, a T-cell marker, does not stain Reed-Sternberg cells. One exception to this rule is in lymphocyte-predominant Hodgkin's disease, in which the large, atypical Reed-Sternberg–like "popcorn cells" often stain for leukocyte common antigen and occasionally L26 (a B-cell marker) but not for Ber H2 (Chapter 159).

20. C Epidermal hyperplasia can be seen in both mycosis fungoides (MF) and in a spongiotic dermatitis of significant duration. Eosinophils are not uncommon in either MF or allergic contact dermatitis. Epidermotropism is characterized by lymphocytes within the epidermis in the absence of significant spongiosis, and this along with lymphocytic atypia is the hallmark of MF (Chapter 158).

21. A (T); B (T); C (T); D (T); E (T) The constellation of flushing, diarrhea, and abdominal pain is known as the carcinoid syndrome, and the tumor responsible is a carcinoid and not a Merkel cell tumor. Most commonly, by the time this syndrome develops, widespread metastases, usually to the liver, have developed. Carcinoid tumors are often located in the small intestine, appendix, and lung. Metastases to the skin are rare, but they may occur, especially when the bronchus is the primary tumor site. Pellagra is due to a deficiency of niacin, which may occur with a carcinoid tumor, both because of decreased absorption of dietary niacin secondary to diarrhea and because the synthesis of niacin is depressed as a result of shunting of tryptophan toward serotonin (Chapters 61 and 161).

22. C Sister Mary Joseph's nodule refers to a periumbilical nodule that may be the first sign of an intraabdominal adenocarcinoma. The stomach, pancreas, and ovary are common primary sites (Chapter 161).

23. B The incidence of metastases of dermatofibrosarcoma protuberans is estimated at 3%. This occurs on average 6 years after the primary excision. The metastases occur in regional lymph nodes or through the bloodstream to lungs, brain, or bone. The best treatment is wide local excision at the time of diagnosis (Chapter 149).

24. B Gingival hypertrophy is common in both acute monocytic leukemia and acute myelomonocytic leukemia, both variants of acute myeloblastic leukemia (AML). Granulocytic sarcoma, or chloroma, is a tumor mass commonly arising in the skin, bone, or lymph nodes that is composed of masses of malignant myeloid precursors seen (1) preceding the development of AML, (2) along with CML, just prior to blast transformation, or (3) in association with known AML (Chapter 160).

PIGMENTATION AND MELANOCYTIC LESIONS

25. B The photograph (see Fig. 25–3) is of a classic Spitz nevus (spindle and epithelioid cell nevus). Note the well-circumscribed, large nests of uniformly atypical melanocytes showing maturation toward the base of the tumor with smaller cells more reminiscent of a usual melanocytic nevus. The overlying epidermis is hyperplastic, with elongation of rete ridges. Clefting above the nests of melanocytes along the dermoepidermal junction is also characteristic of a Spitz nevus. Spitz nevi usually measure less than 1 cm in diameter, whereas nodular melanomas, their histologic look-alikes in a distressingly large number of cases, are often larger than this. They are usually single and occur most commonly on the face and lower extremities of children and young adults (Chapter 150).

26. A Both the Mongolian spot and the blue nevus result from a proliferation of dendritic melanocytes within the dermis that contain melanin pigment. In a blue nevus, the density of these cells is much greater than in the classic Mongolian spot, where they are seen in a low concentration in the lower half of the dermis. The clinical features are quite different; Mongolian spots usually occur on the sacrococcygeal region and consist of an ill-defined patch with a uniformly blue discoloration resembling a bruise. The common blue nevus occurs most often on or near the dorsa of the hands or feet and usually is a small, well-circumscribed nodule with a blue-black or slate-blue color (Chapter 132).

27. C The histologic findings of melasma include increased numbers and activity of melanocytes. These cells are known to show increased formation of melanin pigment and increased transfer of melanin to epidermal keratinocytes and dermal melanophages. There are two types of melasma. In epidermal melasma, which is far easier to treat, the pigment is all epidermal. In the mixed, or dermal, varieties the pigment lies in both the epidermis and dermis or strictly in the dermis, from which it is very difficult to remove (Chapter 132).

28. C Addison's disease results from idiopathic adrenal atrophy, thought to result from an autoimmune process. The damaged adrenal cortex does not respond normally to serum ACTH levels and the pituitary is thereby stimulated to hypersecrete ACTH. As the secretion of ACTH by the pituitary is tied to both the synthesis and secretion of MSH, there is a concurrent increase in serum levels of MSH, which causes an increase in melanocyte activity. This results in increased deposition of melanin, both within epidermal keratinocytes and dermal melanophages (Chapter 132).

29. A Melanocytes are present in usual numbers in both tyrosinase-negative and tyrosinase-positive albinism, but because of an absence of tyrosinase activity in tyrosinase-negative albinism, only premelanosomes (types I and II), types containing no melanin are seen. In tyrosinase-positive albinism, types III and IV melanosomes can occasionally be seen as well, but because of a defect in the synthesis of melanin, the more mature melanosomes are not formed (Chapter 129).

NONINFECTIOUS ERYTHEMATOUS, PAPULOSQUAMOUS DISEASES

30. C Pityriasis rosea histologically resembles a subacute or chronic dermatitis, with mild acanthosis, focal parakeratosis, and areas of spongiosis with intracellular edema and exocytosis of small lymphocytes. The superficial dermis contains a perivascular inflammatory infiltrate of mostly small mononuclear cells, few eosinophils and histiocytes. The two features that distinguish it as pityriasis rosea are exocytosis of erythrocytes in the dermal papillae and dyskeratotic keratinocytes in the epidermis (Chapter 17).

31. B Pustulosis palmaris et plantaris, like the other forms of localized pustular psoriasis, is histologically indistinguishable from generalized pustular psoriasis. Two forms of localized pustular psoriasis—localized acrodermatitis continua of Hallopeau and pustulosis palmaris et plantaris—are clinically characterized by involvement of the palms and soles. The main difference between the two is that in pustulosis palmaris et plantaris, in contrast to acrodermatitis continua of Hallopeau, the acral portion of the fingers and toes is spared (Chapter 27).

32. E This is a rare variant of lichen planus with bullae and erosions on the feet and toes, scarring, and loss of toenails. Cutaneous and oral lesions of lichen planus are also seen, as are patches of atrophic alopecia of the scalp. Ulcerative lichen planus has been associated with an increased risk of squamous cell carcinoma developing at the sites of long-standing lesions (Chapter 20).

33. A Intraepidermal Langerhans cells are increased in early lesions of lichen planus. It is thought that these Langerhans cells process an as yet unknown antigen, leading to a subsequent attraction of T lymphocytes of both CD8 (cytotoxic-suppressor) and CD4 (helper-inducer) subtypes. The initial immune process is thought to be directed against the basal cell layer (Chapter 20).

34. B Direct immunofluorescence demonstrates colloid bodies in approximately 87% of cases of lichen planus. These stain mainly with IgM, although they may also stain with IgG, IgA, C3, and fibrin. Colloid bodies develop from damaged keratinocytes and consist of aggregates of filament bundles that have been discharged into the dermis. Colloid bodies are not specific for lichen planus, since they can be seen in other diseases in which damage is done to the basal keratinocytes (Chapter 20).

35. D The finding of a largely CD8 (cytotoxic-suppressor)–positive lymphocyte population in pityriasis lichenoides et varioliformis acuta (PLEVA) is in contrast to lymphomatoid papulosis, which is largely a CD4 (helper-inducer) lymphocyte–mediated process. Lymphomatoid papulosis shares many immunophenotypic features with a true T-cell lymphoma, such as deletions of normally present surface antigens on T cells. In addition, the atypical cells in lymphomatoid papulosis are Ki1-positive, whereas there are few if any Ki1-positive cells in PLEVA. There is controversy over whether lymphomatoid papulosis belongs to a spectrum of diseases that falls between PLEVA and a true lymphoma. Up to 20% of patients with lymphomatoid papulosis ultimately develop lymphoma (Chapter 23).

36. B The discrete papules of lichen nitidus demonstrate a well-circumscribed lichenoid inflammatory infiltrate of lymphocytes and histiocytes that may extend slightly into the overlying epidermis. The epidermis over the infiltrate is flattened with basal vacuolar change or loss of the entire basal layer. On either side of the infiltrate, the rete ridges extend downward, seeming to "clutch" the "ball" of infiltrate (Chapter 20).

37. A Both actinic reticuloid and PLEVA demonstrate an increase in the ratio of CD8-positive (cytotoxic-suppressor) lymphocytes to CD4-positive (helper-inducer) lymphocytes. Atopic dermatitis, alopecia areata, and mycosis fungoides are CD4-mediated processes (Chapter 23).

NONINFECTIOUS BULLOUS DISEASES OF THE SKIN

38. A Pemphigus vegetans is a variant of pemphigus vulgaris in which increased host resistance leads to the presence of numerous eosinophils, including intraepidermal pustules that consist almost entirely of eosinophils. Bullous pemphigoid classically demonstrates subepidermal pustules filled with eosinophils, but on regeneration of the basal layer, these pustules often appear intraepidermal. Pyoderma vegetans is histologically indistinguishable from pemphigus vegetans and can only be distinguished from the latter with direct immunofluorescence studies, which are negative in pyoderma vegetans (Chapters 74 and 75).

39. 1 (T); 2 (T); 3 (T); 4 (F); 5 (F) Acantholysis in the upper epidermis, usually in the granular layer or just below it, is characteristic of pemphigus foliaceus and pemphigus erythematosus, which may be either an abortive form or early stage of pemphigus foliaceus. Fogo selvagem also shows acantholysis within the upper epidermis, since it is histologically identical to pemphigus foliaceus and has similar antigenic specificity. Pemphigus vulgaris and pemphigus vegetans are characterized by acantholysis in the lower portions of the epidermis (Chapter 74).

40. D Viral infections such as herpes simplex cause degenerative changes in epithelial cells, including ballooning and reticular degeneration. This leads to secondary acantholysis, which usually affects the basal layer and the attachments of these cells with the basement membrane zone. True primary acantholysis results from dissolution of the intercellular cement and intradesmosomal substances. This results in cells falling away from each other and may lead to formation of bullae. The blistering disorders listed, other than herpes simplex, all lead to blister formation by this pathway (Chapter 72).

41. C Eosinophils are not a feature of psoriasis in any location. Although intraepidermal (Kogoj's) pustules are often seen in psoriasis and are of great diagnostic value, they are composed of small collections of neutrophils within a spongiotic upper epidermis. Eosinophilic spongiosis can be seen in all of the other choices in at least one stage in their development (Chapter 27).

42. E A biopsy should not be taken of a vesicular lesion itself if dermatitis herpetiformis is to be conclusively ruled out. Provided that uninvolved skin is sampled, the diagnosis can be made when there are granular deposits of IgA at the dermoepidermal junction. Vesicular lesions do not show this immunofluorescence finding, and even perilesional skin may have negative immunofluorescence (Chapter 79).

43. B The bullous pemphigoid antigen is located within the lamina lucida and is bound specifically to the hemidesmosomes as determined by the peroxidase-antiperoxidase method of immunoelectron microscopy. The bullous pemphigoid antigen has recently been demonstrated to be present within the cytoplasm of the basal keratinocytes as well as within the lamina lucida. This is in contrast to the lupus band test and acquired epidermolysis bullosa, when the electron-dense deposits are located below the lamina lucida (Chapter 75).

DISEASES OF THE CUTANEOUS VESSELS

44. A A defect in proline hydroxylation is due to a deficiency of ascorbic acid and leads to the clinical entity known as scurvy. This is characterized by follicular parakeratosis in association with broken-off "corkscrew hairs," and perifollicular petechiae. Hemorrhage into soft tissue, lower extremity ecchymoses, and bleeding and friable gums may also be seen. These signs are due to the failure of synthesis of normal collagen and to endothelial cell damage, leading to a bleeding diathesis (Chapter 180).

45. B The autoerythrocyte syndrome is an interesting recurrent disorder often seen in people with hysterical personality disorders. Some authors believe the entity to be a factitious process. However, direct immunofluorescence has shown granular IgM and C3 at the dermoepidermal junction as well as properdin and factor B, leading some to favor an immunologic etiology (Chapter 89).

46. A Purpura fulminans usually occurs in children recovering from an infection but may develop spontaneously, and it may occur in adults. It is characterized by the sudden development of large areas of ecchymosis, hypotension, fever, and disseminated intravascular coagulation. Internal organs may also undergo hemorrhagic necrosis as a result of disseminated intravascular coagulation. Although this condition may progress and lead to death, treatment with heparin is often effective. The histologic features of purpura fulminans include dermal and subcutaneous hemorrhagic necrosis with many vessels showing occlusion of their lumina by platelet and fibrin thrombi identical to those seen in coumarin necrosis (Chapter 183).

47. C Purpura pigmentosa chronica shares with stasis dermatitis the features of dermal inflammation, dilated capillaries, extravasation of erythrocytes, and hemosiderin-laden macrophages. The histologic changes of stasis dermatitis usually display a more lobular proliferation of small vessels that extends deeper into the dermis and often shows more pronounced epidermal changes and dermal fibrosis. Although purpura pigmentosa chronica is thought to be the result of a lymphocytic vasculitis, fibrinoid material within vessels is not a feature either of it or of stasis dermatitis (Chapter 26).

48. B Both granuloma faciale and erythema elevatum diutinum show histologic and immunofluorescent evidence of a vasculitis. Granuloma faciale, however, usually shows a separation of the inflammatory infiltrate from the epidermis and pilosebaceous units by a Grenz zone. Also, eosinophils are not characteristically seen in erythema elevatum diutinum, which shows mainly neutrophils, lymphocytes, and histiocytes, whereas eosinophils and neutrophils constitute a large portion of the inflammatory cells in granuloma faciale (Chapter 60).

49. A (F); B (F); C (F); D (T) Both lymphomatoid granulomatosis (angiocentric T-cell lymphoma) and midline granuloma of the face demonstrate markedly atypical mononuclear cells within a background of a polymorphous inflammatory infiltrate. By means of immunoperoxidase studies, both have been identified as T-cell lymphomas. The initial clinical presentation differs in that midline granuloma begins insidiously, at first involving the nasal passages and septum with progression to extensive destruction of the face and late dissemination to cervical and mediastinal lymph nodes, lungs, and the gastrointestinal tract. Lymphomatoid granulomatosis primarily affects the lungs and does so early in the course of the disease (Chapter 159).

50. A (T); B (F); C (T); D (F) Solitary glomus tumors are usually circumscribed and surrounded by a fibrous capsule, whereas glomangiomas do not have a fibrous capsule and possess larger vascular spaces. The glomus cells are more prominent in a solitary glomus tumor, in which the vascular spaces are smaller and less prominent. Finally, multiple small nerve fibers are demonstrated with Bodian stain in the soft tissue surrounding solitary tumors, a finding not found in glomangiomas (Chapter 146).

51. A (T); B (F); C (T); D (F) Kaposi's sarcoma is derived from endothelial cells. As such, it will stain with *Ulex europaeus* and other antibodies that stain endothelial cells from blood vascular and lymphatic derivation. Factor VIII–related antigen also stains some cells within this neoplasm. This antibody marks endothelial cells of blood vascular derivation only. There is some controversy as to which subset of endothelial cells gives rise to this tumor. It is likely that both blood vessel– and lymphatic-derived endothelial cells participate, as do undifferentiated blood vascular endothelial cells. Desmin marks cells of muscular derivation, and S-100 most specifically marks neural cells and melanocytes (Chapters 125 and 146).

52. B Both acute febrile neutrophilic dermatosis and erythema elevatum diutinum demonstrate abundant neutrophils with nuclear dust (leukocytoclasis) in the inflammatory infiltrates that accompany them. Both also lack eosinophils in significant numbers. Either may ulcerate. The feature best used to distinguish between the two is the presence of vasculitis with deposits of eosinophilic fibrinoid material within and around vessel walls in erythema elevatum diutinum. Vasculitis is not present in acute febrile neutrophilic dermatosis (Chapters 38 and 60).

53. D A diagnosis of systemic polyarteritis nodosa (PAN) should never be made on biopsy of skin or muscle alone, given that involvement of these sites is limited to small vessels and the diagnostic feature of systemic PAN is panarteritis of medium-sized and small arteries. Cutaneous lesions of systemic polyarteritis nodosa demonstrate leukocytoclastic vasculitis with necrosis of vessel walls and occlusion by thrombi. Biopsy of a visceral organ such as kidney or clinical studies demonstrating medium-sized vessel involvement are essential for an unequivocal diagnosis. Benign cutaneous polyarteritis nodosa is characterized by cutaneous lesions with similar histologic features, but there is no visceral involvement (Chapter 58).

54. B Hemangiopericytomas are derived from the pericyte, a cell located between the endothelium and adventitia within the walls of capillaries and venules. These cells normally form a discontinuous layer and are completely surrounded by capillary basement membrane. They do not stain with Factor VIII–related antigen or *Ulex europaeus* as would endothelial cells and they are not located only in the wall of the arterial Suquet-Hoyer canal, as are glomus cells (Chapter 146).

55. B Weibel-Palade bodies are seen by electron microscopy as markers of endothelial cell differentiation. Of interest, their numbers are decreased in pyogenic granuloma (lobular capillary hemangiomas). They have also been reported to be diminished in number in other cutaneous vascular proliferations such as Kaposi's sarcoma (Chapter 146).

INFECTIOUS DISEASES OF THE SKIN

56. D "Sulfur granules" refer to the masses of *Actinomyces* organisms that are found in microabscesses surrounded by multinucleated giant cells and histiocytes in the more developed granulomatous stage of actinomycosis. The earlier lesions show diffuse infiltration of neutrophils and resemble acute cellulitis. The most common sites of involvement include the cervicofacial (accounting for more than one half of cases), thoracic, and abdominal areas (Chapter 113).

57. A The histologic features of a cutaneous lesion of sporotrichosis include verrucous hyperplasia of the epidermis, which may contain several intraepidermal abscesses. Within the dermis, there is a dense granulomatous inflammatory infiltrate with numerous giant cells, small granulomas, and collections of neutrophils. The involved lymph nodes and cutaneous nodules in multifocal systemic sporotrichosis often show a characteristic "zonal" arrangement, central suppuration being surrounded by a tuberculoid zone and surrounding this a lymphocytic-plasmacytic infiltrate. Atypical mycobacterial infections, cat-scratch disease, and tularemia infections should be included in the differential diagnosis, since they may show similar features (Chapter 120).

58. A The causative organism in cerebral chromomycosis is *Cladosporium trichoides,* in contrast to the organisms causing cutaneous and subcutaneous chromomycosis, which include *Cladosporium carrionii, Fonsecaea pedrosoi, F. compactum, F. dermatitidis,* and *Phialophora verrucosa*. Both spores and mycelia are seen in the cerebral lesions, as opposed to skin and subcutaneous lesions in which only spores are found. Cerebral lesions can and often do occur without skin lesions (Chapter 120).

59. C Away from the area of ulceration, a primary lesion of syphilis may show the listed features, which are also suggestive of classic secondary syphilis. Pityriasis lichenoides et varioliformis acuta should show epidermal changes as well, including dyskeratotic keratinocytes and extravasation of red blood cells. In addition, the infiltrate should be more lichenoid, and plasma cells are not usually prominent. Tertiary syphilis is characterized by granulomas, seen in both the nodular and gummatous variants of tertiary syphilis (Chapter 108).

60. A (T); B (T); C (T); D (F); E (F) Cowdry type A intranuclear inclusions are acidophilic bodies, approximately one half the diameter of the nucleus surrounded by a clear zone, or halo. Along with multinucleation, they are characteristic of herpesvirus infections. The inclusion is actually coalesced viral nucleoplasm, as these are double-stranded DNA viruses which replicate within the nucleus of infected cells. The varicella-zoster virus, herpes simplex virus, cytomegalovirus, and Epstein-Barr virus are all members of the herpesvirus family. Vaccinia is a complication of vaccination against smallpox, caused by the human cowpox virus, an arthropox virus. This virus forms eosinophilic, intracytoplasmic inclusion bodies, but neither intranuclear inclusions nor multinucleation are seen. Poxviruses, which give rise to infections such as molluscum contagiosum and orf in the skin, may cause intracytoplasmic inclusions but are not present within the nucleus (Chapter 122).

61. A (T); B (T); C (T); D (F) Herpesviruses produce intranuclear Cowdry type A inclusions, and some members of this group (cytomegalovirus) also form intracytoplasmic inclusions. Intracytoplasmic inclusions are seen in poxviral infections, the classic examples being Guarnieri bodies in smallpox infections and Henderson-Patterson or molluscum bodies of molluscum contagiosum. Intranuclear inclusion bodies are difficult to see and few in number but are present in tumors induced by human papillomaviruses. The picornavirus group includes the coxsackieviruses and are RNA viruses that do not form inclusion bodies (Chapter 121).

62. C Malacoplakia is thought to result from an acquired defect in the digestion of phagocytized bacteria. Michaelis-Gutman bodies are diagnostic of malacoplakia, which most commonly involves the urinary and gastrointestinal tracts but may involve the skin. Michaelis-Gutman bodies are cytoplasmic inclusions within histiocytes that have a homogenous or targetoid lamellated appearance and stain strongly with the von Kossa calcium stain, as well as with iron stains and periodic acid–Schiff (PAS). Gram-negative bacteria are also seen within these histiocytes (Chapter 107).

63. C This organism possesses a thick capsule that does not stain with hematoxylin and eosin or PAS. The capsule is made up of acid mucopolysaccharides and therefore stains with methylene blue (purple), Alcian blue (blue), or mucicarmine (red) (Chapter 120).

64. C The presence of a paranuclear kinetoplast limits the choice to the *Leishmania* protozoans. *Klebsiella rhinoscleromatis* is the causative organism in rhinoscleroma, which is in the clinical differential diagnosis of an infectious lesion at this site. Mucocutaneous leishmaniasis is caused by *L. braziliensis* alone. *L. tropica* and *L. mexicana* cause only a cutaneous form of leishmaniasis (Chapter 126).

65. D The kinetoplast is located within large mitochondria, close to the nucleus. It contains abundant DNA, which is why it is histologically visible. The flagellum and its basal body lie at a right angle to the kinetoplast. The flagellum itself is surrounded by an invagination of the plasma membrane and is therefore located extracellularly. When the parasite changes from its amastigote to its promastigote form, this flagellum increases in length to approximately 25 microns (Chapter 126).

66. B Tertiary yaws is characterized by palmar and plantar hyperkeratosis that may be severe enough to cause contractures. Lesions of the mucocutaneous border of the mouth and nose are also characteristic, and this is known as rhinopharyngitis mutilans. Bone lesions may be seen in tertiary yaws as opposed to tertiary pinta and tertiary syphilis. Although hyperkeratotic pitted papules of the palms and soles are classic for secondary syphilis, mucocutaneous lesions and bone lesions are present (Chapter 108).

67. B Acrodermatitis chronica atrophicans is regarded as the late stage of the European variant of borreliosis, which is caused by *Borrelia burgdorferi*. This almost always is seen on the extremities, usually the extensor surfaces. Initially, the lesions are inflammatory, classically appearing red and edematous. This is followed by an atrophic stage, with a flattened, wrinkled, red/brown appearance. Occasionally, fibrous thickening of the skin develops, especially on the dorsal feet, ulnar or tibial region, or as nodules near joints (Chapter 109).

68. A Replication of the varicella-zoster virus occurs almost exclusively within the keratinocytes of the affected epidermis. Electron microscopy has shown that viruses may be found in dermal capillary endothelial cells, axons of nerves, and within dermal macrophages, but only in small numbers. The virus is notorious for remaining latent within dorsal root ganglia with reactivation resulting in spread along sensory nerves to the skin (Chapter 121).

CONNECTIVE TISSUE DISEASES

69. D The syndrome described is the mixed connective tissue disease, which differs from systemic lupus erythematosus in both clinical and laboratory features. The two laboratory features diagnostic of this entity are (1) a high titer of serum antibodies to an extractable nuclear antigen that is ribonuclease-sensitive and (2) direct immunofluorescence findings, including epidermal nuclear staining with IgG in a speckled pattern of normal-appearing skin. A subepidermal "lupus band" may also be seen in the sun-exposed normal skin, but this finding is present in only 20% of such cases (Chapter 24).

70. C The features seen in this biopsy of lupus erythematosus include hyperkeratosis with focal parakeratosis, epidermal atrophy with follicular plugging, and significant liquefactive necrosis of the basal keratinocytes. In the superficial and deep dermis there is a patchy inflammatory infiltrate in both a perivascular and periappendageal distribution. The infiltrate contains predominantly lymphocytes and histiocytes that do not show cytologic atypia. These are features of lupus erythematosus. Lichen planus does not show parakeratosis, and deep dermal and periappendageal inflammation is not characteristic of this entity. Late sclerotic morphea is not suggested, since there is no thickening and homogenization of dermal collagen and because the epidermal changes in this biopsy would not be seen. Polymorphous light eruption should not show liquefactive degeneration of basal keratinocytes. Finally, the lack of cytologic atypia and the presence of the epidermal changes seen are against a diagnosis of lymphoma (Chapters 20, 24, 86, and 98).

71. B The most common manifesting feature of systemic lupus erythematosus is a migratory polyarthritis. Cutaneous lesions occur at the onset of disease in only 20% of cases and are never seen in about 20% of cases. Skin lesions are, of course, characteristic of discoid lupus erythematosus. Both the absence of systemic involvement and serologic studies differentiate this from systemic lupus erythematosus, whereas the histologic findings on biopsy of cutaneous lesions from both differ only in degree (Chapter 24).

INFLAMMATORY DISEASES OF FAT, APPENDAGES, AND CARTILAGE

72. D Alopecia areata is a nonscarring inflammatory alopecia in which there is an excess of miniaturized early anagen or telogen hair structures, normal or atrophic sebaceous glands, and an inflammatory infiltrate consisting predominantly of lymphocytes attacking the hair bulbs in a "swarm of bees" fashion. This infiltrate is made up predominantly of CD4 (helper-inducer phenotype) lymphocytes, and unlike normal hair follicles, the follicles in a lesion of alopecia areata contain intrabulbar Langerhans cells. Androgenic alopecia usually is not inflammatory, but if inflammation is present, it is not peribulbar. Early loss of sebaceous glands is characteristic of pseudopelade of Brocq (Chapters 134 and 135).

73. D Relapsing polychondritis is an inflammatory condition involving cartilaginous tissue throughout the body, including the ear, nasal septum, and joints, whereas chondrodermatitis nodularis helicis involves only the ear, often the apex of the helix, and occasionally the antihelix. A vasculitis is seen in lesions of relapsing polychondritis, and circulating antibodies to type 2 collagen (exclusively seen in cartilage) are present, suggesting an immune mechanism. In contrast, chondrodermatitis nodularis helicis is likely due to poor blood supply, resulting in degeneration of cartilage (Chapter 56).

74. A (F); B (T); C (F); D (T) The findings described are seen both in erythema induratum and in infections. Although granulomas may be seen in chronic erythema nodosum, they are usually tight, well-formed clusters of epithelioid histiocytes, and they lack central caseation. Erythema nodosum is also a septal panniculitis, although the inflammation may extend somewhat into the peripheral fat lobules. Superficial migratory thrombophlebitis does not elicit a granulomatous response, although occasional giant cells may be seen, especially in late stages, with thrombus recanalization. Instead, a single large vein is thrombosed, and the inflammation is centered on this vessel (Chapter 68).

75. B Erythema nodosum may show quite significant involvement of vessels, mainly small vessels and medium-sized veins. If this is significant, it may be difficult to histologically distinguish from benign cutaneous periarteritis nodosa (PAN). An elastic tissue stain can highlight the fact that these medium-sized vessels are veins, not arteries, in erythema nodosum, whereas benign cutaneous PAN shows a necrotizing vasculitis of medium-sized arteries. A renal biopsy is unnecessary unless renal disease suggests systemic PAN. Although an elevated anti-streptolysin-O titer raises the suspicion of erythema nodosum, this is not the best choice of those offered (Chapters 58 and 68).

76. B Although a neutrophilic infiltrate of subcutaneous fat is thought to represent the first stage of Weber-Christian disease, this is rarely seen on biopsy and is not specific for this disease. Foam cells, or fat-laden macrophages resulting from digestion by macrophages of degenerating fat, are quite characteristic of this disease and the most helpful feature. Vasculitis and caseating granulomas are not features of Weber-Christian disease. Extensive fat necrosis with "ghost-like" fat cells are seen in subcutaneous fat necrosis associated with pancreatic disease (Chapter 71).

HISTIOCYTIC PROCESSES

77. D The subacute, transient version of sarcoidosis can generally be diagnosed without biopsy of the erythema nodosum lesions, but if this were done, the histologic findings would be identical to classic erythema nodosum. Tight, well-formed clusters of epithelioid histiocytes typically found in chronic, persistent sarcoidosis are not seen in the acute variant. No other skin manifestations are seen in this syndrome, which tends to resolve within a few months. Lung and ocular involvements are common in the chronic, persistent form of sarcoidosis. Electron microscopic findings of complex laminated bodies and entrapped collagen forming "asteroid bodies" are found within the giant cells seen in older lesions of chronic, persistent sarcoidosis (Chapter 45).

78. A Both sarcoidosis and lupus vulgaris show granulomatous inflammation, and although caseation may occasionally be seen within the granulomas of sarcoidosis, this is much more commonly a feature of lupus vulgaris. Lupus vulgaris also tends to have more marked inflammation and epithelial changes of ulceration, acanthosis, and pseudocarcinomatous hyperplasia. Often, however, only culture study or immunologic testing helps to distinguish the two. A lupus band test is negative in both sarcoidosis and lupus vulgaris (Chapters 45 and 111).

79. A Both cheilitis granulomatosa and cheilitis glandularis contain an inflammatory infiltrate consisting of lymphocytes and plasma cells. Cheilitis granulomatosa usually also contains a tuberculoid inflammatory infiltrate and may even contain tight granulomas resembling sarcoidosis. Cheilitis glandularis contains dilated salivary ducts containing eosinophilic material. Erythema induratum is a panniculitis in which a tuberculoid inflammatory infiltrate is seen (Chapter 138).

80. E Eruptive xanthomas are commonly seen in people with high serum triglycerides and lipids. They may occur in all the subtypes of hyperlipoproteinemia that are associated with high levels of chylomicrons or prebetalipoproteins. This includes types 1, 2b, 3, 4, and 5 (Chapter 176).

81. A (T); B (F); C (T); D (F) These electron microscopic findings are those of Anderson-Fabry disease, which is a sphingolipidosis due to a deficiency in the lysosomal hydrolase α-D-galactosidase A. The lack of this enzyme results in the accumulation of ceramide trihexoside in cells of many organs. The cutaneous lesions associated with this X-linked recessive disorder are multiple small angiokeratomas often located on the lower trunk, hence the name angiokeratoma corporis diffusum. These are not true neoplasms, but angiectasias secondary to vascular damage resulting from deposition of lipid (Chapter 146).

82. C The findings are those of granulomata with small foci of incomplete and complete collagen degeneration surrounded by histiocytes and lymphocytes. Only occasional giant cells are seen. A mucin stain shows increased acid mucopolysaccharides in these areas of collagen degeneration. A close mimic is necrobiosis lipoidica, which, however, demonstrates more multinucleated giant cells; more pronounced vascular changes; extensive degeneration of collagen, often with hyalinization; more deposits of lipid; and fewer deposits of mucin. A rheumatoid nodule also shows degeneration of collagen, but it is found deep within the subcutaneous tissue. A clinical history of rheumatoid disease helps to distinguish rheumatoid nodule from subcutaneous granuloma annulare. Central caseous necrosis is expected in tuberculosis. Acid-fast stains are only occasionally positive (Chapter 47).

DRUG ERUPTIONS AND METABOLIC DISORDERS

83. D Phototoxic reactions represent exaggerated sunburn responses, whereas photoallergic reactions demonstrate histologic changes similar to those seen with a contact dermatitis. A photoallergic reaction has epidermal spongiosis, microvesiculation, a superficial perivas-

cular dermatitis, and exocytosis of lymphocytes. Eosinophils are not necessarily prominent in either reaction nor is vasculitis seen, although enlarged endothelial cells and dermal edema are often present in a phototoxic reaction. Phototoxic reaction has keratinocyte vacuolization and necrosis in addition to dermal edema and endothelial cell swelling (Chapter 83).

84. B The purple-grey coloration in chlorpromazine pigmentation is located predominantly within perivascular dermal macrophages and has the staining properties of melanin. The electron-dense bodies seen on electron microscopy are thought to represent melanin-chlorpromazine complexes that are not metabolized. These are seen in macrophages as well as neutrophils and monocytes of peripheral blood, endothelial cells, pericytes, Schwann's cells, and fibroblasts (Chapter 43).

85. E Penicillamine administration may result in several dermatoses, including anetoderma, elastosis perforans serpiginosa, and pemphigus. The lesions of anetoderma have a diminution or absence of elastic tissue. Penicillamine-induced elastosis perforans serpiginosa lesions are characterized by hyperplasia of elastic fibers, especially in the mid and deep dermis. The fibers display "lateral budding," giving them a sawtooth-like border. Lesions of penicillamine-induced pemphigus are usually identical to those of pemphigus foliaceus, but occasionally pemphigus vulgaris or pemphigus erythematosus–like lesions are seen. Consequently, direct immunofluorescence may demonstrate subepidermal as well as intercellular IgG (Chapter 43).

86. A (T); B (T); C (T); D (T) The biopsy shows epidermal hyperplasia with irregular downward proliferation, referred to as pseudocarcinomatous hyperplasia. There are nuclear changes of "reactive atypia," which are often quite florid, and certainly a well-differentiated squamous cell carcinoma should be considered. Also seen are intraepidermal abscesses filled with neutrophils and eosinophils and a dermal inflammatory infiltrate containing epithelioid histiocytes that appear vaguely granulomatous. The differential diagnosis includes halogen eruptions, such as bromoderma, and deep fungal infections, especially blastomycosis, given the intraepidermal abscesses. In addition, pemphigus vegetans should be considered, although significant acantholysis should also be seen. Pyoderma vegetans should be considered as well in the differential diagnosis. Fungal stains and direct immunofluorescence are occasionally needed to confirm a diagnosis in these cases (Chapters 74 and 120).

87. A (T); B (T); C (T); D (F); E (F) Juvenile colloid milium occurs before puberty, whereas the other two conditions occur in adult life. The juvenile form also differs from the others in the derivation of the colloid material, and this can be seen on a routine hematoxylin and eosin–stained biopsy. The colloid material originates in the epidermis, colloid bodies forming from basal keratinocytes, just as is seen in lichen planus. The colloid material seen in the adult forms originates in the dermis. In all three diseases, the colloid material is periodic acid–Schiff–positive and diastase-resistant. Ultrastructural studies confirm the epidermal derivation of the colloid material in the juvenile form, showing that the colloid consists of whorled bundles of filaments containing cellular organelles, including desmosomes. None of these entities are associated with a plasma cell dyscrasia or monoclonal paraprotein; therefore, electrophoresis studies would not be helpful (Chapter 175).

88. A (T); B (T); C (T); D (T); E (T) The material seen on light microscopy as hyaline in skin biopsies of individuals with hyalinosis cutis et mucosae (lipoid proteinosis) actually consists of true hyaline, seen ultrastructurally as amorphous material produced by dermal fibroblasts; also seen is multiplication of basal laminae, evident around small blood vessels, skin appendages, smooth muscle cells, perineurium, and Schwann's cells. In addition, there is a marked decrease in the size and number of collagen fibrils produced by dermal fibroblasts. Most have a diameter of around 50 nm, compared with the normal size of 70 to 140 nm (Chapter 175).

DEGENERATIVE DISEASES AND THOSE RELATED TO SUNLIGHT AND HEAT

89. B The plaque type of polymorphous light eruption (PMLE) is clinically quite similar to discoid lupus erythematosus (DLE). Both manifest with erythematous, edematous, and slightly indurated plaques in sun-exposed areas. Solar elastosis may or may not be present, since both lesions can be seen in relatively young patients. Discoid lupus erythematosus characteristically demonstrates liquefactive degeneration of the basal keratinocytes, a finding not seen in PMLE. In very early lesions of DLE, however, this may not be a prominent finding, and in these instances, only direct immunofluorescence will help. PMLE does not routinely reveal deposits of immunoglobulin or complement along the dermoepidermal junction, in contrast to DLE (Chapter 86).

90. A The histologic findings in a chronic lymphoid response to an arthropod bite or sting include a dense inflammatory infiltrate that may extend into the subcutaneous fat. There may be quite significant atypia of the lymphocytes with hyperchromasia of nuclei and transformation to large lymphoblasts. These can have irregular nuclear borders and resemble the cells of mycosis fungoides. Giant cell formation with some resemblance to Reed-Sternberg cells of Hodgkin's disease may also be present. The presence of eosinophils and plasma cells within an arthropod reaction may also simulate the polymorphous background of Hodgkin's disease. Lymphomatoid papulosis may also show a dense inflammatory infiltrate that extends deep and contains atypical lymphocytes. The presence of lymphoid follicles in any of these entities favors a benign reactive process. The histology of polymorphous light eruption consists of dermal edema as may be seen in acute arthropod reaction, but the chronic lymphoid response of persistent arthropod bites is absent. In addition, eosinophils are not expected in polymorphous light eruption, and the inflammatory infiltrate is perivascular and less dense (Chapters 86, 91, 156, and 159).

91. C Perforating folliculitis demonstrates a focus of dermal inflammation and degenerating collagen and elastic tissue surrounded by proliferating epithelium that as it proliferates, moves this material to the skin surface. Elastosis perforans serpiginosa is also characterized by transepidermal elimination of elastic fibers that are also found in increased size and number in the upper dermis. There is no degeneration of elastic tissue in Kyrle's disease, and the parakeratotic plug occupying the epidermal invagination does not stain like elastic tissue. Finally, the material that is extruded in reactive perforating collagenosis is degenerated collagen; there are no elastic fibers in the keratotic plug or in the areas of perforation (Chapter 42).

92. C The bullae seen histologically in bullosis diabeticorum are usually subepidermal, although regeneration of the basal layer may result in an intraepidermal bulla. Ultrastructurally, anchoring fibrils are absent with resultant bullae within both the lamina lucida and the sublamina densa (Chapter 72).

93. A (T); B (T); C (T); D (F) Lichen sclerosus et atrophicus classically shows epidermal atrophy with follicular plugging and basilar vacuolar degeneration. Although morphea may show epidermal atrophy, the follicular plugging and basal vacuolar changes are not expected. In addition, a zone of upper dermal edema with homogenization of collagen bundles is present in all but the very early lesions of lichen sclerosis et atrophicus, when a lichenoid inflammatory infiltrate may occupy the superficial dermis. This is not seen in morphea. Loss of elastic fibers within this zone is also a classic sign of lichen sclerosus et atrophicus, whereas elastic tissue is normally present in the upper dermis in lesions of morphea. Thickening and hyperchromasia of collagen bundles is classically found in morphea and may also be seen in old lesions of lichen sclerosus et atrophicus. This feature should therefore not be used alone in distinguishing between the two diseases (Chapter 100).

94. A Actinic reticuloid is a chronic photosensitivity reaction to wavelengths of light that can involve ultraviolet B, ultraviolet A, and visible light. Well-developed lesions histologically mimic mycosis fungoides (MF) with a dense band-like infiltrate in the upper epidermis occasionally seen invading the epidermis. Atypical cells resembling those seen in MF are seen along with histiocytes, eosinophils, and plasma cells, and intraepidermal collections of these atypical cells are indistinguishable from Pautrier's microabscesses. However, actinic reticuloid is benign and reversible. The lymphocytes present are mostly of the T-suppressor (CD8) subset, in contrast to MF, which is T helper-inducer (CD4)–mediated. Earlier lesions have a less characteristic histologic appearance (Chapter 87).

95. E Erythema ab igne occurs most often on the shins, lower back, and buttocks and is due to prolonged exposure to heat such as from heating pads or fireplaces. The histologic features are similar to those of ultraviolet photodamage, with epidermal changes including atypical keratinocytes, either scattered or along the dermoepidermal junction. The classic feature is a marked increase in elastic tissue in the upper and mid-dermis. It differs from photoaging in that there is no homogenization of elastic tissue with loss of fibrous structure (Chapter 93).

GENODERMATOSES

96. B Netherton's syndrome is nearly always inherited autosomal recessively and consists of trichorrhexis invaginata usually associated with ichthyosis linearis circumflexa. However, the initial case reported by Netherton described trichorrhexis invaginata with lamellar ichthyosis. This unusual hair abnormality is clinically characterized by sparse, brittle hair in which the distal portion of the hair shaft invaginates into its proximal portion, resulting in a "ball and cup" configuration (Chapter 163).

97. B The histologic features of keratosis palmaris et plantaris of the Unna-Thost and the Meleda types and those in the Papillon-Lefevre syndrome include marked hyperkeratosis with hypergranulosis, acanthosis, and a superficial dermal inflammatory infiltrate. The differential diagnosis therefore includes lichen simplex chronicus and verruca vulgaris. Epidermolytic hyperkeratosis in palmaris et plantaris is histologically indistinguishable from epidermolytic hyperkeratosis. Psoriasis vulgaris shows a loss of the granular layer, and lichen planus has epidermal changes not seen in keratosis palmaris et plantaris (Chapter 175).

98. A (T); B (T); C (T); D (T); E (F) The histologic features of acrokeratosis verruciformis are nonspecific. They include hyperkeratosis, hypergranulosis, acanthosis, and slight papillomatosis, occasionally resembling "church spires." This, of course, could describe all of the preceding choices except for clear-cell acanthoma, and clinical correlation is required to arrive at the correct diagnosis. Clear-cell acanthoma is characterized by psoriasiform epidermal hyperplasia. The lesional keratinocytes have abundant, pale-staining cytoplasm, containing large amounts of glycogen. Frequently, there is a neutrophilic infiltrate (Chapter 175).

99. B X-linked ichthyosis is due to the lack of steroid sulfatase activity. Steroid sulfatase normally degrades cholesteryl sulfate, a product of Odland's (lamellar) bodies that promotes adhesion of corneocytes. Build-up results in persistent cell cohesion within the stratum corneum and also interferes with desquamation. Ichthyosis vulgaris is due to a defect in the synthesis of filaggrin. Bullous congenital ichthyosiform erythroderma is associated with increased and abnormal keratinization, resulting in abnormal desmosomal attachments and subsequent acantholysis. The basis for lamellar ichthyosis and ichthyosis linearis circumflexa is not known to be due to enzyme deficiencies (Chapter 162).

100. B Immunosuppression has been reported to be the eliciting factor in disseminated superficial actinic porokeratosis (DSAP), which is the most common type of porokeratosis. A marked increase in the incidence of these lesions has been described in patients with organ transplants. More commonly, DSAP is inherited in an autosomal dominant pattern and shows lesions in sun-exposed areas. Histologically, porokeratosis is characterized by a cornoid lamella with clonal proliferation of abnormal keratinocytes in the epidermis just below this parakeratotic column (Chapter 175).

101. E The very severe Ehlers-Danlos type 4 is also known as the arterial form, with an autosomal recessive pattern of inheritance. Death usually occurs in the first or second decade, usually because of rupture of a large gastrointestinal artery. The vessels are weak owing to the lack of normal type 3 collagen, which is not properly secreted by fibroblasts (Chapter 172).

Bibliography

CUTANEOUS NEOPLASMS

Burgdorf WHC, Koester G. Multiple cutaneous tumors: what do they mean? J Cutan Pathol 1992; 19:449–457.
Longacre TA, Smoller BR, Rouse RV. Atypical fibroxanthoma. Multiple immunologic profiles. Am J Surg Pathol 1993; 17:1199–1209.
Requena L, Sangueza OP. Benign neoplasms with neural differentiation: a review. Am J Dermatopathol 1995; 17:75–96.

PIGMENTED LESIONS

Casso EM, Grin-Jorgensen CM, Grant-Kels JM. Spitz nevi. J Am Acad Dermatol 1992; 27:901–13.

PAPULOSQUAMOUS LESIONS

Fox BJ, Odom RB. Papulosquamous diseases: a review. J Am Acad Dermatol 1985; 12:597–624.

NONINFECTIOUS BULLOUS DISEASES

Kroman NJ. Bullous pemphigoid. Dermatol Clin 1993; 11:483–498.
Pazderka-Smith E, Zone JJ. Dermatitis herpetiformis and linear IgA bullous dermatosis. Dermatol Clin 1993; 11:511–526.
Ruiz E, Deng J-S, Abell EA. Eosinophilic spongiosis: a clinical, histologic and immunopathologic study. J Am Acad Dermatol 1994; 30:973–976.
Sams WM Jr, Gammaon WR. Mechanism of lesion production in pemphigus and pemphigoid. J Am Acad Dermatol 1982; 6:431–449.

CUTANEOUS VESSELS

Tappero JW, Conanat MA, Wolfe SF, Berger TG. Kaposi's sarcoma: epidemiology, pathogenesis, histology, clinical spectrum, staging criteria and therapy. J Am Acad Dermatol 1993; 28:371–395.

CONNECTIVE TISSUE DISEASES

Beutner EH, Jablonska S, White DB, et al. Dermatologic criteria for classifying the major forms of cutaneous lupus erythematosus: methods for systemic discriminant analysis and questions on the interpretation of findings. Clin Dermatol 1993; 10:443–456.

INFLAMMATORY DISEASES OF THE HAIR

Mitchell AJ, Krull EA. Alopecia areata: pathogenesis and treatment. J Am Acad Dermatol 1984; 11:763–775.

HISTIOCYTIC PROCESSES

Kerdel FA, Moschella SL. Sarcoidosis: an updated review. J Am Acad Dermatol 1984; 11:1–19.

DRUGS

Wintroub BU, Stern R. Cutaneous drug reactions: pathogenesis and clinical classification. J Am Acad Dermatol 1985; 13:167–179.

DEGENERATIVE DERMATOSES

Patterson JW. The perforating disorders. J Am Acad Dermatol 1984; 10:567–581.
Rahbari H. Histochemical differentiation of localized morphea scleroderma and lichen sclerosus et atrophicus. J Cutan Pathol 1989; 16:342–347.

GENODERMATOSES

Rand RE, Baden HP. The ichthyoses; a review. J Am Acad Dermatol 1983; 8:285–305.
Whiting DA. Structural abnormalities of the hair shaft. J Am Acad Dermatol 1987; 16:1–25.